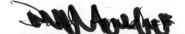
SAUNDERS TEXT AND REVIEW SERIES

BIOCHEMISTRY

ROBERT ROSKOSKI, JR., M.D., Ph.D.

Fred G. Brazda Professor of Biochemistry and Molecular Biology
Louisiana State University Medical Center
New Orleans, Louisiana

W.B. SAUNDERS COMPANY
A Division of Harcourt Brace & Company
Philadelphia London Toronto Montreal Sydney Tokyo

W.B. SAUNDERS COMPANY
A Division of Harcourt Brace & Company

The Curtis Center
Independence Square West
Philadelphia, Pennsylvania 19106

Library of Congress Cataloging-in-Publication Data

Roskoski, Robert.
    Biochemistry / Robert Roskoski.—1st ed.

        p.   cm.

    ISBN 0–7216–5174–7

    1. Biochemistry.   I. Title.

QP514.2.R664   1996

574.19′2—dc20

                                95–1002

BIOCHEMISTRY   ISBN 0–7216–5174–7

Printed in the United States of America.

Last digit is the print number: 9   8   7   6   5   4   3   2   1

To

Joseph E. Weber

Donald F. Steiner

Fritz Lipmann (in memoriam)

PREFACE

This book is designed for students who want to learn biochemistry in the context of molecular medicine. The unique strategy for instruction used in this book was prompted by medical and dental students who expressed interest in learning and applying the principles of biochemistry. This challenge motivated me to collect the 30 principles of biology and biochemistry that are printed inside the front cover. Most of these axioms are familiar to students from previous courses in biology and chemistry. I also formulated eight principles of bioenergetics that describe biochemical reactions. These rules provide guidelines for understanding and analyzing the individual steps that make up metabolic pathways. The principles are numbered for reference, but it is the concept and not an arbitrary number that is important. The identification of unidirectional and bidirectional reactions and the understanding that metabolic pathways are bioenergetically favorable help make sense of what is sometimes regarded as a bewildering series of interconnected metabolic reactions.

The use of the principles of bioenergetics involves an intuitive and qualitative approach based on the structures of so-called high-energy bonds and energy-rich compounds. The energy-rich bond is denoted by the squiggle (~) as introduced by Fritz Lipmann in 1941. The illustrations emphasize the conversion of energy-rich to energy-poor compounds throughout, and repetition will make them second nature to the reader. When energy-rich compounds become familiar, biochemical processes are understood more easily. This approach makes the study of metabolism and molecular biology more comprehensible and deemphasizes rote memorization. I gratefully acknowledge the late Fritz Lipmann for introducing me to the principles of bioenergetics that are used throughout this book. The laws governing oxidation–reduction reactions and decarboxylation reactions add depth and power to this general strategy.

The goal of this book is to help students develop an instinctive basis for understanding intermediary metabolism and macromolecule synthesis and degradation. I have found that students with only a modicum of chemical knowledge can readily and profitably use the high-energy-bond concept to aid in their comprehension of biochemistry. I hope that teachers whose primary interest is not metabolism will find this strategy useful. I have tried to demystify what are sometimes regarded as arcane aspects of metabolism: bioenergetics and structural chemistry help us separate the forest from the trees.

Exceptions in biology abound, and one should not be surprised that anomalies occur in biochemistry. That NADPH is the reductant for biosynthesis holds most but not all of the time. Knowing that this principle holds most of the time, however, helps organize one's thinking. How many exceptions a student wishes to learn may depend on time and motivation. A few important exceptions to general principles are noted. Rare exceptions are not discussed when they are not essential for understanding mainstream metabolism. Although it takes some effort to learn and use the principles, experience shows that, in the long run, they simplify the study of biochemistry. The strategy is not to learn or memorize all the metabolic pathways but to understand the biochemistry of each pathway by using these fundamentals. Both students and faculty have profited from this unique approach. I welcome comments on this tactic from teachers and students and any suggestions for improvement.

I have been privileged to teach undergraduate, graduate, medical, and dental students at the University of Iowa and at the Louisiana State University Medical Center in New Orleans. They have contributed greatly to this book and were quick to point out weaknesses in presentation. The students wanted the principles and not the details. While the detailed description of various biochemical processes is unavoidable, if one understands the principles, the amount of material that has to be memorized (the details) is minimized. Learning is facilitated, moreover, as new reactions are related to familiar principles and prototypical reactions such as those catalyzed by hexokinase or lactate dehydrogenase.

TOPIC SELECTION AND CLINICAL CORRELATIONS

Another goal of this book is to present biochemistry in a clinical context to provide the reader with the information required to understand clinical textbooks and literature at the level of the *New England Journal of Medicine*. Material in this book that is not generally found in university courses of general biochemistry includes enzyme analysis in the diagnosis of diseases, drugs as enzyme inhibitors, and the genetic basis of diseases including cancer. Because of space limitations, some important aspects of medical biochemistry that are found in other basic or clinical sciences were omitted.

The term "noteworthy" as used in this text points out biochemical pearls that are important and occur frequently on examinations. When information is given for general reference or information, that is usually a signal that the material does not have to be committed to memory. Important items in tables are often emphasized by colored type. Clinical correlations are integrated in the text and are set off with icons (▶ ◀). The clinical material is taken from common or celebrated diseases (a celebrated disease is one that may be found on licensing examinations or is often discussed on clinical rounds). Current medical topics, genetics, and drugs are used for illustrative purposes.

ORGANIZATION

Chapters 1 to 6 cover the fundamentals, and Chapters 7 to 14 consider intermediary metabolism. Chapters 15 to 18 include molecular biology, and Chapters 19 to 24 encompass specialized topics of cell biology and signal transduction. Chapter 25, the integration of energy metabolism, considers metabolic regulation, feeding and fasting, and diabetes. The order of the topics, however, can be varied. The reader may profit by referring to material on metabolic regulation in Chapter 25 while studying intermediary metabolism.

CONVENTIONS

The tricarboxylic acid cycle, or citric acid cycle, is called the Krebs cycle in honor of its discoverer and because clinicians rarely use the former terms. The nonsystematic term glyceride is used for the more systematic acylglycerol, again, because clinicians prefer the term glyceride. The Calorie is used as the nutritional unit of energy because of its widespread use in the United States. Extensive use is made of the International System of units, however, and the joule is used as the unit of energy for all calculations involving bioenergetics. Moreover, care was taken to present the correct stereochemistry of isoleucine, threonine, and other chiral compounds in nearly all of the figures using Fischer projection formulas or other standard representations as outlined in *Stereochemistry of Organic Compounds* by E. L. Eliel and S. H. Wilen (1994).

ACKNOWLEDGMENTS

Carol Vartanian edited this book and provided balanced feedback in her friendly and cheerful style. Her thoughtful evaluations contributed to the final organization and presentation. I gratefully acknowledge Dr. Jack D. Herbert, who read the entire text, reviewed the figures, and provided helpful suggestions designed to help both the student and the instructor. I thank Dr. Wayne V. Vedeckis for his evaluation of Chapter 15. I credit Risa Clow, illustrator at the W.B. Saunders Company, and Carol Vartanian for overseeing the art work. William R. Schmitt, Editorial Manager at W.B. Saunders, served as acquisitions editor and guided this process from the planning stages through publication. My spouse, Laura, helped me find innumerable references upon which the text is based.

TO THE STUDENT

One principle that is not listed on the cover, which I give in all of my classes, is that *Biochemistry is fun!*

ROBERT ROSKOSKI, JR.

SUPPLEMENTARY MATERIAL

The material in *Biochemistry Review* (1996) by Robert Roskoski, Jr., and Jack D. Herbert, published by W.B. Saunders Company, supplements this text. *Biochemistry Review* provides a synopsis of each chapter of this book. The synopsis is followed by sample questions, answers, and explanations. Each chapter in *Biochemistry Review* contains a clinical narrative and questions that are designed to develop the use of biochemistry in case analyses. *Biochemistry Review* also contains a comprehensive examination with a randomized selection of biochemical items similar to those encountered in standardized examinations. Its appendix contains hints for studying biochemistry and a glossary of selected biochemical and medical terms that occur in this book and in *Biochemistry Review*. *Biochemistry Review* contains a more extensive discussion of acid-base balance than this book, and it contains sample calculations of pH that do not occur in this text.

A set of 350 color slides of figures from this text is available from the W.B. Saunders Company.

CONTENTS

CHAPTER TWENTY-THREE

CHAPTER TWENTY-FOUR

CHAPTER TWENTY-FIVE

CELLS: THE

UNITS OF LIFE

Advances in biochemical science are at the root of progress in medicine, and the biochemical sciences are essential components of a humanistic education.

—ARTHUR KORNBERG

We are sick because our cells are sick.

—CHRISTIAN DE DUVE

THE SCOPE OF BIOCHEMISTRY

Biochemistry is the study of (1) the molecular composition of living cells, (2) the chemical reactions that biological compounds undergo, and (3) the regulation of these reactions. Biochemistry also includes the study of noncovalent interactions of molecules that relate to cellular and molecular structure and function. Molecular biology, a major branch of biochemistry, is the study of gene structure, function, and regulation.

Biochemistry is a fundamental biological and medical science that provides an understanding of cell biology, microbiology, nutrition, pharmacology, and physiology at the molecular level. The elucidation of mechanisms of disease processes (pathogenesis) is one of the goals of medical biochemistry. Progress is indicated by the numerous articles in the medical literature describing the biochemical and genetic basis of disease. Moreover, biochemical knowledge is useful in the diagnosis and treatment of disease, and tests performed in the clinical chemistry laboratory are used to monitor treatment.

The complexity of living systems is sometimes daunting and bewildering. The large number of components that make up humans and human pathogens adds to the complexity. However, all forms of life are composed of about 50 fundamental building blocks, and the recognition of these compounds greatly simplifies the study of biochemistry.

MAJOR BIOCHEMICAL COMPONENTS OF THE HUMAN BODY

The average human adult body is composed of 55% water, 19% protein, 19% fat, 7% inorganic matter, less than 1% carbohydrate, and less than 1% nucleic acid. Two-thirds of the body mass is cellular. The vast majority of biochemical reactions occur within cells. Cells are suspended in an extracellular matrix to make up tissues and organs.

The two forms of **nucleic acids** are **DNA** (deoxyribonucleic acid) and **RNA** (ribonucleic acid). DNA molecules are large polymers made up of four different mononucleotide building blocks (Figure 1–1). DNA is the genetic material of human cells and most other cells. RNA plays a role in transferring the genetic information from DNA into protein. RNA is the genetic material of some viruses. RNA is a polymer made up of four different mononucleotide building blocks.

Proteins are polymers made up of amino acid residues (Figure 1–1). Twenty genetically encoded amino acids participate in protein synthesis. Proteins play a structural, functional, defensive, and regulatory role in life. **Fats,** or **lipids,** are soluble in organic solvents (ether or chloroform/methanol). A large variety of lipids exists in nature. Fats (triglycerides) serve as a storage form of energy, phospholipids occur in membranes, and steroids occur in membranes and make up the steroid hormones.

Carbohydrates, or **sugars,** are water-soluble compounds that play roles in both energetics and cell and organ structure. Polysaccharides are large carbohydrate polymers made up of building blocks called monosaccharides, the simplest sugar units. Oligosaccharides are compounds made up of a few monosaccharide residues that can be linked to proteins. Oligosaccharides play a functional and structural role in the cellular economy.

CHEMICAL REACTIONS OF LIVING CELLS

Metabolism

Useful energy is generated or used up in many of the chemical reactions that make up metabolism. The term metabolism is derived from a Greek word meaning change. It refers to all the chemical reactions of an organism. *A chemical reaction is a process by which one or more compounds are converted or changed into one or more different compounds.* Let us first consider the example given in Equation 1.1.

$$2\,H_2 + O_2 \rightarrow 2\,H_2O \qquad (1.1)$$

Two molecules of hydrogen react with one molecule of oxygen to produce a different compound, water. The process by which the former are converted into the latter is a chemical reaction. Con-

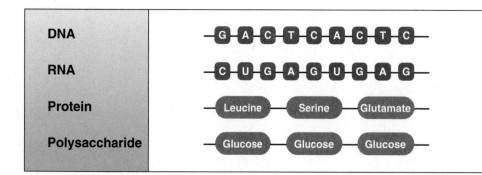

DNA	—G–A–C–T–C–A–C–T–C—
RNA	—C–U–G–A–G–U–G–A–G—
Protein	— Leucine — Serine — Glutamate —
Polysaccharide	— Glucose — Glucose — Glucose —

FIGURE 1–1. Subunit composition of biopolymers. *DNA is made up of four different deoxymononucleotides containing adenine (A), thymine (T), guanine (G), and cytosine (C). RNA is made up of four different mononucleotides containing adenine (A), uracil (U), guanine (G), and cytosine (C).*

sider the biochemical reaction given in Equation 1.2.

ATP + glucose

$$\rightarrow \text{glucose 6-phosphate} + \text{ADP} \qquad (1.2)$$

Here, ATP (adenosine triphosphate) reacts with glucose, a sugar, to produce two different substances: glucose 6-phosphate and ADP (adenosine diphosphate). The phosphorylation of glucose is the first step in the metabolism of glucose.

The chemical reactions making up the metabolism of a living organism are directed along specific sequences called **metabolic pathways.** These reactions are catalyzed by enzymes (protein catalysts), and each participant compound is called a **metabolite.** The product of one enzyme-catalyzed reaction serves as a substrate for the second, and so on. Each biochemical reaction in a metabolic pathway, which can be linear, branched, spiraled, or cyclic, is accompanied by a corresponding energy change. Moreover, metabolic pathways are more than theoretical constructs. For example, *Escherichia coli* grown in a medium containing isoleucine does not produce the enzymes required for isoleucine biosynthesis. In an isoleucine-deficient medium, however, *E. coli* produces each of the enzymes that make up the metabolic pathway that converts precursors to isoleucine, the end product.

Metabolism consists of two subdivisions called catabolism and anabolism. **Catabolism** refers to the conversion of large, complex molecules into smaller, simple metabolites. Some of these reactions produce chemical energy that is captured as ATP. **Anabolism** refers to the conversion of small molecules into large ones during the process of biosynthesis. Anabolic reactions require chemical energy, which is ultimately derived from ATP. Some pathways participate in both catabolic and anabolic reactions. These pathways are called **amphibolic** (Greek *amphi,* "two-sided").

Role of ATP in Metabolism

Besides providing energy for anabolism, ATP (Figure 1–2) serves as the source of the chemical energy used for muscle contraction, cellular motility, ion and metabolite transport, and anabolism. *ATP serves as the common currency of energy exchange in all living systems.* This is a statement of **Lipmann's law** (Fritz Lipmann, 1941) and is a major unifying principle of biochemistry. ATP is the most important biochemical compound in terrestrial life.

THE THREE STAGES OF AEROBIC METABOLISM

The metabolism of cells that use oxygen as an electron acceptor to generate energy is called aer-

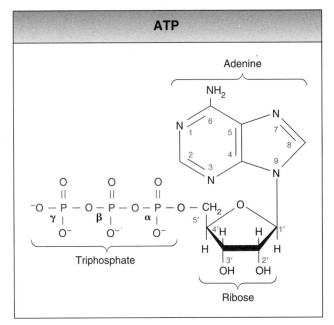

FIGURE 1–2. Structure of ATP (adenosine triphosphate), the common currency of energy exchange. This substance is made up of an adenine ring, ribose, and three phosphates. The carbon atoms in ribose are given prime (') numbers that distinguish them from the atoms in adenine. The phosphorus atoms are designated by Greek letters.

obic. The metabolism of cells that do not use oxygen for energy production is called **anaerobic.** Hans A. Krebs, a physician and biochemist, conceptually divided aerobic metabolism into three stages. His scheme provides an overview of catabolic pathways and energy production. In **stage I,** complex molecules are converted into their building blocks (Figure 1–3). Stage I of aerobic metabolism represents a preparatory stage, and no useful chemical energy is produced for other processes.

In **stage II** of aerobic metabolism, monomeric building blocks are converted to simpler molecules. For example, humans and most bacteria convert hexoses to pyruvate, a three-carbon metabolite. During this process, modest amounts of ATP are generated in oxygen-independent reactions. The conversion of sugars, amino acids, and fatty acids into acetyl coenzyme A constitutes a crucial part of the second stage of metabolism (coenzyme A is an organic metabolite).

In **stage III** of aerobic metabolism, two-carbon acetyl fragments are converted to carbon dioxide and reduced compounds by the Krebs cycle. The Krebs cycle is sometimes called the final common pathway of metabolism. The Krebs cycle makes up a major portion of **catabolism.** Following a series of energy-producing oxidation-reduction reactions, electrons and protons react with oxygen to produce water. Electron transport to oxygen is carried out by humans and other **aerobes.** Electron transport to other acceptors is carried out by **anaerobes.** The oxidation-reduction reactions of electron transport proceed downhill in an energetically fa-

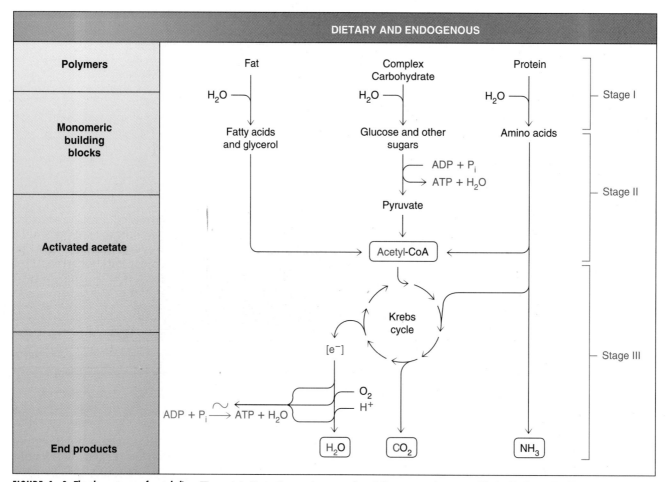

	DIETARY AND ENDOGENOUS	

FIGURE 1–3. The three stages of metabolism. *The catabolic pathways in stages I and II converge on stage III, the Krebs cycle. The Krebs cycle is the final common pathway of metabolism.*

vorable direction and sustain the production of ATP by a process called oxidative phosphorylation.

CELLS, MEMBRANES, AND CELLULAR METABOLISM

Cells are the functional units of living organisms. The **cell theory** of biology states that living cells are derived from other living cells. The human body consists of several hundred different varieties of cells. Cells differentiate into specialized cells that form specific tissues and organs. Each organ system, moreover, may consist of many distinct cell types. The digestive system, for example, is composed of the oral cavity, salivary glands, esophagus, stomach, small bowel, large bowel, liver, gallbladder, and pancreas. Each of these tissues is composed of a number of distinguishable cell types.

Cells from all living organisms are surrounded by a **plasma membrane** that separates the cell interior from the exterior. Cells in higher organisms also contain membranous intracellular organelles and membrane networks. Biological membranes are made up of lipid bilayers and associated pro-

teins. The lipids in membranes are made up of a polar, hydrophilic portion that faces the exterior of each of the two layers of the membrane and a hydrophobic, nonpolar portion projecting into the interior of the membrane (Figure 1–4). Proteins that are embedded in the lipid are called **integral membrane proteins.** Those proteins bound at the surface of a membrane are **peripheral proteins.**

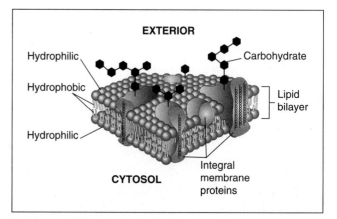

FIGURE 1–4. Topography of a plasma membrane. *Note that the carbohydrate oligosaccharides face the exterior of the cell. The interior of the cell is labeled cytosol.*

Some integral membrane proteins course through the membrane one or more times. Integral membrane proteins subserve several essential cellular functions. For example, integral membrane proteins mediate the transport of several classes of fuel molecules from the cell exterior to interior. These proteins transport specific sugars and specific classes of amino acids. Integral membrane proteins also transport ions.

Membranes function as a barrier between the inside of a cell and its environment and between different intracellular compartments. Membranes separate components that occur in different subcellular compartments. Ions, protons, and most organic compounds do not readily pass through membranes. Most intracellular metabolites are ionized, and the **impermeability** of membranes inhibits the escape of charged substances from cells.

PROKARYOTIC AND EUKARYOTIC CELLS

Cells contain either a nucleus or a nuclear body. These are the chief repositories of the genetic material of the cell and are composed of DNA (about 35% by mass). Specific proteins (60%) and RNA (5%) account for the remaining mass of the nucleus or the nuclear body.

Living organisms consist of two major classes based on the nature of the nucleus: (1) prokaryotes and (2) eukaryotes. **Prokaryotes** lack a well-defined nucleus (*pro,* "before"; *karyon,* "kernel" or "nucleus"). **Eukaryotes** have a well-defined nucleus surrounded by a nuclear membrane (*eu,* "normal"). Animals, plants, and protists make up the eukaryotes. The protists are unicellular organisms that include algae, fungi (including yeast), and protozoa. Pathogenic (Greek *pathos,* "disease"; *genesis,* "producing") organisms include some bacteria (prokaryotes), viruses, and protozoa (eukaryotes).

CELLULAR LOCALIZATION OF METABOLIC PROCESSES

The structure of eukaryotic cells varies from organism to organism and from tissue to tissue within an organism. Besides the well-defined nucleus and nuclear membrane, eukaryotic cells have extensive intracellular membrane-bounded organelles and membrane systems (Figure 1–5). Metabolic compartmentation is much more pronounced in eukaryotes than in prokaryotes. Only rare prokaryotes possess any intracellular membranes, and the amount is very modest.

All cells are enveloped by a **plasma membrane,** the boundary between the cell interior and exterior. Intracellular components differ from those of the extracellular milieu. The plasma membrane contains ATP-dependent transport systems, for example, that maintain ionic gradients between the cell's interior and exterior. The continuous

aqueous phase of the cytoplasm is the **cytosol,** where many biochemical processes are localized (Table 1–1). Moreover, the **nucleus** is the site of DNA-directed processes, including DNA replication and DNA-directed RNA biosynthesis.

Mitochondria, the chemical powerhouses of the cell, are the major site of ATP production (Table 1–1) and contain the components of stage III of metabolism. The electron transport chain, which transfers electrons from reducing agents sequentially to molecular oxygen, is located in the inner mitochondrial membrane. Mitochondria are the site of greater than 95% of oxygen consumption in humans.

The occurrence of oxidative catabolic reactions and ATP biosynthesis in a specialized organelle (the mitochondrion) has several advantages. The reducing equivalents from most catabolic reactions are produced in the mitochondrion and can be transferred directly to the electron transport chain. The catabolic reactions of the mitochondrion can be regulated independently of anabolic reactions in other compartments. Specialized metabolic functions occur in specific locations in the cell, and a division of labor results.

Lysosomes are small, membrane-enclosed organelles containing many different degradative enzymes, some of which are listed in Table 1–1. The hydrogen ion concentration within the lysosome is acidic (pH 5) compared with that of the remainder of the cytosol (pH 7). Specific ATP-dependent reactions are responsible for generating this acidic differential.

▶ More is known about the role of lysosomes in cell pathology than about any other organelle. Lysosomes are involved directly or indirectly in any disease process in which there is cell death, cell involution, or cell injury. Moreover, more than 20 different diseases are due to a deficiency in a lysosomal enzyme activity. Because of each enzyme deficiency, the substrate of the defective or missing enzyme accumulates in the lysosomes. The organelles become enlarged, and crowding interferes with cell function.

Defects in lysosomal enzymes for a special class of phospholipids called sphingolipids are associated with specific diseases. Tay-Sachs disease (hexosaminidase A) and Niemann-Pick disease (sphingomyelinase), for example, are caused by defects in specific hydrolases. In gout, the underlying disease is due to an accumulation of urate. The lysosomes become damaged and leak their digestive enzymes into the cell, thereby resulting in cellular and tissue injury. ◀

Peroxisomes are organelles associated with peroxide metabolism. Peroxisomes contain **catalase,** an enzyme that catalyzes the following reaction:

$$H_2O_2 \rightarrow H_2O + \tfrac{1}{2} O_2 \qquad (1.3)$$

Hydrogen peroxide (H_2O_2) is toxic, and its metabolism must be restricted as much as possible to a specialized compartment of the cell.

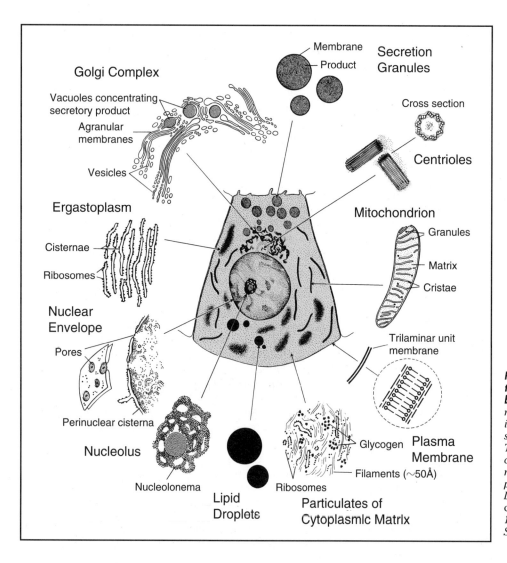

Golgi Complex
Vacuoles concentrating secretory product
Agranular membranes
Vesicles

Membrane
Product

Secretion Granules

Cross section

Centrioles

Ergastoplasm
Cisternae
Ribosomes

Mitochondrion
Granules
Matrix
Cristae

Nuclear Envelope
Pores

Trilaminar unit membrane

Perinuclear cisterna

Nucleolus

Nucleolonema

Lipid Droplets

Glycogen
Ribosomes

Plasma Membrane
Filaments (~50Å)

Particulates of Cytoplasmic Matrix

FIGURE 1-5. A cell is illustrated at the center of the diagram as it appears by light microscopy. Around the periphery are representations of the intracellular organelles as observed by electron microscopy. The ergastoplasm of the light microscopist is now called the rough endoplasmic reticulum. Reproduced, with permission, from D. W. Fawcett: Bloom and Fawcett: A Textbook of Histology, 11th ed., Philadelphia, W.B. Saunders Company, 1986, p. 2.

TABLE 1-1. Metabolic Properties of Animal Cell Components

Component	General Properties	Associated Biochemical Processes	Percent Volume	Number per Cell
Cytosol	Nonsedimentable	Glycolysis, gluconeogenesis, glycogenesis, glycogenolysis, pentose phosphate pathway; fatty acid, steroid, purine, pyrimidine, and protein synthesis (free ribosomes), copper-zinc superoxide dismutase	54	1
Lysosome	Wastebasket of the cell	Cathepsins (degrade several classes of proteins), DNAse, RNAse, hexosaminidase A, and sphingomyelinase	1	300
Mitochondrion	Powerhouse of the cell, major site of ATP formation	Krebs cycle, β-oxidation of fatty acids, oxidative phosphorylation, pyruvate dehydrogenase activity, and manganese superoxide dismutase	22	1700
Nucleus	Repository and expression of genes	DNA replication, RNA synthesis and processing	6	1
Peroxisome	Hydrogen peroxide metabolism	Catalase and peroxidase	1	400
Plasma membrane	Boundary between cell exterior and interior	Sodium-potassium ATPase, insulin and glucagon receptors, glucose translocase, and γ-glutamyl transpeptidase	1	1
Smooth endoplasmic reticulum	Complex lipid biosynthesis	Phospholipid synthesis, steroid hydroxylation, and cytochrome P-450 activity	6	1
Rough endoplasmic reticulum and Golgi complex	Synthesis of membrane proteins and proteins for export	Protein synthesis and processing	9	1

The **endoplasmic reticulum** (endoplasmic, "inside the cell"; reticulum, "network") is an extensive membrane system found in eukaryotic cells that is involved in many metabolic processes (Table 1–1). The **rough endoplasmic reticulum** is studded with ribosomes (Figure 1–5). The cisternae of the endoplasmic reticulum form the spaces between surrounding membranes. Proteins destined for export from the cell or for insertion into membranes are generally synthesized in the rough endoplasmic reticulum and occur transiently in cisternae. These proteins are transported to the Golgi complex, where further processing occurs. Processing can involve cleavage of the protein into smaller segments, the addition of one or more carbohydrate residues, or many other chemical modifications.

HUMAN CHROMOSOMES

When a human cell divides, homogeneous chromatin condenses to form rod-shaped bodies called chromosomes (Greek *chroma*, "color"; *soma*, "body"). Each eukaryotic species has a characteristic chromosomal anatomy and number called a **karyotype.** Genes lie in a linear order along the chromosomes. Each gene has a characteristic position, or locus. The map of the chromosomal location of the genes is characteristic of each species.

The somatic cells of humans contain 46 chromosomes or 23 pairs (Figure 1–6B). Of these, 22 pairs are alike in males and females and are called **autosomes.** The remaining pair are the **sex chromosomes,** denoted XX in females and XY in males. Each pair of autosomal chromosomes (not including the X and Y chromosome pairs) carries matching genetic information. One member of each pair is inherited from the mother, and the other from the father. With modern molecular techniques, it is possible to determine which of the two chromosomes was obtained from each parent and grandparent.

The inheritance of genes located on autosomes is designated as autosomal, and the inheritance of genes on the X chromosome is called X-linked. If one copy of a gene is sufficient for expression of an individual's phenotype, or observable trait, such a gene is called **dominant.** If two copies of a gene are required for expression of an individual's phenotype, such a gene is called **recessive.**

Alternative forms of a gene are called **alleles.**

▶ Sickle cell anemia is inherited as an **autosomal recessive** trait. Both alleles must be of the sickle cell variety for the phenotypic expression of anemia. If only one allele is of the sickle cell type and the other allele is normal, or wild type, the individual is phenotypically normal. This characteristic defines the recessive nature of the disorder. Familial hypercholesterolemia is an **autosomal dominant** trait. Only one allele is required for the expression of hypercholesterolemia. Hemo-

philia, a blood clotting disorder, is a **sex-linked trait.** Because males possess only one X chromosome, males with the hemophilia gene are affected. Females have two X chromosomes. Even if one of them contains a hemophilia gene, expression of the normal allele produces a normal phenotype. ◀

Chromosomes during mitosis consist of two **chromatids** joined at the **centromere** (Figure 1–6A). The centromere divides the chromosome into two arms designated **p** (for petite or small) and **q** for the long arm. Chromosomes are numbered from 1 to 22 based upon size, with 1 being the largest and 22 being the smallest. Arms of individual chromosomes are designated by the chromosome number and a p or q: 7q refers to the long arm of chromosome 7; 11p refers to the short arm of chromosome 11. The long arm and the short arm of each chromosome have a specific dye-staining pattern and morphology. In some cases, the location of a gene in a specific band is known, and this is expressed as numerals after the p or q. The gene for Tay-Sachs disease, for example, is located on chromosome 15q23-q24. The first number of the doublet 23 refers to a location on major band 2 on the long arm of chromosome 15, and the 3 or 4 refers to sub-bands on the main band. The numbering of bands begins on the center of the chromosome (centromere) and extends toward each end (**telomere**). The relative position of the centromere determines whether a chromosome is **metacentric, submetacentric,** or **acrocentric** (Figure 1–6A).

▶ The **Philadelphia chromosome** (denoted Ph[1]) occurs in about 95% of individuals with chronic myelogenous leukemia (abnormal proliferation of white blood cells). Ph[1] is an abbreviated chromosome 22 that results from the reciprocal translocation of segments between chromosomes 22 and 9 (Figure 1–6C). ◀

There are several identical copies of DNA per mitochondrion and thousands per cell. A unique feature of **mitochondrial DNA** is its maternal inheritance. Mitochondria from the sperm do not persist in the offspring. ▶ A few rare genetic diseases are linked with mitochondrial DNA. The diseases are transmitted maternally, and no affected males transmit the disease. Affected individuals may be male or female. One example of this variety of disease is Leber hereditary optic neuropathy (LHON), a rare but celebrated disorder. ◀

THE CELL CYCLE AND MITOSIS

Humans begin development as a fertilized ovum (**zygote**); a zygote is a diploid cell from which all cells of the body ($\approx 10^{14}$) are derived by hundreds of cell divisions, or mitoses. DNA synthesis and cell division are key events in the cell cycle. The four stages of the cell cycle include G_1, S, G_2, and M (Figure 1–7). G_1 and G_2 are gaps or growth phases. G_1 is the gap between the previous cell

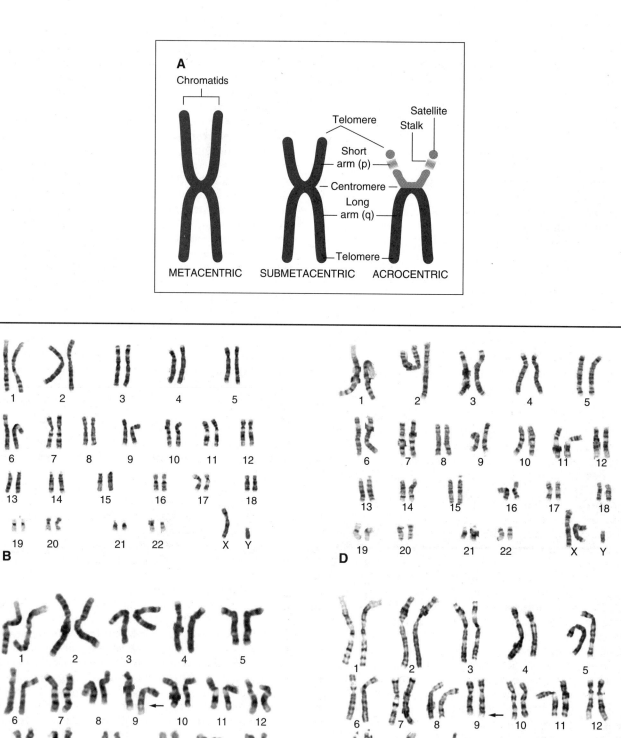

FIGURE 1–6. Chromosome morphology and karyotype. *Chromosomes in the initial stage of mitosis are made up of duplicated parent DNA molecules that are paired as chromatids bound at a centromere. A. Metacentric, submetacentric, and acrocentric chromosomes. B. Normal male (46XY). C. Philadelphia chromosome (translocation from 22q to 9q) in a female. D. Klinefelter syndrome (47XXY). E. Trisomy 21 (Down syndrome). Courtesy of Y. S. Kao and T. van Brunt, Louisiana State University Medical Center.*

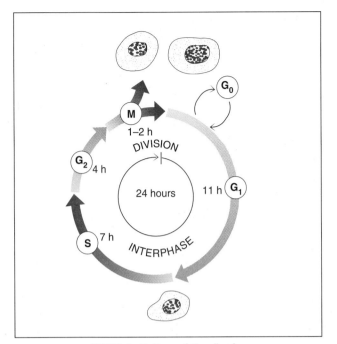

FIGURE 1-7. Stages of the cell cycle.

division (cytokinesis) and the beginning of DNA synthesis. S refers to the DNA *synthesis* phase. G_2 is the gap between DNA replication and nuclear division. M refers to *mitosis*, during which all pairs of duplicated chromosomes separate into the two daughter cells. G_1, S, and G_2 make up interphase. Interphase in human cells in culture lasts for about 23 hours, and mitosis occurs in 1–2 hours. The rate of cell division in humans ranges from 16 hours to months. The duration of G_1 is variable and depends upon the cell type. Slowly dividing cells are said to enter a G_0 phase of the cell cycle.

When a cell enters mitosis, each of its chromosomes consists of a pair of identical sister chromatids joined at the centromere. During mitosis, one chromatid of each chromosome is distributed to each daughter cell. The four stages of mitosis include (1) prophase, (2) metaphase, (3) anaphase, and (4) telophase (Figure 1–8). At the completion of mitosis, each of the daughter cell's chromosomes consists of one DNA molecule. Each molecule will be duplicated during the S phase of the cell cycle.

MEIOSIS

Meiosis is the type of cell division that reduces the diploid number (2N) of chromosomes to the haploid number (1N) of the gamete (egg or sperm). Meiosis is more complex than mitosis because meiosis involves two successive divisions. Each of the 2N chromosomes is duplicated as sister chromatids, 4N in number, before the first meiotic division. The chromosome number is reduced to 2N during the first meiotic division. During the second

meiotic division, the chromatids of each of the haploid number of chromosomes separate to form gametes (Figure 1–8).

Chromosomal Abnormalities

▶ The possession of three copies of human chromosome 21 (trisomy 21) results in **Down syndrome** and is the most common abnormality (1 in 1000 live births) of the number of autosomes in live-born infants (Figure 1–6E). The incidence of Down syndrome increases with the age of the mother. The normal female somatic cell contains two X chromosomes, and the normal male somatic cell contains an X and a Y chromosome. The presence of only one X chromosome (XO) results in **Turner syndrome,** characterized by a female phenotype with short stature, webbed neck, failure to develop secondary sex characteristics, and abnormal ovaries. The presence of an extra X chromosome (XXX) occurs in clinically normal females. The occurrence of one Y chromosome and at least two X chromosomes (XXY, XXXY, XXXXY) produces **Klinefelter syndrome** (Figure 1–6D). The affected individual is phenotypically male with tall stature, poorly developed secondary sex characteristics, and testicular atrophy. ◀

MICROORGANISMS AS AGENTS OF DISEASE

Diversity of Bacteria

More than 2500 bacterial species are known. Of these, only a small fraction produce human disease. Bacteria exhibit metabolic diversity in the biochemical strategies used to produce ATP. Some bacteria are **aerobes** and reduce oxygen by processes similar to those used by mitochondria. Other bacteria, such as *Streptococcus,* are unable to reduce oxygen. Fuel molecules are converted to simpler molecules, such as lactate, by fermentation reactions. These microbes are called **anaerobes.** Still other bacteria, such as *E. coli,* can survive under either aerobic or anaerobic conditions and are called **facultative anaerobes.** Some species of *Clostridium* are killed by oxygen. Such microbes are called **obligate anaerobes.**

Classification of Bacteria

Bacteria with the shape of a sphere are called **cocci,** and those with the shape of a rod are called **bacilli.** A **vibrio** is made up of a curved rod with a flagellum at one end. A **spirillum** is a spiral or screw-shaped bacterium (Figure 1–9). These morphological terms are applied to both genera and families of bacteria.

One of the traditional ways to classify bacteria is by the **Gram stain,** first described by Christian

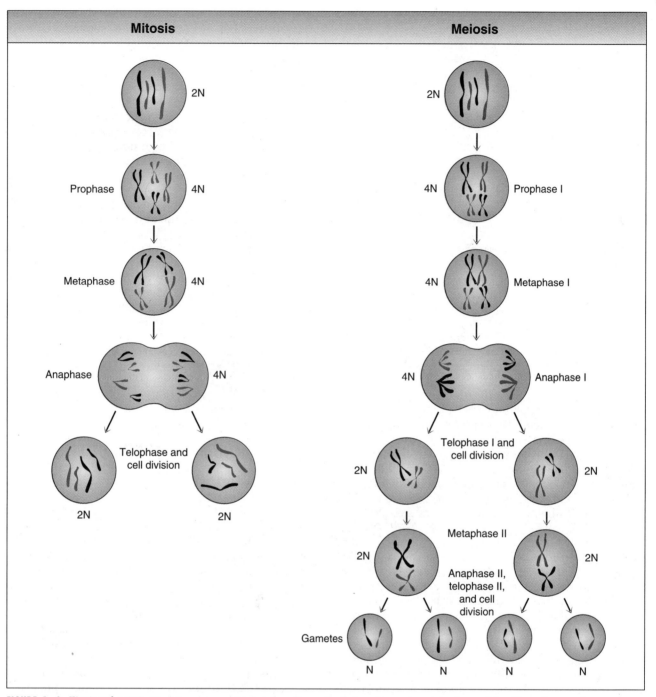

FIGURE 1–8. Mitosis and meiosis. *Crossing over, which involves the reciprocal exchange between chromatids of homologous chromosomes, occurs during prophase I of meiosis. Crossing over is a form of genetic recombination. For simplicity, the number of chromosomes illustrated is 4 and not 23. The haploid content of chromosomes is indicated by N. Adapted, with permission, from J. D. Watson, M. Gilman, J. Witkowski, and M. Zoller,* Recombinant DNA, *2nd ed. New York, W. H. Freeman and Company, 1992, p. 8.*

Gram in 1884. **Gram-positive** bacteria can take up and retain an iodine complex of the basic dye, crystal violet. **Gram-negative** bacteria are unable to retain this complex. Most spore-forming bacilli and cocci are gram-positive. *E. coli,* other enterobacteria (bacteria that inhabit the gut), and pseudomonads (bacteria that occur singly [Greek *monos,* "single"]) are gram-negative. Distinct Gram-staining properties are produced by differences in the cell wall that surrounds the plasma membrane

of the cell (Figure 1–10). Gram-positive bacteria exhibit a uniform but thick cell wall. In contrast, gram-negative bacteria exhibit a thinner cell wall with two layers. To know the identity of an infectious agent as gram-positive or gram-negative is helpful in diagnosis and for prescribing classes of antibiotics.

▶ Table 1–2 provides a list of selected gram-positive human pathogens. *Streptococcus mutans* produces dental caries, or tooth decay, by generat-

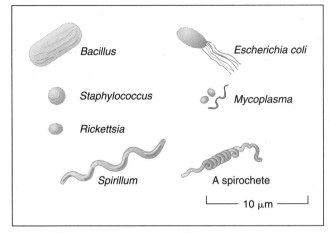

FIGURE 1–9. Several varieties of bacteria drawn to scale.

TABLE 1–2.   Pathogenic Gram-Positive Bacteria

Group/Pathogen	Principal Disease
Endospore-forming bacteria	
Clostridium tetani	Tetanus
Lactic acid bacteria	
Streptococcus mutans	Dental caries
Streptococcus pneumoniae	Meningitis, middle ear infections, pneumonia
Streptococcus pyogenes	Glomerulonephritis, pharyngitis, rheumatic fever
Nocardioform bacteria	
Corynebacterium diphtheriae	Diphtheria
Mycobacterium tuberculosis	Tuberculosis
Staphylococci	
Staphylococcus aureus	Pneumonia, wound infections

ing lactic acid from glucose. The lactic acid dissolves tooth enamel, leading to caries. Table 1–3 provides a list of selected gram-negative human pathogens. The best understood of all organisms, *E. coli,* is a member of this category. *E. coli,* which is a physiological inhabitant of the large bowel, can also be pathogenic.

Spirochetes are helix-shaped bacteria with endoflagella (Figure 1–9). *Treponema* includes many pathogenic strains, including that which produces syphilis (*T. pallidum*). The rickettsiae are obligate intracellular parasites. When compared with other bacteria, rickettsiae are smaller, have a longer generation time, and require an exogenous energy supply for growth. Rickettsiae are the causative agents of typhus and Rocky Mountain spotted fever.

Protozoa are unicellular eukaryotes. These include *Entamoeba histolytica,* the causative agent of amebic dysentery. Protozoa are also the agents responsible for African sleeping sickness (*Trypanosoma gambiense*) and malaria (*Plasmodium falciparum, Plasmodium ovale,* and *Plasmodium vivax*). ◄

ORGANIZATION OF BACTERIAL CELLS

Prokaryotes such as *E. coli* (gram-negative) and *Streptococcus pneumoniae* (gram-positive) are small, unicellular organisms about 1 μm in diameter and 2 μm in length. Prokaryotes contain a plasma membrane that may be surrounded by a cell wall and by a capsule (Figure 1–10). Motile bacteria contain external flagella. Mesosomes are localized membrane infoldings that arise near the site of cell division. Mesosomes probably partici-

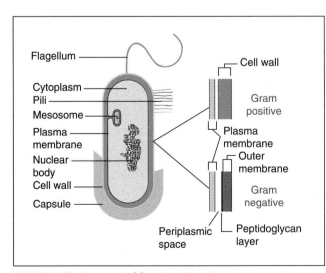

FIGURE 1–10. A prototypical bacterium. *Not all structures are present in all bacteria. The enlargements on the right represent details of gram-positive and gram-negative bacteria. The cell wall of the gram-positive bacterium contains appreciable peptidoglycan. Adapted, with permission, from B. A. Freeman.* In Burrows Textbook of Microbiology, *22nd ed. Philadelphia, W.B. Saunders Company, 1985, p. 23.*

TABLE 1–3.   Pathogenic Gram-Negative Bacteria

Group/Pathogen	Principal Disease
Aerobic rod-shaped bacteria	
Bordetella pertussis	Whooping cough
Legionella pneumophila	Legionnaires disease
Pseudomonas aeruginosa	Burn infections, pneumonia, urinary tract infections
Chlamydia	
Chlamydia pneumoniae	Atypical pneumonia
Enteric bacteria	
Escherichia coli	Diarrhea, urinary tract infections
Salmonella typhosa	Typhoid fever
Salmonella typhimurium	Diarrhea
Shigella dysenteriae	Dysentery
Facultatively anaerobic rod-shaped bacteria	
Campylobacter jejuni	Diarrhea
Helicobacter pylori	Gastritis and peptic ulcer
Haemophilus influenzae	Meningitis, middle ear infections, pharyngitis, pneumonia
Vibrio cholerae	Cholera
Neisseria	
Neisseria gonorrhoeae	Conjunctivitis, gonorrhea, pelvic inflammatory disease
Neisseria meningitidis	Meningitis, pharyngitis, pneumonia

TABLE 1–4. Classification of Viruses

Group	Viruses	Disease
DNA Virus*		
Adenovirus	Adenoviruses	Upper and lower respiratory infections, conjunctivitis, diarrhea
Hepatitis virus	Hepatitis virus B	Acute, chronic, and inapparent infection; hepatocellular carcinoma
Herpesvirus	Herpes simplex	Genital herpes, "cold sore"
	Epstein-Barr (EB) virus	Infectious mononucleosis, Burkitt lymphoma
	Varicella-zoster virus	Chickenpox, shingles
Poxvirus	Variola virus	Smallpox
	Vaccinia virus	Smallpox vaccine reaction
RNA Virus†		
Orthomyxovirus	Influenza viruses	Influenza
Paramyxovirus	Measles (rubella) virus	Measles
	Measles (rubeola) virus	German measles
	Mumps virus	Parotitis, orchitis, meningitis
Picornavirus	Poliovirus	Poliomyelitis
	Rhinovirus, echovirus	Upper respiratory infections
Retrovirus	Human T-cell lymphotropic viruses (HTLV)	Human T-cell leukemia (I, II)
	Human immunodeficiency virus (HIV)	Acquired immunodeficiency syndrome (AIDS)

* The DNA viruses in this table have double-stranded DNA as the genome.

† The RNA viruses in this table have single-stranded RNA as the genome. Retroviruses have two identical single-stranded RNA molecules per virus particle.

pate in the formation of a transverse septum during cell division. Bacteria divide by **binary fission.** This process occurs without chromosome condensation or spindle formation.

Because prokaryotes lack appreciable intracellular membranes and organization, the various metabolic pathways occur in a single intracellular compartment. Some metabolic processes require the participation of a membrane. For example, oxidative phosphorylation, which requires mitochondrial membranes in eukaryotic cells, uses the plasma membrane in prokaryotes for the same purpose. Several reactions involved in complex lipid metabolism occur in the plasma membrane of prokaryotes but use internal membranes (endoplasmic reticulum) of eukaryotes.

NEED FOR SUBCELLULAR COMPARTMENTATION IN EUKARYOTES

The division of labor in eukaryotic cells is necessary in part because of their large volume. Eukaryotic cells are much larger than prokaryotic cells. A representative eukaryotic cell ($20~\mu m \times 20~\mu m \times 20~\mu m = 8000~\mu m^3$) has a volume 5000 times that of a representative prokaryotic cell ($2~\mu m \times 1~\mu m$ diameter $= 1.6~\mu m^3$). The dispersion of enzymes and metabolites that occurs uniformly throughout this volume of eukaryotic cytoplasm has the potential to decrease the flux of compounds through metabolic pathways.

The localization of related functions in organelles promotes biochemical efficiency. Such specialization eliminates the necessity for diffusion of intermediates through relatively long distances. There is evidence, moreover, that enzymes of metabolic pathways form complexes in cells that are not apparent in the laboratory. Complex formation is postulated to result in the channeling of substrates from one enzyme active site to the next. The aggregate of enzymes of a metabolic pathway is called a **metabolon.**

VIRUSES

Viruses are infectious agents that are incapable of independent replication. Viruses require living cells for reproduction. Viruses exist for animal, plant, and bacterial cells. Virus particles are made of nucleic acid (either DNA or RNA), protein, and occasionally a lipid membrane. Viruses are simpler than other obligate intracellular parasites such as rickettsiae. Viruses are classified as DNA or RNA viruses based upon the nature of the genetic nucleic acid composition (Table 1–4). RNA viruses replicate by RNA-dependent RNA biosynthesis. RNA viruses do not go through a DNA stage in their replication cycle. Retroviruses, in contrast, are RNA viruses that synthesize DNA during their replication cycle. The DNA serves as a template for genomic RNA biosynthesis. HIV (human immunodeficiency virus), the causative agent of AIDS (acquired immunodeficiency syndrome), is an example of a retrovirus.

SELECTED READINGS

Becker, W.M., and D.W. Deamer. *The World of the Cell,* 2nd ed. Menlo Park, California, Benjamin/Cummings, 1991.

Fawcett, D.W. *Bloom and Fawcett: A Textbook of Histology,* 11th ed. Philadelphia, W.B. Saunders Company, 1986.

Krebs, H.A., and H.L. Kornberg. *Energy Transduction in Living Matter.* Berlin, Springer-Verlag, 1957.

Samuelson, J., and F. von Lichtenberg. Infectious disease. *In* R.S. Cotran, V. Kumar, and S.L. Robbins (eds.) *Robbins Pathologic Basis of Disease,* 5th ed. Philadelphia, W.B. Saunders Company, 1995, pp. 305–377.

Singer, S.J., and G.L. Nicholson. The fluid mosaic model of the structure of cell membranes. Science 175:720–731, 1972.

Stanier, R.Y., J.L. Ingraham, M.L. Wheelis, and P.R. Painter. *The Microbial World,* 5th ed. Englewood Cliffs, New Jersey, Prentice-Hall, 1986.

Thompson, M.W., R.R. McInnes, and H.F. Willard. *Genetics in Medicine,* 5th ed. Philadelphia, W.B. Saunders Company, 1991.

CHAPTER TWO

VITAMINS, MINERALS, AND NUTRITION

Scientific research consists in seeing what everyone else has seen, but thinking what no one else has thought.

—ALBERT SZENT-GYORGYI

In addition to inspiring them with the desire to carry on research, it is necessary in the training of young scientists to give them a good background of the knowledge that has already been obtained.

—LINUS PAULING

ELEMENTS FOUND IN HUMANS

Organic and Inorganic Elements

Humans are made up of about 20 of the 92 naturally occurring elements. The elements form salts (minerals), or they combine to form biomolecules. Biomolecules range from low-molecular-mass metabolites ($\approx 30-1500$) to macromolecules (proteins, nucleic acids, and glycogen) with molecular masses of millions. The chemical elements found in humans can be classified as (1) elements that make up organic matter and water, (2) abundant minerals, and (3) trace minerals. Because the human body is about 55% water by mass, oxygen and hydrogen predominate. **Carbon, hydrogen,** and **nitrogen** are the chief components of biomolecules. **Oxygen** is the most prevalent element in humans and accounts for greater than half of the mass of humans (Table 2–1). Sulfur occurs in proteins and some complex carbohydrates.

Sodium is the principal extracellular cation, and **potassium** is the chief intracellular cation (Table 2–1). While humans can conserve sodium, there is an obligatory loss of potassium in the urine of about 40 milliequivalents per day (mEq/d). This loss must be considered in determining the fluid and electrolyte solutions used for intravenous therapy. A **mole** is the mass of a compound or element that contains Avogadro's number of particles. An **equivalent** is a mole divided by the absolute value of the electrical charge per particle; a **milliequivalent** is one-thousandth of an equivalent.

An equivalent of potassium (charge $+1$) is the same as the atomic mass (39.1 g). A milliequivalent of potassium is 39.1 mg. An equivalent of calcium (charge $+2$) is 40.08 g/2 = 20.04 g. **Chloride** is the predominant extracellular anion. Intracellular anions include biochemical metabolites and proteins.

Calcium is the most abundant mineral in humans (Table 2–1). Although calcium is predominantly extracellular (as a 2 mM solution and as solid hydroxyapatite in bones and teeth), calcium plays an important regulatory role within cells. Changes in the intracellular concentration of calcium trigger muscle contraction and other cellular processes. **Magnesium** is widely distributed in the body. ▶ Preeclampsia or eclampsia is a condition that may occur during pregnancy and is associated with edema, hypertension, proteinuria (protein in the urine), and seizures. Women experiencing these seizures are often treated with intramuscular injections of magnesium sulfate. ◀

All of the elements listed in Table 2–1, except **fluoride,** are essential. An **essential** substance is one whose intake is required for life. A deficiency of any of the elements listed in Table 2–1 (except fluoride) leads to disease or even death. Although not strictly essential, fluoride enhances well-being. Fluoride is found in the bones and teeth and increases their hardness. The chief mineral in bones and teeth is hydroxyapatite. **Hydroxyapatite** is a calcium phosphate–calcium hydroxide complex that is described by the formula $Ca_{10}(PO_4)_6(OH)_2$. The substitution of fluoride for hydroxide results

TABLE 2–1.   Elements of the Human Body

Element	Symbol	Mass in 70-Kg Human	Comments
Organic matter and water			
Oxygen	O	45.5 kg	Found in organic chemicals and water
Carbon	C	12.6 kg	Found in organic chemicals
Hydrogen	H	7.0 kg	Found in organic chemicals and water
Nitrogen	N	2.1 kg	Found in nucleic acids and amino acids
Phosphorous	P	0.7 kg	Found in nucleic acids and many metabolites; constituent of bones and teeth
Sulfur	S	0.175 kg	Found in proteins and connective tissue
Abundant minerals			
Calcium	Ca	1050 g	Constituent of bones and teeth; intracellular second messenger; triggers exocytosis and muscle contraction
Potassium	K	245 g	Principal intracellular cation; obligatory loss of 40 mEq/d in urine
Sodium	Na	105 g	Principal extracellular cation
Chloride	Cl	105 g	Major extracellular anion; activates amylase
Magnesium	Mg	35 g	Cosubstrate for ATP and other nucleotide reactants; a calcium antagonist
Fluoride	F	8 g	Increases hardness of bones and teeth; excess produces dental fluorosis
Trace minerals			
Iron	Fe	3000 mg	Found in hemoglobin, myoglobin, cytochromes, iron-sulfur proteins; deficiency leads to a microcytic anemia
Zinc	Zn	2300 mg	Cofactor for carbonic anhydrase, carboxypeptidase, and cytosolic superoxide dismutase
Copper	Cu	100 mg	Component of cytochrome a, a_3 and cytosolic superoxide dismutase
Manganese	Mn	20 mg	Cofactor for mitochondrial superoxide dismutase
Cobalt	Co	5 mg	Component of vitamin B_{12}
Molybdenum	Mo	Trace	Component of xanthine dehydrogenase in purine metabolism and aldehyde oxidase in catecholamine metabolism
Iodine	I	Trace	Required for production of thyroid hormones T_4 and T_3; hyperthyroidism is treated with radioiodine
Selenium	Se	Trace	Component of glutathione peroxidase.

in fluorapatite, or $Ca_{10}(PO_4)_6F_2$. Fluorapatite is harder and more resilient than hydroxyapatite. The fluoride content of water varies greatly. Some sources contain only trace amounts, and some well water or springs may contain several milligrams per liter. The optimal intake of fluoride per day in adult humans is 1–2 mg, and an optimal fluoride content is about 1 mg per liter. One milligram per liter is one part per million (ppm).

▶ The daily intake of several milligrams of fluoride chronically (months to years) can produce **fluorosis.** One of the signs of fluorosis is mottled or dark teeth. Bones and teeth become brittle in people with fluorosis. **Osteoporosis** is a disease of demineralization or decalcification of the bones. It is more prevalent in older women than in men. High doses of fluoride (50 mg/d) intermittently, along with other agents including calcium, estrogen, and vitamin D, are being evaluated as treatments for osteoporosis. ◀

Most of the **iron** in humans is complexed as an organic compound called heme. About two-thirds is found in the hemoglobin of the red blood cells, or erythrocytes; hemoglobin is the chief oxygen transport protein in the circulation. Iron absorption by the intestine is regulated because excess iron is toxic. Iron is transported by **transferrin,** a glycoprotein produced by liver. The **total iron binding capacity** is a clinical measure of the amount of transferrin in the serum. **Ferritin,** a protein that can bind up to 4000 iron atoms per molecule, is the cellular storage form of iron with a wide tissue distribution. **Hemosiderin** is an insoluble iron aggregate that is derived from ferritin. ▶ Too much iron in the tissues is toxic and leads to **hemochromatosis.** ◀

Adult women are prone to iron deficiency owing to blood loss during menstruation. ▶ **Iron deficiency anemia** is a prevalent nutritional disorder in the United States. It is also common in children but is rare in adult men. The erythrocytes in iron deficiency anemia are smaller than normal, thereby accounting for the designation of **microcytic anemia** (Greek *mikros,* "small"; *kytos,* "a hollow" or "cell"). ◀

Cobalt is a metal ion found in trace amounts in humans. *The only known role of cobalt in biochemistry is as a constituent of vitamin B_{12}.* Vitamins are organic molecules that cannot be synthesized in humans, are essential for health, and must be taken in the diet in small amounts (milligram to microgram amounts). Vitamin B_{12} is an intricate organic molecule (Figure 2–1) that participates in carbon-transfer reactions.

The role of **iodide** in human metabolism is to serve as a component of thyroid hormone. The active components include tetraiodothyronine (T_4) and triiodothyronine (T_3) (Figure 2–2). Iodide is an

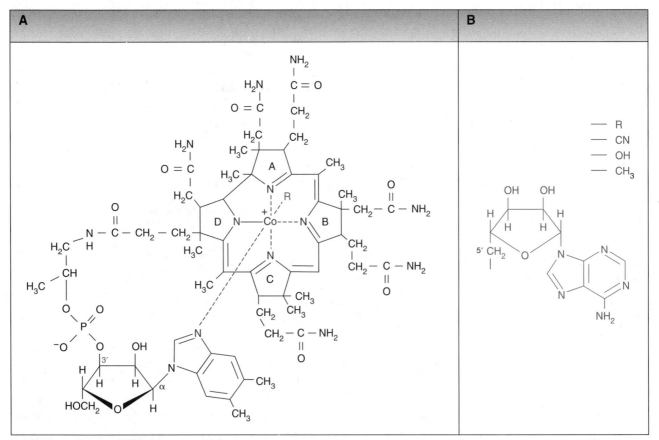

FIGURE 2–1. Structure of vitamin B_{12}. A. *Vitamin B_{12} has two components: the corrin ring system (A–D) and 5,6-dimethylbenzimidazole ribonucleotide covalently attached to ring D. B. The R group in the over-the-counter form of the vitamin is —CN. In the coenzyme form, R is a methyl group (CH_3—) or a 5'-deoxyadenosyl-group. Note that B_{12} contains cobalt, and the structure of B_{12} is intricate.*

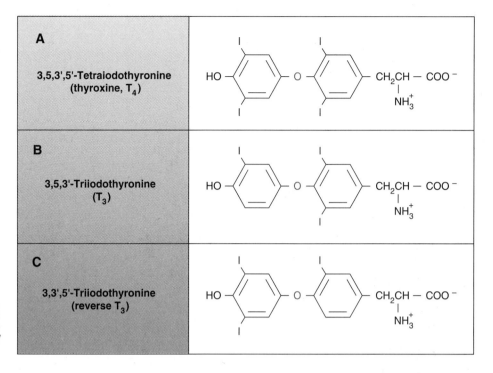

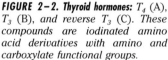

FIGURE 2–2. Thyroid hormones: T_4 (A), T_3 (B), and reverse T_3 (C). These compounds are iodinated amino acid derivatives with amino and carboxylate functional groups.

essential component in the diet. ▶ The water of some areas of the earth, especially inland and away from the sea, lacks iodide. Individuals with inadequate iodide intake develop an enlargement of the thyroid gland called a **goiter.** To provide adequate intake of this mineral, proprietary table salt or sodium chloride contains added iodide. This is called iodized salt.

A deficiency of thyroid hormone results in **hypothyroidism.** Hypothyroidism in children results in growth defects and subnormal central nervous system development. The disorder is called **cretinism,** and it is treated with oral tetraiodothyronine. Adults may develop hypothyroidism or **myxedema.**

Adults may also develop **hyperthyroidism.** This may be associated with an enlarged thyroid gland (goiter), oculopathy (eye disorder), and an increased metabolic rate. This illness in adults is called **Graves disease** (after the physician who described it). Graves disease is generally due to diffuse enlargement and overactivity of the thyroid gland. The ailment is treated with radioiodine (^{131}I). ^{131}I emits both x rays and γ rays (high-energy electromagnetic radiation). The thyroid gland cells concentrate the radioiodine and are destroyed by the radioactivity. Such individuals often develop hypothyroidism because of the destruction of too much tissue. The complication of hypothyroidism is easily treated with oral thyroid hormone. ◀

The functions of other trace elements are listed in Table 2–1.

Toxic Elements in the Environment

Including the 20 or so elements essential for life, the earth's crust and atmosphere contain 92 natu-rally occurring elements. This number excludes the elements created by physicists with atomic numbers greater than 92. Almost all the natural elements (except actinium, protactinium, and radium) are found in humans. ▶ The intake of excess lead can result in **lead poisoning,** especially in children (Chapter 24). Lead is present in air, water, soil, and food. The use of nonleaded gasoline fuels has decreased the lead content of air. The use of lead in plumbing is now banned in the United States, but lead can still get into the drinking water from old water pipes.

One of the products of the radioactive decay of uranium (a natural element) is radon. **Radon,** a radioactive gas, is a fission product of terrestrial uranium and seeps from the earth's surface into buildings. Radon, which emits helium nuclei or α-particles, is alleged to be an important cause of lung cancer in humans. The gas, which decomposes by radioactive decay into polonium, binds to aerosol particles and deposits in the tracheobronchial tree and irradiates the lungs. ◀

NATURE OF CHEMICAL BONDS

Five types of chemical bonds are important in determining the structure of biological molecules: (1) covalent, (2) ionic (salt bridges), (3) hydrogen, (4) hydrophobic, and (5) van der Waals.

Covalent bonds, which are composed of a pair of electrons, are strong (≈ 400 kJ or 100 kcal/mol) and account for the stability of carbohydrates, fats, proteins, nucleic acids, and other biomolecules. Covalent bonds are depicted as paired dots or, more commonly, as lines (Figure 2–3). Double bonds are depicted by two lines. The representa-

A Water	H:Ö:H = H — O 　　　　　　　　　| 　　　　　　　　　H
B Methane	H 　　| H:C:H = H — C — H 　　Ḧ　　　| 　　　　　　　H
C Formaldehyde	H 　\ :C::O = 　C = O 　/　　　　　/ 　H　　　　H
D Octanoic acid	H H H H H H H ⦂O H:C:C:C:C:C:C:C:Ċ: = H — C — C — C — C — C — C — C — C H H H H H H H Ö:H *or* ⌇⌇⌇⌇⌇⌇⌇ COOH

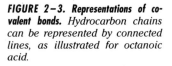

FIGURE 2–3. Representations of covalent bonds. *Hydrocarbon chains can be represented by connected lines, as illustrated for octanoic acid.*

tion of a molecule that cannot be portrayed by a single valence structure but can be embodied as a hybrid of two or more structures in which all of the atomic nuclei remain in the same position is called **resonance.** Figure 2–4 depicts the resonance hybrids of benzene, an aromatic compound. The chemical bonds linking the carbon atoms of benzene are hybrid bonds. They are not single bonds part of the time and double bonds part of the time but are intermediate in character all of the time. Phosphate can also be represented by alternative and equivalent resonance hybrids. Covalent bonds are strong and stable. In contrast, the bonds listed below are weak and can break and re-form at physiological temperatures.

Hydrogen bonds are formed by the sharing of a hydrogen atom between electronegative oxygen atoms, nitrogen atoms, or a combination of the two (Figure 2–5). The hydrogen atom is covalently

linked to one of the atoms of the pair (the hydrogen bond donor) and interacts electrostatically with the second (the hydrogen bond acceptor). The strength of hydrogen bonds is dependent upon direction. Although individually weak (8–20 kJ or 2–5 kcal/mol), formation of a large number of these bonds promotes stability. **Salt bridges,** or **ionic bonds** (Figure 2–6), that result from electrostatic attraction between positively and negatively charged species are weaker ($\approx$ 20–40 kJ or 5–10 kcal/mol) than covalent bonds.

Hydrophobic ("water-fearing") **bonds** are nonpolar bonds between hydrocarbon-containing compounds (Figure 2–6). It is energetically favorable to sequester hydrocarbons in hydrophobic domains and minimize their contact with polar water molecules in solution. Although individually weak, formation of a large number of hydrophobic bonds results in a stable structure. **Van der Waals bonds**

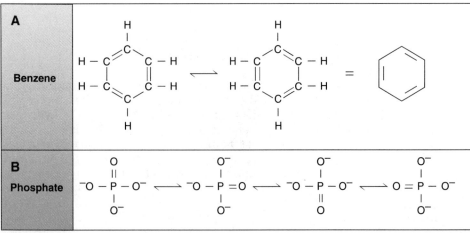

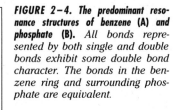

FIGURE 2–4. The predominant resonance structures of benzene (A) and phosphate (B). *All bonds represented by both single and double bonds exhibit some double bond character. The bonds in the benzene ring and surrounding phosphate are equivalent.*

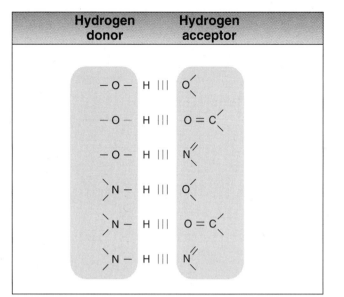

Hydrogen donor	Hydrogen acceptor

FIGURE 2–5. Hydrogen bonds.

are the result of the mutual interaction of electrons and nuclei of molecules. These result from the electrostatic attraction of the nuclei of one molecule for the electrons of another. Hydrophobic and van der Waals bonds are weak ($\approx$ 4 kJ or 1 kcal/mol).

FUNCTIONAL GROUPS OF ORGANIC COMPOUNDS

In considering metabolic reactions, it is important to delineate the chemistry of the participating

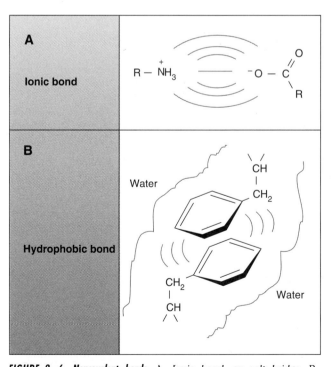

FIGURE 2–6. Noncovalent bonds. A. *Ionic bond, or salt bridge.* B. *Hydrophobic bond. Hydrophobic interactions between two aromatic groups are illustrated.*

functional groups. Identifying the precise bonds that are made and broken during chemical transformations aids in understanding biochemical processes. The main functional groups of biomolecules (Table 2–2) are familiar from organic chemistry.

Hydrocarbons, made up of hydrogen and carbon, generally constitute a part of the structure of most biomolecules. For example, some amino acid side chains are nonpolar hydrocarbons. Lipids, including fat-soluble vitamins, are largely hydrocarbon in nature.

The oxygen of an **alcohol,** the nitrogen of an **amine,** and the sulfur of a **thiol** group contain a free electron pair and are nucleophiles (Table 2–2). Much of the chemistry of these compounds can be explained by the reaction of this electron pair with an electrophilic center. The oxygen atoms of phosphate and carboxylate can also function as nucleophiles.

The **carbonyl group** is a prominent reagent in biochemical reactions (Table 2–2). The carbonyl group occurs in sugars as either an **aldehyde** or **ketone. Carboxylic acids** occur in fatty acids (fatty acids contain a hydrocarbon side chain attached to a carboxylic acid). Octanoic acid, illustrated in Figure 2–3, is an example of a medium-chain fatty acid. Carboxylic acids at physiological hydrogen ion concentrations exist as the charged anion or carboxylate as indicated in the following equation:

$$R - COOH \rightleftarrows R - COO^- + H^+ \qquad (2.1)$$

Carboxylic acid $\leftrightarrows$ carboxylate + proton

Even though the term acid is used to describe a biomolecule, it is usually the anionic or salt form that is present in solution under physiological conditions.

The linkage of a carboxylate (1) with an alcohol results in an **ester,** (2) with an amino group results in an **amide,** and (3) with a thiol results in a **thioester** (Table 2–2); water is eliminated in these three processes. The combination of fatty acids with the alcohol glycerol results in triglyceride (triacylglycerol). The combination of a carboxylate with a phosphate yields an **acyl-phosphate.** This is an acid anhydride (two acids combined with the elimination of the elements of water).

Most biomolecules contain more than one functional group. For example, molecules that contain two or three carboxylate groups are important metabolites. These are known as dicarboxylic and tricarboxylic acids. The addition of an alcohol to a carboxylate-containing molecule produces a hydroxy acid. The addition of a ketone group to a carboxylate-containing molecule yields a keto acid (Table 2–2).

Phosphate and **phosphate derivatives** are essential for all forms of life. The combination of two molecules of phosphate with the elimination of the elements of water yields **pyrophosphate** (Table 2–2). The condensation of an alcohol with phosphate yields a **phosphate ester.** The combination

TABLE 2–2. Functional Groups in Biomolecules

Group	Structure	Group	Structure
Hydrocarbons			
Alkyl group	$CH_3(CH_2)_n$	Acetal	$R-\overset{OR''}{\underset{OR'}{C}}-H$
Alkene	$C=C$		
Aromatic group	(benzene ring)	Dicarboxylate	$^-O-\overset{O}{C}-\overset{H}{\underset{H}{C}}-\overset{H}{\underset{H}{C}}-\overset{O}{C}-O^-$
Ether	$R-O-R'$	**Phosphates**	
Alcohol	$R-\ddot{O}H$	Inorganic phosphate (P_1)	$HO-\overset{O}{\underset{O^-}{P}}-O^-$
Amine	$R-\ddot{N}H_2$		
Guanidine	$R-\underset{H}{N}-C\overset{NH}{\underset{NH_2}{}}$	Pyrophosphate (PP_1)*	$HO-\overset{O}{\underset{O^-}{P}}-O-\overset{O}{\underset{O^-}{P}}-OH$
Sulfur derivatives			
Thiol or sulfhydryl group	$R-\ddot{S}H$	Phosphomonoester	$R-O-\overset{O}{\underset{O^-}{P}}-O^-$
Disulfide	$R-S-S-R'$		
Thioether	$R-S-R'$	Phosphodiester	$R-O-\overset{O}{\underset{O^-}{P}}-O-R'$
Sulfate ester	$R-O-\overset{O}{\underset{O}{S}}-O^-$	Bisphosphate	$^-O-\overset{O}{\underset{O^-}{P}}-O-\overset{H}{\underset{H}{C}}-\overset{H}{\underset{H}{C}}-O-\overset{O}{\underset{O^-}{P}}-O^-$
Carbonyl groups	$-C\overset{O}{}$		
Aldehyde	$R-C\overset{O}{\underset{H}{}}$	Trisphosphate	$^-O-\overset{O}{\underset{O^-}{P}}-O-C-C-C-O-P-O^-$ ... $^-O-P=O$
Ketone	$R-C\overset{O}{\underset{R}{}}$		
Carboxylic acid	$R-C\overset{O}{\underset{OH}{}}$	Disphosphate*	$R-O-\overset{O}{\underset{O^-}{P}}-O-\overset{O}{\underset{O^-}{P}}-O^-$
Ester	$R-C\overset{O}{\underset{OR'}{}}$		
Amide	$R-C\overset{O}{\underset{NH_2}{}}$	Trisphosphate*	$R-O-\overset{O}{\underset{O^-}{P}}-O-\overset{O}{\underset{O^-}{P}}-O-\overset{O}{\underset{O^-}{P}}-O^-$
Thioester*	$R-C\overset{O}{\underset{SR}{}}$		
Multifunctional compounds		Phosphoenol group*	$\overset{COO^-}{\underset{CH_2}{C}}-O-\overset{O}{\underset{O^-}{P}}-O^-$
Hydroxy acid	$R-\overset{OH}{\underset{H}{C}}-C\overset{O}{\underset{OH}{}}$	Phosphoramidate*	$R-\underset{H}{N}-PO_3^{2-}$
Keto acid	$R-\overset{O}{C}-C\overset{O}{\underset{OH}{}}$	Acyl-phosphate*	$R-C\overset{O}{\underset{OPO_3^{2-}}{}}$
Hemiacetal	$R-\overset{OH}{\underset{OR'}{C}}-H$		

* Energy-rich compound

of phosphate with two molecules of alcohol yields a **phosphodiester.** The connection of two molecules of phosphate with a molecule containing two alcohols yields a **bisphosphate.** The attachment of three molecules of phosphate to a molecule containing three alcohols yields a **trisphosphate.**

We noted in Chapter 1 that adenosine triphosphate (ATP) is an extraordinary substance in biochemistry and biology. This compound contains three phosphate groups linked in series to each other (Figure 1–2). These compounds are called **triphosphates.** ATP contains two acid anhydride bonds and one phosphate ester bond linking the phosphate to the alcohol of ribose. Adenosine diphosphate (ADP) contains two phosphate groups linked together, accounting for the term **diphosphate.**

The combination of phosphate with an amino group with the elimination of water yields a **phosphoramidate** (Table 2–2). Creatine phosphate is an example of such a compound. The combination of phosphate with the enol oxygen of enolpyruvate results in **phosphoenolpyruvate,** an important compound in carbohydrate metabolism.

Although there is immense diversity in all forms of life, about 50 fundamental compounds constitute the major mass of living organisms. These include 20 amino acids used in protein synthesis; the five bases that are found in DNA and RNA; glucose, ribose, deoxyribose, and other sugars; glycerol; several fatty acids; and a few other pivotal metabolites. Besides the fundamental building blocks, a few hundred other metabolites constitute the bulk of compounds with which biochemists are concerned.

BIOCHEMICAL ISOMERS

Isomers are compounds containing the same atoms in different arrangements. Chemical isomers, for example, glyceraldehyde 3-phosphate and dihydroxyacetone phosphate, have different functional groups (Figure 2–7). The former is an aldehyde and the latter a ketone, but each has the molecular formula $C_3H_5O_6P^{-2}$. Geometric isomers, or *cis-trans* isomers, differ in the arrangement of their substituent groups with respect to a rigid double bond. Examples include maleate and fumarate (Figure 2–7).

Organic compounds that contain carbon atoms with four different substituents are asymmetrical and can exist in two different isomeric forms called stereoisomers. Glyceraldehyde contains one asymmetrical carbon atom (C^2) and exists in two forms that are nonsuperimposable mirror images called enantiomers (Figure 2–8). Each stereoisomer exhibits optical activity, and the stereoisomers rotate the plane of polarized light in opposite directions.

D-Glyceraldehyde and L-glyceraldehyde represent standard compounds to which optical isomers are compared. Those with the configuration of D-glyceraldehyde are given a D-designation, and those with the L-configuration are given an L-designation. The small capital L or D refers to the configuration and not to the direction in which these compounds rotate the plane of polarized light. Compounds that rotate the plane of polarized light to the left are called levorotary and are designated l- or (−). Compounds that rotate the plane of polarized light to the right are called dextrorotary and are designated d- or (+). Because of these ambiguities, chemists have devised a rigorous stereochemical nomenclature denoted by R (rectus, or right) and S (sinister, or left) and priorities of substituents based on mass. L-Glyceraldehyde has the S configuration, and D-glyceraldehyde has the R configuration. Because the biochemical literature continues to refer to D-glucose and L-amino acids, this scheme is not considered further.

Compounds with asymmetrical carbon atoms can be regarded as occurring in left- and right-handed

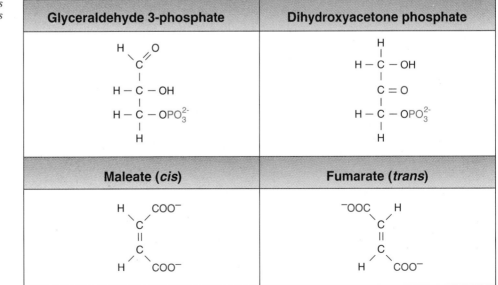

FIGURE 2–7. Isomers. Cis *means same side, and* trans *means other side.*

Glyceraldehyde 3-phosphate	Dihydroxyacetone phosphate
(structure)	(structure)
Maleate (*cis*)	**Fumarate (*trans*)**
(structure)	(structure)

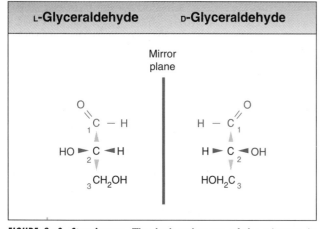

FIGURE 2–8. Stereoisomers. *The hydroxyl group of the L-isomer in this Fischer projection points to the left with the aldehyde on the top. The hydroxyl group of the D-isomer points to the right with the aldehyde on the top. In Fischer projections, the horizontal bonds are directed toward the front and the vertical bonds are directed toward the rear.*

forms, and such compounds are called chiral compounds (Greek *chiros*, "hand"). The asymmetrical atom or center is called the chiral center. Compounds with carbon atoms that contain three different substituents are precursors of chiral molecules, or prochiral molecules.

Most biomolecules contain chiral carbon atoms. *Amino acids that occur in proteins correspond to L-glyceraldehyde and have the L-configuration. Most sugars in nature correspond to D-glyceraldehyde at the reference carbon and have the D-configuration.*

CLASSES OF BIOCHEMICAL REACTIONS

Categories of Reactions

The conversion of one or more compounds into other compounds is the result of a **chemical reaction.** The large number of biochemical reactions can be classified into six major categories. (1) Oxidation-reduction reactions involve the transfer of electrons from a donor to an acceptor. (2) Transferase reactions involve the transfer of part of a molecule from a donor to an acceptor. (3) Hydrolysis reactions (lysis by water) involve the cleavage of a bond of a molecule with the formation of products that contain the elements of water. (4) Lyase reactions involve the conversion of a reactant into two products that contain one more double bond than occurs in the reactant (or the reverse reaction). (5) Isomerase reactions involve the conversion of one type of isomer to another. (6) Ligase reactions involve the combination of two molecules that is driven by ATP or an equivalent source of chemical energy.

Oxidation refers to the loss of electrons; **reduction** refers to the acquisition of electrons. In the following reaction,

$$A + B^+ \rightleftharpoons A^+ + B \qquad (2.2)$$

A is the **electron donor, reducing agent,** or **reductant.** B^+ is the **electron acceptor, oxidizing agent,** or **oxidant.** The electron donor (A) becomes oxidized (A^+); the electron acceptor (B^+) becomes reduced (B). The reductant (A) becomes oxidized as it loses an electron, and the oxidant (B^+) becomes reduced as it gains an electron.

Transferase reactions involve the transfer of a part of a molecule from a donor to an acceptor, as illustrated by the following:

$$A - B + C \rightleftharpoons A + B - C \qquad (2.3)$$

There are many classes of transferase reactions in metabolism, including phosphotransferase, aminotransferase, and acyltransferase reactions.

Hydrolysis reactions are among the most common reactions in biochemistry. They are a specialized case of transferase reaction in which the hydroxyl group of water functions as the acceptor. Hydrolysis reactions are characterized by the addition of the elements of water across a chemical bond with the attendant cleavage or lysis of the bond, as illustrated by the following:

$$A - B + H_2O \rightarrow A - OH + HB \qquad (2.4)$$

Lyase reactions are characterized by the splitting of one molecule into two molecules, with the formation of an additional double bond. Lyase reactions also include the combination of two molecules to form one molecule with the loss of a double bond. The dehydration of malate to produce fumarate and the reverse hydration are illustrated in Figure 2–9. Note that water adds to fumarate, but the molecule is not cleaved in the process. A hydration reaction thus differs from a hydrolysis reaction.

Isomerase reactions involve the conversion of one isomer into another. An isomerase catalyzes the conversion of glyceraldehyde 3-phosphate to dihydroxyacetone phosphate (Figure 2–7). In other cases, a molecule with the D-configuration is converted into the isomer with the L-configuration.

Ligase reactions involve the combination of two molecules to form a single molecule that is accompanied by the expenditure of the phosphate bond energy of ATP or an equivalent compound (Figure 2–10). Ligate means tie together.

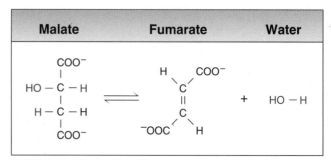

FIGURE 2–9. A lyase reaction. *This reaction involves the formation of a new double bond in fumarate in the forward direction (toward the right) or the loss of a double bond in the reverse direction.*

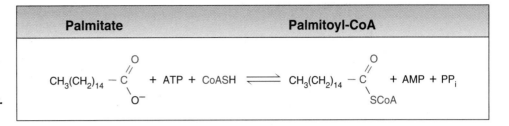

FIGURE 2–10. Synthesis of palmitoyl-CoA, a ligase reaction.

Analysis of Metabolic Reactions

To achieve a genuine understanding of metabolism is one of the goals of this book. That each step falls into one of a half-dozen types of reaction greatly simplifies this analysis. Understanding is facilitated by identifying the functional groups in the reactant and product molecules, by determining where bonds are cleaved and formed, and by noting the bioenergetics of the process (as described in Chapter 5).

As an introduction to this strategy, we consider the functional groups that characterize vitamins. The water-soluble vitamins that are found in numerous coenzymes participate in many biochemical reactions in metabolism. Although the structure of many of these vitamins is intricate, the identification of the reactive portion of the coenzyme is usually sufficient for an understanding of the process, and committing the whole structure to memory is not required except under special circumstances.

INTRODUCTION TO NUTRITION AND VITAMINS

▶ Nutrition is an important factor in health and in the cause and management of several varieties of disease. Obesity, osteoporosis, diabetes, iron deficiency anemia, and dental caries are a few examples of disorders in which nutrition plays at least an ancillary role. Essential hypertension may be reduced by decreasing the intake of sodium. Hypertension may be caused by too much sodium and aggravated by obesity. The role of cholesterol, triglyceride, saturated fats, and polyunsaturated fats in the development of atherosclerosis is a major focus of contemporary nutritional and medical research. Coronary heart disease and cerebral, renal, and peripheral artery disease account for more than half the deaths in the United States today. Health authorities agree that the maintenance of ideal weight promotes health. ◀

Humans require several complex organic molecules and several inorganic minerals in their diet. Food supports cell and tissue growth, development, maintenance, and repair, and food satisfies energy requirements. There are six categories of nutrients: (1) water, (2) minerals, (3) protein, (4) fats, (5) carbohydrates, (6) and vitamins.

Vitamins are low-molecular-mass organic compounds (< 1500 Da) that cannot be synthesized by humans or are synthesized in inadequate amounts (i.e., niacin). Vitamins must be obtained from an exogenous source (such as the diet, bacterial flora in the gut, or by injection) for the maintenance of optimal health. Vitamins are important because they play a central role in metabolism. Vitamins are divided into water-soluble and fat-soluble groups, the fat-soluble vitamins being vitamins A, D, E, and K, and the water-soluble vitamins being the B vitamins (thiamine or B_1, riboflavin or B_2, niacin or B_3, pantothenate or B_5, pyridoxine or B_6, cobalamin or B_{12}), ascorbate or vitamin C, folate, and biotin.

▶ Grave vitamin deficiencies are uncommon in the United States. However, individuals with alcoholism frequently have serious vitamin deficiencies. Whether the association of alcoholism with vitamin deficiencies is related to poor dietary intake or is a manifestation of alcoholism is uncertain. Mild-to-moderate vitamin deficiencies can be found in many population groups, such as the elderly and the poor. ◀

The **recommended dietary allowance** (RDA) is the daily level of intake of essential nutrients considered in the judgment of the Food and Nutrition Board of the National Research Council of the United States to be adequate to meet the nutritional need of practically all healthy persons. When no deficiency symptoms are known to occur in the general population, such as with vitamin E, the RDA is defined as the normal intake in the American diet. The recommended dietary allowance may be inadequate for individuals with infectious disease, fever, or another anomaly.

Table 2–3 provides a list of vitamins, some of their biochemical functions, and the names of their deficiency states. The biochemical functions can be reviewed after each process is described in later chapters. Only those deficiency states with distinctive clinical manifestations have received names.

WATER-SOLUBLE VITAMINS

Thiamine

The reactive portion of thiamine pyrophosphate is the carbon between the sulfur and nitrogen of the thiazole ring (Figure 2–11). This carbon reacts as a negatively charged carbanion (a nucleophile) with various carbonyl groups (electrophiles) to

TABLE 2–3. Major Characteristics of Vitamins

Vitamin	Cofactor	Deficiency State	Biochemical Functions	Comments
Water-soluble group				
Thiamine (B₁)	Thiamine pyrophosphate	Beriberi	Oxidative decarboxylation; pyruvate dehydrogenase; α-ketoglutarate dehydrogenase; transketolase	
Riboflavin (B₂)	FAD FMN		Oxidation-reduction reactions	
Niacin	NAD⁺, NADP⁺	Pellagra	Hydride-transfer reactions	Some derived from tryptophan metabolism
Pantothenate	Coenzyme A, 4′-phosphopantetheine		Acyl transfer; cofactor of acyl carrier protein	Widely distributed, and isolated deficiency unknown
Pyridoxine (B₆)	Pyridoxal phosphate		Transamination, decarboxylation, and dehydration reactions	Deficiency in infants produces seizures
Cobalamin (B₁₂)	5′-Deoxyadenosylcobalamine, methylcobalamine	Pernicious anemia	Methylmalonyl-CoA mutase 5-Methyl-THF homocysteine methyltransferase	B₁₂ = extrinsic factor; not found in plants
Biotin			Acetyl-CoA carboxylase; propionyl-CoA carboxylase; pyruvate carboxylase	
Folate	Tetrahydrofolate		One-carbon transfer; thymidylate synthase; purine biosynthesis	
Ascorbate (C)	Ascorbate	Scurvy	Prolyl and lysyl hydroxylases (collagen); dopamine β-hydroxylase	Antioxidant
Fat-soluble group				
A, retinol		Night blindness	Forms 11-*cis*-retinal with rhodopsin	Antioxidant, promotes differentiation
D	1,25-Dihydroxyvitamin D₃	Rickets in children, osteomalacia in adults	Calcium and phosphate metabolism	25-Hydroxylation in liver, 1-hydroxylation in kidney
E, tocopherol		Selected neural degeneration	Unknown	Antioxidant
K		Bleeding disorders	Blood-clotting factors II, VII, IX, and X; calbindin; protein C and protein S	Mediates formation of protein γ-carboxyglutamate residues

form an alcohol derivative. Thiamine pyrophosphate plays an important role in decarboxylation reactions and two-carbon transfer reactions (Table 2–3).

▶ Thiamine deficiency produces **beriberi.** An early symptom of beriberi is a peripheral neuropathy with decreased sensitivity to temperature, touch, and vibration in the arms and legs. **Dry beriberi** is characterized by neuromuscular symptoms, including muscle atrophy and weakness. **Wet beriberi** is similar but with the additional sign of edema. Beriberi is prone to occur in individuals with a carbohydrate-rich, low-thiamine diet. The

intake of polished rice as the main food staple without a thiamine supplement is a characteristic diet that promotes beriberi. Although thiamine is abundant in rice and other whole grains, it is concentrated in the grain husks that are stripped off by the rice-polishing process. ◀

Riboflavin

Riboflavin consists of isoalloxazine linked to the five-carbon sugar alcohol called ribitol (Figure

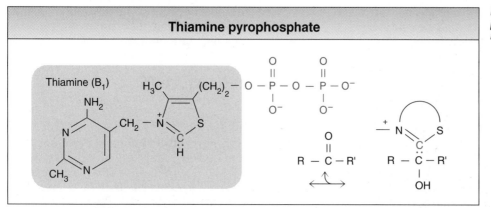

FIGURE 2–11. Thiamine pyrophosphate, *the coenzyme form of thiamine, or vitamin B₁.*

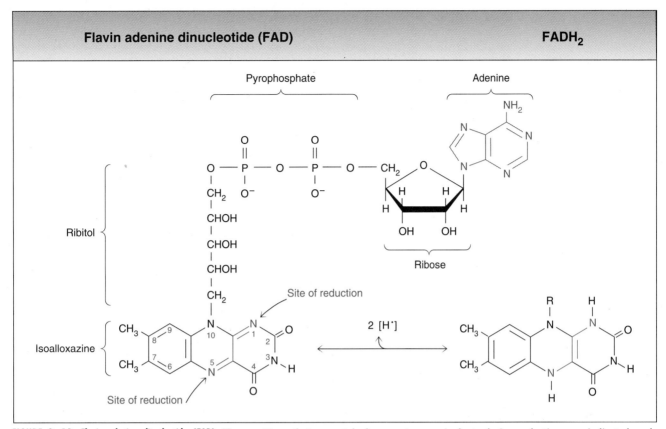

FIGURE 2–12. Flavin adenine dinucleotide (FAD). *The positions that accept hydrogen atom equivalents during reduction are indicated and correspond to N^1 and N^5.*

FIGURE 2–13. NAD⁺ (nicotinamide adenine dinucleotide) and NADP⁺ (nicotinamide adenine dinucleotide phosphate). *The reduction of the nicotinamide group by the hydride ion occurs at C^4. The addition of the negatively charged hydride to the positively charged nucleotide results in the formation of an uncharged derivative. The addition of the hydride occurs stereospecifically from above the ring (the A face) or from below (the B face), depending upon the enzyme that catalyzes the specific reaction.*

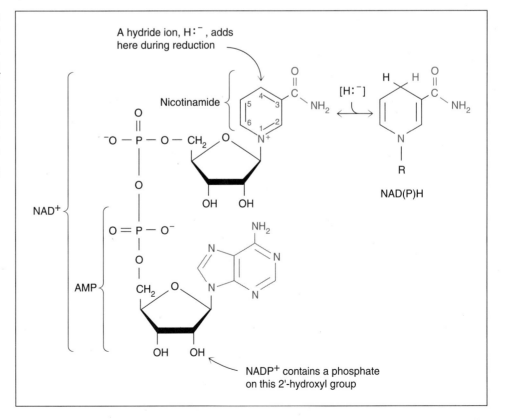

2–12). When phosphate is attached to the ribitol of riboflavin, the compound is called flavin mononucleotide (FMN). When the ribitol group of riboflavin is linked to adenine via a pyrophosphate and ribose, the compound is flavin adenine dinucleotide (FAD). FMN and FAD play a key role in many oxidation-reduction reactions. ▶ Riboflavin occurs widely, and a deficiency of only riboflavin is rare. Lesions of the skin, mouth, and tongue result. ◀

Niacin

Niacin is the generic name for nicotinic acid and nicotinamide (Figure 2–13). The nicotinamide coenzymes play a pivotal role in oxidation-reduction reactions of metabolism. NAD$^+$ is a common oxidant in catabolic reactions, and NADPH is a common reductant in anabolic reactions. NAD$^+$ and NADP$^+$ function as hydride ion (H:$^-$, two electrons and one proton) acceptors; NADH and NADPH function as hydride ion donors. ▶ Niacin deficiency produces **pellagra.** The symptoms include the three D's: dermatitis, diarrhea, and dementia. Sometimes a fourth D, death, is added. Because all cells in humans require niacin, the symptoms of pellagra cannot be explained simply. *It is noteworthy that NAD$^+$ can be formed during the metabolism of the amino acid tryptophan by a complex series of reactions* (Figures 13–25 and 13–26). Niacin is a vitamin because the extent of synthesis from tryptophan is inadequate to prevent the occurrence of pellagra. Nicotinic acid has been used as a pharmacological agent for lowering plasma cholesterol. ◀

Pantothenate

The vitamin pantothenate is formed from pantoic acid and β-alanine (Figure 2–14). The coenzyme form of pantothenate is coenzyme A, or the coenzyme of *acyl*ation. The reactive group in coenzyme A is the thiol group. The prefix of *pan*tothenic acid refers to its widespread occurrence in nature, just as a *pan*demic is a worldwide epidemic. Human pantothenate deficiency diseases occur rarely, if ever.

Vitamin B$_6$: Pyridoxine

Vitamin B$_6$ consists of three related pyridine derivatives: **pyridoxine, pyridoxamine,** and **pyridoxal** (Figure 2–15). Pyridoxal phosphate combines with its proteins through a Schiff base or aldimine linkage, and the Schiff base is involved in the chemistry of nearly all of this vitamin's reactions. It is noteworthy, however, that **glycogen phosphorylase** contains pyridoxal phosphate, and it is the phosphate (which functions as an acid) and not the Schiff base that is important. ▶ B$_6$ is widely available, and a specific deficiency syndrome has not been described. In well-known cases in the 1950s, however, infants in the United States were inadvertently fed milk formulas that lacked vitamin B$_6$ and these infants developed seizures. Because several central nervous system neurotransmitters require pyridoxal phosphate for their synthesis, a deficiency of B$_6$ has been postulated to produce irritability, nervousness, and depression. The antituberculosis drug isoniazid forms an inactive complex with pyridoxal phosphate. It is common to prescribe pyridoxine for individuals receiving isoniazid to prevent an iatrogenic ("caused by treatment") vitamin deficiency. ◀

Vitamin B$_{12}$

Vitamin B$_{12}$ contains cobalt and a corrin ring (Figure 2–1). **Transcobalamin I, II,** and **III** are plasma transport proteins for vitamin B$_{12}$. Vitamin

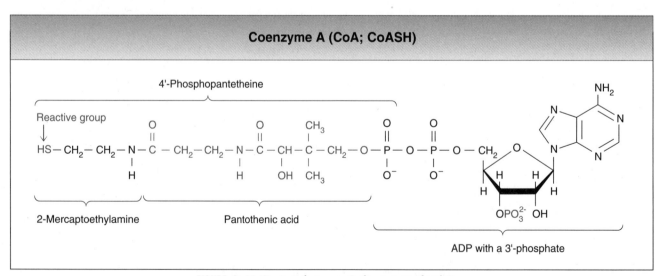

FIGURE 2–14. Structure of coenzyme A, the coenzyme of acylation.

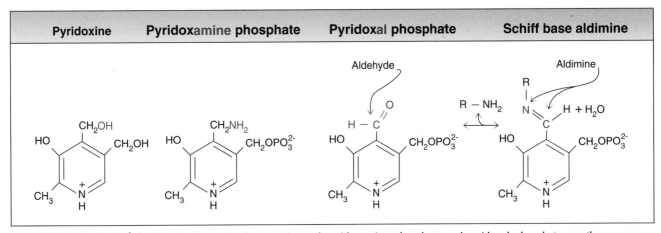

FIGURE 2-15. Vitamin B₆ derivatives. *Pyridoxine is the vitamin, and pyridoxamine phosphate and pyridoxal phosphate are the coenzyme forms.*

B_{12} is stored in liver as methylcobalamin, adenosyl-cobalamin, and hydroxy cobalamin, and liver is a good dietary source of the vitamin. The commercial form of B_{12} in over-the-counter vitamin preparations is cyanocobalamin. The coenzyme forms of B_{12} are methylcobalamin and 5'-deoxyadenosylcobalamin. These coenzyme forms contain a carbon-cobalt bond. The reader should master the two B_{12}-dependent reactions (Table 2-3) when they are encountered (Figures 11-12 and 13-35).

▶ Vitamin B_{12} deficiency in humans results in **pernicious anemia.** Pernicious means highly injurious or destructive; if untreated, B_{12} deficiency is lethal. Erythrocytes in pernicious anemia are 25-50% larger than normal, and B_{12} deficiency produces a macrocytic ("large cell") anemia. Neutrophils are also hypersegmented. Loss of vibratory sensation, paresthesias ("tingling"), and ataxia are due to the development of peripheral neuropathy. Elevated serum lactate dehydrogenase and aspartate aminotransferase levels (Chapter 4) result from destruction of deformed cellular elements in the bone marrow. Serum bilirubin can be slightly elevated.

Classic pernicious anemia is not due to inadequate intake of the vitamin but rather to deficiency in absorption of B_{12}. A glycoprotein, called **intrinsic factor,** produced by the stomach, combines with dietary vitamin B_{12}, extrinsic factor, to form a complex. The complex is absorbed in the ileum. In the absence of intrinsic factor, vitamin B_{12} is not absorbed. The symptoms of pernicious anemia can take several years to develop after the production of intrinsic factor ceases. Usually, the reason for the cessation of production of intrinsic factor is unknown. Pernicious anemia is treated by monthly injections of the vitamin.

The vitamin is synthesized exclusively by microorganisms; plants do not contain the vitamin unless contaminated by bacteria. Vegans may develop pernicious anemia owing to inadequate intake. The bacteria of the large bowel contain vitamin B_{12}, but humans are unable to absorb it be-cause the bacteria are distal to the stomach (source of intrinsic factor) and the ileum (site of absorption). Individuals with stomach cancer may develop pernicious anemia because the diseased stomach fails to produce adequate amounts of intrinsic factor. ◀

Folate

In dietary and cellular folate (Figure 2-16), the glutamyl group is covalently attached to five to seven additional glutamyl residues. An enzyme in the gut (with the inappropriate name of conjugase) catalyzes the hydrolytic removal of these additional glutamyl residues prior to absorption. Folate is transported loosely bound to albumin. Folate is converted to 5,6,7,8-tetrahydrofolate during two reactions catalyzed by dihydrofolate reductase. Tetrahydrofolate carries one-carbon atoms in various states of oxidation. These include methyl (CH_3-),

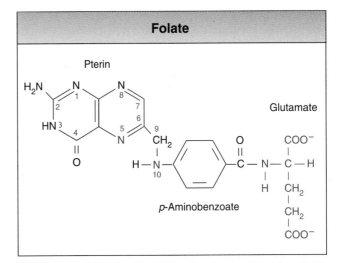

FIGURE 2-16. Folate. *Pterin refers to 2-amino-4-oxopteridine. Pteridine is the ring system that is illustrated. The functional portions of the molecule include N^5 and N^{10}.*

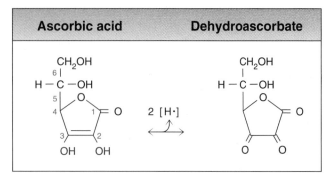

FIGURE 2–17. Ascorbic acid, or vitamin C. *Either of the two hydroxyl groups on C^2 or C^3 can release a proton at physiological pH, accounting for the compound's acidity and name of ascorbic acid.*

methylene ($—CH_2—$), methenyl ($—CH=$), and formyl ($—CHO$) groups. These one-carbon groups are attached to N^5 or N^{10} or both.

The interrelationship of B_{12} and folate metabolism is complex. ▶ Individuals with pernicious anemia develop both anemia and central nervous system lesions. Folate corrects the anemia but not the neuropathology. The anemia is reversible but not the nervous system disorder. Folate is omitted from proprietary vitamins or included in small amounts to avoid masking the symptoms of pernicious anemia, which prompt individuals to seek medical attention. The advisability of limiting folate in proprietary vitamins is debatable because many people have marginally adequate folate intake. Folate deficiency during pregnancy is postulated to produce neural tube defects, and folate is often prescribed for pregnant women. Folate deficiency, similar to B_{12} deficiency, produces **megaloblastic anemia** and hypersegmented polymorphonuclear leukocytes. ◀

Vitamin C (Ascorbate)

Vitamin C is a six-carbon sugar derivative (Figure 2–17) that participates in hydroxylation reactions. Most animals can synthesize ascorbate. The two common exceptions are humans and guinea pigs. ▶ The deficiency of ascorbate produces **scurvy,** which is associated with an abnormal skel-

eton in children, presumably related to collagen abnormalities. In adults, hemorrhages called ecchymoses and petechiae, weakness, swollen gingiva, and loose teeth develop. Normal stores of vitamin C in humans last for 3–4 months. Long periods without fresh fruit or a source of vitamin C led to the scurvy that developed during long sea voyages in earlier centuries. ◀

Biotin

Biotin (Figure 2–18) is a vitamin synthesized by bacteria. Biotin serves as a carrier of activated carbon dioxide. Spontaneous biotin deficiency occurs rarely, if ever, in humans. The daily biotin requirement is small (≈ 20 $\mu g/d$), and intestinal microbes synthesize sufficient amounts that can be absorbed without additional nutritional sources. Egg white contains a protein called avidin that binds biotin very tightly (very avidly). Cooking egg white denatures avidin and abolishes the biotin-binding activity.

FAT-SOLUBLE VITAMINS

Vitamin A

The precursor of vitamin A in vegetables is β-carotene, a yellow pigment. β-Carotene is a polyisoprenoid hydrocarbon that consists of two molecules of retinal (without the oxygen atoms) joined tail to tail (Figure 2–19). Vitamin A, or **retinol,** is an alco*hol* (hence the name retin*ol*). Other retinol derivatives include **retin*al*** (containing an aldehyde) and **retinoic acid.** Polyisoprenoids, including vitamin A, are derivatives of isoprene or 2-methyl-1,3-butadiene (Figure 2–20). Retinol is stored in the liver as retinyl palmitate, an ester formed from retinol and the 16-carbon fatty acid. Retinol is released from the liver following its hydrolysis from retinol ester. Retinol is transported to cells as a complex with a plasma protein called **retinol binding protein.**

In the rod cells of the retina, which are responsible for vision in dim light, all-*trans*-retinal is con-

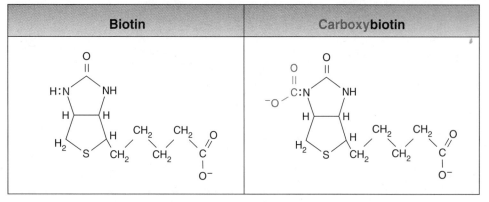

FIGURE 2–18. Biotin and carboxybiotin. *The side chain of biotin is covalently linked to proteins via an amide linkage.*

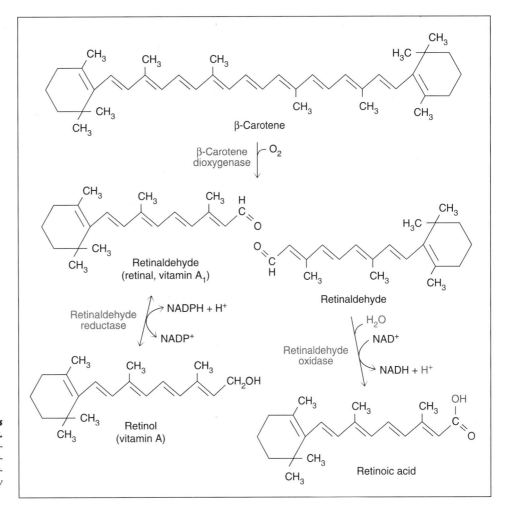

FIGURE 2–19. *β-Carotene and its conversion to vitamin A derivatives. These reactions occur in intestinal mucosal cells. These substances enter the lymphatic chylomicrons and are taken up by the liver.*

verted to 11-*cis* retinal (Figure 2–21). Rhodopsin is the combination of opsin and 11-*cis* retinal. Opsin is an integral membrane protein. 11-*cis* Retinal combines with opsin in the dark. Light converts 11-*cis* retinal into the all-*trans* isomer. The conversion alters the conformation, or three-dimensional structure, of opsin in a millisecond, initiating reactions that generate an impulse in an adjacent target nerve cell. After a minute or so, the all-*trans* retinal dissociates from opsin and undergoes an isomerization reaction to form the 11-*cis* compound. The cycle repeats. Retinal also plays a role in vision in the cone cells of the retina.

▶ Vitamin A is stored in the liver; deficiencies can develop only over prolonged periods of inadequate intake or because of fat malabsorption. The participation of retinal in the visual cycle of rod cells explains the symptoms of night blindness. Vitamin A is required for the maintenance of healthy epithelial cells. Severe vitamin A deficiency leads to the production of abnormal epithelial tissues (keratinization). Keratinization of the cornea, called **xerophthalmia,** leads to an opaque cornea and blindness. Although vitamin A deficiency is rare in the United States, it is a leading cause of blindness worldwide. β-Carotene is an antioxidant and may trap reactive oxygen radicals in tissues. Retinoic acid also plays a role in the regulation of gene expression (DNA-directed RNA synthesis). Vitamin A has been implicated as an agent that protects individuals from the development of cancer. β-Carotene may play an important role in reducing the risk of lung cancer, especially in people who smoke tobacco.

Large amounts of vitamin A are toxic. Toxicity can occur when pharmacological amounts are prescribed to treat acne. Symptoms of vitamin A toxicity include bone pain, scaly dermatitis, hepatosplenomegaly, and diarrhea. ◀

Vitamin D

Vitamin D is the precursor of a hormone called calcitriol; calcitriol is a compound with three hy-

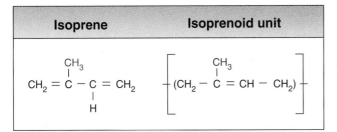

FIGURE 2–20. *Isoprene and the isoprenoid unit.*

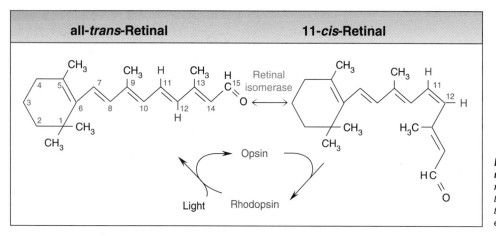

FIGURE 2–21. The participation of retinal in the visual cycle. *Following rhodopsin's interaction with light, the 11-cis-retinal is converted into the all-trans-isomer by photoisomerization.*

droxyl groups, a triol, that influences calcium metabolism. A **hormone** is a substance that is produced and released by synthetic cells and carried by the circulation to target cells where the hormone produces its physiological effects. 7-Dehydrocholesterol, an endogenous human metabolite, is a precursor of **calcitriol.** 7-Dehydrocholesterol is a steroid that contains four rings designated as A, B, C, and D (Figure 2–22).

7-Dehydrocholesterol undergoes a photolytic isomerization reaction that opens the B ring to form **cholecalciferol,** or **vitamin D_3** (Figure 2–22). Cholecalciferol reacts with oxygen and NADPH to form 25-hydroxycholecalciferol, $NADP^+$, and water. 25-Hydroxycholecalciferol, which is the predominant form of vitamin D in the circulation and liver stores, undergoes a second hydroxylation reaction at the 1-position to form calcitriol, the active compound (Figure 2–22). 25-Hydroxycholecalciferol can also undergo hydroxylation at the 24-position to form an inactive compound. The ratio of the conversion to the active and inactive compounds is physiologically regulated. Note that the photoisomerization occurs in the skin, the 25-hydroxylation in the liver, and the 1-hydroxylation in the kidney.

▶ When individuals are exposed to adequate light, there is little or no dietary requirement for vitamin D. Moreover, dairy products are fortified with vitamin D, and deficiency is rare. Most vitamin D deficiency syndromes result from fat malabsorption or from severe liver or kidney disease. Humans without kidneys cannot form adequate calcitriol. Serum calcium levels in these individuals can be regulated by hemodialysis.

Calcitriol plays a role in calcium and phosphate metabolism. A deficiency of this substance in children results in **rickets.** Rickets is characterized by the formation of osteoid matrix that is improperly mineralized, resulting in soft, pliable bones. Inadequate intake of vitamin D or a lack of exposure to adequate sunlight produces rickets. Inadequate light might occur in cloudy regions with limited periods of sunlight, such as winter in temperate climates. The deficiency of vitamin D in adults leads to **osteomalacia.** Osteomalacia is also characterized by the development of soft bones.

Vitamin D, calcium, estrogen, and fluoride have all been suggested as possible modalities in the treatment of osteoporosis. The efficacy of these agents, alone and in combination, is under investigation. Osteoid is lacking in osteoporosis but not in osteomalacia due to vitamin D deficiency. Osteoporosis is common in the elderly, especially in women, whereas osteomalacia is rare. The intake of 10–100 times the RDA may cause vitamin D toxicity. The content of vitamin D in dairy products has been decreased in the United States since the 1950s because children developed frank toxicity. ◀

Vitamin E

Vitamin E includes several related **tocopherols.** These compounds are isoprenoids with a 6-hydroxylchromane ring (Figure 2–23). ▶ Vitamin E deficiency results in the degeneration of the posterior columns of the spinal cord and nerve cells of the dorsal root ganglia. Vitamin E is the least toxic of the fat-soluble vitamins. ◀ *Vitamin E appears to prevent the peroxidation of polyunsaturated fatty acids that occur in membranes throughout the body.* Besides vitamin E, β-carotene serves as an antioxidant in membranes. Vitamin C, which is hydrophilic, is postulated to act as an antioxidant in solution.

Vitamin K

Vitamins of the K group are polyisoprenoid-substituted naphthoquinones (Figure 2–24). Vitamin K_1 is found in plants; it is converted by bacteria in the gut of animals to vitamin K_2. The natural forms of vitamin K are absorbed with other lipids. Menadione, a water-soluble medicinal agent, is absorbed without bile salts. Several proteins that participate in blood clotting and in calcium metabolism undergo vitamin K–dependent modifications (Figure 18–20).

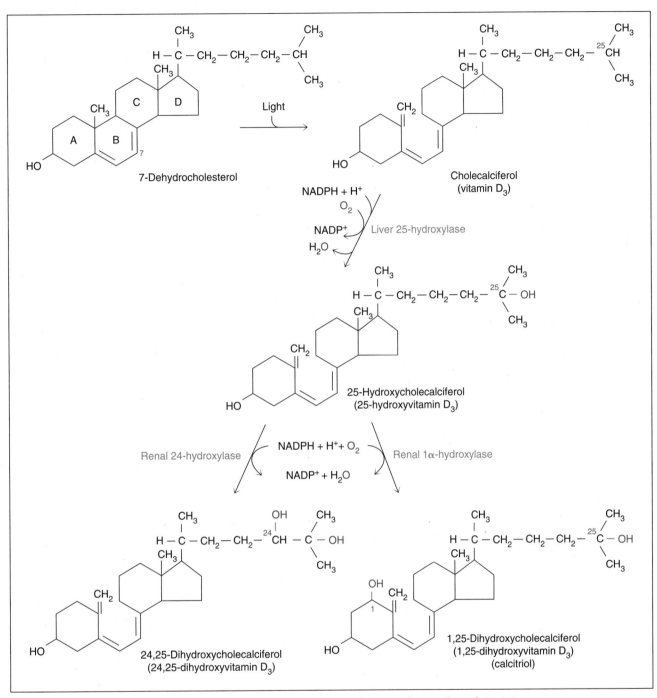

FIGURE 2–22. *Conversion of 7-dehydrocholesterol to the active and inactive forms of vitamin D.*

FIGURE 2–23. *α-Tocopherol. The chromane ring contains an iso-prenoid side chain attached at C^2. The side chain is a saturated hydrocarbon.*

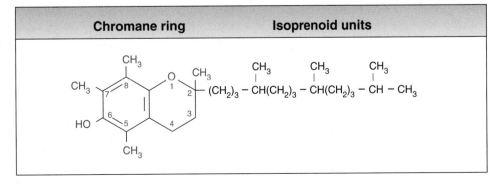

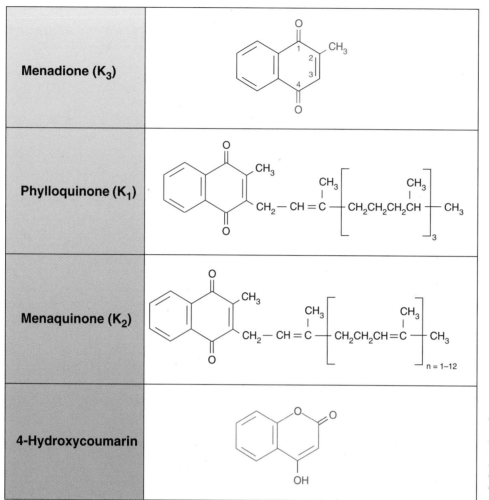

Menadione (K$_3$)	
Phylloquinone (K$_1$)	
Menaquinone (K$_2$)	
4-Hydroxycoumarin	

FIGURE 2–24. Structure of compounds with vitamin K activity and a vitamin K antagonist. Phylloquinone from plants has one double bond in the side chain, and menaquinone, synthesized by bacteria and found in animals, has one double bond per five-carbon fragment.

▶ Vitamin K deficiency in adults can be caused by fat malabsorption. Vitamin K deficiency occurs occasionally in newborns. Vitamin K does not cross the placental barrier; newborns lack bacterial flora, and milk is not a good source of vitamin K. Symptoms in adults or infants include easy bruising or frank hemorrhaging.

The formation of intravascular clots (thrombi) is deleterious to health. Formation of a thrombus in the coronary circulation (coronary thrombosis) produces vascular occlusion, ischemia (inadequate blood supply), and necrosis (tissue death). This results in a myocardial infarction (ischemic necrosis or tissue death due to the lack of oxygen) or a heart attack. Development of deep vein thrombosis (in the legs, for example) can result in a pulmonary embolus (the thrombus is carried by the circulation to the right heart and into the pulmonary arterial tree with subsequent ischemia).

Thromboembolic diseases are sometimes treated with anticoagulants (Chapter 24) that are vitamin K antagonists. 4-Hydroxycoumarin is an example of such an agent (Figure 2–24). Several laboratory tests are used to determine the function of various portions of the blood-clotting cascade. The one that most directly tests the vitamin K status and the action of vitamin K antagonists is the prothrombin time. ◀

DIETARY ESSENTIALS

Essential nutrients are those that cannot be synthesized in adequate amounts (if at all) and are required in the diet. These essentials are listed in Table 2–4. Essential **amino acids** can be represented by the mnemonic PVT TIM *HALL* ("Private Tim Hall"). The italicized histidine and arginine indicate that their essential nature in humans has not been rigorously established. Histidine and arginine may be required in growing children but not in adults. The most devastating worldwide nutritional problem is protein-calorie deficiency in children, and this disorder is called **marasmus. Kwashiorkor** develops in children with adequate energy but insufficient protein intake.

Linoleate and **linolenate** are essential fatty acids (Figure 2–25). They cannot be synthesized and are therefore required in the diet. Linoleate serves as a precursor of prostaglandins and related compounds. The functions of linolenate are a puzzle. **Minerals** cannot be synthesized, and required min-

TABLE 2-4.   Essential Human Nutrients

Amino Acids	Fatty Acids	Vitamins	Minerals	Other
		Water-soluble	*Abundant*	
Phenylalanine	Linoleic	Thiamine (B_1)	Sodium	Water
Valine	Linolenic	Riboflavin (B_2)	Potassium	Energy
Threonine		Niacin	Phosphate	
Tryptophan		Pyridoxine (B_6)	Magnesium	
Isoleucine		Pantothenate	Calcium	
Methionine		Folate	Chloride	
Histidine*		Cobalamin (B_{12})		
Arginine†		Ascorbate (C)	*Trace*	
Leucine		Biotin†	Chromium	
Lysine		Myoinositol†	Cobalt‡	
			Copper	
			Iodine	
		Fat-soluble	Iron	
		A	Molybdenum	
		D	Selenium	
		E	Zinc	
		K	Fluoride§	

* Essential in infants.
† Human requirement not rigorously established.
‡ As vitamin B_{12}.
§ Promotes stronger teeth and bones; essential character not established.

erals are therefore dietary essentials. The role of minerals in human metabolism is given in Table 2-1. **Carbohydrates** are a common and abundant source of food energy. Individuals on a carbohydrate-free or carbohydrate-deficient diet develop a condition called **ketosis.** Carbohydrates are not strictly essential, since all carbohydrates can be synthesized from dietary amino acids.

CALORIC AND ENERGY EXPENDITURE

The Calorie is the standard unit for nutrition in the United States (but not the world), and the Calorie is used in the nutrition sections in this book. The Calorie (capital C) of the nutritionist represents 1000 calories (lowercase c) or 1 kilocalorie of the biochemist. The joule is the preferred energy unit for science and the standard throughout the world. The joule is also the standard unit for biochemical calculations in the United States and is so used in this book. Note that 1 kilogram (kg) is 2.2 pounds (lb), and 1 Calorie is 4.184 kilojoules (kJ). (Multiplying Calories by 4 to obtain kilojoules is sufficiently accurate for most purposes.)

Body weight in adults is determined by the balance between energy expended and energy consumed. If more calories are ingested than consumed, body weight (as adipose tissue) increases. Energy expenditure varies considerably among individuals. Energy expenditure is generally greater in children than adults, males than females, young adults than elderly, and pregnant women than nonpregnant. Energy requirements increase during fever and following injury or physical stress such as surgery. Energy expenditure is increased by activity.

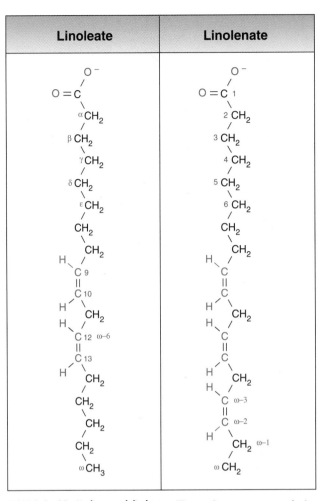

FIGURE 2-25. Linoleate and linolenate. *The carbon atoms are designated by Greek letters in linoleate and by Roman numbers in linolenate. The former is in the ω6 family of fatty acids and linolenate is in the ω3 family of fatty acids. The omega numbering system starts from the noncarboxylate, or ω, end of the molecule.*

Calculation of Caloric Energy Requirements of Adults

The **basal metabolic rate (BMR)** is the energy necessary for maintaining basal physiological activities (cardiac output, brain activity, renal output, body temperature, and respiratory function). A rule of thumb for the energy requirement for basal metabolism is 25 kcal/kg/d (or 100 kJ/kg/d). A formula for calculating approximate energy requirements in healthy adults is provided in Table 2-5. The energy required for activity above basal metabolism can be much greater than indicated in the table for those in active occupations. The approximate energy requirement for a 70-kg individual with moderate activity is estimated as follows:

$$70 \text{ kg} \times 25 \text{ kcal/kg} = 1750 \text{ kcal} \qquad (2.5)$$

$$0.4 \times 1750 \text{ kcal} = 700 \text{ kcal}$$

$$\text{Total requirement} = 2450 \text{ kcal or Calories}$$

TABLE 2–5. Daily Energy Requirements for Adults

Daily energy = basal metabolic rate (BMR) + activity Expenditure
BMR = weight (kg) × 25 Calories*
Activity: Modest = 0.3 × BMR
Moderate = 0.4 × BMR
Heavy = 0.5 × BMR

* 1 Calorie of the nutritionist = 1 kilocalorie (4.184 kilojoules); 1 kilogram = 2.2 pounds.

Energy Sources

The main sources of metabolic energy include carbohydrates, lipids, and proteins. The energy derived from each is given in Table 2–6, and these values are used frequently by health care providers. In assessing caloric intake, alcohol consumption must be determined because this substance provides metabolic energy. Although essential, vitamins, minerals, and water are not sources of energy.

▶ **Obesity** is one of the most prevalent nutritional disorders in the United States. Obesity is the accumulation of excess calories as fat or triglyceride. The definition of excess is inexact in the medical and nutritional literature. A weight 20% greater than the average weight for a given height in women and in men is an approximate definition of obesity. Obesity is a serious problem because it is associated with an increased incidence of diabetes, hypertension, cardiovascular disease, cancer, cholelithiasis (gallstone), and arthritis. Obesity may involve 10–20% of North Americans between the ages of 20 and 75. The diagnosis of obesity can usually be made by visual inspection. More objective measurements include height and weight. In contrast to the ease of diagnosis, the underlying mechanisms and treatment are fraught with difficulty for both the individual and the health care provider. When energy expenditure exceeds energy intake, weight loss follows. ◀

Excess Calories in the obese are stored as adipose tissue. The energy equivalent of a pound of adipose tissue is about 3500 Calories. This is equivalent to 15,000 kJ/pound or 32,000 kJ/kg. The energy values of adipose tissue are based on a

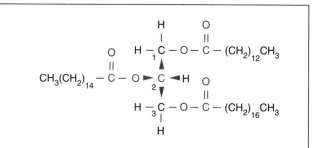

FIGURE 2–26. Triglyceride (triacylglycerol). *Note that the central carbon bears four different substituents and is chiral. The 16-carbon palmitate is attached to sn-2, which is the designation for stereospecific nomenclature.*

value of 85% fat, 15% water, and negligible carbohydrate and protein per pound of adipose tissue.

$$1 \text{ lb} \times 454 \text{ g/lb} \times 0.85 \times 9 \text{ Cal/g} \approx 3500 \text{ Cal} \quad (2.6)$$

When energy expenditure exceeds energy intake by about 3500 Calories, a loss of one pound in body weight occurs. Triglyceride (Figure 2–26) is the major storage form of metabolic fuel in humans.

WATER AS AN ESSENTIAL NUTRIENT

Humans can live without oxygen for only a matter of minutes. Water is the next most essential requirement for life. Death from dehydration follows within several days without fluid intake. Death can occur sooner when there is excessive water loss because of diarrhea, emesis, or sweating. The massive diarrhea of cholera, for example, can kill in 8 hours.

Water balance describes the condition that exists when fluid intake is equivalent to output. Representative values for water balance are given in Table 2–7. Wide variations in fluid intake in the normal range are possible. Compensating changes in the urinary output maintain balance under physiological conditions. **Metabolic water** is produced when protons, electrons, and oxygen react during stage III of metabolism (Figure 1–3).

TABLE 2–6. Metabolic Calories Derived from Foodstuffs

Class	Calories per gram
Carboydrate	4
Ethanol	7
Fat	9
Protein	4

TABLE 2–7. Representative Values for Fluid Intake and Output in Humans

Volume	mL
Intake	
Food and beverage	2300
Metabolic	300
Total	2600
Output	
Expired air	800
Feces	200
Perspiration	400
Urine	1200
Total	2600

► Urolithiasis (kidney stone) results from the precipitation of calcium, phosphate, oxalate, or urate. Whatever the cause or mechanism of renal calculus formation, high fluid intakes are recommended for those individuals who have or are at risk for urolithiasis. Fluid intake to ensure a daily urine volume of 2–3 liters is used in the treatment of urolithiasis. ◄

THE JUDICIOUS DIET

The RDA of foodstuffs should be met with a variety of foods. The RDA for proteins in adults is 56 g/d, whereas that for children, per kilogram, is about twice that for adults. Foods vary in protein quality. This variation reflects the proportion of essential amino acids contained in them and their digestibility. Animal proteins are of higher quality than plant proteins. It is recommended that 10–15% of caloric intake be derived from protein.

The dietary protein content is rather constant. The relative amount of carbohydrate and fat, however, varies considerably. The caloric energy derived from the average North American diet in 1988 was as follows: protein, 15%; carbohydrate, 40%; and fat, 45%. The caloric value of saturated fat in the typical diet represents about 15% of the total intake. The U.S. Surgeon General's Report on Nutrition and Health (1988) outlines prudent dietary recommendations to avoid diseases and disabilities that may be related to diet. These recommenda-

FIGURE 2–27. The food guide pyramid. Adapted, with permission, from S. Welsh, C. Davis, and A. Shaw. Nutrition Today 12:23, November/December 1992.

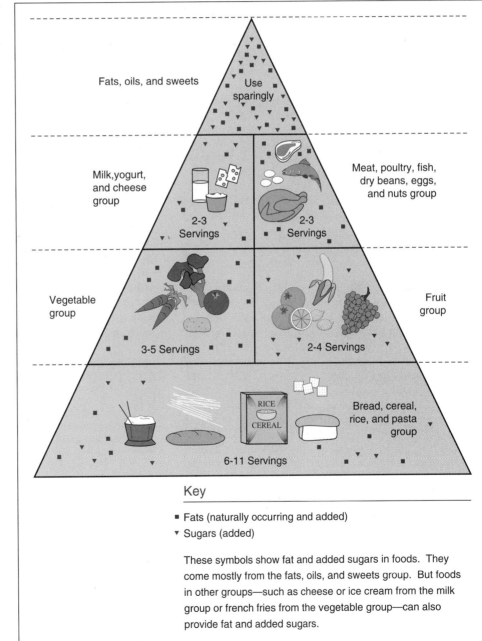

Fats, oils, and sweets — Use sparingly

Milk, yogurt, and cheese group — 2-3 Servings

Meat, poultry, fish, dry beans, eggs, and nuts group — 2-3 Servings

Vegetable group — 3-5 Servings

Fruit group — 2-4 Servings

Bread, cereal, rice, and pasta group — 6-11 Servings

Key

■ Fats (naturally occurring and added)

▼ Sugars (added)

These symbols show fat and added sugars in foods. They come mostly from the fats, oils, and sweets group. But foods in other groups—such as cheese or ice cream from the milk group or french fries from the vegetable group—can also provide fat and added sugars.

tions are as follows: protein, 15%; fat, 30%; and carbohydrate, 55%. It is recommended that less than 10% of total calories be obtained from saturated fatty acids and less than 10% be from polyunsaturated fatty acids. Intake of complex carbohydrate (starch) should be increased; less than 10% of the caloric intake should be derived from refined sugars such as sucrose. The specified number of servings of the foodstuffs shown in Figure 2–27 conforms to these recommendations.

The U.S. Department of Agriculture and the U.S. Department of Health and Human Services recommend that the intake of dietary cholesterol should be less than 300 mg/d and that of sodium should be less than 2.4 g/d. ▶ Higher sodium intake is a possible causative factor or aggravating factor in the development and sustenance of arterial hypertension. The first step in the treatment of essential hypertension is sodium restriction. Successful weight reduction in obese individuals decreases arterial pressure and sometimes results in normal pressure. ◀

Almost all dietary carbohydrate is of plant origin. Dietary carbohydrate can be divided into available (absorbable) and unavailable (fiber) varieties. Some types of fiber have a high capacity for water absorption and increase the bulk of the stool. ▶ Epidemiological studies suggest that colon cancer and diverticulitis are decreased by fiber intake, and 20–30 grams of fiber per day has been recommended. Other types of fiber absorb bile acids, the chief metabolite of cholesterol, and such fiber may be helpful in lowering blood cholesterol levels. ◀

SUMMARY

Oxygen is the most abundant element by mass in humans, and calcium is the predominant mineral. Cobalt is a constituent of vitamin B_{12}, and iodine is a component of thyroid hormone. Five types of chemical bonds determine the structure of biological molecules: (1) covalent, (2) ionic, (3) hydrogen, (4) hydrophobic, and (5) van der Waals bonds. Covalent bonds are strong and are responsible for the stability of the molecules of life. Most biomolecules contain multiple functional groups. Many biochemicals contain carbon atoms with four different substituents that can be attached in alternative forms that are nonsuperimposable mirror images. Amino acids that occur in proteins correspond to L-glyceraldehyde and have the L-configuration. Most sugars in nature correspond to D-glyceraldehyde and have the D-configuration at the reference carbon.

Humans must be supplied with complex organic molecules in addition to many inorganic minerals. Vitamins are low-molecular-mass organic compounds (< 1500 Da) that cannot be synthesized by humans or are synthesized in inadequate amounts (i.e., niacin). Thiamine deficiency produces beri-

beri. Riboflavin and niacin derivatives participate in oxidation-reduction reactions. Niacin deficiency is called pellagra. Pantothenate forms part of coenzyme A and participates in acyl transfer reactions. Pyridoxal phosphate (a B_6-derivative) forms aldimine or Schiff-base linkages with proteins.

Vitamin B_{12}, which contains cobalt, plays a role in carbon-transfer reactions. A deficiency of intrinsic factor, produced in the stomach, eliminates B_{12} absorption in the ileum and results in pernicious anemia. Folate plays a key role in one-carbon metabolism. B_{12} and folate deficiency produce a macrocytic anemia. Vitamin C participates in hydroxylation reactions. The skeletal abnormalities in scurvy are likely due to a deficiency of collagen hydroxylation. Biotin participates in carbon dioxide fixation reactions.

Vitamins A, D, E, and K are the fat-soluble vitamins. Vitamin A participates in the visual cycle. Vitamin D functions in calcium metabolism. The vitamin must be hydroxylated in the 24-position in the liver and the 1-position in the kidney to become functional. Vitamin D deficiency in children produces rickets, and in adults, osteomalacia. β-Carotene and vitamins C and E are antioxidants. Vitamin K is required for the biosynthesis of blood clotting factors. Excess intake of the fat-soluble vitamins is toxic. In contrast, the water-soluble vitamins can be excreted and are nontoxic.

The essential amino acids in humans include those in the mnemonic PVT TIM HALL: phenylalanine, valine, threonine, tryptophan, isoleucine, methionine, histidine, arginine, leucine, and lysine. The essential fatty acids include linoleate and linolenate. After oxygen, water is the second most essential substance required for human life. The U.S. Surgeon General's Report on Nutrition and Health (1988) recommends a diet of about 15% protein, 30% fat, and 55% carbohydrate. Others recommend that dietary cholesterol be less than 300 mg/d and sodium less than 2.4 g/d.

SELECTED READINGS

Chapuy, M.C., M.E. Arlot, F. Duboeuf, J. Brun, B. Crouzet, S. Arnaud, P.D. Delmas, and P.J. Meunier. Vitamin D_3 and calcium to prevent hip fractures in elderly women. New England Journal of Medicine 327:1637–1642, 1992.

DeLuca, H.F. The vitamin D story: A collaborative effort of basic science and clinical medicine. FASEB Journal 2:224–236, 1988.

Food and Nutrition Board of the National Academy of Sciences. *Recommended Daily Allowances,* 10th ed. Washington, D.C., National Academy of Sciences, 1989.

Kane, J.P. The judicious diet. In J.B. Wyngaarden, L.H. Smith, Jr., and J.C. Bennett (eds.). *Cecil Textbook of Medicine,* 19th ed. Philadelphia, W.B. Saunders Company, 1992, pp. 39–42.

Merrill, A.H., Jr., and J.M. Henderson. Disease associated with defects in vitamin B_6 metabolism or utilization. Annual Review of Nutrition 7:137–156, 1987.

Parrott-Garcia, M., and D.A. McCarron. Calcium and hypertension. Nutrition Reviews 42:206–213, 1984.

The Surgeon General's Report on Nutrition and Health. Washington, D.C., U.S. Department of Health and Human Services (DHHS) Publication No. 88-50211, 1988.

CHAPTER THREE

AMINO ACIDS

AND PROTEINS

Making a discovery is such a wonderful thing. It's like falling in love and getting to the top of the mountain all in one.

—MAX PERUTZ

The term protein is derived from Greek *protos* meaning "first" or "primary." Proteins function as catalysts, receptor and effector molecules, transport molecules, antibodies, contractile elements, and hormones. Proteins serve a structural role within the cell as the cytoskeleton, and they provide a matrix for bone, connective tissue, muscle, and teeth. They are informational macromolecules, where information is defined as sequence of amino acids. The sequence of amino acids in a protein is analogous to the sequence of the letters of the alphabet, which give information as words and sentences. The amino acid sequence of proteins is determined by the nucleotide sequence of DNA.

Proteins are polymers of α-amino acids. There are 20 common amino acids that are genetically encoded and serve as precursors for protein biosynthesis on ribosomes. Some of these amino acid residues are modified after biosynthesis (post-translational modification). About 19% of the mass of the human body is protein. It is noteworthy that **collagen,** a connective tissue component, is the most abundant protein by mass in humans. Amino acids also have functions other than serving as building blocks for proteins. Thyroid hormone, for example, is an iodinated amino acid derivative (Figure 2–2), and amino acids function as neurotransmitters.

pH AND THE HENDERSON-HASSELBALCH EQUATION

Ionization of Water

Water makes up more than half the mass of humans and is an essential nutrient. Water dissociates into a proton and hydroxyl group:

$$H_2O \rightleftharpoons H^+ + OH^- \qquad (3.1)$$

Pure water forms a 55.6 molar (M) solution (1000 g/L ÷ 18 g/mol). Moreover, the concentration of hydrogen and hydroxyl ions in pure water is expressed as follows:

$$[H^+] = [OH^-] = 10^{-7}\ M \qquad (3.2)$$

The concentrations of OH^- and H^+ are in reciprocal relationship to each other. When $[H^+]$ increases, $[OH^-]$ decreases, and vice versa. The product of their concentrations is 1×10^{-14}.

$$[H^+] \times [OH^-] = 1 \times 10^{-14} \qquad (3.3)$$

When $[H^+] = 1 \times 10^{-4}\ M$, for example, then $[OH^-] = 1 \times 10^{-10}\ M$.

The **pH** is defined by the following expression:

$$pH = -\log_{10} [H^+] \qquad (3.4)$$

At neutrality (when $[H^+] = [OH^-]$),

$$pH = -\log [10^{-7}] \qquad (3.5)$$
$$= -(-7) = +7$$

Buffers

The pH of blood is maintained at 7.4 ± 0.05, and the intracellular pH is close to this value.

$$7.4 = -\log [H^+] \qquad (3.6)$$
$$3.98 \times 10^{-8}\ M = [H^+]$$

The maintenance of blood and cellular pH near 7.4 is aided by the action of buffers. Buffers are substances that diminish the change in pH when acid or alkali is added. Buffers are composed of weak acids and their salts or weak bases and their acids. The physiologically important buffers in blood, saliva, and other body fluids, in order of their effectiveness as buffers, are (1) H_2CO_3—HCO_3^-, (2) $H_2PO_4^-$—HPO_4^{2-}, and (3) protein—protein$^-$.

The **Henderson-Hasselbalch** equation (3.7) provides a convenient way to describe and think about buffers and pH:

$$pH = pK_a + \log \frac{[\text{unprotonated compound}]}{[\text{protonated compound}]} \qquad (3.7)$$

or equivalently

$$pH = pK_a + \log [\text{salt}]/[\text{acid}] \qquad (3.8)$$

The pH is the negative logarithm of the molar concentration of the hydrogen ion, and the pK_a is the pH at which the concentration of the protonated species is equal to that of the unprotonated species.

For the phosphate buffer system near physiological pH (≈ 7),

$$H_2PO_4^- \rightleftharpoons H^+ + HPO_4^{2-} \qquad (3.9)$$
$$pH = pK_a + \log [HPO_4^{2-}]/[H_2PO_4^-]$$

When $[HPO_4^{2-}] = [H_2PO_4^{1-}]$, the concentration of the protonated form equals that of the unprotonated form, and their ratio is 1.

$$pH = pK_a + \log 1 \qquad (3.10)$$
$$pH = pK_a$$
$$(\text{Recall } \log 1 = 0)$$

For phosphate at physiological ionic strength, the $pK_a = 6.8$. The pK_a is the pH at which the concentration of salt (unprotonated form) and acid (protonated form) is identical. Having the pK_a, we can calculate the pH when the concentrations of HPO_4^{2-} and $H_2PO_4^-$ are known. At a given pH, we can calculate the ratios of the two forms. For example, when $[HPO_4^{-2}]/[H_2PO_4^-] = 10$, then

$$pH = 6.8 + \log 10 \qquad (3.11)$$
$$= 6.8 + 1$$
$$= 7.8$$

When $[HPO_4^{2-}]/[H_2PO_4^-] = 0.1$, then

$$pH = 6.8 + \log 0.1 \qquad (3.12)$$
$$= 6.8 - 1.0$$
$$= 5.8$$

The carbon dioxide/bicarbonate buffer system is more intricate. The CO_2 system can be expressed as follows:

$$CO_2 + H_2O \rightleftharpoons H_2CO_3 \qquad (3.13)$$

$$H_2CO_3 \rightleftharpoons H^+ + HCO_3^-$$

$$pH = 6.1 + \log \frac{[HCO_3^-]}{[CO_2 + H_2CO_3]} \qquad (3.14)$$

The pK_a of the CO_2 system at physiological ionic strength is 6.1. The bicarbonate/carbon dioxide system is coupled. The total acid consists of carbonic acid (H_2CO_3) plus dissolved carbon dioxide (CO_2). This approach accounts for the two terms in the denominator of the Henderson-Hasselbalch equation. At pH 7.4, the ratio of salt to acid, or $[HCO_3^-]/[CO_2 + H_2CO_3]$, is about 20.

STRUCTURES OF AMINO ACIDS

Let us consider the identity and structures of the 20 genetically encoded amino acids. The amino acids that are found in proteins are α-amino acids. Except for glycine, which lacks a chiral carbon atom

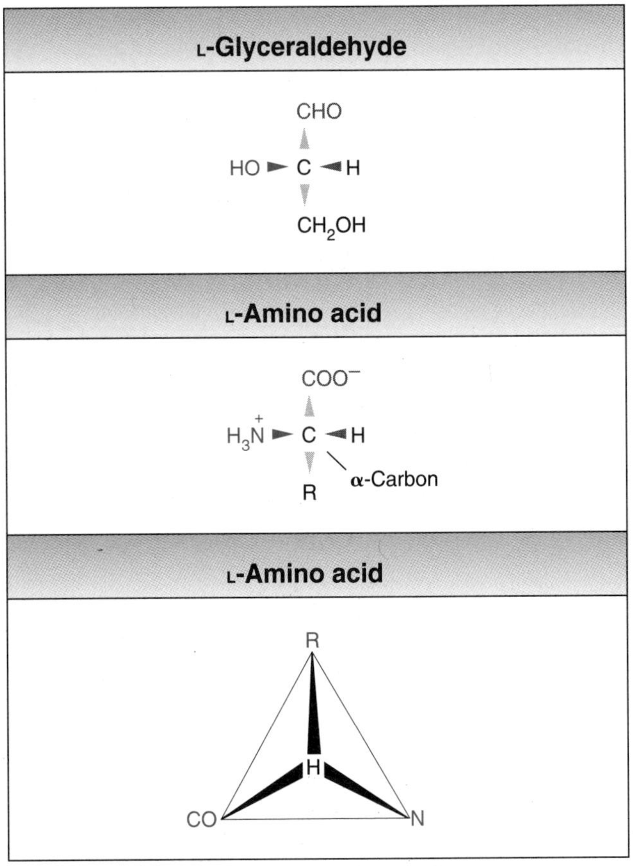

L-Glyceraldehyde

CHO

HO ► C ◄ H

CH_2OH

L-Amino acid

COO^-

$H_3\overset{+}{N}$ ► C ◄ H

R α-Carbon

L-Amino acid

R

H

CO   N

FIGURE 3–1. Amino acid structure. *Amino acids that occur in proteins have the L-configuration of L-glyceraldehyde. Carbon atoms have a valence of four and are found at the center of a tetrahedron with the four substituents at the four corners. With the hydrogen atom linked to the asymmetric α-carbon at the top of a tetrahedron, the carbonyl group (CO), the R group, and the amino group (N) have the indicated locations and spell "CORN."*

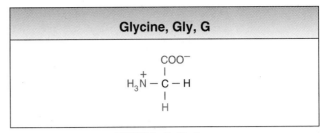

Glycine, Gly, G

COO^-

$H_3\overset{+}{N} - C - H$

H

FIGURE 3–2. Glycine.

(a carbon atom with four different substituents), the amino acids found in proteins possess the L-**configuration** (the absolute form corresponds to L-glyceraldehyde) as illustrated in Figure 3–1. The four different substituents include a carboxyl group, an amino group, hydrogen, and a characteristic side chain called the R group (R formerly referred to radical; R has now taken on a meaning of its own that refers to the side chain).

Glycine is the simplest of the amino acids. Glycine contains a positively charged amino group, a negatively charged carboxyl group, and two hydrogens attached to the α-carbon (Figure 3–2). Glycine is named after its sweet taste (glyco-, "sugar"). It is noteworthy (for examinations) that glycine is the only common amino acid that lacks an asymmetric carbon atom. There are four common amino acids with hydrocarbon side chains. **Alanine** contains three carbon atoms (Figure 3–3). **Valine,** which contains five carbon atoms, has an R group that is branched. **Leucine,** which contains six carbon atoms, has an R group that also is branched. **Isoleucine** is an isomer of leucine that contains a methyl group on the β-carbon atom. Note that isoleucine contains two chiral carbon atoms. The R groups of these four amino acids tend to form hydrophobic bonds and to exist in the interior of proteins away from water.

There are three **aromatic amino acids.** The aromatic groups are attached to the three-carbon alanyl group. **Phenylalanine,** as the name implies, consists of a phenyl group attached to alanine (Figure 3–4). **Tyrosine** possesses a hydroxyl group in the aromatic ring, making it a phenol derivative. The hydroxyl group of certain protein-tyrosine residues can be phosphorylated. **Tryptophan** contains the indole ring attached to the alanyl side chain. Aromatic amino acids are hydrophobic and tend to occur in the interior of proteins.

Two amino acids contain **sulfur. Cysteine,** which contains three carbon atoms, possesses a thiol group (Figure 3–5). The oxidized dimer is known as **cystine.** Cysteine is the form of the amino acid that is incorporated into proteins during synthesis, whereas cystine is the form found in blood. **Methionine** is the second common amino acid that contains a sulfur atom (Figure 3–6). Methionine, which provides methyl groups for metabolism, is the initiating amino acid during protein biosynthesis. Methionine tends to occur in the interior of proteins such as the amino acids with the hydrocarbon side chains.

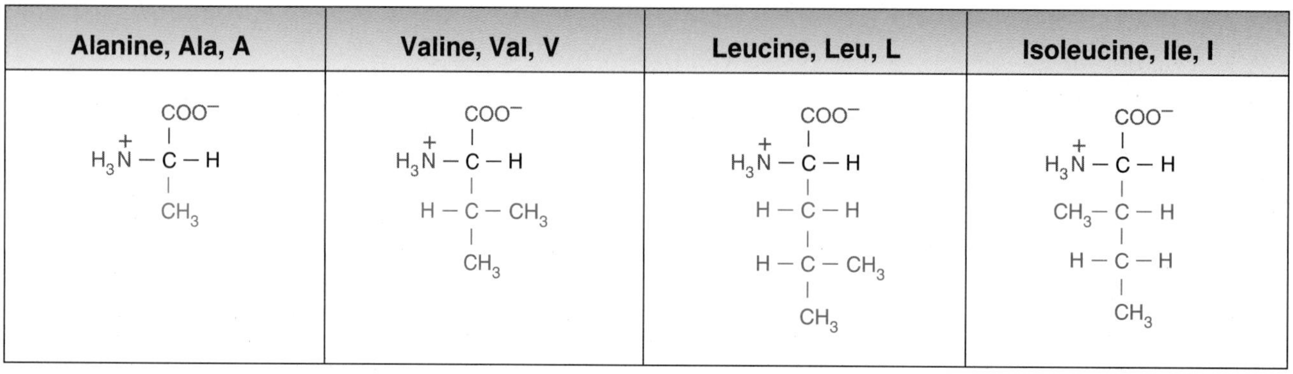

Alanine, Ala, A	Valine, Val, V	Leucine, Leu, L	Isoleucine, Ile, I

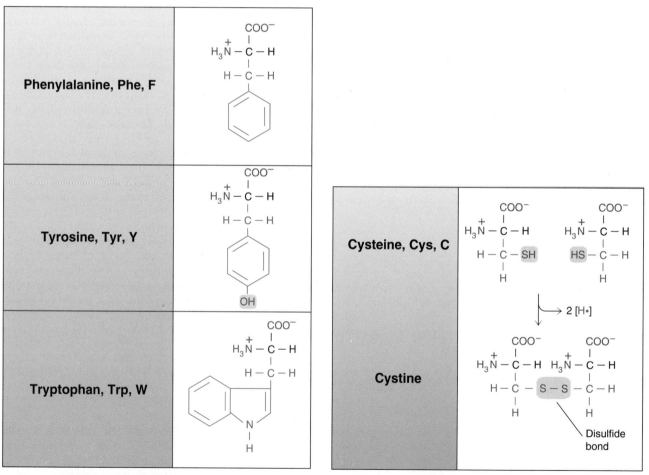

FIGURE 3–3. Amino acids with hydrocarbon side chains.

Phenylalanine, Phe, F	
Tyrosine, Tyr, Y	
Tryptophan, Trp, W	

FIGURE 3–4. The three aromatic amino acids.

Cysteine, Cys, C	
Cystine	

Disulfide bond

FIGURE 3–5. Cysteine and cystine.

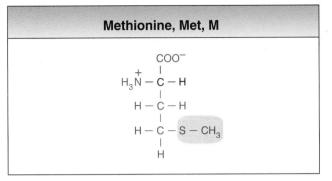

Methionine, Met, M
$$\begin{array}{c} COO^- \\ | \\ H_3\overset{+}{N} - C - H \\ | \\ H - C - H \\ | \\ H - C - S - CH_3 \\ | \\ H \end{array}$$

FIGURE 3–6. Methionine. *The carbon-sulfur-carbon functional group is a thioether.*

Four amino acids are dicarboxylic acids or their derivatives. **Aspartate** (four carbon atoms) and **glutamate** (five carbon atoms) contain carboxylate R groups that bear a negative charge at physiological pH (Figure 3–7). The carboxylates can act as proton acceptors, and the acids can act as proton donors. These two side chains can form ionic bonds, and they can also function as hydrogen bond acceptors. **Asparagine,** first isolated from asparagus, and **glutamine** contain polar amide R groups. The carbonyl group can function as a hydrogen bond acceptor, and the amido group can function as a hydrogen bond donor. These four hydrophilic residues tend to occur on the exterior surface of proteins. Free glutamate and glutamine play a central role in amino acid metabolism. Glutamate, moreover, is the most prevalent excitatory neurotransmitter in the central nervous system.

Three amino acids contain basic, nitrogen-containing, polar side chains. **Lysine** is a six-carbon amino acid that contains a second amino group that is bound to the ϵ-carbon (Figure 3–8). **Arginine** contains a guanidinium group attached to the five-carbon amino acid skeleton. Both lysine and arginine side chains are positively charged at physiological pH. Both can form ionic bonds, and both hydrophilic groups tend to occur on the surface of proteins. **Histidine** contains an imidazole group bound to alanine. The R group of histidine has a pK$_a$ value near 7, and histidine is the only

amino acid with this property. At physiological pH, a portion of the residues is uncharged and a portion is charged. Histidine is hydrophilic and tends to occur on the surface of proteins. The nitrogens of the imidazole ring are good nucleophiles and good proton acceptors. Because of its favorable reactivity, histidine occurs in the active site of many enzymes.

Two amino acids contain aliphatic hydroxyl groups. **Serine** is a three-carbon amino acid containing an alcohol side chain (Figure 3–9). **Threonine** is a four-carbon amino acid that contains a hydroxyl group. These hydrophilic amino acids tend to occur on the exterior surface of proteins in contact with water. *Serine is the most commonly phosphorylated residue in proteins, threonine is second, and tyrosine is third.* The active site of many enzymes contains serine but not threonine. Note that threonine contains two chiral carbon atoms.

The last of the genetically encoded amino acids is a cyclic amino acid named **proline** (Figure 3–10). Note that the nitrogen atom of proline is linked to two carbon atoms. Proline is a hydrocarbon and is therefore expected to be hydrophobic. Because of its cyclic structure, proline often occurs at turns in the polypeptide chain of proteins, and proline does not occur in the interior of proteins as frequently as leucine or valine.

To conclude, glycine lacks a chiral carbon atom. Two amino acids, isoleucine and threonine, contain two chiral carbon atoms. Amino acids may be designated by a three-letter or a single-letter abbreviation (Table 3–1).

IONIC STATES OF AMINO ACIDS

The pK$_a$ of a group is the pH value at which the concentration of the protonated group equals that of the unprotonated group. The pK$_a$ of the α-carboxyl group of the common amino acids is about 2 and that of the α-amino group is about 10. The α-carboxyl group of an amino acid is negatively charged, and the α-amino group is positively charged at physiological pH. At physiological pH, the common amino acids exist as a **dipolar ion,** or

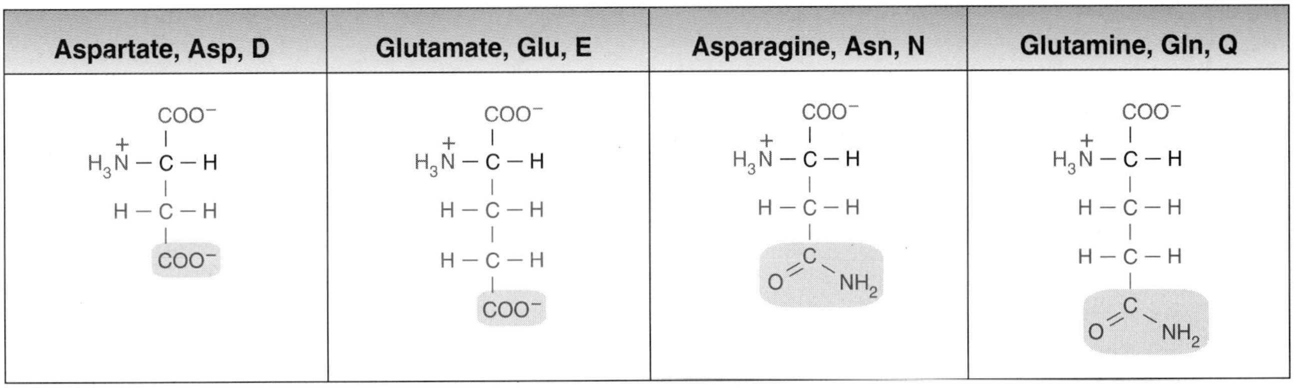

Aspartate, Asp, D	**Glutamate, Glu, E**	**Asparagine, Asn, N**	**Glutamine, Gln, Q**
$$\begin{array}{c} COO^- \\ | \\ H_3\overset{+}{N} - C - H \\ | \\ H - C - H \\ | \\ COO^- \end{array}$$	$$\begin{array}{c} COO^- \\ | \\ H_3\overset{+}{N} - C - H \\ | \\ H - C - H \\ | \\ H - C - H \\ | \\ COO^- \end{array}$$	$$\begin{array}{c} COO^- \\ | \\ H_3\overset{+}{N} - C - H \\ | \\ H - C - H \\ | \\ O{=}C{-}NH_2 \end{array}$$	$$\begin{array}{c} COO^- \\ | \\ H_3\overset{+}{N} - C - H \\ | \\ H - C - H \\ | \\ H - C - H \\ | \\ O{=}C{-}NH_2 \end{array}$$

FIGURE 3–7. The dicarboxylate family of amino acids.

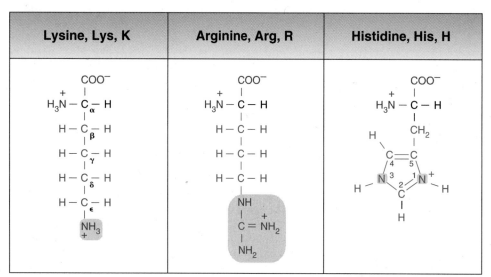

FIGURE 3-8. Three basic amino acids.

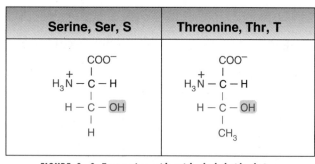

FIGURE 3-9. Two amino acids with alcohol side chains.

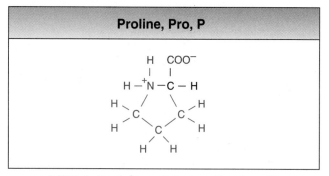

FIGURE 3-10. Proline, an imino or cyclic amino acid.

TABLE 3-1.   pK$_a$ and Hydropathy Values of Amino Acids

Amino Acid	Three-letter Abbreviation	One-letter Abbreviation	pK$_a$ of R Group	Hydropathy Value
Alanine	Ala	A		1.8
Arginine	Arg	R	≈ 12	−4.5
Asparagine	Asn	N		−3.5
Aspartate	Asp	D	4.4	−3.5
Asparagine or aspartate	Asx	B		
Cysteine	Cys	C	8.5	2.5
Glutamine	Gln	Q		−3.5
Glutamate	Glu	E	4.4	−3.5
Glutamine or glutamate	Glx	Z		
Glycine	Gly	G		−0.4
Histidine	His	H	6.5	−3.2
Isoleucine	Ile	I		4.5
Leucine	Leu	L		3.8
Lysine	Lys	K	10	−3.9
Methionine	Met	M		1.9
Phenylalanine	Phe	F		2.8
Proline	Pro	P		−1.6
Serine	Ser	S		−0.8
Threonine	Thr	T		−0.7
Tryptophan	Trp	W		−0.9
Tyrosine	Tyr	Y	10	−1.3
Valine	Val	V		4.2

Memory hints: F, *f*enylalanine; N, asparagi*n*e; R, a*r*ginine; Y, t*y*rosine; W, t*w*yptophan.

zwitterion (^+H_3N—R—COO^-). The pK$_a$ value for various R groups is given in Table 3-1. The carboxylates of aspartate and glutamate are anionic, and the basic groups of lysine and arginine are cationic at physiological pH values. The ionic forms of leucine, glutamate, and lysine are illustrated in Figure 3-11.

PEPTIDE BONDS

Peptides

The combination of an α-amino group of one amino acid with the carboxyl group of a second amino acid, with the elimination of water, results in the formation of a **peptide bond** (Figure 3-12). The resulting compound is a **dipeptide**. A **tripeptide** contains three amino acid residues, an **oligopeptide** contains several, and a **polypeptide** contains many amino acid residues. The peptide bond is planar (Figure 3-13). The carbonyl and substituted amide groups occur in a plane, and rotation about the C—N bond is prohibited, limiting the conformations that a polypeptide chain may assume.

Angiotensin and the Control of Arterial Pressure

Angiotensin is a peptide of great clinical significance. The renin-angiotensin system plays a pivotal role in sodium metabolism and the regulation of arterial pressure. Liver synthesizes **angiotensinogen,** a protein that occurs in blood. A circulating proteolytic enzyme, **renin,** catalyzes the hydrolysis of angiotensinogen to produce a precursor decapeptide called angiotensin I and a large protein fragment (Figure 3-14). **Angiotensin converting enzyme** (ACE) catalyzes the conversion of angiotensin I to angiotensin II, an octapeptide having great activity. Angiotensin II and III produce vasoconstriction to elevate the arterial pressure, and they promote the synthesis of a steroid hormone called aldosterone that promotes sodium retention. ► ACE inhibitors are commonly used for the treatment of hypertension and congestive heart failure. Captopril and enalapril are two examples of ACE inhibitors (Figure 20-6). ◄

Proteins

Proteins are polypeptides consisting of many amino acid residues. An average polypeptide chain in a protein contains about 500 amino acid residues; a few contain more than 2000 amino acid residues. The molecular masses of single polypeptide chains range from about 5000 to 300,000 Da. To determine the approximate number of amino acids in a protein, divide the molecular mass by 110 (or 100 for a less accurate estimate). This value (110 Da) approximates the average molecular mass of an amino acid residue in an average protein.

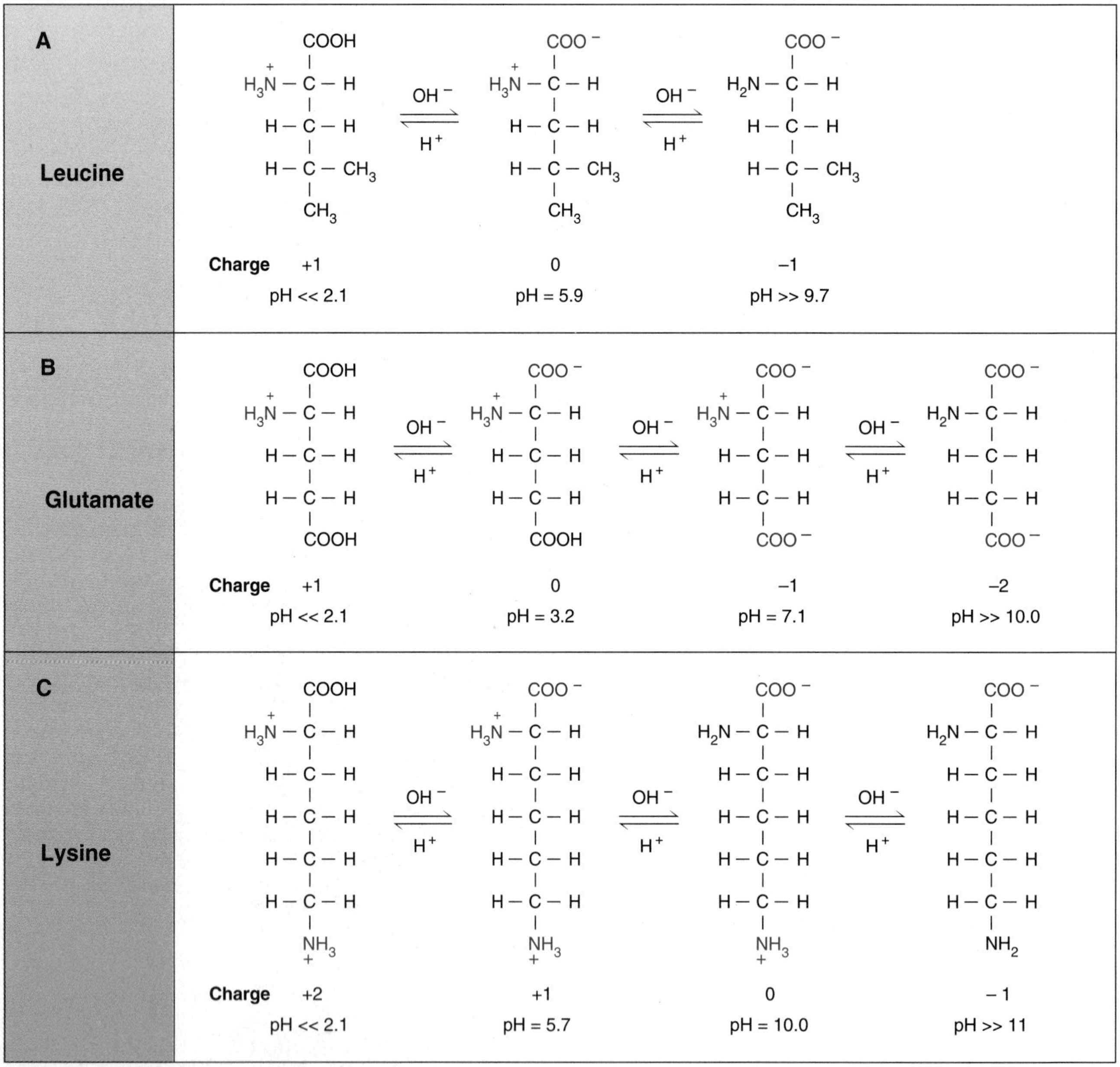

FIGURE 3–11. Ionic forms of (A) leucine, (B) glutamate, and (C) lysine at the indicated pH values. *The R group of leucine is uncharged. At pH 7, the R group of glutamate bears a negative charge, and that of lysine bears a positive charge.*

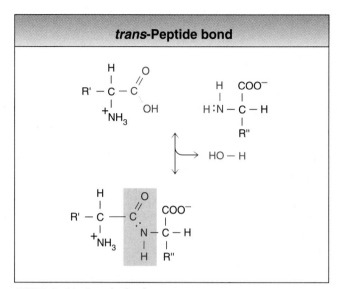

FIGURE 3–12. Peptide bond. *The peptide bond is a substituted amide bond. The large substituents can be* cis *or* trans. *In most peptides, the* trans *configuration predominates. Switching the hydrogen atom and the CH(R″)COO⁻ attached to nitrogen produces the* cis *configuration.*

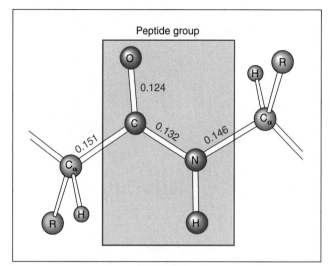

FIGURE 3–13. Peptide bond. *The peptide bond is planar. The distances are given in nanometers (nm); 1 nm = 1 × 10⁻⁹ m.*

FIGURE 3–14. Generation and structures of angiotensins I, II, and III.

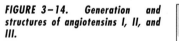

Angiotensinogen	Asp - Arg - Val - Tyr - Ile - His - Pro - Phe - His - Leu - Leu - Protein
Renin ⌐ H₂O ↓ ⌐ Leu - Protein	
Angiotensin I	Asp - Arg - Val - Tyr - Ile - His - Pro - Phe - His - Leu
Angiotensin converting enzyme (ACE) ⌐ H₂O ↓ ⌐ His - Leu	
Angiotensin II	Asp - Arg - Val - Tyr - Ile - His - Pro - Phe
Aminopeptidase ⌐ H₂O ↓ ⌐ Asp	
Angiotensin III	Arg - Val - Tyr - Ile - His - Pro - Phe

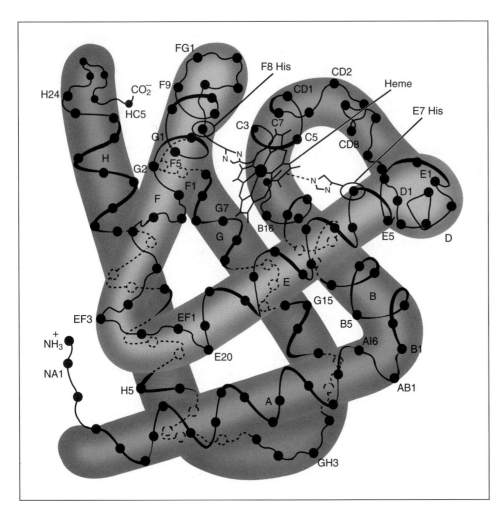

FIGURE 3–15. Myoglobin. *Large dots represent α-carbon positions. A–H designate the eight helices, and AB, CD, etc., represent the residues that connect the two designated helices. Numbers represent specific residues in the helix or connecting region. (Adapted, with permission, from R. E. Dickerson. In H. Neurath (ed.). The Proteins, 2nd ed., Vol. 2. New York, Academic Press, 1964, p. 634.)*

Proteins consist of one or more polypeptide chains. **Myoglobin,** an intracellular oxygen storage protein containing heme, consists of a single polypeptide chain and is a monomer (Figure 3–15). ► Myoglobin is released from the myocardium following an infarction, and its presence in blood aids in the differential diagnosis of an infarction and unstable angina pectoris. Unstable angina pectoris is cardiac pain that occurs at rest and is due to inadequate coronary blood supply. ◄ Hemoglobin, the oxygen-transport protein in erythrocytes, is a tetramer consisting of two α-chains and two β-chains, denoted as $\alpha_2\beta_2$ (Figure 3–16).

PROTEIN STRUCTURE

Primary Structure

The structure of proteins is considered hierarchically at four levels: primary, secondary, tertiary, and quaternary. The primary structure refers to the sequence of amino acids and the nature and position of any covalently attached derivatives. Peptides have directionality with an amino group at one end and a carboxyl group at the other. The amino or carboxyterminal groups may be modified.

By convention, structures are written with the amino terminus on the left and carboxyl terminus on the right.

Insulin is a hormone that is produced in the β-cells of the islets of Langerhans in the pancreas. Insulin consists of an A chain with 21 residues and a B chain with 30 residues (Figure 3–17). There are two interchain disulfide bonds and one intrachain disulfide bond. Each disulfide bond arises from the oxidation of two cysteine residues.

► **Diabetes mellitus** is due to a deficiency of insulin or the lack of an insulin effect (insulin resistance). Hyperglycemia (elevated blood glucose concentration) is a characteristic feature of the disease. Early-onset (type I) and late-onset (type II) disorders have different clinical pictures. Severe diabetes mellitus is associated with the triad of polydipsia (excessive thirst and fluid intake), polyphagia (great food intake), and polyuria (large urine output).

Early-onset disease is usually treated with insulin injection. Until the 1980s, insulin was isolated from pigs or cattle. These hormones are effective in humans, but they differ slightly in primary structure from human insulin, and there is the possibility, observed occasionally, that the hormones are immunogenic and elicit an antibody response. To

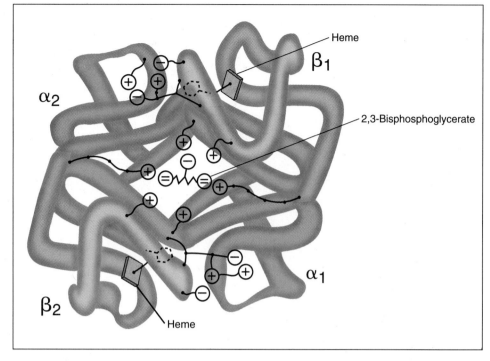

FIGURE 3–16. Binding of 2,3-bis-phosphoglycerate (2,3-BPG) to hemoglobin. *The β-subunits are closer to the viewer. The central cavity of deoxyhemoglobin is lined with positive charges that form ionic bonds with the negative charges of the carboxylate and phosphates of 2,3-BPG, which stabilizes deoxyhemoglobin. Each of the four subunits contains heme, but only those of the β-chain are visible. (Reproduced, with permission, from R. E. Dickerson. X-ray studies of protein mechanisms. Annual Review of Biochemistry 41:819, 1972.)*

avoid this potential problem, genetic engineering was used to produce authentic human insulin in bacteria. Late-onset diabetes is due to insulin resistance and does not usually require treatment by insulin injection. Most individuals with late-onset diabetes are obese, and weight reduction is usually associated with a greater response to endogenous insulin. Because of the importance of diabetes in clinical medicine, it is considered in several relevant sections of this book. ◄

Secondary Structure

The secondary structure of a protein refers to motifs of hydrogen bonding. There are two major classes of secondary structure. The first to be described, the **α-helix,** refers to a helix stabilized by hydrogen bonding between a carbonyl group of one peptide bond (residue n) and the N—H group of the peptide bond of residue n + 4 (Figure 3-18). The α-helix has 3.6 residues per turn. The

closed loop from the N—H nitrogen, the peptide chain, the carbonyl oxygen, and the hydrogen-bonding hydrogen contains 13 atoms. The α-helix is known as the 3.6_{13}-helix. The **rise** per residue along the helix is 0.15 nm (1.5 Å); the **pitch** of the helix or rise per turn is 0.54 nm (5.4 Å) (3.6 residues per turn × 0.15 nm/residue). As much as 80% of a protein can be α-helical; only one protein in 25 lacks any α-helix.

The second class of secondary structure to be described was called the **β-pleated sheet.** Here, >N—H and >C=O (carbonyl) groups from residues far apart on the polypeptide chain or even residues on a different polypeptide chain form hydrogen bonds. The polypeptide chains that make up the β-pleated sheets are called β-strands. β-Strands are fully stretched from their amino to carboxyl terminus. Two varieties of β-pleated sheet are recognized based on the polarity of the polypeptide chains. When the chains are going in the same direction from the amino to carboxyl end of the molecule, the structure is a **parallel β-pleated**

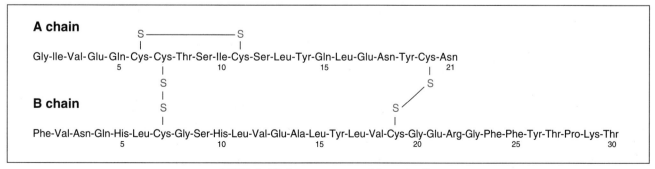

A chain

S————————S
| |
Gly-Ile-Val-Glu-Gln-Cys-Cys-Thr-Ser-Ile-Cys-Ser-Leu-Tyr-Gln-Leu-Glu-Asn-Tyr-Cys-Asn
     5 | 10   15 | 21
                S   S
                |
B chain   S   S
                |
Phe-Val-Asn-Gln-His-Leu-Cys-Gly-Ser-His-Leu-Val-Glu-Ala-Leu-Tyr-Leu-Val-Cys-Gly-Glu-Arg-Gly-Phe-Phe-Tyr-Thr-Pro-Lys-Thr
     5   10   15   20   25   30

FIGURE 3–17. Primary structure of human insulin.

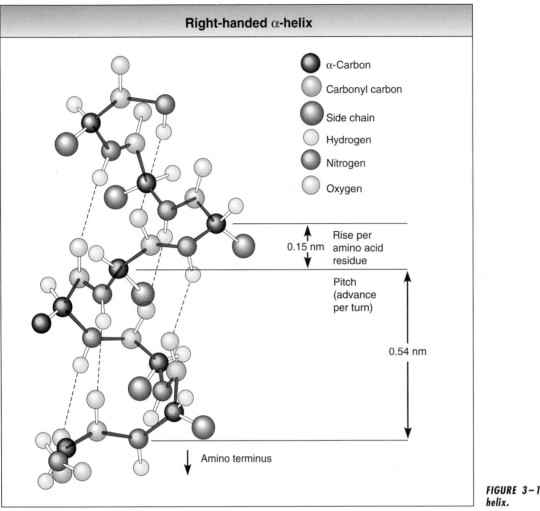

FIGURE 3–18. A right-handed α-helix.

sheet (Figure 3–19). When the participating chains are going in opposite directions with respect to the amino and carboxyl termini, the structure is an **antiparallel β-pleated sheet.** Both parallel and antiparallel β-sheets are pleated, i.e., the α-carbon atoms are successively a little above and below the plane of the sheet.

Reversal in the direction of the polypeptide chain occurs with the formation of a **β-bend.** This configuration involves the formation of a loop in which a residue's carbonyl group forms a hydrogen bond with the amide NH group of the residue three positions farther (n + 3) along the polypeptide chain (Figure 3–20). β-Bends are 3.0_{10} helices (three residues per turn with 10 atoms in a loop). Between a quarter and a third of a protein's structure is made of turns and loops. Glycine occurs in the majority of β-bends.

Many recurring structural motifs occur in a variety of proteins. Some of these have to do with the interconnections of α-helices and β-sheets. Some of these common motifs and super-secondary structures are illustrated in Figure 3–21.

Coil is a term for none-of-the-above forms of secondary structure. Coils are as stable as any other type of structure considered thus far; they are just

more difficult to describe. Although frequently described as random coil, their structure is anything but random.

Tertiary Structure

The tertiary structure of a protein refers to the three-dimensional arrangement of the atoms of the molecule in space. For a monomeric protein such as myoglobin (Figure 3–15), the tertiary structure is the highest order of structure. Myoglobin consists of eight stretches of α-helix labelled A through H; the junctions are denoted AB, BC, CD, etc.

Quaternary Structure

The quaternary structure refers to the manner in which subunits of a multimeric protein interact. During the oxygenation of hemoglobin, a tetrameric protein, the subunits move relative to each other. This aspect of structure is the quaternary structure. The amino acid sequences of the subunits of a protein can be the same, similar, or completely

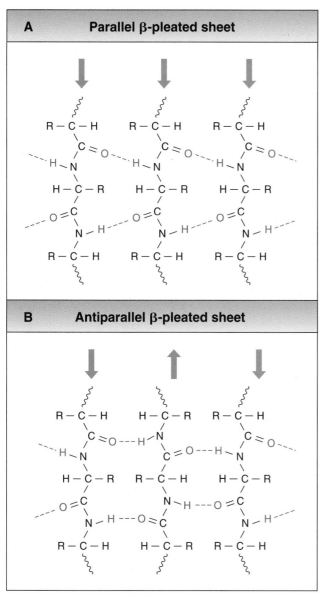

A   Parallel β-pleated sheet

B   Antiparallel β-pleated sheet

FIGURE 3–19. β-pleated sheet. A. Parallel. B. Antiparallel.

sible for maintaining the active conformation include covalent bonds, salt bridges, hydrogen bonds, hydrophobic bonds, and van der Waals bonds. The contributions of the latter four in maintaining the active conformation vary among proteins. The charged R groups of amino acids are seldom buried in the interior of proteins unless they are serving a special function. Proline disrupts secondary structure (α-helix and β-sheet) and is good at forming turns. Glycine also occurs in a large fraction of turns.

When proteins are exposed to extremes of pH such as the acid pH (≈ 1.5) of the stomach, high temperature (60 °C or greater), or treatment with charged detergents such as sodium dodecylsulfate (found in household detergents), the native conformation is destroyed and a **denatured** structure results. The native state corresponds to one or a few active conformations, while the denatured state may be associated with multiple but inactive conformations. Heating and detergent treatments are often used to kill bacteria and viruses in the home, hospital, and clinic.

Protein Folding and Chaperones

The sequence of amino acids in a polypeptide chain determines the structure and properties of the protein. **Anfinsen's law** states that the secondary, tertiary, and quaternary structures are determined by the primary structure (PRINCIPLE 6 OF BIOCHEMISTRY). The substitution of an amino acid by a similar one, e.g., the replacement of leucine by valine, may not be of great consequence. Substitution

different. Subunit interactions are similar to those of a protein interior and involve hydrophobic bonds, ionic bonds, and side chain and backbone hydrogen bonds. β-Sheet hydrogen bonds between strands in opposite subunits are also common. In hemoglobin, the subunit contacts can shift back and forth between two different stable positions.

The definition of **domains** is imprecise. Domains may refer to independent and stable folding units analogous to subunits. The mean domain size consists of 200 amino acid residues; the range is from about 40 to 400.

ANFINSEN'S LAW AND PROTEIN STRUCTURE

Native Versus Denatured Structure of Proteins

The physiologically active conformation of a protein is called the **native** structure. Forces respon-

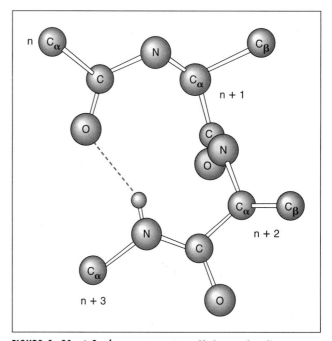

FIGURE 3–20. β-Bend, or reverse turn. Hydrogen bonding occurs between residue n and n + 3. Two residues are not involved in hydrogen bonding. Proline predominates at position n + 1 and glycine predominates at position n + 3.

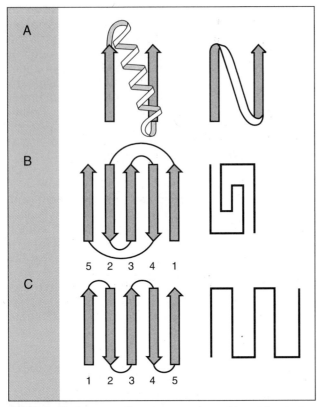

FIGURE 3–21. Super-secondary structures observed in proteins. A. *β-α-β unit.* B. *Greek key motif.* C. *β-Meander.*

by unlike residues, however, can result in a protein with greatly different properties. ▶ Substitution of valine for glutamate at position 6 (from the amino terminus) in the β-chain of human hemoglobin, for example, produces **hemoglobin S** (sickle cell hemoglobin). Deoxygenated sickle cell hemoglobin assumes an abnormal conformation and is poorly soluble under physiological conditions. This leads to hemolysis and the circulatory abnormalities of **sickle cell anemia.** ◀

Chaperones are proteins that aid in protein folding during synthesis, but they are not responsible for the stability of the final product. There are several classes of chaperones, and they occur in the cytosol, in various organelles, and in bacteria. Many chaperones are heat shock or stress proteins, but they have other functions under physiological conditions. Chaperones bind to hydrophobic patches and stabilize intermediates during folding. Chaperones prevent the aggregation of incompletely folded proteins by precluding adventitious contacts between exposed hydrophobic regions. The energy requirements of chaperones can be substantial, and more than 120 ATP molecules can be expended during the folding of a single polypeptide chain.

The condensation of amino acids to form proteins results in the loss of all the α-amino and α-carboxyl groups of a polypeptide chain except for a free amino terminus and a free carboxyl terminus; the amino and carboxyl groups in peptide bond linkage do not contribute to a protein's electrostatic charge. The R groups make the predominant contribution to the ionization state of a protein. When the amino acids occur in proteins, various interactions can alter pK_a values, so that ranges are usually given for the side chains as they occur in proteins. The pK_a values of an R group in a protein can be altered by two or more pH units compared with that of the free amino acid.

HYDROPATHY PROFILES AND PROTEIN STRUCTURE

The tendency of the R group of an amino acid to form a hydrophobic bond, determined experimentally, is called hydropathy (Table 3–1). The hydropathic index of a protein is the sum of the hydropathies of nine or so consecutive residues versus the residue sequence number. When the hydropathic index of the protein chymotrypsinogen was compared with the three-dimensional structure established by x-ray crystallography, the positive (more hydropathic) regions were found on the interior of the protein, and the negative regions were found on the protein's exterior (Figure 3–22). Similar results have been observed with other proteins. This finding suggests that hydrophobic forces play a major role in determining the tertiary structure of proteins.

When the primary structure of a protein is established, an analysis of the hydropathic index can be informative. For example, the hydropathy plot often reveals the existence of hydrophobic transmembrane regions of integral membrane proteins. The finding of a stretch of 20 or so amino acids with a positive hydropathy index is consistent with the existence of a transmembrane domain. Several plasma membrane receptors exhibit seven transmembrane segments, and these domains are observed in the hydropathy plots.

ZINC FINGER AND LEUCINE ZIPPER PROTEINS

Zinc finger proteins accommodate from 2 to about 35 related domains that contain zinc. Each domain contains about 30 residues, including 2 cysteines, 2 histidines, and several hydrophobic amino acid residues. The zinc atom is bound to the two cysteine and two histidine residues. The determination of the structure of zinc fingers by nuclear magnetic resonance (NMR) indicates that each "finger" consists of two antiparallel β-strands and an α-helix. The zinc atom connects these three components (Figure 3–23). Zinc finger proteins often bind to DNA. Examples of zinc finger proteins include the glucocorticoid and estrogen steroid hormone receptors. In some proteins, all four zinc-binding amino acids are cysteine, and a second class of zinc finger results.

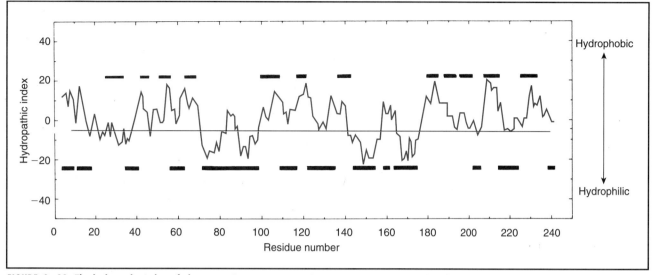

FIGURE 3–22. The hydropathy index of chymotrypsinogen, a pancreatic enzyme. *A positive hydropathic index signifies a hydrophobic region of the polypeptide chain, and a large negative value signifies a hydrophilic region. Upper bars denote the protein's interior regions, and lower bars show the protein's exterior regions, as established by x-ray crystallography. After J. Kyte and R. F. Doolittle. A simple method for displaying the hydropathic character of protein.* Journal of Molecular Biology *157:111, 1982.*

Another important type of DNA binding protein possesses leucine zippers. These proteins contain domains with leucine repeats at every seventh residue for 28 to 35 residues. The leucine residues occur at the same relative position of an α-helix (3.6 residues per turn, or about 7 residues per two turns of the helix). It is postulated that two such domains of a protein form an interdigitated connection that binds two such proteins together as illustrated in Figure 3–24. The leucine zipper, first postulated for DNA binding proteins, does not interact directly with DNA. Some proteins may contain both zinc fingers and leucine zippers.

SUMMARY

Proteins are polymers of α-amino acids. The most prevalent protein in humans is collagen. The amino acids found in proteins possess the L-configuration. Glycine lacks a chiral carbon atom. Two amino acids, isoleucine and threonine, contain two chiral carbon atoms. The combination of the amino group of one amino acid with the carboxyl group of a second amino acid (minus water) produces a peptide bond. Peptide bonds are planar, and rotation about the carbon-nitrogen bond is restricted.

The pK_a of a group is the pH value at which the

FIGURE 3–23. The zinc finger domain of a protein. A. The two-dimensional structure of the zinc binding domain that prompted the term "zinc finger." B. Finger domains consist of antiparallel β-sheets and an α-helix. C. The binding of zinc finger proteins to DNA. The ribbons represent the exterior of the DNA double helix, and the lines connecting the ribbons represent bases.

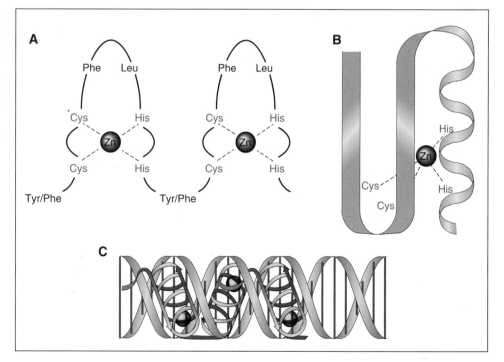

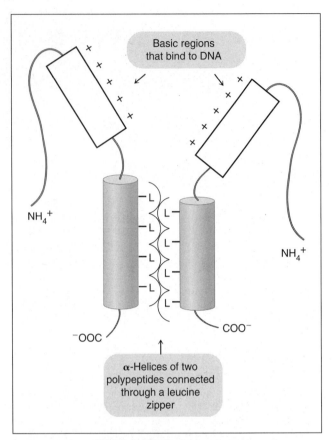

FIGURE 3–24. The leucine zipper.

concentration of the protonated group equals that of the unprotonated group. pH is defined as follows: $pH = -\log_{10} [H^+]$. The pH of blood is 7.4. Buffers are substances that diminish the change in pH when acid or alkali is added to a solution. The physiologically important buffers in blood, saliva, and other body fluids, in order of their effectiveness as buffers, are (1) H_2CO_3—HCO_3^-, (2) $H_2PO_4^-$—HPO_4^{2-}, and (3) protein—protein⁻. The Henderson-Hasselbalch equation is given by the following expression: $pH = pK_a + \log [salt]/[acid]$.

The amino acids that bear negatively charged R groups at physiological pH include aspartate and glutamate. Amino acids that bear positively charged R groups at physiological pH include arginine and lysine. Some imidazole groups of histidine are positively charged and others are neutral at physiological pH.

The primary structure of a protein refers to the sequence of amino acids and the nature and position of any covalently attached derivatives. The secondary structure refers to patterns of hydrogen bonding. There are two major classes of hydrogen-bonded structures associated with secondary structure. The α-helix is stabilized by hydrogen bonding between a carbonyl group of one peptide bond (residue n) and the N—H group on the peptide bond of residue n + 4. The β-pleated sheet is stabilized by hydrogen bonding between residues that are far apart in the primary structure. When the polypeptide chains are going in the same direction, the structure is parallel. When the chains are going in opposite directions, the structure is antiparallel. β-Bends often connect two β-strands to form the antiparallel sheet. Two residues in a β-bend do not form hydrogen bonds.

The tertiary structure is the three-dimensional structure. This is the highest order of structure in myoglobin, a monomeric protein. The quaternary structure of a multimeric protein such as hemoglobin refers to subunit interactions. Anfinsen's law states that the primary structure determines a protein's secondary, tertiary, and quaternary structures. The hydropathy plots of a protein suggest regions of a protein that are buried or are on the surface. These plots often reveal segments of a protein that can pass through membranes.

Zinc fingers are regions of a protein that consist of two histidines and two cysteines bound to zinc. These regions consist of two β-strands and an α-helix. Proteins that contain such domains often bind to DNA. Leucine zippers contain four or five leucine residues that are separated by seven residues (two turns of an α-helix). The leucine zippers interdigitate to form dimers. Some proteins contain both zinc fingers and leucine zippers.

SELECTED READINGS

Jennings, M.L. Topography of membrane proteins. Annual Review of Biochemistry 58:999–1027, 1989.

Kyte, J., and R.F. Doolittle. A simple method for displaying the hydropathic character of protein. Journal of Molecular Biology 157:105–132, 1982.

Landschulz, W.H., P.F. Johnson, and S.L. McKnight. The leucine zipper: A hypothetical structure common to a new class of DNA binding proteins. Science 240:1759–1764, 1988.

Lee, M.S., G.P. Gippert, K.V. Soman, D.A. Case, and P.E. Wright. Three-dimensional solution structure of a single zinc finger DNA-binding domain. Science 245:635–637, 1989.

Perutz, M. *Protein Structure: New Approaches to Disease and Therapy.* New York, W.H. Freeman & Company, 1992.

Richardson, J.S. The anatomy and taxonomy of protein structure. Advances in Protein Chemistry 34:167–339, 1981.

CHAPTER FOUR

ENZYMES

I have never known a dull enzyme.
—ARTHUR KORNBERG

GENERAL PROPERTIES OF ENZYMES

An enzyme is a protein catalyst. A protein is a polypeptide made up of amino acid residues, and a **catalyst** is a substance that alters the rate of a chemical reaction. The molecules that enzymes operate on are called **substrates,** and the molecules that result are **products.** Enzymes are required for nearly all cellular reactions. The conversion of carbon dioxide and water to carbonic acid (equation 4.1) occurs slowly without an enzyme. **Carbonic anhydrase** catalyzes this reaction *in vivo* to ensure that the process proceeds rapidly enough to meet physiological needs. The example of carbonic anhydrase is unusual because the uncatalyzed reaction proceeds at a measurable rate under physiological conditions, whereas most biochemical reactions do not proceed at a detectable rate at physiological temperature and pH values without a catalyst.

$$CO_2 + H_2O \rightleftharpoons H_2CO_3 \qquad (4.1)$$

Perhaps the most impressive property of enzymes is the extent by which they increase the rates of reactions. The rate of a catalyzed reaction ranges from 10^3- to 10^{11}-fold greater than that of an uncatalyzed reaction. A catalyst accelerates the rate by decreasing the **free energy of activation** of a reaction (Figure 4–1). The free energy of activation is denoted by $\Delta G\ddagger$ (where G refers to the American physicist J. Willard Gibbs). A catalyst increases the rate at which a thermodynamically feasible reaction attains its equilibrium without altering the position of the equilibrium.

Enzymes fall into two general classes. Some enzymes are **simple proteins** that contain only amino acid residues. Examples include the digestive enzymes trypsin, chymotrypsin, and elastase. Other enzymes are **complex proteins** that contain amino acid residues and a non–amino acid cofactor. The complete, active enzyme is called a **holoenzyme,** and it is made of a protein portion **(apoenzyme)** and **cofactor.** The apoenzyme is inactive.

$$\text{Holoenzyme} \rightleftharpoons \text{apoenzyme} + \text{cofactor} \qquad (4.2)$$

A metal ion can serve as a cofactor for an enzyme. Zinc ion, for example, is a cofactor for carbonic anhydrase. Cofactors such as pyridoxal phosphate (Figure 2–15), which are tightly held by the enzyme, are called **prosthetic groups.** Many coenzyme forms of the water-soluble vitamins serve as cofactors for many enzyme-catalyzed reactions. Coenzymes differ from prosthetic groups in that coenzymes diffuse to and from the enzyme during each reaction cycle, whereas prosthetic groups remain bound to the enzyme. This distinction is not absolute, since a compound that serves as a coenzyme for one enzyme can serve as a prosthetic group for another enzyme.

Evidence from x-ray crystallography shows that enzymes possess an **active site** that is a small portion of the entire protein. The active site is responsible for binding the **substrates** and for operating chemically on the substrates to catalyze their transformation to **products.** Besides the active, or catalytic, site some enzymes possess an allosteric, or regulatory, site. The **allosteric site** is not at the active site or the substrate binding site but is elsewhere on the protein (Figure 4–2). The allosteric site is where regulatory molecules called allosteric effectors bind to the enzyme and alter the enzyme's conformation and activity. Allosteric molecules can increase (positive effectors) or decrease (negative effectors) the rate of an enzyme-catalyzed reaction. The response depends upon the enzyme and the effector. An enzyme can possess more than one allosteric site, and a single enzyme can have both positive and negative regulatory sites.

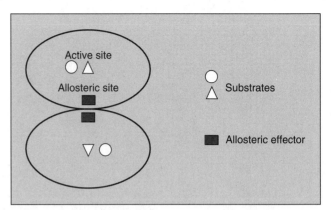

FIGURE 4–2. *An enzyme with an active site and a regulatory, or allosteric, site. These sites represent small portions of the entire protein.*

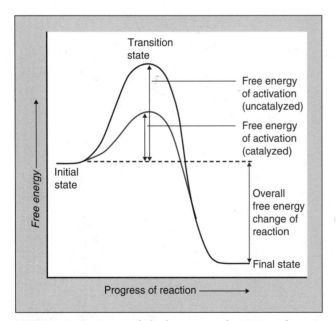

FIGURE 4–1. *Comparison of the free energy of activation of a catalyzed and uncatalyzed reaction. The free energy of activation is related exponentially to the reaction rate, and a small change in the free energy of activation corresponds to a large change in reaction rate.*

TABLE 4-1.   Enzyme Classification

Class	Reaction
Major Classes	
Oxidoreductases	Transfer hydrogen; act on oxygen or peroxide
Transferases	Transfer various groups
Hydrolases	Cleave a bond in a molecule (lysis by water) with the formation of two products
Lyases	Convert one reactant into two products that contain one more double bond than occurs in the reactant
Isomerases	Catalyze racemase, epimerase, intramolecular transferase reactions
Ligases	Catalyze ATP-dependent condensation reactions
Selected Subclasses	
Hydratases	Add water to double bond; lyases
Kinases	Transfer phosphoryl group from ATP; transferases
Mutases	Move phosphoryl group intramolecularly; isomerases
Phosphorylases	Cleave a bond in a molecule (lysis by phosphate) with the formation of two products; transferases
Synthases	ATP-independent synthesis (e.g., UDP-Glc* + glycogen$_n$ → glycogen$_{n+1}$ + UDP), glycogen synthase; transferases
Synthetases	ATP-dependent synthesis; ligases

* UDP-Glc, uridine diphosphate glucose.

Enzymes are organized into six classes based upon the type of reaction that they catalyze (Table 4-1 and Chapter 2). The distinction between synthetases and synthases, enzyme subclasses, is sometimes difficult to comprehend. Both enzymes catalyze biosynthetic reactions. **Synthetases** catalyze ATP-dependent condensation reactions. **Synthases** catalyze biosynthetic reactions that do not directly involve ATP or related nucleoside triphosphates.

ENZYME KINETICS

The study of the rates of reactions is the science of kinetics. Enzyme kinetics is the study of the rates of enzyme-catalyzed reactions. For many chemical reactions, the rate is proportional to the concentration of a reactant (A) as expressed by the following:

$$\text{Velocity} = k_1[A]^1 = k_1[A] \qquad (4.3a)$$

$$\text{Velocity} = k_0[A]^0 = k_0 \qquad (4.3b)$$

where k_1 is the **first-order** rate constant and [A] is the concentration of A. If the velocity is independent of the concentration of A, the exponent is zero and the reaction is described as a **zero-order** reaction whose rate is equal to k_0.

In an enzyme-catalyzed reaction, there is an increase in reaction velocity with an increase in substrate concentration. Often, a plot of velocity as a function of substrate concentration yields a **rectangular hyperbola** (Figure 4-3). At increasingly higher substrate concentrations, the increase in activity is progressively smaller. *Such data show that enzymes exhibit saturation.* Saturation means that substrates interact with a set number of catalytic molecules and are converted into products. In an uncatalyzed process, the reaction would increase indefinitely as reactant concentration increased. At low concentrations, an increase in the substrate concentration leads to a linear, or first-

order, increase in the rate of an enzyme-catalyzed reaction. At very high concentrations, an increase in substrate concentration leads to a very small increase in the rate of an enzyme-catalyzed reaction with zero-order kinetics (the velocity is independent of substrate concentration).

Michaelis-Menten Equation

Consider the enzyme-catalyzed conversion of substrate (S) to product (P).

$$S \rightleftharpoons P \qquad (4.4)$$

We evaluate an expression called the Michaelis-Menten equation that relates the velocity of the enzyme-catalyzed reaction to two kinetic constants with the following properties. Under defined conditions and specific amounts of enzyme, an enzyme exhibits a **maximum velocity** (V_{max}), which is approached as a limiting value as the substrate concentration increases. The K_m **(Michaelis constant)** is the substrate concentration at half the maximal velocity ($V_{max}/2$) as illustrated in Figure 4-3. The

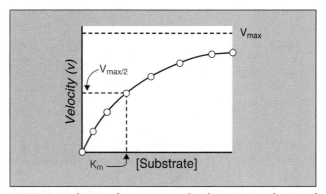

FIGURE 4-3. The rate of an enzyme-catalyzed reaction as a function of substrate concentration. *The curve is a rectangular hyperbola. The K_m is the substrate concentration which corresponds to a reaction velocity that is one-half of the maximal velocity or $V_{max}/2$.*

Michaelis-Menten equation is given by the following expression.

$$v = \frac{V_{max}[S]}{K_m + [S]} \qquad (4.5)$$

This equation was derived by Leonor Michaelis, an enzymologist, and Maude Menten, a pediatrician. The Michaelis-Menten equation is valuable because it provides a tool for understanding enzymatic reactions.

When $v = V_{max}/2$, the reader should verify the result that $K_m = [S]$; we noted that the K_m is the substrate concentration at $V_{max}/2$. It is instructive to use the Michaelis-Menten equation to calculate some reaction velocities under the following conditions. Set the V_{max} at 100 μmol/min and the K_m at 1 mM. Then calculate the velocity (v) at the following substrate concentrations: 0.1 mM, 1 mM, 10 mM, 100 mM, and 1000 mM. Notice that there is a large change in reaction velocity in going from 0.1 mM to 1 mM, and there is a small change in velocity in going from 100 mM to 1000 mM.

Lineweaver-Burk Equation

It is difficult to determine the K_m and V_{max} from a rectangular hyperbola. A common procedure for establishing the kinetic constants is by a **Lineweaver-Burk,** or double reciprocal, equation. Take the reciprocal of the Michaelis-Menten equation to obtain the following:

$$\frac{1}{v} = \frac{K_m + [S]}{V_{max}[S]} = \frac{K_m}{V_{max}[S]} + \frac{[S]}{V_{max}[S]} \qquad (4.6)$$

$$\frac{1}{v} = \frac{K_m}{V_{max}}\left(\frac{1}{[S]}\right) + \frac{1}{V_{max}} \qquad (4.7)$$

Lineweaver-Burk equation

This equation can be compared with the following equation for a straight line, where b is the intercept on the y-axis and m is the slope.

$$y = mx + b \qquad (4.8)$$

In the Lineweaver-Burk equation, $1/V_{max}$ is the y-intercept, or b, and K_m/V_{max} is the slope, or m.

When the reciprocal of the substrate concentration (1/S) is plotted versus the reciprocal of the velocity (1/v), results similar to those in Figure 4–4 are obtained. The value of $1/V_{max}$ is obtained by extrapolation to the y-axis, and the maximal velocity corresponds to the velocity at an infinite substrate concentration ($1/\infty = 0$). The plot also yields $-1/K_m$. Because this is a reciprocal plot, note that a larger V_{max} corresponds to a smaller value of the ordinate (y-axis). Similarly, a larger K_m corresponds to a less negative value of the abscissa (along the x-axis). Note that the x-intercept and $-1/K_m$ are negative, and K_m is positive (a substrate concentration cannot be negative).

The Michaelis constant is made up of rate con-

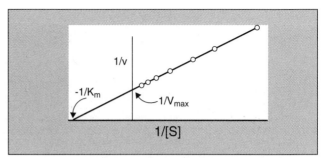

FIGURE 4–4. A double reciprocal, or Lineweaver-Burk, plot.

stants for the formation of the enzyme-substrate complex and the decomposition of the complex to form enzyme and product or substrate. The Michaelis constant is generally not equal to the dissociation constant of an enzyme for the substrate (the dissociation constant is the concentration of substrate when half the enzyme is free and half is occupied with substrate under nonturnover conditions). It is difficult to measure the dissociation constant of an enzyme for a substrate, and this procedure is not considered here. The Michaelis constant is a property of each enzyme and is generally near the physiological concentration of the substrate.

A comparison of the Michaelis constants for hexokinase and glucokinase for glucose is informative. Hexokinase is found in all human cells, including liver, and has a Michaelis constant for glucose of about 30 μM. Glucokinase is found in liver, and it has a Michaelis constant for glucose of 10 mM. At the concentrations of glucose in the hepatic portal vein postprandially (several millimolar), hexokinase is operating at its maximal velocity. In contrast, glucokinase is not saturated and can metabolize more glucose as the substrate concentration increases.

Specificity Constant

The **turnover number** of an enzyme, or the k_{cat}, is the maximal number of molecules of substrate converted to product per active site per unit time when the enzyme is fully complexed with substrate. This value is calculated from the maximal velocity. The k_{cat} for catalase is 4×10^7 per second and that for chymotrypsin is 100 per second. The turnover number per mole of enzyme is a zero-order rate constant because it does not depend upon substrate concentration.

Some enzymes, such as hexokinase, can catalyze the conversion of several different substrates to products. The k_{cat}/K_m value, or **specificity constant,** of the various substrates can be compared. That substrate with the highest value is the best substrate for the enzyme, accounting for the name specificity constant. The rate of any reaction is limited by the rate at which reactant molecules collide. The diffusional limiting rate for a bimolecular reaction is 10^8 to 10^9 $M^{-1}s^{-1}$. The ratio of k_{cat}/K_m is a first-order rate constant. The product of k_{cat}/K_m and the substrate concentration (at subsaturating levels) gives the rate of the enzyme-catalyzed reaction. This rate is proportional to the substrate concentration and is therefore designated first order. Enzymes that have ratios of k_{cat}/K_m near 10^8 to 10^9 $M^{-1}s^{-1}$ (close to the maximum allowed by the rate of diffusion) have achieved catalytic perfection. Triose phosphate isomerase, an enzyme of the glycolytic pathway, is an enzyme that has this attribute. Most enzymes, however, have specificity constants that are below this value.

ENZYME INHIBITION

Irreversible Inhibitors

The study of enzyme inhibitors is important to gain an understanding of enzymes and the action of several drugs used in therapeutics. Enzyme inhibitors can be classified as reversible or irreversible. An **irreversible** enzyme inhibitor reacts with an enzyme and forms a stable complex. As a result, the enzyme is permanently inactivated or at best is slowly reactivated (requiring hours or days for reversal). Usually the irreversible inhibitor forms a covalent bond with the enzyme. This typically involves a reaction of the inhibitor with an amino acid residue in the enzyme's active site.

The reaction of aspirin with cyclooxygenase represents one example of the action of an irreversible enzyme inhibitor. **Cyclooxygenase** catalyzes the first reaction in the biosynthesis of prostaglandins from arachidonate (Figure 12–35). **Aspirin** acetylates an active site serine (Figure 4–5). This chemical modification is stable and leads to irreversible inhibition. New cyclooxygenase must be synthesized to regain activity. ▶ Aspirin is used as an anti-inflammatory, antipyretic, and analgesic drug. Aspirin is also used prophylactically to inhibit platelet aggregation and coronary thrombosis. ◀

Reversible Inhibitors

Reversible enzyme inhibition does not involve covalent modification. Reversible inhibitors work by a variety of mechanisms that can be distinguished by **steady-state enzyme kinetics.** The velocity of an enzyme reaction is measured at several substrate concentrations without and with fixed concentrations of inhibitor. The data are plotted as the reciprocal of the substrate concentration versus the reciprocal of the velocity. The key value to examine on such a Lineweaver-Burk plot is the V_{max}.

In **competitive inhibition,** the inhibitor and a substrate cannot bind to the enzyme simultaneously because they bind to the same enzyme forms. Competitive inhibitors are structural analogues of the substrate whose concentration is being varied. With a competitive inhibitor, the V_{max} is unchanged (Figure 4–6). At infinite substrate concentration (obtained by extrapolation), the inhibitor does not affect enzyme activity. The substrate overrides the effect of the inhibitor and accounts for the term competitive. Competitive inhibitors have an effect on the slope of the double reciprocal plot but not on the y-intercept ($1/V_{max}$). The apparent K_m becomes larger with increasing inhibitor concentration.

In **noncompetitive inhibition,** the inhibitor can bind to the free enzyme and to the enzyme-substrate complex. Increasing the concentration of substrate does not override the binding of inhibitor to the enzyme, and the V_{max} is decreased. Noncompetitive inhibitors have an effect on both the slope and the y-intercept of the double reciprocal plot. The Michaelis constant for the substrate is not changed (Figure 4–6).

In **uncompetitive inhibition,** the inhibitor can bind only to the enzyme-substrate complex (Figure 4–6). It is not easy to imagine how this might occur with an enzyme with a single substrate, but uncompetitive inhibition occurs with multisubstrate enzymes that bind substrates and inhibitors in an obligatory order. Note that the slopes are unchanged, the y-intercepts increase (the V_{max} values decrease), and the Michaelis constants decrease ($-1/K_m$ becomes more negative).

FIGURE 4–5. Irreversible inhibition of cyclooxygenase by aspirin.

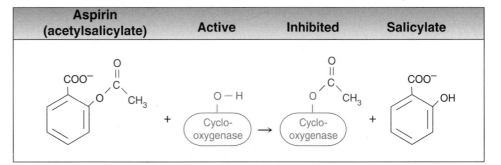

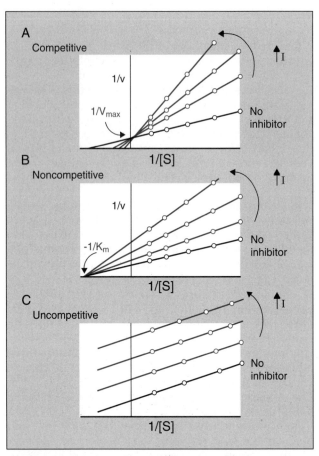

FIGURE 4–6. Three types of reversible enzyme inhibition. A. *Competitive inhibition.* B. *Noncompetitive inhibition.* C. *Uncompetitive inhibition.*

Drugs as Enzyme Inhibitors

Many therapeutic agents, including aspirin, exert their pharmacological effect by acting as enzyme inhibitors. Those drugs that resemble the substrate of an enzyme-catalyzed reaction are competitive inhibitors with respect to that substrate (and noncompetitive inhibitors with respect to the other substrates). ▶ One commonly prescribed class of drugs is the angiotensin converting enzyme (ACE) inhibitors, which are widely used in the treatment of hypertension and congestive heart failure. This enzyme catalyzes the proteolytic cleavage of angiotensin I to angiotensin II (Figure 3–14). Angiotensin II elevates arterial pressure. Captopril and enalapril are two examples of competitive ACE inhibitors. Both agents contain proline (Figure 20–6), and proline is an important substrate binding determinant.

Lovastatin and mevinolin are commonly prescribed as cholesterol lowering agents for various forms of hypercholesterolemia. The rate-limiting step in the pathway for cholesterol biosynthesis is catalyzed by hydroxymethylglutaryl coenzyme A reductase (HMG-CoA reductase) illustrated in Figure 12–18. Both lovastatin and mevinolin resemble hydroxymethylglutaryl coenzyme A and are com-

petitive inhibitors when HMG-CoA is the varied substrate. ◀

MULTISUBSTRATE REACTIONS

Thus far we have considered enzyme reactions with a single substrate and a single product. These are called uni uni reactions and represent a minority of the reactions that occur in metabolism. For multisubstrate reactions, reactants are designated A, B, C, D . . . for the uni, bi, ter, and quad reactant substrates. The products are designated P, Q, R, S . . . The Michaelis-Menten equations are similar to the one already considered, but the complexity increases considerably.

Let us consider bi reactant, bi product reactions that are illustrated by the following:

$$A + B \rightleftharpoons P + Q \qquad (4.9)$$

The reaction might be ordered with A combining with the enzyme (E) before B. The release of products might also be ordered with P dissociating from the enzyme before Q. This scheme is an example of an **ordered-sequential** reaction. Such reactions are diagrammed in the following fashion:

$$
\begin{array}{ccccc}
A & B & & P & Q \\
\downarrow & \downarrow & & \uparrow & \uparrow \\
\hline
\end{array}
$$
$$
E \qquad EA \qquad (EAB \rightleftharpoons EPQ) \qquad EQ \qquad E
$$
$$(4.10)$$

The reaction might be random (either A or B could combine with the enzyme, and either P or Q could dissociate from the enzyme). This reaction is an example of a **random-sequential** reaction. This type of reaction is depicted in the following diagram:

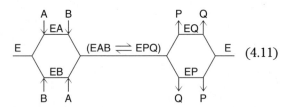

$$(4.11)$$

A **ping-pong** mechanism is a third major type of bimolecular reaction, depicted in the following diagram. E′ indicates that the enzyme exists in a chemically modified form.

$$
\begin{array}{cccc}
A & P & B & Q \\
\downarrow & \uparrow & \downarrow & \uparrow \\
\hline
\end{array}
$$
$$
E \quad (EA \rightleftharpoons E'P) \quad E' \quad (E'B \rightleftharpoons EQ) \quad E
$$
$$(4.12)$$

Aspartate aminotransferase is an example of an enzyme that uses a ping-pong mechanism. E represents enzyme with bound pyridoxal phosphate, and E′ is enzyme with pyridoxamine phosphate (Figure 2–15).

FACTORS THAT CONTRIBUTE TO THE RATE ENHANCEMENT OF ENZYMES

Many factors produce the remarkable rate enhancement that is characteristic of enzymes, but not all are operative for a given enzyme. By using **proximity** and **orientation,** substrates bind to the enzyme so that the catalytic amino acid residues of the enzyme are near the atoms and bonds of the substrate undergoing change. Sometimes an amino acid residue forms a covalent bond with the substrate during catalysis. **Covalent catalysis** is a special case that involves the proximity of an enzyme and substrate and the appropriate orientation of the reactive groups.

Binding of the substrates can produce a conformational change in the enzyme called **induced fit.** To illustrate, a hand and glove are complementary. Placing a hand in a folded glove is analogous to induced fit; the substrate (hand) produces a change in the conformation of enzyme (changes the shape of the glove). Changes in the conformation can strain or distort the substrate and promote the formation of the transition state. **Strain** and **distortion** of the substrates produced by the enzyme can explain the large size of the enzyme compared with the size of the active site.

Only one, two, or three residues participate in reactions at the active site; additional residues can participate in binding the substrate to the enzyme. Cofactors and prosthetic groups generally occur at the active site. The active site of the enzyme can furnish amino acid residues that are proton donors or proton acceptors. **General acid** or **general base catalysis** can occur alone or in concert with other actions. Histidine, lysine, aspartate, and glutamate are residues that can function in general acid-base catalysis. Metal ions can participate in enzymatic catalysis in many ways. Metal ions can act by binding substrates and orientating them for reaction, and they can stabilize the substrates electrostatically. Metals can interact with water and promote the reaction of hydroxyl groups. They can act in much the same way as a proton. Metals can have charges greater than that of a proton, and metal ions are sometimes called **superacids.**

Catalysis can be mediated by **transition-state binding.** Enzymes can bind the transition state with greater affinity than they bind either the substrate or products. The transition state is an intermediate in a chemical reaction. The enzyme can act by binding substrate and forcing the substrates to assume the structure of the transition state and thereby accelerate the reaction. Transition state analogues have been synthesized by enzymologists, and such analogues bind tightly to the enzyme and are powerful inhibitors.

BIOCHEMICAL MECHANISM OF SERINE PROTEASES

Serine proteases are enzymes that have serine in their active site. These enzymes, which include trypsin, chymotrypsin, and elastase, act by a similar mechanism. The substrate specificities of these three pancreatic digestive enzymes, which are listed in Table 4–2, are determined by their structures. In trypsin, for example, the active-site serine is located next to a binding pocket that contains anionic aspartate, which attracts lysine and arginine of the substrate. The binding pocket of chymotrypsin is hydrophobic and interacts favorably with phenylalanine, tyrosine, or tryptophan of the substrate. Elastase's binding pocket is shallow and binds small nonpolar residues, particularly alanine.

Let us consider the catalytic mechanism for chymotrypsin (Figure 4–7). The combination of serine 195, histidine 57, and aspartate 102 of chymotrypsin is called a **catalytic triad.** (Numbers refer to the position of the amino acid residue in the protein, starting at the amino terminus.) Serine 195 is positioned by proximity and orientation to carry out a nucleophilic attack. The reaction also involves covalent and general acid catalysis. Catalytic triads occur in these three proteases and other serine proteases, including several blood clotting factors.

REGULATION OF ENZYME ACTIVITY

The activity of enzymes in the cell is subject to a variety of regulatory mechanisms. The amount of enzyme can be altered by increasing or decreasing its synthesis or degradation. Enzyme **induction** refers to increased biosynthesis, and enzyme **repression** refers to decreased biosynthesis. Enzyme activity can also be altered by **covalent modification.** Phosphorylation of specific serine residues by protein kinases increases or decreases catalytic activity, depending upon the enzyme (Figure 4–8). Proteolytic cleavage of proenzymes (chymotrypsinogen, trypsinogen, proelastase, clotting factors) converts an inactive form to an active form.

Enzyme activity can also be regulated by noncovalent **allosteric mechanisms** (PRINCIPLE 8 OF BIOCHEMISTRY). Isocitrate dehydrogenase is an enzyme in the Krebs cycle that is activated by ADP. ADP is not a substrate or a substrate analogue. ADP binds to a site distinct from the active site called the **allosteric site.** Allosteric regulation is common, and the changes in activity in response to allo-

TABLE 4–2.   Substrate Specificity for Selected Serine Proteases

Protease	Recognized Amino Acid Residue
Chymotrypsin	Phenylalanine, tyrosine, tryptophan, hydrophobic residues
Elastase	Alanine
Trypsin	Lysine and arginine

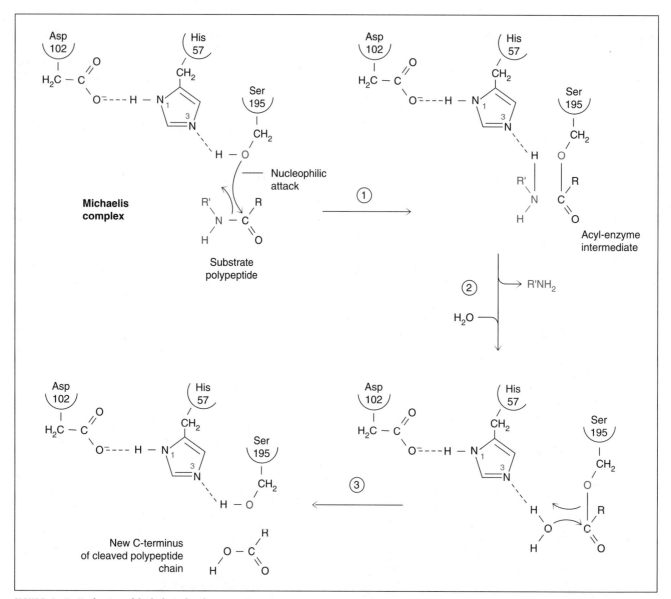

FIGURE 4–7. Mechanism of hydrolysis by chymotrypsin. *(1) After the substrate binds to the enzyme to form a Michaelis complex, the oxygen atom of serine attacks the carbonyl group to form an acyl-enzyme intermediate that is linked covalently to the enzyme. The imidazole ring of histidine takes up the proton from serine and donates it to the amino group of the substrate to form one product. This proton transfer is aided by aspartate, which is hydrogen bonded to histidine. (2) The peptide chain containing the liberated amino group is released from the enzyme and is replaced by water. (3) The hydroxyl group of water attacks and releases the acyl group from the enzyme by hydrolysis. Histidine combines with the proton of the water in the active site to facilitate this process. The acyl group is released from the enzyme, and histidine donates a proton to the serine group to complete the reaction.*

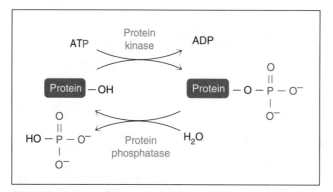

FIGURE 4–8. Protein kinase and phosphoprotein phosphatase reactions.

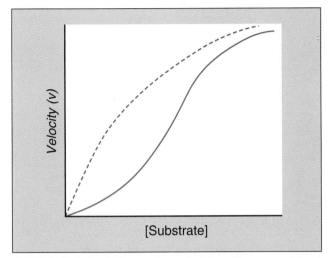

FIGURE 4–9. A sigmoidal curve observed with positive cooperativity. *A rectangular hyperbola (broken line) is illustrated for comparison.*

steric effectors make physiological sense—called the molecular logic of the cell (PRINCIPLE 9 OF BIO-CHEMISTRY). When it is realized that one of the primary functions of the Krebs cycle is to provide reducing equivalents for ATP biosynthesis, then we can rationalize Krebs cycle regulation by ADP. When the concentration of ATP is decreased, the concentration of ADP increases and serves as a signal to activate ATP formation. ADP regulates one of the early reactions of the Krebs cycle (isocitrate dehydrogenase) and promotes greater activity. Besides activation, some enzymes are subject to **allosteric inhibition.**

Some enzymes fail to conform to simple saturation kinetics and do not exhibit a rectangular hyperbola when velocity is measured as a function of substrate concentration. In the most common case, a sigmoidal curve is observed (Figure 4–9). *A sigmoidal curve is the sine qua non for positive cooperativity.* **Positive cooperativity** is the situation in which the binding of one substrate (or ligand) makes it easier for the second to bind. This increased binding is reflected by the increasing slope on the initial portion of the sigmoidal curve when compared with decreasing slope of a rectangular hyperbola. Positive cooperativity is often associated with allosterism, but these are independent

phenomena. Allosteric enzymes and proteins often, but not invariably, exhibit positive cooperativity. A sigmoidal binding curve does not show that an enzyme has an allosteric site distinct from an active site.

CLINICAL SIGNIFICANCE OF ENZYMES

▶ Besides the central role of enzymes in biochemistry, the activity of enzymes in the serum provides information of value in the diagnosis of various diseases. Most of the enzymes in serum do not perform a physiological function and are released into the circulation during the normal turnover of tissue. Under pathological conditions, the serum levels can increase. Following an infarction, for example, the affected cells release their enzymes into the circulation. The pattern or profile of serum enzyme activity is related to the disease process and to the cells or organs affected. We consider the activities of the commonly measured serum enzymes and some diagnostic clues that these provide.

Transaminases

Glutamate-oxaloacetate transaminase (GOT), or **aspartate aminotransferase (AST),** catalyzes the reversible transfer of the amino group from glutamate to oxaloacetate to form α-ketoglutarate and aspartate (Figure 4–10). GOT is released from many diseased cells into serum as SGOT. SGOT is elevated in liver disease and following a myocardial infarction. The serum level has diagnostic value. It can be moderately elevated (fivefold) in people with cirrhosis and obstructive liver disease (a stone blocking the bile duct). It can become very high (25-fold) in people with viral hepatitis.

Glutamate-pyruvate transaminase (GPT), or alanine aminotransferase (ALT), catalyzes the reversible transfer of the amino group from glutamate to pyruvate (Figure 4–11). Glutamate-pyruvate transaminase has most of the properties noted for glutamate-oxaloacetate transaminase. SGPT is also elevated during liver disease and following a myocardial infarction.

FIGURE 4–10. The glutamate-oxaloacetate transaminase reaction.

Glutamate	Oxaloacetate		α-Ketoglutarate	Aspartate

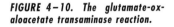

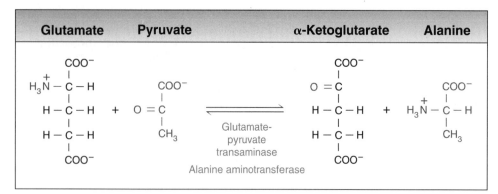

FIGURE 4–11. The glutamate-pyruvate transaminase reaction.

Phosphatases

Alkaline phosphatase is present in many tissues including liver and bone. Alkaline phosphatase catalyzes the hydrolysis of phosphate from a variety of phosphate esters.

$$RO-PO_3^{2-} + H_2O \rightarrow RO-H + HO-PO_3^{2-} \qquad (4.13)$$

The enzyme was so named because of its high pH optimum (pH 8–9). Alkaline phosphatase in bone probably plays a role in calcium phosphate deposition. This enzyme is often elevated in many bone disorders including Paget disease and osteomalacia (Table 2–3). The invasion of bone by cancer from a primary tumor located elsewhere (such as breast, lung, or prostate) occurs by metastasis and can lead to an elevation of alkaline phosphatase. Obstructive liver disease also elevates alkaline phosphatase. Moreover, there is a physiological elevation of alkaline phosphatase during adoles-

cence that is associated with growth of the skeleton. Dentists can use the adolescent elevation of alkaline phosphatase to choose the optimal timing for orthodontic procedures.

Acid phosphatase also catalyzes the reaction given by equation 4.13. As its name implies, acid phosphatase exhibits an acid pH optimum (pH 5–6), and it is a lysosomal enzyme. Elevation of acid phosphatase occurs with metastatic carcinoma of the prostate. Normal prostate does not release significant acid phosphatase into the bloodstream, whereas metastatic prostate tissue does.

Transferases

γ-Glutamyl transpeptidase (GGT) catalyzes a reaction between glutathione, a tripeptide, and an amino acid to form a γ-glutamyl amino acid and cysteinylglycine (Figure 4–12). This enzyme is a

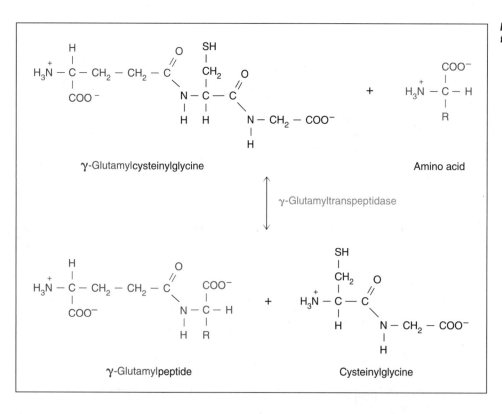

FIGURE 4–12. The γ-glutamyl transpeptidase reaction.

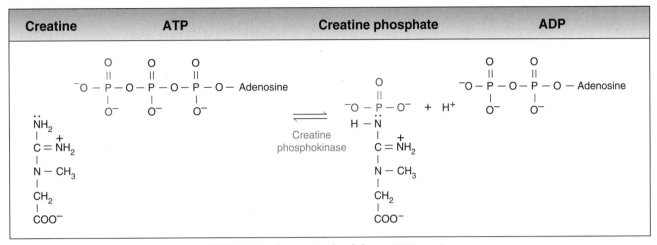

FIGURE 4-13. The creatine phosphokinase (CPK) reaction.

sensitive indicator of liver disease and can be elevated in alcoholism when there are no other serum enzyme abnormalities.

Creatine phosphokinase (CPK) is important in energy metabolism (Figure 4–13). It is found in heart, skeletal muscle, and brain. It is the first cardiac enzyme whose activity is elevated following a myocardial infarction; the enzyme is elevated in about half of the affected people 6 hours after the initial insult. CPK is also elevated in people with Duchenne muscular dystrophy. Lung lacks this enzyme. An individual with chest pain may be suffering from a myocardial infarction, pulmonary infarction, or (rarely) both. Either disorder can occur with (or without) changes in the electrocardiogram (ECG). In a pulmonary infarction, there can be elevations of SGOT, lactate dehydrogenase, and β-hydroxybutyrate dehydrogenase but not of CPK. In myocardial infarction, there can be elevation of all four activities.

Amylase

Amylase catalyzes the hydrolysis of starch and glycogen. Amylase is produced by the pancreas and salivary gland and is elevated during acute pancreatitis. Abdominal pain and an elevation of amylase are consistent with the existence of pancreatitis. Modest elevations in amylase can occur with inflammation of the salivary gland such as that produced by mumps.

Dehydrogenases

Lactate dehydrogenase (LDH) catalyzes the reversible interconversion of lactate and pyruvate (Figure 4–14). Lactate dehydrogenase occurs in all human cells. This enzyme can be elevated following a myocardial infarction and during many liver diseases. Its activity can also be increased during hemolytic anemia when erythrocytes are degraded more rapidly than normally.

β-Hydroxybutyrate dehydrogenase catalyzes the oxidation of β-hydroxybutyrate by NAD^+ (Figure 4–15). The enzyme is present in most human cells. Hydroxybutyrate dehydrogenase activity is elevated following a myocardial infarction, and the elevation follows that of CPK and SGOT (Figure 4-16).

Isozymes

Isozymes (isoenzymes) are different but closely related protein molecules that catalyze the same reaction. Many isozyme studies have relied upon different electrophoretic migration patterns that permit the separation of isoenzyme forms. A common mechanism for the production of isoenzymes arises from different combinations of polypeptide subunits. The practical application of isozymes permits a determination of their tissue of origin.

In the case of **lactate dehydrogenase,** the heart isozyme differs from the liver isozyme. LDH is a tetrameric enzyme made up of two types of subunits: H (for heart) and M (for muscle). These two subunits can be combined in five different ways (Table 4–3). Because lactate dehydrogenase might be released owing to either liver disease or heart disease, establishing the tissue of origin aids in diagnosis.

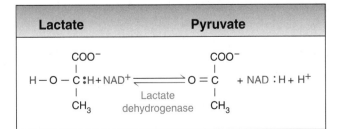

FIGURE 4-14. The lactate dehydrogenase reaction. NAD$^+$ represents nicotinamide adenine dinucleotide.

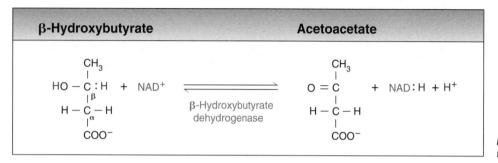

β-Hydroxybutyrate	Acetoacetate

FIGURE 4–15. The β-hydroxybutyrate dehydrogenase reaction.

The time course of the LDH isozyme profile over a few days following a myocardial infarction can also be informative. LDH_1 and LDH_2 (the cardiac forms) can be elevated from 12 to 48 hours after the initial insult. A myocardial infarction refers to heart cell death, and heart failure refers to the inability of the heart to adequately maintain cardiovascular output. The two are independent, and an infarction can occur without heart failure, and vice versa. The LDH_5 can increase after 48 hours, indicating liver congestion secondary to congestive heart failure. In right heart failure, blood accumulates in the venous side of the circulation and causes liver engorgement. As a result, liver cells release LDH_5.

Two gene products correspond to creatine phosphokinase: M (for muscle) and B (for brain). Creatine phosphokinase also occurs as a dimer, and three isozyme forms therefore are possible: CPK_1 (BB), CPK_2 (MB), and CPK_3 (MM). CPK_1 (BB) occurs in brain, CPK_2 (MB) occurs in heart, and CPK_3 (MM) occurs in muscle. The activity of plasma CPK_2 is the cornerstone for the diagnosis of a myocardial infarction because of its abundance in heart and absence from other cells. It may be elevated after 4 hours, and its activity may increase from two- to ten-fold after 16–24 hours. ◀

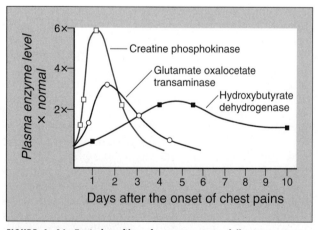

FIGURE 4–16. Typical profiles of serum enzymes following a myocardial infarction (heart attack, coronary thrombosis).

SUMMARY

An enzyme is a protein catalyst. A catalyst accelerates a reaction by decreasing the free energy of activation of the reaction. Enzymes do not alter the equilibrium of a reaction. A holoenzyme is made up of an apoenzyme and cofactor. A tightly bound cofactor is a prosthetic group. That portion of an enzyme that binds substrates and converts them to products is called the active site. Allosteric effectors are molecules that alter enzyme activity binding to the enzyme at a site distinct from the active site called the allosteric site. The activity of an enzyme can also be altered by covalent modification.

Enzymes exhibit saturation kinetics, and the plot of the velocity versus substrate concentration is usually a rectangular hyperbola. When the plot of the velocity versus substrate concentration is sigmoidal, then the process exhibits positive cooperativity. Irreversible inhibitors commonly form a covalent bond with an enzyme and thereby permanently inactivate it. Reversible inhibitors bind noncovalently to enzymes, and their characteristics are determined by steady-state enzyme kinetics. Competitive inhibitors bind to the same site of the enzyme as the varied substrate. Their effects can be overcome at high substrate concentrations. They do not alter the V_{max}. Noncompetitive inhibitors do not bind to the same site as the varied substrate, and their effects cannot be overcome at high substrate concentrations.

Enzymes perform their catalytic function by a variety of mechanisms such as general acid-base catalysis, covalent catalysis, induced fit, strain, and

TABLE 4–3. Lactate Dehydrogenase Isozymes

Type	Composition*	Location
LDH_1	HHHH	Myocardium and red blood cell
LDH_2	HHHM	Myocardium and red blood cell
LDH_3	HHMM	Brain and kidney
LDH_4	HMMM	
LDH_5	MMMM	Liver and skeletal muscle

* H = heart, M = muscle.

binding of the transition state. Trypsin is a serine protease that cleaves on the carboxyl side of lysine and arginine (basic amino acids). Serine, histidine, and aspartate form a catalytic triad that participates in the process. The serine residue forms a covalent bond with a peptide carbonyl group during the reaction.

SELECTED READINGS

Fersht, A. *Enzyme Structure and Mechanism,* 2nd ed., New York, W.H. Freeman & Company, 1985.

Segel, I.H. *Enzyme Kinetics.* New York, John Wiley & Sons, 1975.

Sovel, B.E. Acute myocardial infarction. *In* J.B. Wyngaarden, L.H. Smith, Jr., and J.C. Bennett (eds.). *Cecil Textbook of Medicine,* 19th ed. Philadelphia, W.B. Saunders Company, 1992, pp. 304–318.

Tietz, N.W. *Textbook of Clinical Chemistry.* Philadelphia, W.B. Saunders Company, 1986.

Walsh, C. *Enzymatic Reaction Mechanisms.* New York, W.H. Freeman & Company, 1979.

Weisiger, R.A. Laboratory tests in liver disease. *In* J.B. Wyngaarden, L.H. Smith, Jr., and J. C. Bennett (eds.). *Cecil Textbook of Medicine,* 19th ed. Philadelphia, W.B. Saunders Company, 1992, pp. 760–763.

CHAPTER FIVE

BIOENERGETICS AND OXIDATION-REDUCTION REACTIONS

More and more clearly it appears that in all cells a tendency exists to convert the major part of available oxidation-reduction energy into phosphate bond energy.

—FRITZ LIPMANN

Bioenergetics is the study of energy changes accompanying biological processes. Bioenergetics aids in our understanding of the intricacies of metabolism. One goal and achievement of bioenergetics is to predict whether a biochemical process can occur. The oxidation-reduction energy of catabolism is converted to the phosphate-bond energy of ATP; this metabolic strategy occurs during stages II and III of aerobic metabolism (Figure 1–3). ATP energizes innumerable group transfer reactions in anabolism and catabolism.

FREE ENERGY CHANGE AS A CRITERION OF FEASIBILITY

The Gibbs free energy is the most important thermodynamic function used in biochemistry. *For any real or feasible process, the Gibbs free energy change (ΔG) is negative; the system has more free energy in the initial state than in the final state.*

$$\Delta G = G_{final} - G_{initial} \quad (5.1)$$

All feasible reactions occur with a negative free energy change (ΔG). When the free energy change is zero, the reaction or process is at equilibrium. These important results are summarized as follows.

$\Delta G < 0$ (process is feasible and is **exergonic**)   (5.2a)

$\Delta G = 0$ (equilibrium conditions prevail, and process is **isoergonic**)   (5.2b)

$\Delta G > 0$ (process is not feasible and is **endergonic**)   (5.2c)

STANDARD FREE ENERGY CHANGE AND THE EQUILIBRIUM CONSTANT

The *standard* free energy change is related to the equilibrium constant. Consider the following general chemical reaction:

$$A + B \rightleftharpoons C + D \quad (5.3)$$

By convention, the components on the left side are called reactants and those on the right side are called products. The following equation illustrates the logarithmic relationship between the standard free energy change and the equilibrium constant:

$$\Delta G^\circ = -RT \ln K_{eq} \quad (5.4)$$

R, called the gas constant or temperature-energy coefficient, relates temperature to energy (Table 5–1). R has the value of 8.314 J K^{-1}mol^{-1}, and T is the absolute temperature in degrees Kelvin. Equation 5.4 is a most important result and describes the standard free energy change as a function of the equilibrium constant (and vice versa).

The standard free energy change (ΔG°) for the reaction $A + B \rightleftharpoons C + D$ is the free energy change that accompanies the conversion of A and B into C

TABLE 5–1. Units of Energy and Mass and the Values of Some Physical Constants

Avogadro's number (N_A)
  $N_A = 6.022 \times 10^{23}$ mol^{-1}
Calorie (cal)
  1 calorie is the energy required to heat 1 g of water from 14.5°C to 15.5°C
  1 calorie = 4.184 J
Faraday ($\mathscr{F}$)
  1 $\mathscr{F} = N_A$ electron charges
  1 $\mathscr{F} = 96.485$ kJ V^{-1} or 23 kcal V^{-1}
Gas constant, or temperature-energy coefficient (R)
  R = 8.314 J K^{-1} mol^{-1}
  R = 1.987 cal K^{-1} mol^{-1}
Joule (J)
  1 J = 0.239 calories
  1 kilojoule (kJ) = 1000 J
Kelvin temperature (T) scale (K)
  0 K = absolute zero
  273 K = 0°C
Molar solution
  A molar (M) solution consists of 1 mole of a substance in 1.00 liter of solution.
  mM, millimolar, 1×10^{-3} M; μM, micromolar, 1×10^{-6} M; nM, nanomolar, 1×10^{-9} M; pM, picomolar, 1×10^{-12} M; fM, femtomolar, 1×10^{-15} M
Mole
  A mole is Avogadro's number of molecules. The molecular mass corresponds to the sum of the masses of the elements that make up the molecule. An equivalent is the molecular mass divided by the absolute value of the charge (1, 2, 3)

and D under standard conditions. We now define standard conditions. Because most biochemical reactions of interest occur in aqueous solution, the concentrations of reactants and products under standard conditions are taken to be 1 M (1 mol/L).

The value for water, however, is set to 1.00 and not 55.6 (1000 g/L ÷ 18 g/mol water = 55.6 mol water/L, where 18 is the molecular mass of water and 1000 g is the mass of 1 L of water). It is inconvenient to use 1 M as a standard concentration for water because it is far from the physiological concentration. The uniform use of 1.00 for unit concentration of water does not affect differences in free energy change.

To summarize, the standard free energy change of a chemical process is the Gibbs free energy change during the conversion of reactants to products when all components (except water) are present at 1 M concentration. The concentrations of these components remain constant during the conversion.

The temperature is an important thermodynamic parameter and must be specified. Biochemical reactions are usually studied at 25°C (298 K), 30°C (303 K), or 37°C (310 K). However, most thermodynamic data were collected at 25°C, and values in this book correspond to this temperature. These values, moreover, are close to those at 37°C. The free energy change of many biochemical reactions is affected by pH. Because most biochemical reactions occur near neutrality (pH 7.0), this pH value is used for the biochemical standard state and this convention is denoted by the prime (') as in $\Delta G^{\circ\prime}$,

$\Delta G'$, or K_{eq}'. Thus, $[H^+] = 1 \times 10^{-7}$ M is given an activity of one. The term for the free energy change (not standard free energy change) at pH = 7.0 is $\Delta G'$.

The standard free energy change is a logarithmic function of the equilibrium constant:

$$\Delta G^{\circ\prime} = -RT \ln K_{eq}' \qquad (5.5)$$

The equilibrium constant (K_{eq}') for the following reaction at 25°C and pH 7.0 is 14.66.

$$\text{Isocitrate}^{-3} \rightleftharpoons \text{citrate}^{-3} \qquad (5.6)$$

The standard free energy change can then be calculated in the following fashion:

$$\Delta G^{\circ\prime} = -8.314 \text{ JK}^{-1}\text{mol}^{-1} \times 298 \text{ K} \times \ln 14.66 \quad (5.7)$$

$$\Delta G^{\circ\prime} = -8.314 \text{ JK}^{-1}\text{mol}^{-1} \times 298 \text{ K} \times 2.685$$

$$\Delta G^{\circ\prime} = -6653 \text{ J mol}^{-1}$$

The equilibrium constant is greater than one, and the standard free energy change is negative. Under standard conditions (1 M in reactants and products), the reaction will proceed to the right with the formation of citrate.

Table 5–2 gives the relationship between equilibrium constants (K_{eq}) and standard free energy changes (ΔG°) at 25°C or 298 K. The reader should be able to verify the values; it is not necessary to memorize them. Note that when the equilibrium constant is greater than one, the standard free energy change is negative. Under standard conditions, reactants are converted to products. When the equilibrium constant is less than one, the standard free energy change is positive.

It is the free energy change ($\Delta G'$) and not the standard free energy change ($\Delta G^{\circ\prime}$) that determines whether a chemical or physical process can occur. The free energy change is influenced by the concentrations of the reactants and products. It is common, however, to use the standard free energy changes ($\Delta G^{\circ\prime}$) for qualitative analyses of biochemical reactions, and the procedure for calculating free energy changes from standard free energy changes is not considered in this book. That the use of standard free energy changes is only an approximation when used under physiological conditions, however, must be remembered.

TABLE 5–2. Relationship Between the Standard Free Energy Change and the Equilibrium Constant at 25°C

	ΔG°	
K_{eq}	kJ/mol	kcal/mol
1000	−17.1	−4.09
100	−11.4	−2.73
10	−5.69	−1.36
1	0	0
0.1	+5.69	+1.36
0.01	+11.4	+2.73
0.001	+17.1	+4.09

STANDARD FREE ENERGY CHANGE AS A STATE FUNCTION

Standard free energy changes depend only on the initial and final states of a system. If we know the free energy change associated with each portion of a chemical process or pathway, we can calculate the free energy change for the entire process, since the free energy changes are state functions. We can add or subtract chemical reactions and their corresponding free energy changes. The free energy of hydrolysis of many biochemical compounds has been measured. This information can be used in the analysis of many phosphotransferase reactions as follows:

In the hydrolysis of glucose 6-phosphate,

Glucose 6-phosphate + $H_2O \rightarrow$ glucose + P_i;
$$\Delta G^{\circ\prime} = -13.8 \text{ kJ mol}^{-1} \quad (5.8)$$

Under standard conditions (1 M glucose 6-phosphate, 1 M glucose, 1 M phosphate) in aqueous solution, the reaction proceeds to the right and free energy is liberated ($G^{\circ\prime}_{products} - G^{\circ\prime}_{reactants} = -13.8$ kJ/mol). The free energy of the reactants is greater than that of the products. We can recast the reaction and standard free energy change in the following manner.

Glucose + $P_i \rightarrow$ glucose 6-phosphate + H_2O
$$\Delta G^{\circ\prime} = +13.8 \text{ kJ/mol} \quad (5.9)$$

For the reaction shown in equation 5.9 to proceed from left to right requires the input of energy ($\Delta G^{\circ\prime}$ is opposite in sign to that in the reverse direction shown in equation 5.8). The free energy of hydrolysis of adenosine triphosphate (ATP) is −30.4 kJ/mol. The reactions and their corresponding standard free energy changes ($\Delta G^{\circ\prime}$) can be added.

		$\Delta G^{\circ\prime}$ (kJ/mol)
Glucose + P_i	$\rightarrow$ glucose 6-phosphate + H_2O	+13.8
ATP + H_2O	$\rightarrow$ ADP + P_i	−30.4
Glucose + ATP	$\rightarrow$ glucose 6-phosphate + ADP	−16.6

$$(5.10)$$

From the thermodynamic data of two reactions, we can calculate the standard free energy change at pH 7 ($\Delta G^{\circ\prime}$) for a third reaction. These calculations indicate that the reaction in equation 5.10 will proceed from reactants to products under standard conditions.

From the standard free energy of hydrolysis of glucose 6-phosphate and the standard free energy for the conversion of glucose 1-phosphate to glucose 6-phosphate, we can calculate the standard free energy of hydrolysis of glucose 1-phosphate.

Glucose $\rightarrow$ glucose	$\Delta G^{\circ\prime}$ (kJ/mol)
1-phosphate 6-phosphate	-6.32
Glucose $\rightarrow$ glucose	
6-phosphate +	-13.8
+ P_i	
H_2O	
Glucose $\rightarrow$ glucose	
1-phosphate +	-20.1
+ P_i	
H_2O	(5.11)

Several procedures can be used to determine the standard free energy change of a reaction. Two of the most important include calculations based on (1) the equilibrium constant and (2) differences in the standard reduction potentials. We next consider standard reduction potentials.

OXIDATION-REDUCTION REACTIONS

In Chapter 2, we defined oxidation as the loss of electrons and reduction as the gain in electrons. Oxidation-reduction reactions represent the main source of biochemical energy. The energy from the oxidation of carbohydrates and lipids sustains the biochemical reactions required for life. There are four varieties of biological oxidation-reduction reactions.

Four Types of Oxidation-Reduction Reactions

First, electrons can be transferred directly from donor to acceptor. For example, equation 5.12 depicts an oxidation-reduction reaction where an electron is transferred from the ferrous iron of a protein called cytochrome b to the ferric iron of cytochrome c:

Cytochrome b (Fe^{+2}) + cytochrome c (Fe^{+3}) $\rightleftharpoons$

cytochrome b (Fe^{+3}) + cytochrome c (Fe^{+2}) (5.12)

Cytochrome b is the reducing agent, and cytochrome c is the oxidizing agent. The cytochromes are proteins that contain iron complexed with heme, and cytochromes participate in electron transfer reactions.

Second, electrons can be transferred with protons in a process formally equivalent to the transfer of hydrogen atoms.

$$A + 2 H^+ + 2 e^- \rightarrow AH_2 \qquad (5.13)$$

A represents the oxidizing agent or electron acceptor. The reduction of FAD (flavin adenine dinucleotide) is an example of a substance that undergoes reduction by the equivalent of two protons and electrons or two hydrogen atoms (Figure 2–12).

Third, electrons can be transferred as the hydride ion ($H:^-$) as shown in equation 5.14. NAD^+ is the oxidant.

$$NAD^+ + H:^- \rightarrow NADH \qquad (5.14)$$

The structure of NAD^+ and the oxidation-reduction reaction of the nicotinamide ring are shown in Figure 2–13.

Fourth, there can be a direct reaction between a reductant (AH) and molecular oxygen. One way that this can occur is illustrated by equation 5.15.

$$AH + O_2 + BH_2 \rightarrow AOH + H_2O + B \quad (5.15)$$

Oxidation and reduction reactions occur simultaneously, and one does not occur without the other. However, it is convenient to deal with oxidation-reduction reactions in terms of **half reactions.** Instead of tabulating information on reactions between innumerable oxidants and reductants, we can compare each half reaction with a reference reaction and then consider any pair of half reactions of interest.

Half Reactions

By convention, *half reactions are written as reductions;* hence the term **reduction potential.** This distinction is lost with the ambiguous term redox potential. Electrons are accepted by the oxidizing reagent. Recall that reactants are written on the left side and the products on the right side of a chemical equation. We will use the term reduction potential to emphasize the reduction process; an electron is written on the left side of the equation as a reactant. The reactant in both of the following examples is reduced.

$$A^+ + e^- \rightarrow A \qquad (5.16a)$$

$$B^+ + e^- \rightarrow B \qquad (5.16b)$$

The reference standard for oxidation-reduction reactions is the hydrogen electrode, and its half reaction is written as follows:

$$2 H^+ + 2 e^- \rightarrow H_2 \qquad 0.00 \text{ V} \qquad (5.17)$$

By convention, the concentration of H^+ is 1 M and hydrogen gas is present at 1 atmosphere of pressure. The reaction is assigned a standard reduction potential of zero volts (V). The standard conditions for the other components are 1 M concentration of solute at atmospheric pressure in aqueous solution. If a compound under standard conditions can donate its electrons to the hydrogen reference electrode in an external circuit, the standard reduction potential of this compound is negative. If a compound under standard conditions accepts electrons from the standard reference electrode from the external circuit, the standard reduction potential of this compound is positive. A convenient way to remember this convention is that electrons bear a negative charge. Compounds with a tendency to donate electrons have a negative reduction potential.

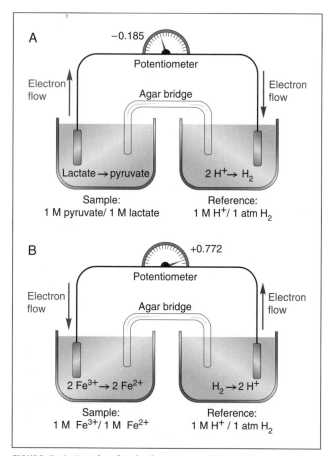

FIGURE 5-1. *Procedure for the determination of the standard reduction potentials of* **(A)** *pyruvate/lactate and* **(B)** *ferric/ferrous half cells. The salt-agar bridge allows for the flow of counterions.*

Most biochemical reactions of interest occur at physiological pH. Like the standard conditions for free energy changes, biochemists have adopted pH 7.0 as a reference state. When standard reduction potential values are given at pH 7.0, these are denoted $\mathscr{E}^{\circ\prime}$ ($\mathscr{E}^{\circ}$ designates a standard reduction potential and the prime indicates pH 7.0).

Electrons flow to the more positive half cell. By convention, the difference in the electrical potential ($\Delta\mathscr{E}$) of the acceptor minus the donor is positive during electron transfer. A difference in reduction potential that is positive corresponds to a negative free energy change, and both are associated with thermodynamically feasible reactions. The procedure used for measuring the standard reduction potential is illustrated in Figure 5-1. The sample half cell contains the oxidized and reduced species at a concentration of 1 M; the reference half cell contains 1 M H^+ (pH 0.0) and is in equilibrium with H_2 at 1 atmosphere pressure. The standard reduction potential of the standard hydrogen electrode is defined as 0.00 V. Electrons flow from the negative half cell to the positive half cell. For the pyruvate/lactate half cell, electrons flow from it to the hydrogen electrode. The pyruvate/lactate standard reduction potential is therefore negative. The potentiometer records a value of -0.185 V.

For the Fe^{+3}/Fe^{+2} half cell, electrons flow from the standard hydrogen electrode to Fe^{+3}/Fe^{+2}. The Fe^{+3}/Fe^{+2} standard reduction potential is therefore positive. The potentiometer records a value of $+0.772$ V.

STANDARD REDUCTION POTENTIALS

Direction of Electron Transfer

Each oxidant in a half reaction has a characteristic electron affinity.

$$\text{Oxidized form} + n\ e^- \rightarrow \text{reduced form}^{-n} \qquad (5.18)$$

The greater the tendency to donate electrons and act as a reducing agent, the more negative is the reduc-

TABLE 5-3. Standard Reduction Potentials of Some Biological Reactants

Half Reaction	$\mathscr{E}^{\circ\prime}$(pH 7), V
Acetate$^-$ + CO_2 + 2 H^+ + 2 e^- → pyruvate$^-$ + H_2O	-0.700
Succinate^{-2} + CO_2 + 2 H^+ + 2 e^- → α-ketoglutarate^{-2} + H_2O	-0.670
3-Phosphoglycerate^{-3} + 3 H^+ + 2 e^- → glyceraldehyde 3-phosphate^{-2} + H_2O	-0.570
RCOO$^-$ + 4 H^+ + 4 e^- → RCH_2OH + OH^-	-0.436
Urate + 2 H^+ + 2 e^- → xanthine + H_2O	-0.360
Cystine + 2 H^+ + 2 e^- → 2 cysteine	-0.340
Pyruvate$^-$ + CO_2 + H^+ + 2 e^- → malate^{-2}	-0.330
O_2 + e^- → O_2^-	-0.330
NAD^+ + H^+ + 2 e^- → NADH	-0.320
$NADP^+$ + H^+ + 2 e^- → NADPH	-0.320
Lipoate$^-$ + 2 H^+ + 2 e^- → dihydrolipoate$^-$	-0.290
Acetoacetyl-CoA + 2 H^+ + 2 e^- → β-hydroxybutyryl-CoA	-0.238
FAD + 2 H^+ + 2 e^- → $FADH_2$	-0.220
Acetaldehyde + 2 H^+ + 2 e^- → ethanol	-0.197
Dihydroxyacetone phosphate^{-2} + 2 H^+ + 2 e^- → glycerol phosphate^{-2}	-0.190
FMN + 2 H^+ + 2 e^- → $FMNH_2$	-0.190
Pyruvate^{-1} + 2 H^+ + 2 e^- → lactate^{-1}	-0.185
Oxaloacetate^{-2} + 2 H^+ + 2 e^- → malate^{-2}	-0.175
α-Ketoglutarate^{-2} + NH_3 + 3 H^+ + 2 e^- → glutamate^{-1} + H_2O	-0.140
Acrylyl-CoA + 2 H^+ + 2 e^- → propionyl-CoA	-0.015
GSSG + 2 H^+ + 2 e^- → 2 GSH (glutathione)	-0.010
Methylene blue + 2 H^+ + 2 e^- → leucomethylene blue	0.011
Fumarate^{-2} + 2 H^+ + 2 e^- → succinate^{-2}	0.031
Metmyoglobin (Fe^{+3}) + e^- → myoglobin (Fe^{+2})	0.046
Dehydroascorbate + 2 H^+ + 2 e^- → ascorbate	0.058
Cytochrome b (Fe^{+3}) + e^- → cytochrome b (Fe^{+2})	0.075
Coenzyme Q + 2 H^+ + 2 e^- → QH_2	0.100
Adrenodoxin (Fe^{+3}) + e^- → adrenodoxin (Fe^{+2})	0.150
Dihydrobiopterin + 2 H^+ + 2 e^+ → tetrahydrobiopterin	0.150
Methemoglobin (Fe^{+3}) + e^- → hemoglobin (Fe^{+2})	0.170
Crotonyl-CoA + 2 H^+ + 2 e^- → Butyryl-CoA	0.190
Cytochrome a (Fe^{+3}) + e^- → cytochrome a (Fe^{+2})	0.210
Cytochrome c (Fe^{+3}) + e^- → cytochrome c (Fe^{+2})	0.254
O_2 + 2 H^+ + 2 e^- → H_2O_2	0.295
H_2O_2 + H^+ + e^- → $OH^{\cdot}$ + H_2O	0.380
Fe^{+3} + e^- → Fe^{+2}	0.772
$\frac{1}{2}$ O_2 + 2 H^+ + 2 e^- → H_2O	0.818
O_2^- + e^- + 2 H^+ → H_2O_2	0.940
$\frac{1}{2}$ H_2O_2 + H^+ + e^- → H_2O	1.350
$OH^{\cdot}$ + H^+ + e^- → H_2O	2.330

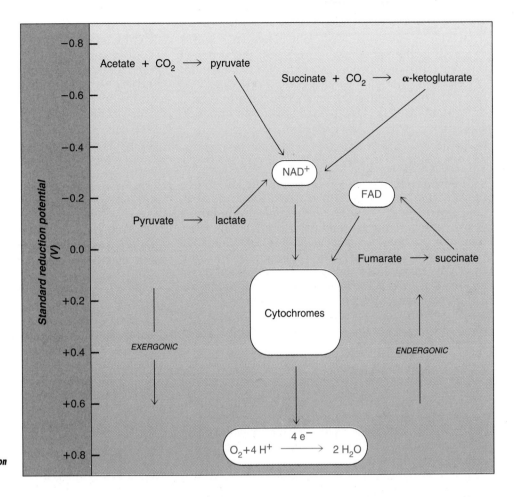

FIGURE 5–2. *The direction of electron flow of biochemical metabolites.*

tion potential. The standard reduction potentials for a variety of half reactions are given in Table 5–3. Electrons tend to go from the compound with the more negative reduction potential to the one with the less negative reduction potential. The compound with the more positive reduction potential accepts electrons and is reduced. Notice that the standard reduction potential for oxygen is highly positive. Oxygen has little tendency to donate electrons and act as a reducing agent.

The following general properties of oxidation-reduction reactions recur throughout biochemistry and bioenergetics. Electrons are passed from fuel molecules listed at the top of Table 5–3 to NAD^+, to cytochromes, and to strong oxidants such as oxygen. Note that common metabolic fuels such as pyruvate and α-ketoglutarate are strong reductants (Table 5–3). Also note that the standard reduction potential of NAD^+ occurs between fuel molecules and the cytochromes. These generalizations are presented diagrammatically in Figure 5–2.

Lactate Dehydrogenase Reaction

The lactate dehydrogenase reaction is a prototype of many oxidation-reduction reactions in biochemistry. Pyruvate, a ketone, is reduced by NADH to produce lactate, an alcohol, and NAD^+. The net

reaction is given in the following chemical equation.

$$
\begin{array}{ccc}
COO^- & & COO^- \qquad (5.19)\\
| & & |\\
C{=}O & \rightleftharpoons & HO{-}C{-}H\\
| & & |\\
CH_3 & & CH_3\\
\text{Pyruvate} & & \text{L-Lactate}\\
+ & & +\\
NADH + H^+ & & NAD^+
\end{array}
$$

The reaction can be divided into its component half reactions:

$$
\begin{array}{ccc}
COO^- & & COO^- \qquad\qquad (5.20)\\
| & & | \qquad\qquad \mathscr{E}^{\circ\prime}\;(V)\\
C{=}O & \rightleftharpoons & HO{-}C{-}H \qquad -0.19\\
| & & |\\
CH_3 & & CH_3\\
\text{Pyruvate} & & \text{L-Lactate}\\
+ & & \\
2\,H^+ \;+\; 2\,e^- & &
\end{array}
$$

$$
\begin{array}{ccc}
NAD^+ & & NADH \qquad (5.21)\\
+ & \rightleftharpoons & + \qquad\quad -0.32\\
2\,H^+ \;+\; 2\,e^- & & H^+
\end{array}
$$

Under standard conditions, the electrons will be donated by the compound with the more negative standard reduction potential ($\mathscr{E}^{\circ\prime}$) to the compound with the more positive standard reduction potential ($\mathcal{E}°'$). The lower reaction is subtracted from the upper reaction. Subtracting the lower equation is the same as (1) reversing the order of the reactants and products of the lower equation, (2) changing the sign of the potential to $+0.32$ V, and (3) then adding the chemical equations and the potentials. The result is illustrated in equation 5.22.

$$\text{Pyruvate}^{-1} + \text{NADH} + \text{H}^+$$
$$\rightleftharpoons \text{lactate}^{-1} + \text{NAD}^+ \quad \Delta\mathcal{E}°' = +0.13 \text{ V} \quad (5.22)$$

By convention, a positive value for the difference in reduction potentials corresponds to actual electron flow. Under standard biochemical conditions (1 M reactants and products and pH 7.0), the reaction will proceed from reactants to products as written in equation 5.22. The reduction of a ketone by NADH to produce an alcohol is a favorable reaction. *The lactate dehydrogenase reaction serves as a prototype for oxidation-reduction reactions of aldehydes and ketones with pyridine nucleotides;* we will refer to this prototypical reaction often during our study of biochemistry.

Standard Free Energy Change

Any real reaction occurs with a negative free energy change. By convention, a positive value in the difference of the reduction potentials ($\Delta\mathcal{E}$) is associated with a feasible change. Then the following relationship obtains.

$$\Delta G°' = -n\mathcal{F}\,\Delta\mathcal{E}°' \quad (5.23)$$

Where n is the number of moles of electrons transferred, $\mathcal{F}$ is the energy-voltage coefficient, or faraday constant (96.485 kJ [V equivalent]$^{-1}$). $\Delta\mathcal{E}°'$ is the difference in the standard reduction potentials. This equation has wide applicability in bioenergetics. It converts voltage to energy and vice versa. This expression describes the relationship between the standard free energy change and the difference in the standard reduction potentials. Besides the equilibrium constant, standard free energy data are obtained from the difference of standard reduction potentials. For the lactate dehydrogenase reaction under standard conditions,

$$\Delta G°' = -2 \times 96.485 \text{ kJ V}^{-1}\text{ mol}^{-1} \times 0.13 \text{ V} \quad (5.24)$$

$$\Delta G°' = -25.1 \text{ kJ mol}^{-1} \quad (5.25)$$

The reaction is exergonic; the equilibrium greatly favors the formation of products. To convert voltage to energy per mole, multiply the voltage by n times the faraday constant. To convert energy per mole to voltage, divide the energy by n times the faraday constant.

OXYGEN, SUPEROXIDE, PEROXIDE, AND HYDROXYL FREE RADICALS

Chemical Properties of Oxygen

The importance of oxygen, water, and food (energy) to human well-being is widely recognized. Of these three essentials, deprivation of oxygen most rapidly leads to death.

▶ Impairment of oxygen delivery by the pathological occlusion of blood vessels results in serious disease. Brain damage or death due to strokes and disability or death due to coronary artery occlusion occur frequently in humans. Brain cells survive only 3–5 minutes without oxygen; brain cells die when anoxic conditions last longer. Heart, liver, and kidney cells can survive from 30 minutes to 2 hours without oxygen. In contrast, skeletal muscle, fibroblasts, and skin cells can survive several hours without oxygen. ◀

Let us consider the properties of oxygen that allow it to abstract electrons readily from other substances. Molecular oxygen is electron deficient and can be depicted as shown below, where the dots refer to electrons.

$$:\!\ddot{\text{O}}\!:\!\dot{\text{O}}\!:$$

Each oxygen atom lacks a complete octet of electrons. The oxygen molecule, moreover, contains two unshared electrons. The complete reduction of oxygen to form water can be formally indicated as shown in equation 5.26. The x's indicate electrons derived from hydrogen. The reduction of molecular oxygen to water involves four electrons and four protons.

$$:\!\ddot{\text{O}}\!:\!\ddot{\text{O}}\!: \qquad \overset{\displaystyle\cdot\cdot}{\text{O}}\overset{x}{\text{O}}\text{H} \qquad H\overset{x}{\text{O}}\text{O}\!:$$
$$\qquad\qquad\quad \overset{x}{\text{H}} \qquad\qquad \cdot\cdot$$

$$H\overset{x}{\text{O}}H \qquad H\overset{x}{\text{O}}H$$

$$O_2 + 2 H_2 \rightarrow 2 H_2O \quad (5.26)$$

Oxygen is a good oxidizing agent because it is electron deficient. Oxygen is also electronegative and has a strong tendency to attract electrons to it (to oxidize other substances). Oxygen has little tendency to give up its electrons. The oxidation of water to form molecular oxygen is highly endergonic.

Reactive Oxygen Intermediates

The reaction of oxygen with a single electron results in the formation of the superoxide anion radical (Figure 5–3). Superoxide formation can occur by the spontaneous (nonenzymatic) reaction of oxygen with ferrous ion, other metals, or reactive oxidation-reduction metabolites. Superoxide is a reactive substance that can cause the modification of cellular proteins, nucleic acids, and lipids in membranes, and it is therefore toxic. **Superoxide dismutase** catalyzes the conversion of two superoxide anions (and two protons) to oxygen and hydrogen peroxide (Figure 5–3). A dismutation is a reaction in which two identical molecules are converted into different substances. Here, one molecule of superoxide is oxidized and the other is

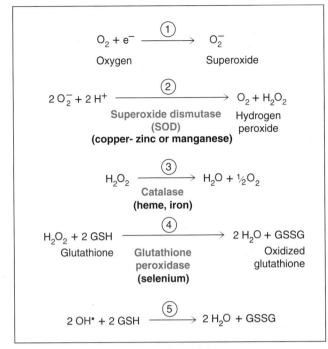

FIGURE 5-3. Superoxide and peroxide metabolism. *Glutathione is a tripeptide made up of γ-glutamylcysteinylglycine. The –SH group contributed by cysteine serves as reductant.*

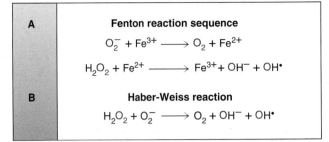

FIGURE 5-4. Generation of hydroxyl free radicals. *A. The two-step production of hydroxyl free radicals involving ferrous and ferric iron is called the Fenton reaction. B. The one-step production of hydroxyl free radicals involving peroxide and superoxide is called the Haber-Weiss reaction.*

reduced. Peroxides result from the reaction of oxygen with two electrons.

Superoxide dismutase plays a pivotal role in protecting against oxygen toxicity. Superoxide dismutases are found in all aerobes and are absent from obligate anaerobes. Human cells contain two types of dismutase. The cytosolic enzyme consists of two identical subunits, both of which contain an atom of copper and an atom of zinc. The mitochondrial enzyme contains two manganese atoms per monomeric protein. Bacterial superoxide dismutase also contains two manganese atoms.

▶ A familial form of amyotrophic lateral sclerosis (Lou Gehrig disease), a degenerative brain disorder, is reported to be due to an abnormality of cytosolic or copper-zinc superoxide dismutase. Superoxide forms in cells and tissues following ischemia and reperfusion. The intravenous injection of superoxide dismutase is being tested clinically following coronary occlusion to decrease the possible toxicity of superoxide following such pathological insults. ◀

The two-electron reduction of molecular oxygen produces hydrogen peroxide. Hydrogen peroxide is a reactive substance that can modify cellular macromolecules, and it is toxic. Hydrogen peroxide is converted to oxygen and water by catalase or by glutathione peroxidase (Figure 5-3).

▶ Hydrogen peroxide solutions are used as disinfectants and for the treatment of wound infections. Hydrogen peroxide is also generated by leukocytes and macrophages that kill invading bacteria. ◀

A third toxic oxygen derivative is the hydroxyl free radical. The hydroxyl free radical is more

reactive and toxic than superoxide and peroxide. The hydroxyl free radical can be formed through a reaction of hydrogen peroxide with ferrous iron by the **Fenton reaction.** It is also formed by the reaction of superoxide with hydrogen peroxide by the **Haber-Weiss** reaction (Figure 5-4). In addition, the hydroxyl free radical can be formed by the radiolysis of water produced by cosmic rays, x-rays, and other energetic electromagnetic radiation. The hydroxyl free radical reacts with and modifies cellular macromolecules. It can be destroyed by its reaction with ascorbate, β-carotene, or vitamin E. These actions may play a role in the beneficial and protective antioxidant effects of these vitamins. The hydroxyl free radical can also be destroyed by its reaction with glutathione (Figure 5-3). A summary of the toxic reactions of oxygen and its metabolites is given in Figure 5-5.

Hypoxia

▶ Hypoxia is a term that denotes insufficient oxygenation of cells. This condition can result from a variety of causes. Asthma, emphysema, and pulmonary edema are common causes of hypoxia. Impaired energy production can lead to cellular injury and death. The role of oxygen in ATP production is discussed in Chapter 9.

Atmospheric air contains 20% oxygen. Hypoxia can be treated with 100% oxygen. Breathing 100% oxygen, however, can lead to undesirable oxidative processes under unusual circumstances. The treatment of premature infants (< 44 weeks' gestation) with 100% oxygen is sometimes necessary for their survival. This treatment can lead to visual impairment later in life in the form of retrolental fibroplasia, an eye disorder that is thought to be due to aberrant angiogenesis in the developing eye. As often happens, trade-offs must be considered in therapeutics. ◀

BACTERICIDAL ACTIONS OF LEUKOCYTES

Toxic Oxygen Metabolites

Leukocytes engulf and degrade microorganisms during inflammatory reactions. This process in-

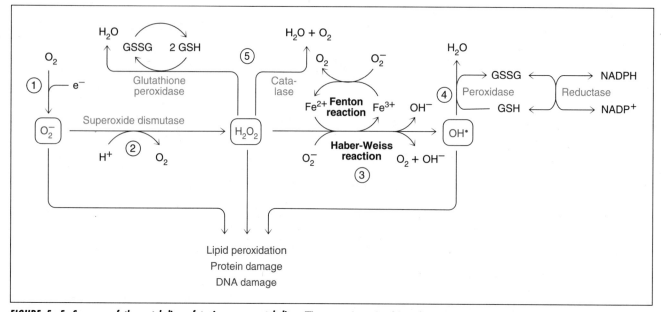

FIGURE 5–5. Summary of the metabolism of toxic oxygen metabolites. *The equations in this scheme are not all balanced. (1) The one-electron reduction of molecular oxygen produces superoxide anion. (2) Superoxide dismutase catalyzes the formation of hydrogen peroxide. (3) The two mechanisms that convert peroxide to hydroxyl free radicals in cells are the Fenton reaction and the Haber-Weiss reaction. (4) The hydroxyl free radical can be destroyed by reacting with glutathione. (5) Peroxide can be destroyed by reacting with glutathione, or it can be converted to oxygen and water in a reaction mediated by catalase.*

volves the generation of toxic oxygen metabolites, phagocytosis, and the lysosomal degradation of the microbe. A burst of oxygen consumption accompanies this response as molecular oxygen is con-

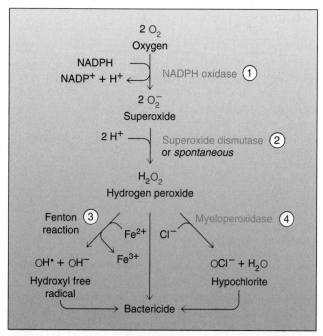

FIGURE 5–6. Oxygen-dependent bactericidal mechanisms. *(1) NADPH oxidase, a membranous enzyme, catalyzes the reduction of oxygen to superoxide anion. (2) Superoxide is converted to hydrogen peroxide. Hydrogen peroxide is bactericidal. (3) Hydrogen peroxide is converted to a hydroxyl free radical by the Fenton reaction. The hydroxyl free radical is bactericidal. This conversion can also occur by the Haber-Weiss mechanism. (4) Myeloperoxidase catalyzes the conversion of peroxide and chloride ion to form hypochlorite. Hypochlorite is a reactive oxygen species that is bactericidal.*

verted to superoxide. This reaction is catalyzed by a leukocytic enzyme called **NADPH oxidase.** This enzyme is located in the plasma membrane or in the invaginated plasma membrane that combines with the lysosome to form a phagolysosomal derivative. Superoxide forms hydrogen peroxide nonenzymatically or in a reaction catalyzed by superoxide dismutase. Hydrogen peroxide can act directly on bacteria, or hydrogen peroxide can be converted to hypochlorite or the hydroxyl free radical (Figure 5–6). These agents are bactericidal.

Chronic Granulomatous Disease

▶ Granuloma is a type of inflammation. Chronic granulomatous disease, a rare disorder, is due to a deficiency of NADPH oxidase (Figure 5–6). Enzyme activity depends upon two plasma membrane and two cytosolic proteins. About half the cases are X-linked (those due to a deficiency of the membrane proteins), and half are autosomal recessive (those due to a deficiency of the cytosolic proteins). Affected individuals develop recurrent bacterial infections during the first 2 years of life. Treatment is symptomatic.

The neutrophils of individuals with chronic granulomatous disease exhibit normal motility and phagocytosis. The neutrophils are unable to generate superoxide anion, and they are unable to kill catalase-positive microbes. Paradoxically, catalase-positive bacteria are overwhelmed by the peroxide that is produced by neutrophils, and catalase-negative bacteria are peroxide producers and are less sensitive to peroxide. Catalase-positive bacteria that are cultured from infected sites in affected individuals include gram-positive and gram-negative bacteria (Tables 1–2 and 1–3) such as *Staphylococcus aureus, Shigella, Salmonella,* and *Escherichia coli.* Catalase-negative bacteria (not found in infected sites) include *Streptococcus* and *Haemophilus influenzae.* ◄

SUMMARY

Energy is defined as the ability to perform work or to produce heat. The Gibbs free energy change is the most useful criterion of whether a given biochemical process can occur. The free energy change (ΔG) represents the free energy of the products minus that of the reactants. The criteria are illustrated as follows.

$\Delta G < 0$ (process is feasible and is exergonic)

$\Delta G = 0$ (at equilibrium and process is isoergonic)

$\Delta G > 0$ (process is not feasible and is endergonic)

Standard free energies and chemical reactions can be added or subtracted. The results give the standard free energy change of the resulting process.

The less the affinity for electrons, the greater is the tendency that a substance will donate its electrons and act as a reducing agent, and the more negative is the reduction potential. Superoxide is generated by the one-electron reduction of oxygen. Superoxide is converted to oxygen and hydrogen peroxide in a reaction catalyzed by superoxide dismutase. Cytosolic superoxide dismutase contains copper and zinc. Mitochondrial superoxide dismutase contains manganese. Peroxides are formed by the two-electron reductions of molecular oxygen. Hydrogen peroxide is destroyed by catalase (which occurs in the peroxisome) and by glutathione peroxidase (which occurs in the cytosol). Glutathione peroxidase contains selenium as cofactor. Hydroxyl free radicals can be formed by a reaction of peroxide with ferrous iron (the Fenton reaction) or by a reaction of peroxide with superoxide (the Haber-Weiss reaction). Leukocytes generate superoxide in a reaction catalyzed by NADPH oxidase. Superoxide is converted to hydrogen peroxide. Myeloperoxidase is a leukocytic enzyme that catalyzes the conversion of peroxide to hypochlorite. Peroxide, hypochlorite, and hydroxyl free radicals are bactericidal.

SELECTED READINGS

Baehner, R.L. The phagocytic systems and associated diseases. *In* R.E. Behrman (ed.). *Nelson Textbook of Pediatrics.* Philadelphia, W.B. Saunders Company, 1992, pp. 563–570.

Cadenas, E. Biochemistry of oxygen toxicity. Annual Review of Biochemistry 58:79–110, 1989.

Naqui, A., B. Chance, and E. Cadenas. Reactive oxygen intermediates in biochemistry. Annual Review of Biochemistry 55:137–166, 1986.

Tinoco, I., Jr., K. Sauer, and J.C. Wang. *Physical Chemistry, Principles and Applications in Biological Sciences.* New York, Prentice-Hall, 1986, Chapters 2–6.

CHAPTER SIX

PRINCIPLES OF

METABOLISM

The primary aim of research must not just be more facts and more facts, but more facts of strategic value.

—PAUL WEISS

CLASSIFICATION OF ENERGY-RICH AND ENERGY-POOR COMPOUNDS

We now consider the free energy of hydrolysis of several important biological compounds. We make a transition from the formalism of bioenergetics to a structurally based approach toward understanding biochemical reactions. The standard free energy of hydrolysis of ATP (to ADP and P_i) and that of several other compounds is about -30 kJ/mol (about -7 kcal/mol) or even more negative. These compounds are **energy rich** and exhibit a **high group transfer potential** (Table 6–1). Those compounds with a standard free energy of hydrolysis less negative than -30 kJ/mol such as glucose 6-phosphate are **energy poor** and exhibit **low group transfer potential.** The former set of compounds contains a hydrolyzable **high-energy bond,** and the latter set contains a hydrolyzable **low-energy bond.** Thus, these terms refer to the standard free energy differences between the products and reactants of a hydrolysis reaction. The use of -30 kJ/mol for the standard free energy of hydrolysis as the division between high-energy and low-energy compounds is empirical. The concept of the high-energy bond is powerful and simplifies the study of biochemistry and molecular biology.

The group transfer potential is defined as the negative of the free energy of hydrolysis.

Standard group transfer potential

$$= -\Delta G°' \text{ of hydrolysis} \quad (6.1)$$

Group transfer potential

$$= -\Delta G' \text{ of hydrolysis} \quad (6.2)$$

The transfer to water (hydrolysis) provides a standard for use in comparing reactions. The more positive the group transfer potential (the more negative the standard free energy of hydrolysis), the greater is the tendency to transfer the group to an acceptor. This is analogous to the use of standard reduction potentials in establishing the relative tendency of a group of compounds to donate electrons in oxidation-reduction reactions. Having data on the transfer of (1) groups from several donors to water or (2) electrons from several compounds to hydrogen provides the means for establishing the direction of (3) group transfer or (4) electron transfer among various donor-acceptor molecules.

Table 6–2 lists compounds that exhibit high and low group transfer potentials. Two classes of oxygen ester are denoted as special oxygen esters. Aminoacyl-tRNAs and acylcarnitines are oxygen monoesters that invariably possess high group transfer potential. Ordinary oxygen esters with phosphate, sulfate, or carboxylate, on the other hand, are energy-poor compounds with a low group transfer potential. Special phosphodiesters involving nucleotide bonds in DNA and RNA are energy rich. Ordinary phosphodiesters, for example, those occurring in complex lipids, are energy poor.

Energy-Rich Compounds

Phosphoenolpyruvate is an important intermediate in glucose metabolism, and its hydrolysis is illustrated in Figure 6–1 (this is an appropriate time to review the structures of biomolecules given in Table 2–2). The "squiggle" ($\sim$) is the symbol for an energy-rich linkage. (Lipmann coined this colorful term.) Part of the driving force for this reaction is the conversion of the enol form of pyruvate to the more stable keto form by tautomerism. **Tautomers** are isomers that differ in the position of a bonded hydrogen atom. The exceptional energy richness of phosphoenolpyruvate has some unusual biochemical consequences. This is the only example where the acceptor substrate (pyruvate) cannot be phosphorylated directly by ATP.

Both carbamoyl phosphate and 1,3-bisphosphoglycerate are **acylphosphates,** and both are **mixed-acid anhydrides.** To form the anhydride of two acids, the elements of water are removed. Acid anhydrides are divided into two categories. **Mixed-**

TABLE 6–2. Energy-Rich and Energy-Poor Compounds

General Class	Examples
Energy rich	
Cyclic phosphodiester	Cyclic 3′,5′-adenosine monophosphate (cyclic AMP)
Glycoside diphosphate	UDP-glucose
Mixed-acid anhydride	1,3-Bisphosphoglycerate, carbamoyl phosphate
Nucleotide phosphodiester	RNA, DNA
Phosphoenolpyruvate	Phosphoenolpyruvate
Phosphoramidate (P–N)	Phosphocreatine
Simple acid anhydride	ATP, ADP
Special oxygen ester (2)	Acylcarnitine, aminoacyl-tRNA
Sulfonium derivative	S-Adenosylmethionine
Thioester	Acetyl coenzyme A
Energy poor	
Amide	Glutamine
Glycoside	Glycogen, lactose
Ordinary oxygen ester	Glucose 6-phosphate
Peptide bond	Glutathione, insulin
Phosphodiester	Phosphatidylcholine

TABLE 6–1. Classification of Compounds That Participate in Group Transfer Reactions

Class	$\Delta G°'$ of Hydrolysis	
	kJ/mol	*kcal/mol*
Energy-rich compound	-30 or more negative	-7 or more negative
High group transfer potential		
High-energy bond		
Energy-poor compound	0 to -30	0 to -7
Low group transfer potential		
Low-energy bond		

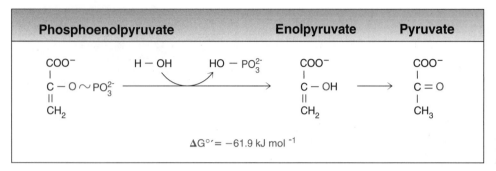

FIGURE 6-1. Hydrolysis of phospho-enolpyruvate. *The squiggle denotes the high-energy bond.*

acid anhydrides are composed of two different types of acids (for example, a carboxylic acid and phosphoric acid yield an acylphosphate). **Simple acid anhydrides** are made up of the same type of acid (for example, two molecules of phosphoric acid). The hydrolysis reaction involving the high-energy bond of carbamoyl phosphate, a mixed-acid anhydride, is given in the following equation:

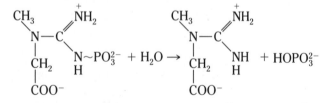

Carbamoyl phosphate   Carbamic acid   (6.3)

$$\Delta G^{\circ\prime} = -51.5 \text{ kJ/mol}$$

The products are carbamic acid and phosphoric acid (at physiological pH, the hydroxyl group of carbamic acid loses its proton and becomes ionized). Essentially all mixed-acid anhydrides in biochemical systems, whatever the identity of the acids, are energy rich in nature. Acid anhydrides involving sulfate, for example, are energy rich. These structural considerations enable one to deduce the energy-rich nature of new or unfamiliar compounds that contain an acid anhydride bond.

Phosphoramidates, which contain a P~N linkage, are energy rich. The hydrolysis of **phosphocreatine** to yield creatine and phosphate is illustrated in equation 6.4. Phosphocreatine serves as a storage form of energy-rich phosphate bonds in skeletal muscle, cardiac muscle, and brain.

Creatine phosphate   Creatine   (6.4)

$$\Delta G^{\circ\prime} = -41.3 \text{ kJ/mol}$$

Cyclic phosphodiesters are energy-rich compounds. Cyclic AMP and cyclic GMP are two regulatory molecules that activate their corresponding protein kinases. The hydrolysis reaction is illus-

trated in equation 6.5, and the squiggle identifies the high-energy bond.

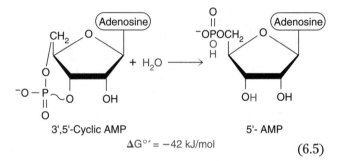

3',5'-Cyclic AMP   5'-AMP

$$\Delta G^{\circ\prime} = -42 \text{ kJ/mol}$$ (6.5)

An ester is the anhydride of an acid and alcohol. The anhydride between two alcohols and an acid is a diester (Table 2-2).

ATP is the historical prototype of a high-energy compound, and ATP's importance in the energy economy of the cell is emphasized throughout this book. The hydrolysis reactions of ATP are illustrated in Figure 6-2. *ATP possesses two high-energy bonds, and each is a simple acid anhydride of phosphoric acid.* The hydrolysis of 5'-AMP is accompanied by a standard free energy change of only -9.6 kJ mol^{-1}. 5'-AMP is a phosphomonoester and is a low-energy compound. The standard free energy changes are affected by magnesium ion, ionic strength, and pH. The values given in Figure 6-2 for ATP are for the metal-free nucleotide. The standard free energy of hydrolysis of ATP with 1 mM free magnesium ion concentration is -30.4 kJ/mol. The values for the hydrolysis of the magnesium complexes of ADP and AMP are less certain.

In contrast to ordinary oxygen esters, thioesters are energy-rich compounds. **Thioesters** are the anhydride of a thiol (–SH) group and an acid. Acids in biochemical systems include carboxylic acids (RCOOH). The hydrolysis reaction is given in equation 6.6.

$$\underset{CH_3}{\overset{\overset{\displaystyle O}{\|}}{C}}\text{~SCoA} + H_2O \rightarrow \underset{CH_3}{\overset{\overset{\displaystyle O}{\|}}{C}}\text{—OH} + \text{HSCoA} \qquad (6.6)$$

Acetyl-CoA   Acetic acid

$$\Delta G^{\circ\prime} = -35.1 \text{ kJ/mol}$$

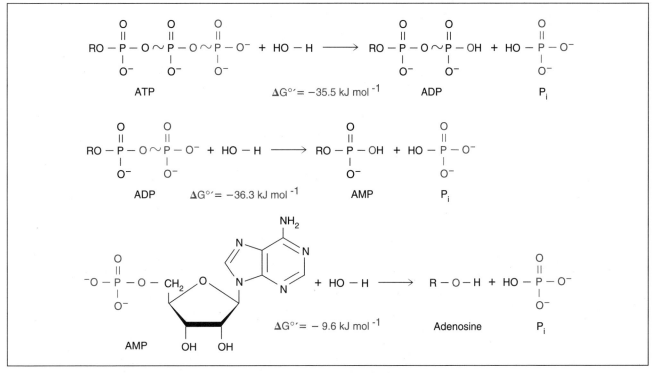

FIGURE 6-2. Hydrolysis of ATP.

The functional group of coenzyme A is the thiol group (–SH), and this is the most important characteristic to remember (Figure 2–14).

Glycoside diphosphates are energy rich and possess two high-energy bonds. The hydrolysis of one such compound, uridine diphosphate glucose (UDP-glucose), is illustrated in Figure 6–3. Note that UDP-glucose contains two high-energy bonds and UDP contains one high-energy bond.

The **special phosphodiester bonds** of RNA and of DNA exhibit a standard free energy of hydrolysis around −30 kJ/mol (Figure 6–4). The standard free energy of hydrolysis is not as high as that of cyclic AMP or cyclic GMP. Hydrolysis can occur on either

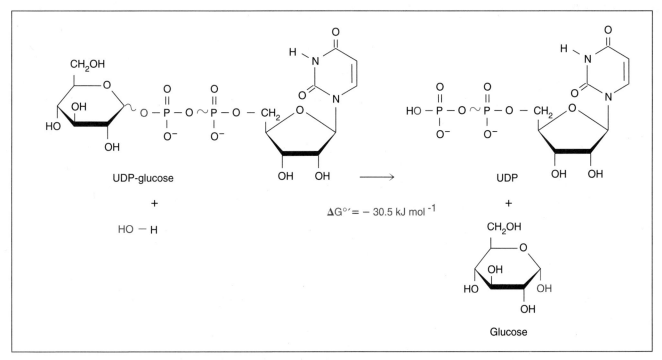

FIGURE 6-3. Hydrolysis of uridine diphosphate glucose (UDP-glucose), a glycoside diphosphate.

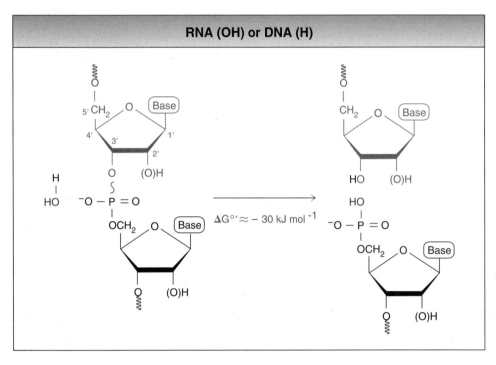

RNA (OH) or DNA (H)

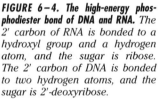

$\Delta G^{\circ\prime} \approx -30$ kJ mol^{-1}

FIGURE 6–4. The high-energy phosphodiester bond of DNA and RNA. The 2' carbon of RNA is bonded to a hydroxyl group and a hydrogen atom, and the sugar is ribose. The 2' carbon of DNA is bonded to two hydrogen atoms, and the sugar is 2'-deoxyribose.

side of the phosphate to yield either the 3'- or 5'-phosphate in the product. The total number of high-energy bonds associated with a single phosphodiester bond, however, is one. Enzymatic hydrolysis of cyclic AMP or cyclic GMP yields the 5' derivative. It is unclear why the free energy of hydrolysis of RNA and DNA exceeds that of other phosphodiesters such as those that occur in lipids.

Special oxygen esters are formed from the combination of an alcohol and an acid with the removal of the elements of water. Amino acids cova-

lently linked to the 3'- or 2'-hydroxyl group of ribose at the 3' end of transfer RNA (tRNA) form the energy-rich aminoacyl-tRNA. The hydrolysis of this special oxygen ester is shown in Figure 6–5. Acylcarnitine derivatives of fatty acids are energy rich and participate in the transport of these substances across the inner mitochondrial membrane. The energy richness of this class of compounds permits the reversible interconversion with the energy-rich thioesters of fatty acids and coenzyme A. The hydrolysis reaction of acetylcarnitine, a special oxygen ester, is illustrated in equation 6.7.

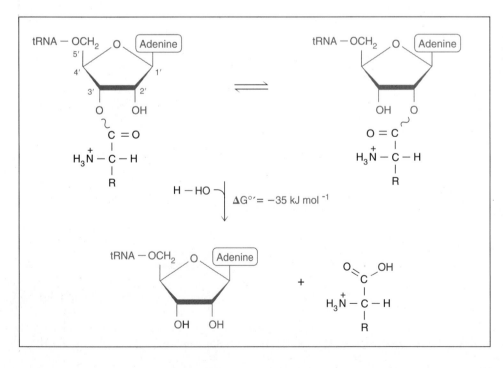

$\Delta G^{\circ\prime} = -35$ kJ mol^{-1}

FIGURE 6–5. The high-energy bond of aminoacyl-tRNA. The isomerization reaction between the two hydroxyl groups is nonenzymatic.

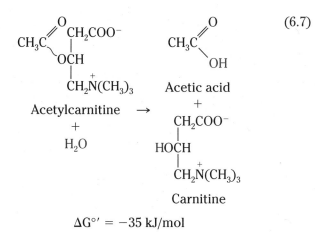

(6.7)

Acetylcarnitine → Acetic acid + Carnitine

$\Delta G°' = -35$ kJ/mol

Energy-Poor Compounds

Most biochemical substances not specifically mentioned in the previous section are energy-poor compounds with low group transfer potential. These include ordinary oxygen esters (other than acylcarnitine and aminoacyl-tRNA, the two energy-rich types mentioned earlier). 1,3-Bisphosphoglycerate, shown in equation 6.8, contains two phosphate groups with different standard free energies of hydrolysis. The first is energy rich, and the second is energy poor. The analysis of the hydrolysis of this compound illustrates many principles and conventions outlined in this chapter.

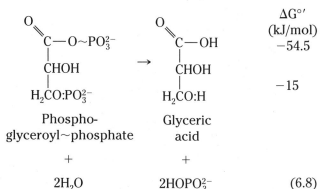

Phospho-glyceroyl~phosphate + 2H₂O → Glyceric acid + 2HOPO₃²⁻

(6.8)

The functional group of C^1 is an acylphosphate (a mixed-acid anhydride involving a carboxylic and phosphoric acid). This is an energy-rich linkage. This is in contrast to the functional group at C^3, which is an ester made from an alcohol (ROH) and phosphoric acid and which is energy poor. To emphasize the differences in the standard free energy of hydrolysis of the two phosphates, the compound is sometimes called phosphoglyceroyl~phosphate. The term 1,3-bisphosphoglycerate lacks this distinction.

That free energies of hydrolysis are altered by the pH, ionic strength, free magnesium concentration, and concentrations of reactants and products that are not 1 M justifies the use of approximate values under most circumstances. One need not memorize standard free energies of hydrolysis.

Knowing that a particular compound is energy rich and another energy poor is usually sufficient for practical considerations using the PRINCIPLES OF BIOENERGETICS. Knowing that a standard free energy of hydrolysis more negative than −30 kJ/mol is associated with an energy-rich compound suffices as a first approximation. The use of values for the free energy of hydrolysis of ATP of −30 kJ/mol, of phosphoenolpyruvate of −60 kJ/mol, and of creatine phosphate and 1,3-bisphosphoglycerate of intermediate values is generally adequate for analysis.

PRINCIPLES OF BIOENERGETICS

Counting High-Energy Bonds

Armed with the concept of the high-energy bond, the feasibility of many biochemical reactions can be intuitively grasped and understood. Based upon the chemical structures of reactants and products, moreover, one can make valid predictions about the feasibility of transferase reactions. Using the concept of energy-rich and energy-poor compounds enables us to predict which reactions are or are not energetically favorable. The general precepts for using the number of high-energy bonds are denoted as FIVE PRINCIPLES OF BIOENERGETICS that are given on the inside front cover, and these principles are discussed in the following paragraphs. Three additional principles are discussed at the end of this section.

The five statements of special principles of transferase reactions given subsequently have wide utility. Their application greatly simplifies the study of biochemistry. On the basis of the structures of reactants and products, we can analyze most group transfer reactions encountered in biochemistry. Frequent use will reinforce these principles.

PRINCIPLE 1.   When an equal number of energy-rich bonds occur in the reactants and products, the transferase reaction is functionally isoergonic and can proceed in either direction. The reaction catalyzed by creatine phosphokinase illustrates PRINCIPLE 1 (equation 6.9).

ATP + creatine ⇌ ADP + creatine phosphate

High-energy bonds	1	0	1	1

(6.9)

ATP contains two simple acid anhydride bonds that are energy rich in nature. ADP contains one simple acid anhydride bond, and creatine phosphate contains one energy-rich P–N (phosphoramidate) linkage. The number of bonds with high group transfer potential on the left side of the chemical equation equals those on the right side. The reaction can proceed in either direction, depending upon the physiological conditions. When the concentration of ADP increases (by depletion of ATP), then phosphocreatine reacts with ADP to regenerate ATP. When ATP is regenerated, then creatine is phosphorylated to produce creatine phosphate. The function of creatine phosphate in cells is to maintain a high ratio of ATP to ADP.

The only exception to PRINCIPLE 1 involves the pyruvate kinase reaction depicted in equation 6.10.

$$\text{ADP} + \begin{array}{c}\text{phosphoenol-}\\\text{pyruvate}\end{array} \rightarrow \text{ATP} + \text{pyruvate}$$

| High-energy bonds | 1 | 1 | 2 | 0 |

$$(6.10)$$

Even though the relative energy richness of the reactants and products is the same, the reaction proceeds to the right. This exception is a consequence of the extraordinarily high group transfer potential (very negative standard free energy of hydrolysis) of phosphoenolpyruvate (Table 6–3).

PRINCIPLE 2. When the number of energy-rich bonds is greater in the reactants than in the products, the reaction is exergonic and the conversion of reactants to products is favored. The reaction catalyzed by hexokinase (equation 6.11) illustrates PRINCIPLE 2.

$$\text{ATP} + \text{glucose} \rightarrow \text{ADP} + \begin{array}{c}\text{glucose}\\\text{6-phosphate}\end{array}$$

| High-energy bonds | 2 | 0 | 1 | 0 |

$$(6.11)$$

ATP contains two energy-rich bonds, and ADP contains one high-energy bond. Glucose 6-phosphate is an ester and is energy poor in nature. The reaction toward products is favored in this and all analogous cases, and the reverse reaction does not occur to a physiologically significant extent.

TABLE 6–3. Standard Free Energy of Hydrolysis of Selected Compounds at 25°C and pH 7.0 (in kJ mol⁻¹)

Compound	Products	$\Delta G^{\circ\prime}$
Acetyl-CoA	Acetate⁻ + H⁺ + CoA	− 35.1
Asparagine	Aspartate⁻ + NH₄⁺	− 15.1
ADP	AMP + Pᵢ	− 36.3
AMP	Adenosine + Pᵢ	− 9.6
ATP (1 mM free Mg²⁺)	ADP + Pᵢ	− 30.4
ATP	ADP + Pᵢ	− 35.5
ATP	AMP + PPᵢ	− 37.4
1,3-Bisphosphoglycerate	3-Phosphoglycerate + Pᵢ	− 54.5
Carbamoyl phosphate	Carbamate + Pᵢ	− 51.5
Creatine phosphate	Creatine + Pᵢ	− 43.1
N^{10}-Formyltetrahydrofolic acid	Formate⁻ + H⁺ + tetrahydrofolic acid	− 25.9
Glucose 1-phosphate	Glucose + Pᵢ	− 20.9
Glucose 6-phosphate	Glucose + Pᵢ	− 13.8
Glycerol phosphate	Glycerol + Pᵢ	− 9.2
Maltose (or glycogen)	2 Glucose	− 6.7
Phosphoenolpyruvate	Pyruvate + Pᵢ	− 61.9
Pyrophosphate (PPᵢ)	2 Pᵢ	− 33.4
Succinyl-CoA⁻	Succinate⁻² + H⁺ + CoA	− 43.5
Sucrose	Glucose + fructose	− 29.3
UDP-glucose	Glucose + UDP	− 30.5
Valyl-tRNA⁺	Valine + tRNA + H⁺	− 35.1

Data from Metzler, D.M. *Biochemistry*. New York, Academic Press, 1977, pp. 168–169.

PRINCIPLE 3. When the number of energy-rich bonds is greater in the products than in the reactants, the reaction is endergonic, and the conversion of products to reactants is favored. This is equivalent to PRINCIPLE 2 except that, in this case, the products contain more high-energy bonds than do the reactants. The synthesis of uridine diphosphate glucose (equation 6.12) provides an example of this situation.

$$\text{UTP} + \begin{array}{c}\text{glucose}\\\text{1-phosphate}\end{array} \rightleftharpoons \begin{array}{c}\text{UDP-}\\\text{glucose}\end{array} + \text{PP}_i$$

| High-energy bonds | 2 | 0 | 2 | 1 |

$$(6.12)$$

UTP, similar to ATP, contains two energy-rich bonds; glucose 1-phosphate contains a low-energy bond. UDP-glucose contains two high-energy bonds (the phosphate anhydride and the glycosidic diphosphate bond), and pyrophosphate contains one high-energy bond as the acid anhydride. The reaction as written is endergonic, and according to PRINCIPLE 3, conversion of the products to reactants is favored. In the physiological situation, pyrophosphatase catalyzes the hydrolysis of PPᵢ to pull the reaction toward the right.

PRINCIPLE 4. When the number of energy-poor bonds in the reactants and products of a transferase reaction is the same (no energy-rich bonds), the reaction is functionally isoergonic and can proceed in either direction. The interconversion of glucose 6-phosphate (a low-energy compound) and glucose 1-phosphate (a low-energy compound) as catalyzed by phosphoglucomutase (equation 6.13) illustrates PRINCIPLE 4.

$$\begin{array}{c}\text{Glucose}\\\text{6-phosphate}\end{array} \rightleftharpoons \begin{array}{c}\text{glucose}\\\text{1-phosphate}\end{array}$$

| Low-energy bonds | 1 | 1 |

$$(6.13)$$

The phosphoglucomutase reaction is readily reversible. The direction of the reaction depends upon the concentrations of reactant and product in this functionally isoergonic reaction.

PRINCIPLE 5. The hydrolysis of energy-rich or energy-poor compounds is exergonic and thermodynamically favored. The following two examples are illustrative. Cyclic AMP contains an energy-rich linkage. A family of enzymes (phosphodiesterases) catalyzes the hydrolysis of cyclic AMP to 5′-adenosine monophosphate (equation 6.5). 5′-Adenosine monophosphate contains an energy-poor linkage. The hydrolysis to adenosine and phosphate is the favored direction of the reaction (Figure 6–2). The reverse reactions do not occur to a physiologically meaningful extent. Stage I of aerobic metabolism involves the hydrolysis of fuel molecules to simpler biochemical building blocks (Figure 1–3). These reactions are exergonic and proceed without the input of exogenous chemical energy.

Oxidation-Reduction Reactions

Three additional PRINCIPLES OF BIOENERGETICS exist. Decarboxylation reactions are exergonic (PRINCIPLE 6). Simple oxidation-reduction reactions are bidirectional and functionally isoergonic (PRINCIPLE 7). Simple oxidation-reduction reactions are like those between cytochrome *b* and cytochrome *c* (equation 5.12) and between pyruvate and NADH (equation 5.19). Simple oxidation-reduction reactions do not involve molecular oxygen, a simultaneous decarboxylation, or the formation of a carboxylic acid. Finally, the reactions of organic substances with oxygen, as illustrated in equation 5.15, are exergonic and unidirectional (PRINCIPLE 8).

FOUR REACTIONS OF ATP

ATP undergoes a variety of chemical reactions. For example, ATP transfers its terminal phosphoryl group to acceptor substrates. This is the most common reaction that ATP undergoes (Figure 6–6, I). In the special case in which the phosphoryl group is transferred to water, ATP hydrolysis occurs. At the completion of the type I reactions, ADP and the phosphorylated compound (or P_i) result. In the second type of reaction, the α-phosphorus atom undergoes attack, inorganic pyrophosphate is displaced, and the adenylyl group is transferred (Figure 6–6, II). In the third type of reaction, ATP serves as a pyrophosphoryl donor (Figure 6–6, III), and 5′-AMP is the leaving group. In this reaction, ATP represents activated pyrophosphate. In the fourth type of reaction, the 5′ carbon undergoes attack by methionine to yield *S*-adenosylmethionine (AdoMet); the triphosphate chain is displaced (Figure 6–6, IV) and undergoes hydrolysis to P_i and PP_i prior to release from the enzyme. We will consider these reactions in order.

Type I Reactions: Transfer of the Phosphoryl Group

Let us consider the reaction of glucose and ATP catalyzed by hexokinase (Figure 6–7). The hydroxyl group at C^6 of glucose is the nucleophile, and this hydroxyl group attacks the terminal phosphorus atom of ATP. ADP is displaced, and glucose 6-phosphate is formed. *Note that the phosphoryl group or phosphorylium ion (PO_3^{1-}) is transferred and not the phosphate group ($-OPO_3^{2-}$).* This distinction is often a source of confusion, and the term "phosphate transfer," although commonly used, is imprecise.

The hexokinase reaction proceeds with a decrease in the number of energy-rich bonds (from two to one), the reaction is exergonic, and the formation of products is favored (PRINCIPLE 2 OF BIOENERGETICS). Such reactions are common in biochemistry. The hexokinase reaction is a prototype reaction for the transfer of the phosphoryl group from ATP to an acceptor to form a low-energy phosphate ester.

Type II Reactions: Adenylyl Transfer and the Pyrophosphate Split

Transfer of the adenylyl group to an acceptor and the displacement of intact inorganic pyrophosphate is the second most common class of reaction undergone by ATP. This class of reaction was first described in fatty acid metabolism (Figure 6–8).

The combination of two reactions (equations 6.14 and 6.15) provides an example of the use of coupled reactions in metabolism. The utilization of a product (PP_i) formed in one reaction (6.14) as a substrate in a subsequent highly exergonic reaction (6.15) serves to draw the former reaction forward. The overall process (equation 6.16) is exergonic. Pyrophosphate is a common intermediate in a two-step process. The only significant reaction of PP_i in human cells is that of hydrolysis. This biochemical strategy is employed to convert an unfavorable process into a favorable process.

		$\Delta G^{\circ\prime}$ (kJ/mol)	
ATP (2~)	O‖RC~SCoA (1~)		
+	+		
RCOOH $\rightleftharpoons$	AMP	+ 4.7	(6.14)
+	+		
CoASH	PP_i (1~)		
$PP_i + H_2O \rightarrow$	$2P_i$	− 33.4	(6.15)
ATP	O‖RC~SCoA		
+	+		
RCOOH $\rightarrow$	AMP	− 28.7	(6.16)
+	+		
CoASH	$2\,P_i$		
+			
H_2O			

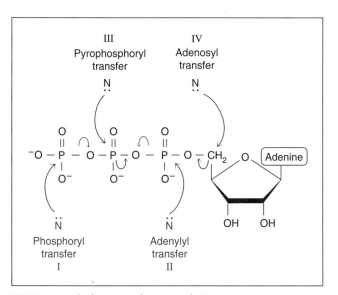

FIGURE 6–6. The four types of reactions of ATP. *N represents a nucleophile with its electron pair.*

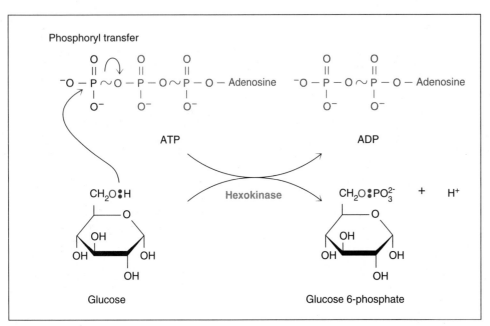

FIGURE 6–7. The hexokinase reaction. *Note that the reaction involves a phosphoryl transfer (PO_3^{1-}) and not a phosphate transfer (PO_4^{2-}).*

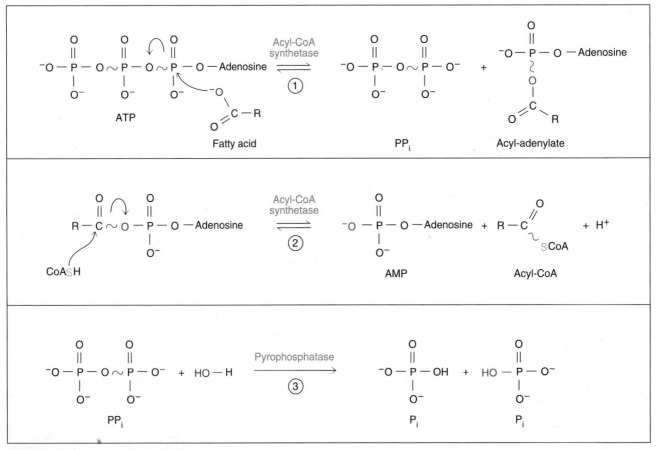

FIGURE 6–8. The synthesis of fatty acyl–CoA. *Steps (1) and (2), which are functionally isoergonic, are catalyzed by a single enzyme. Step (3), an exergonic hydrolysis, is catalyzed by pyrophosphatase.*

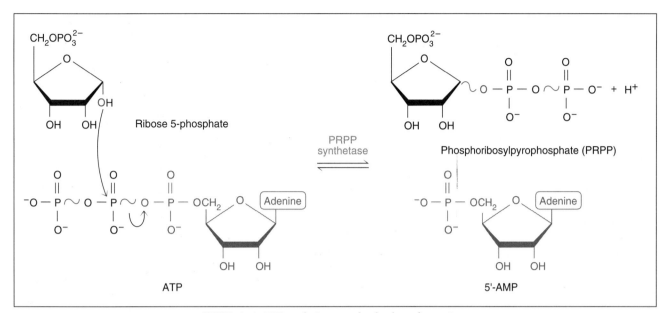

FIGURE 6–9. *PRPP synthesis, a pyrophosphoryl transfer reaction.*

Because of its frequent occurrence in all classes of organisms, the general nature of pyrophosphate formation and hydrolysis is an important principle of biochemistry (PRINCIPLE 14 OF BIOCHEMISTRY). The purpose of generating and hydrolyzing pyrophosphate is to provide additional energy for pulling a chemical process forward. Besides fatty acid activation, this strategy is employed in nucleotide activation for DNA and RNA biosynthesis and in amino acid activation for protein synthesis.

The utility of pyrophosphate cleavage also provides an explanation for the use of ATP and not ADP as the major source of chemical energy. The difference is that ATP can simultaneously form an adenylated compound and generate pyrophosphate. The hydrolysis of pyrophosphate can thus provide an additional source of free energy to pull other reactions forward. Although ADP contains a high-energy bond, ADP cannot function in this fashion.

Type III Reactions: Transfer of the Pyrophosphoryl Group

In type III reactions, the pyrophosphoryl group is transferred to an acceptor. For example, ATP transfers its pyrophosphoryl group to ribose 5-phosphate to yield phosphoribosyl-1-pyrophosphate, or PRPP (Figure 6–9). The high ratio of ATP/AMP provides the physiological driving force for producing PRPP.

Type IV Reaction: S-Adenosylmethionine Biosynthesis

The predominant type IV reaction of ATP (Figure 6–10) involves the biosynthesis of S-adenosylmeth-ionine (AdoMet). This complicated reaction is catalyzed by **S-adenosylmethionine synthetase.** The reactants include ATP, methionine, and water. The products include S-adenosylmethionine, PP_i, and P_i. Pyrophosphate hydrolysis provides energy to pull the synthesis of S-adenosylmethionine forward. S-Adenosylmethionine contains an activated methyl group and is an important methyl donor in various biosynthetic processes.

ENERGY CHARGE

The energy charge plays an important conceptual role in understanding metabolic regulation. The energy charge is defined in equation 6.17.

$$\text{Energy charge} = \frac{[\text{ATP}] + 0.5\,[\text{ADP}]}{[\text{ATP}] + [\text{ADP}] + [\text{AMP}]} \quad (6.17)$$

The energy charge reflects the molar fraction of the total adenine nucleotide pool (ATP + ADP + AMP) that contains high-energy bonds. The factor of 0.5 before ADP reflects ADP's high-energy bond content as one half that of ATP. This feature is illustrated in equation 6.18.

$$\text{ADP} \rightleftharpoons \tfrac{1}{2}\,\text{ATP} + \tfrac{1}{2}\,\text{AMP} \quad (6.18)$$

The number of high-energy bonds in the reactants and products in this reaction is the same (AMP is adenylic acid, or adenylate). The equilibrium constant of this isoergonic reaction, catalyzed by adenylate kinase, is near unity.

The range of possible values for the energy charge is from 0 (all AMP) to 1 (all ATP). Under physiological conditions in all organisms and cells, the energy charge value hovers around 0.85. Regulatory enzymes respond to the energy charge in a way that reflects the molecular logic of the cell.

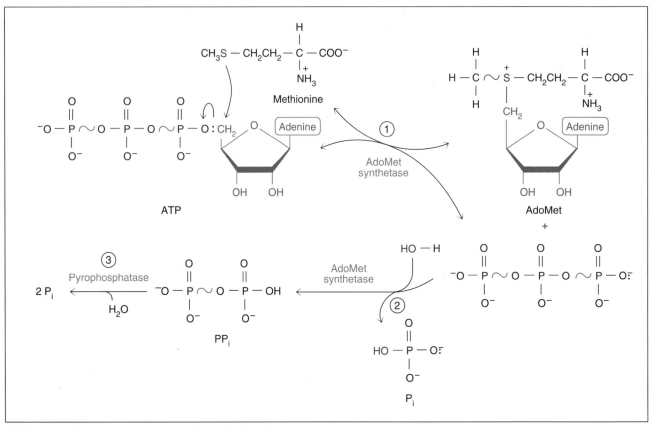

FIGURE 6-10. The synthesis of S-adenosylmethionine (AdoMet). *The combined reaction (1-3) occurs with the loss of one high-energy bond and is exergonic.*

Ample metabolic fuel and a resulting high-energy charge favors anabolic or biosynthetic reactions. Under conditions of low-energy charge, the catabolism or breakdown of fuels is favored to provide chemical energy for regenerating ATP and the energy charge. Many enzymes are regulated by the concentrations of ATP, ADP, or AMP. ATP inhibits regulatory enzymes that result in the synthesis of more ATP (Figure 6-11). ADP or AMP often acti-

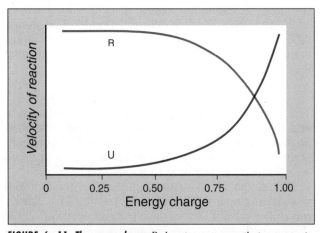

FIGURE 6-11. The energy charge. *R denotes enzymes that* regenerate *ATP and the energy charge, and U denotes enzymes that use the energy charge.*

vates the same enzymes to promote the attainment of a high-energy charge. These properties make up the molecular logic of the cell. Maintenance of the energy charge is an important regulatory principle in bioenergetics and biochemistry.

PHOSPHORYLATION OF PURINE AND PYRIMIDINE NUCLEOSIDES

Although ATP plays a central role in energy metabolism, other nucleotides are essential in the biochemistry of cells. There are two major classes of nucleotides based upon the structure of the planar, aromatic base: **purines** and **pyrimidines** (Figure 6-12). The purine bases include **adenine** (found in ATP) and **guanine.** The commonly occurring pyrimidines include **uracil, thymine,** and **cytosine.** When attached to ribose 5′-phosphate, these substances make up the ribonucleotides. When attached to 2′-deoxyribose-5′-phosphate, the compounds are deoxyribonucleotides. The structures and nomenclature of the ribonucleoside monophosphates and the deoxyribonucleoside monophosphates are given in Figure 6-13.

Pyrimidine and purine nucleotides are synthesized as nucleoside monophosphates (described in Chapter 14). The bioenergetics of the formation of diphosphates and triphosphates is straightforward.

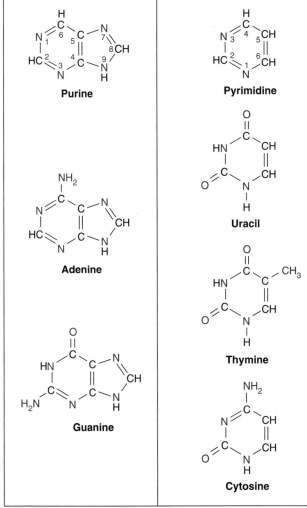

FIGURE 6–12. *Purine and pyrimidine bases and the numbering systems.*

In contrast to the family of enzymes that mediates the phosphorylation of the nucleoside monophosphates, a single enzyme with broad specificity catalyzes the phosphorylation of the diphosphates. **Nucleoside diphosphokinase** catalyzes the formation of the nucleoside diphosphates according to the following equation, where NTP represents any of the physiological nucleoside triphosphates.

$$\text{ATP}(2\sim) + \text{NDP}(1\sim) \rightleftharpoons \text{ADP}(1\sim) + \text{NTP}(2\sim) \quad (6.20)$$

The number of high-energy bonds (3~) is the same on both sides of the equation. The reaction is isoergonic (PRINCIPLE 1 OF BIOENERGETICS). The high ratio of ATP/ADP in cells promotes the formation of the nucleoside triphosphate. All the enzymes that catalyze the phosphorylation of nucleoside monophosphates and diphosphates require magnesium ion for activity because the substrates and products are metal-nucleotide complexes.

The specificity of the monophosphate kinases and nucleoside diphosphokinase is broader than indicated because many derivatives of the naturally occurring bases serve as substrates. ▶ For example, AZT (3'-*azido*-2',3'-dideoxy*thymidine*), a drug used in the treatment of AIDS (*acquired immunodeficiency syndrome*) in humans, is converted to the triphosphate *in vivo*. ◀

Specific nucleotides are associated with the biosynthesis and metabolism of various classes of biochemical compounds. UTP, for example, plays an important role in glycogen, glycoprotein, and glycolipid biosynthesis. GTP serves as a source for some of the energy in protein biosynthesis. CTP and cytidine derivatives play an important role in the biosynthesis of complex lipids. The role of activated nucleotides in DNA and RNA biosynthesis was noted in the beginning of this section. These interrelationships are illustrated in Figure 6–14. As the common currency, ATP distributes energy payments.

ATP AND ENERGY EXCHANGE: LIPMANN'S LAW

ATP plays a central role in cellular metabolism: ATP is formed from ADP and P_i during the catabolism of fuel molecules (Figure 1–3). ATP provides the chemical energy that can be used for chemical, osmotic, and mechanical work. Lipmann introduced the concept of the high-energy bond and the use of the squiggle (~) to denote it. All forms of life (plants, animals, and microorganisms) use ATP as the fundamental unit of biochemical energy. There are no exceptions to this principle, and this principle assumes the status of a law.

The standard free energy of hydrolysis of ATP is between that of 1,3-bisphosphoglycerate (1,3-bisphosphoglycerate + H_2O → 3-phosphoglycerate + P_i) and glucose 6-phosphate (Table 6–3). ADP can accept the phosphoryl group (PO_3^{1-}) from donors with a higher group transfer potential, and

The conversion of the physiological nucleoside monophosphates to the diphosphates is catalyzed by a family of four enzymes. These enzymes catalyze the phosphorylation of (1) AMP and dAMP; (2) GMP and dGMP; (3) CMP, dCMP, and UMP; and (4) dTMP. The first enzyme is named **adenylate kinase.** Its activity is higher in most cells than that of the other three enzymes. This greater activity is related to the large flux of adenine nucleotides in metabolism. The reaction catalyzed by this family of enzymes is given in the following chemical equation, where NMP is a nucleoside monophosphate and NDP is the corresponding nucleoside diphosphate:

$$\text{ATP}(2\sim) + \text{NMP}(0\sim) \rightleftharpoons \text{ADP}(1\sim) + \text{NDP}(1\sim) \quad (6.19)$$

The bioenergetics of the reactions catalyzed by this family of enzymes is identical. The number of high-energy bonds (2~) is the same on both sides of the equation. The reaction is isoergonic (PRINCIPLE 1 OF BIOENERGETICS). The high ratio of ATP/ADP in cells promotes the formation of the nucleoside diphosphate.

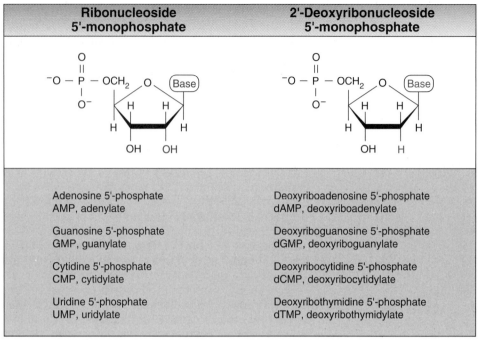

FIGURE 6–13. *The generic structure and nomenclature of the ribonucleoside 5'-monophosphates and the deoxyribonucleoside 5'-monophosphates.*

ATP can readily transfer the phosphoryl group to acceptors with lower group transfer (Figure 6–15).

The criterion for describing ATP as a high-energy compound is its standard free energy of hydrolysis. The simple hydrolysis of ATP, however, generates only heat. To perform chemical and mechanical work, other energy changes are required before the formation of ADP and P_i from ATP and water. In muscle contraction, the hydrolysis of ATP leads to the formation of an energized contractile protein (myosin). This energized molecule participates in the transduction from chemical into mechanical energy. In providing energy for biosynthetic reactions, energy-rich intermediates are formed. The activated intermediates react to form products. The net hydrolysis of ATP to ADP and P_i or to AMP and PP_i occurs during the overall process. ATP

reacts to produce an energized protein or molecule that is now able to further react. It must be emphasized that *the source of energy for most metabolic transformations does not result directly from a simple hydrolysis of ATP.* Moreover, ATP is able to function as the universal currency of exchange because it exists in cells at concentrations that are far removed from hydrolytic equilibrium.

HIGH-ENERGY BOND AND GROUP ACTIVATION

The combination of acetate with coenzyme A through a high-energy thioester bond confers a high group transfer potential on the acetyl group. Acetyl-CoA can then react with an acceptor to form

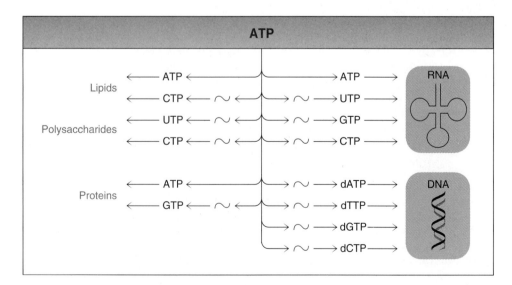

FIGURE 6–14. *Role of nucleotides in metabolism. The chemical energy of ATP is used directly for biosynthesis, or the energy of ATP is transferred to other nucleotides to energize biosynthetic reactions.*

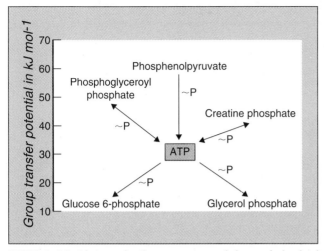

FIGURE 6–15. *Adenine nucleotides as acceptors and donors of phosphoryl groups. The group transfer potential lies between that of several energy-rich phosphoryl donors and energy-poor products.*

an acetyl derivative and the coenzyme A leaving group. Coenzyme A is said to "activate" the acetyl group, and acetyl-CoA is sometimes called "active" acetate. This same principle and terminology are applicable to the other groups that participate in the formation of the energy-rich bonds. Aminoacyl-tRNAs, for example, represent activated amino acids that are used in protein biosynthesis.

SUMMARY

Compounds whose standard free energy of hydrolysis is −30 kJ/mol and more negative are energy rich. Compounds whose standard free energy of hydrolysis is less negative than −30 kJ/mol are energy poor. Examples of energy-rich compounds include phosphoenolpyruvate, mixed-acid anhydrides (made up of two different acids), simple acid anhydrides (made up of a single kind of acid), thioesters, phosphoramidates (compounds with a P–N bond), and glycoside diphosphates. Aminoacyl-tRNAs and acylcarnitines are special oxygen monoesters that invariably possess high group transfer potential. Most other compounds are energy-poor compounds.

ATP is an example (and the prototype) of a high-energy compound. ATP contains two acid anhydride bonds that are energy rich. The standard free energy of hydrolysis of ATP to ADP and P_i is about −30 kJ/mol. With physiological concentrations of reactants and products, the actual free energy change ranges from about −45 to −60 kJ/mol. ATP also contains a low-energy phosphate bond, a phosphate ester.

Transferase reactions that proceed without a loss of high-energy bonds are functionally isoergonic. The sole exception to this rule is an inability of ATP to phosphorylate pyruvate to give phosphoenolpyruvate and ADP. Transferase reactions that proceed with a loss of high-energy bonds are exergonic. Moreover, hydrolysis reactions are exergonic. The high-energy bond is said to activate the energy-rich compound. Acetyl-CoA, for example, is "active" acetate.

ATP undergoes four types of reactions. In the most common variety, the phosphoryl group of ATP is transferred to an acceptor substrate. In another common variety, an adenylate derivative forms and pyrophosphate is released. The pyrophosphate split is important and accounts for the universality of ATP, and not ADP, as the fundamental nucleotide of bioenergetics. The energy charge is the ratio of $[ATP] + \frac{1}{2}[ADP]$ divided by the total adenine nucleotide concentration ($[ATP] + [ADP] + [AMP]$). Cells in diverse organisms maintain the energy charge at about 0.85.

Lipmann's law states that ATP is the universal energy donor in plants, animals, and bacteria. Lipmann's law is the cornerstone of bioenergetics. ATP is the most important biochemical in nature. Adenylate kinase and related nucleoside monophosphate kinases catalyze the conversion of nucleoside monophosphates to nucleoside diphosphates. Nucleoside diphosphate kinase catalyzes the reaction of ATP with a nucleoside diphosphate acceptor to yield the nucleoside triphosphate. ADP is converted to ATP by substrate level or electron transport phosphorylation.

SELECTED READINGS

Bridger, W.A., and J.F. Henderson. *Cell ATP*. New York, John Wiley & Sons, 1983.

Lipmann, F. Metabolic generation and utilization of phosphate bond energy. Advances in Enzymology 1:99–162, 1941.

Lipmann, F. The ATP-phosphate cycle. Current Topics in Cellular Regulation 18:301–311, 1981.

Roskoski Jr., R., Fritz Lipmann (1899–1986): An appreciation. Trends in Biochemical Sciences 12:136–138, 1987.

CHAPTER SEVEN

GLYCOLYSIS AND THE PENTOSE PHOSPHATE PATHWAY

Attitudes rather than knowledge are conveyed by the distinguished teacher.

—HANS A. KREBS

When Hans Krebs in 1925 appeared at Berlin-Dahlem in the Kaiser-wilhelminstitute of Biology, he was a modest thoughtful youth, very intelligent and already wise in spite of his youth. Nearly 40 years later I met him in Dublin at an important meeting. Few scientists were more famous. How civilized he is, I thought, if I compared him, even with myself.

—OTTO WARBURG

Fuel molecules such as carbohydrates and fats are oxidized, and the resulting chemical energy is used to sustain the formation of ATP (Figure 7–1). Fuel molecules also furnish reducing equivalents (NADPH) that are used for the cell's anabolic reactions. There are two major pathways for catabolizing glucose in humans: the **glycolytic pathway** and the **pentose phosphate pathway.** The glycolytic pathway is the most widespread and important pathway for glucose metabolism in nature. Glycolysis refers to the breakdown (lysis) of sugars (glyco is a generic prefix for sugar).

Glucose serves as a ready source of chemical energy for humans. Glucose is converted to pyruvate in 10 steps by glycolysis. During this process, two molecules of ATP are formed from energy-rich phosphate compounds by substrate level phosphorylation. **Substrate level phosphorylation** involves the generation of ATP enzymatically by processes that are independent of an electron transport chain and oxygen (Chapter 9). The fates of pyruvate and NADH differ during aerobic (in the presence of oxygen) and anaerobic (in the absence of oxygen) conditions. During anaerobic glycolysis, pyruvate is reduced to lactate. Under aerobic conditions, pyruvate is oxidized to carbon dioxide and water.

CARBOHYDRATE CHEMISTRY

Monosaccharides and Disaccharides

Carbohydrates are polyhydroxy aldehydes or ketones. Formulas representing various forms of D-glucose, the most prevalent sugar in nature, are shown in Figure 7–2. It is significant that glucose,

in its β-configuration, is very stable. The six-membered ring lacks strain, and the hydroxyl groups are far apart. The open-chain and the ring structures are in equilibrium, and the forms can readily interconvert without an enzyme. The predominant forms ($>99\%$) of glucose and glucose derivatives are cyclic.

The structure of the β-anomer of D-glucose should be mastered. The hydroxyl groups of the β-anomer of glucose alternate above and below the ring in regular fashion. A convenient depiction of glucose consists of a six-membered ring (five carbons and one oxygen) with C^6 and its hydroxyl group above the ring (Figure 7–2B). The hydroxyl groups alternate from top (C^6) to bottom in regular fashion: C^4 (bottom), C^3 (top), C^2 (bottom), and C^1 (top, as the β-anomer). If the configuration of the hydroxyl on C^1 is below the ring, then the α-anomer results (Figure 7–2C). **Anomers** are isomers that differ in configuration at the anomeric carbon of the hemiacetal linkage (for example, α-D-glucose and β-D-glucose) or hemiketal linkage (for example, α-D-fructose and β-D-fructose).

Galactose is the isomer of glucose that differs by the hydroxyl configuration about C^4, and mannose differs at C^2 (Figure 7–3). Galactose and mannose are epimers of glucose. **Epimers** are isomers that differ in configuration at one chiral carbon atom exclusive of the anomeric hemiacetal or hemiketal linkage.

The aldehyde groups of glucose, mannose, and galactose are easily oxidized by copper in alkaline solution. These compounds are therefore designated as reducing sugars. The disaccharides **lactose, maltose,** and **isomaltose** form aldehyde groups from hemiacetal groups (Figure 7–4) that make them reducing sugars. *Sucrose, in contrast, is not a reducing sugar.* The hemiacetal group of glucose and hemiketal group of fructose form an acetal bond. The absence of a hemiacetal group makes sucrose a nonreducing sugar in alkaline copper solution, and this is a noteworthy property. Trehalose is also a nonreducing sugar.

Diabetes Mellitus

▶ Thomas Willis (the discoverer of the arterial circle of Willis at the base of the brain) remarked that the urine of the diabetic tastes as if imbued with the "spirits of honey." Fortunately, organic chemists have developed other procedures for the determination of glucose (the honey-like substance) in urine. Glucosuria is now determined by a colorimetric reaction involving glucose oxidase (a plant enzyme). This colorimetric analysis is based upon the following reactions.

$$\text{Glucose} + O_2 \xrightarrow{\text{Glucose oxidase}} \text{gluconolactone} + H_2O_2 \quad (7.1)$$

$$H_2O_2 + \text{chromogen} \rightarrow \text{colored compound} + H_2O \quad (7.2)$$

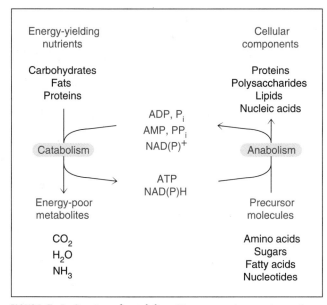

FIGURE 7–1. Overview of metabolism. *The exergonic reactions of catabolism sustain ATP, NADH, and NADPH formation. ATP and NADPH provide energy and reducing equivalents for the endergonic reactions of anabolism.*

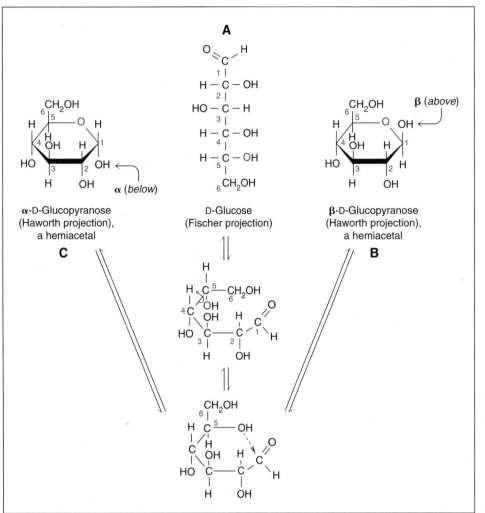

FIGURE 7-2. Structure of D-glucose.
A. *The Fischer projection formula illustrates the open-chain form of glucose. The hydroxyl group on C^5 forms a bond with the carbonyl group on C^1, and a stable six-membered ring results. This combination generates a hemiacetal with a new chiral carbon atom at C^1. The hydroxyl group on C^1 occurs with the (B) β- or (C) α-configuration.*

The first reaction is catalyzed by glucose oxidase; the second reaction is nonenzymatic. Glucosuria occurs in diabetes mellitus when the blood sugar levels exceed the renal threshold for glucose reabsorption. Urinalysis for glucose is an important screening test in routine health examinations and during hospitalization.

A triad of complications of diabetes mellitus includes retinopathy, nephropathy, and neuropathy. Elevated blood and tissue levels of glucose contribute to these and other complications. Better control of hyperglycemia seems to be associated with fewer complications. Glucose, which exists in solution chiefly as the unreactive hemiacetal, does not have a great propensity to react with and modify proteins. The ring form of glucose, however, is in equilibrium with the more reactive open-chain, or aldehyde, form of glucose. The ε-amino groups of lysine residues and the free amino terminus of proteins can be glycosylated nonenzymatically (Figure 7–5). The formation of such derivatives may contribute to the common complications of diabetes mellitus. The chronically high blood and tissue levels of glucose may promote the modification of critical proteins in retina, kid-

ney, peripheral nerves, and other cells. Such protein modifications are postulated to contribute to the complications of diabetes mellitus.

The extent of glycosylation of hemoglobin can be conveniently monitored and used to assess the control of hyperglycemia. Analysis of hemoglobin A (the *A*dult form of hemoglobin) reveals the existence of minor components called hemoglobin A_1. Hemoglobin A_1 forms by the nonenzymatic modification of hemoglobin A by glucose (Figure 7–5). Glycosylation has only minor effects on normal hemoglobin function.

Glycosylation occurs continuously within the red cell, and the extent of glycosylation reflects the average glucose concentration to which the cell is exposed during its 120-day life span. Measurement of glycosylated hemoglobin content provides a clinically useful means to assess the degree of hyperglycemia that existed over the previous several weeks. HbA_1 in normal individuals (without diabetes mellitus) makes up about 6% of total hemoglobin. Individuals with controlled diabetes (blood glucose levels < 10 mM, or 180 mg/dL) have levels of hemoglobin A_1 of about 9% of total hemoglobin. Those with less well con-

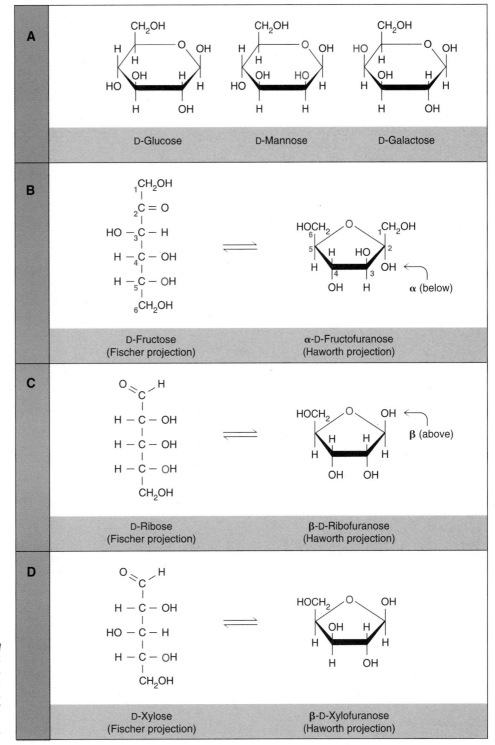

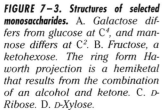

FIGURE 7-3. Structures of selected monosaccharides. A. *Galactose differs from glucose at C^4, and mannose differs at C^2. B. Fructose, a ketohexose. The ring form Haworth projection is a hemiketal that results from the combination of an alcohol and ketone. C. D-Ribose. D. D-Xylose.*

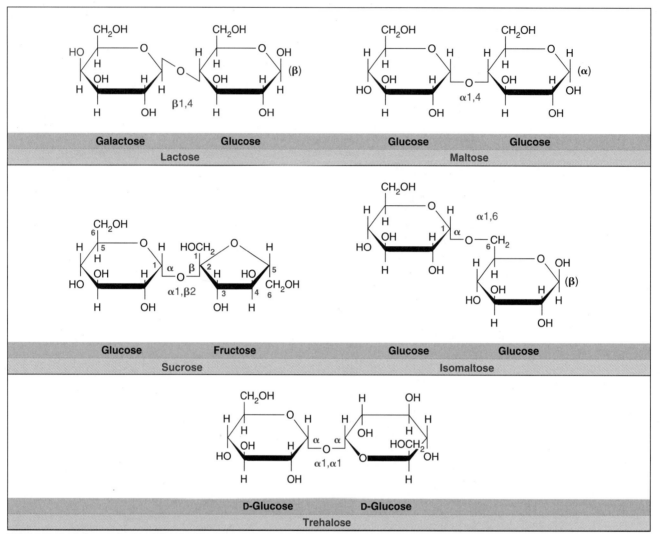

FIGURE 7–4. Structures of selected disaccharides. *The Greek letters to the right of lactose, maltose, and isomaltose indicate the location and configuration of the reducing hemiacetal groups.*

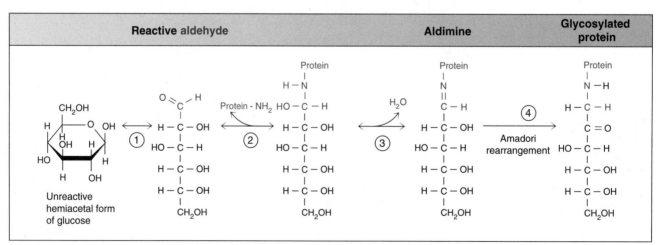

FIGURE 7–5. Nonenzymatic reaction of glucose with proteins.

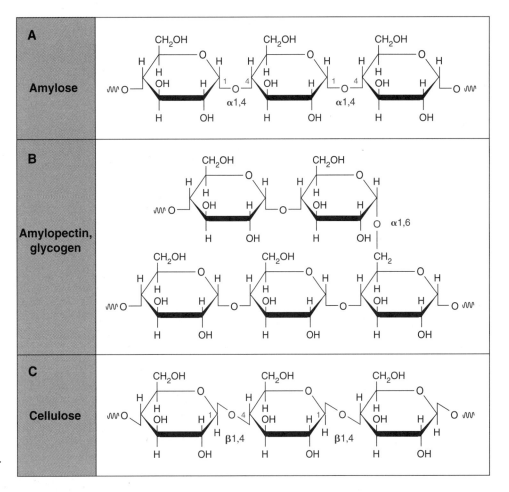

FIGURE 7–6. A. Amylose. B. Amylopectin and glycogen. C. Cellulose.

trolled diabetes have greater than 9% hemoglobin A_1. ◄

Polysaccharides

Starch is a polymer of D-glucose that is made in plants. Although its structure consists of monomeric repeats, nutritionists regard starch as a **complex carbohydrate.** Glucose and sucrose are **simple carbohydrates.** Starch is found in many plants and plant products such as flour. Starch has two components: amylose and amylopectin. **Amylose** is a straight-chain polymer that consists of D-glucosyl units linked by α-1,4-glycosidic bonds (Figure 7–6A). **Amylopectin** has a tree-like structure with straight-chain portions linked by α-1,4-glycosidic bonds and many branches that are linked by α-1,6-glycosidic bonds (Figure 7–6B). The branches occur every 20 or so residues.

Glycogen has a structure like that of amylopectin with straight-chain portions with branches. Glycogen has a greater degree of branching (about every 12 residues) and a greater molecular mass (1 million Da) than amylopectin (100,000 Da). Glycogen is only a minor component of the human diet. Most of the glycogen that is found in animal tissues degrades postmortem. Oysters are one of the few sources of dietary glycogen for humans.

Cellulose is another polymer of glucose that is synthesized by plants. Cellulose consists of long straight chains that are linked by β-1,4-glycosidic bonds (Figure 7–6C). Since humans lack an enzyme that will hydrolyze the β-1,4-glycosidic bonds of polysaccharides, cellulose cannot be digested and absorbed. Cellulose is a component of fiber (nondigestible carbohydrate) in the diet. Fiber aids intestinal motility and acts as a stool softener. Note that a change in the configuration about the glycosidic bond from α to β has profound consequences on the biochemical and physiological properties of these isomers (amylose versus cellulose).

CARBOHYDRATE DIGESTION

Digestive Enzymes

The digestion of carbohydrates involves their hydrolysis into monosaccharides (stage I of metabolism, Figure 1–3). Carbohydrate digestion occurs in the mouth and small intestine. Monosaccharides, and not disaccharides or higher polymers, are absorbed into the bloodstream from the gut. The liver plays a pivotal role in the metabolism of absorbed carbohydrate. Liver cells take up and metabolize fructose, galactose, glucose, and mannose.

Salivary glands secrete α-**amylase** (also called ptyalin), which initiates the hydrolysis of starch and glycogen. This enzyme is an endoglycosidase that hydrolyzes internal α-1,4-glycosidic bonds; this enzyme does not attack α-1,6-glycosidic bonds (Figure 7–7). When the food reaches the stomach and encounters gastric acid at pH 1.5, the activity of α-amylase is abolished by acid denaturation. The pH of the small intestine is made alkaline by secretions from the pancreas and liver. Carbohydrate digestion continues in the small intestine as catalyzed by pancreatic amylase, also an α-amylase. Both forms of amylase are activated by chloride, the chief extracellular anion (Table 2–1).

α-Amylase hydrolyzes starch into maltose, maltotriose (a trimer of glucose bonded by two α-1,4-glycosidic bonds), and oligosaccharides of about eight residues in length called dextrins. **Dextrinases** of the small intestine catalyze the hydrolysis of dextrins from the nonreducing end to form glucose. Disaccharidases, which include **maltase, isomaltase, sucrase, lactase,** and **trehalase,** act on the smaller carbohydrates to liberate monosaccharides from the corresponding substrates. Sucrose and lactose are not digested until they reach the small intestine. Except for the amylases, the other enzymes of carbohydrate digestion listed in Table 7–1 are anchored to the plasma membrane of the brush border of the cells of the small intestine.

The major monosaccharides that result from digestion include glucose, galactose, and fructose. There are two types of monosaccharide transporter that mediate the entry of these sugars into

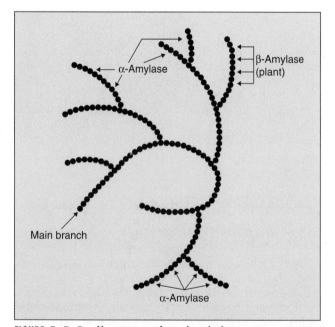

FIGURE 7–7. Tree-like structure of starch and glycogen. *These are digested in humans by α-amylase, an endoglycosidase that cleaves interior α-1,4 bonds. β-Amylase is a plant enzyme that cleaves disaccharide residues sequentially from substrate.*

TABLE 7–1. Enzymes for Carbohydrate Digestion

Enzyme	Source	Substrate	Products
α-Amylase	Salivary gland, pancreas	Starch, glycogen	Oligosaccharides
Dextrinase	Small intestine	Dextrins	Glucose
Isomaltase	Small intestine	α-1,6-Glucosides	Glucose
Lactase*	Small intestine	Lactose	Galactose, glucose
Maltase	Small intestine	Maltose	Glucose
Sucrase	Small intestine	Sucrose	Fructose, glucose
Trehalase	Small intestine	Trehalose	Glucose

*Lactase deficiency produces lactose intolerance.

the cell. One protein cotransports sodium and glucose or galactose into the epithelial cell. Another protein transports fructose without sodium cotransport. These sugars are released into the extracellular space by facilitated diffusion (Table 22–2) and enter the circulation.

Malabsorption

▶ Malabsorption is defined as any disorder involving impaired absorption of carbohydrate, fat, protein, or vitamins. D-Xylose absorption is used as a screening test when carbohydrate malabsorption is suspected. D-Xylose is absorbed by the glucose transport system. After oral administration, xylose blood levels are measured after 1 hour. Alternatively, xylose excretion in the urine is quantified. Because free xylose is poorly catabolized, 20% or more is excreted in the urine, in normal people, within 5 hours after oral administration.

Failure to absorb dietary lactose is common in adults throughout the world. This condition is not due to malabsorption but to lactase deficiency and the inability to hydrolyze lactose. Individuals with lactase deficiency avoid milk products to escape the gastrointestinal symptoms (abdominal distention, pain, diarrhea) that accompany this disorder. However, individuals with lactase deficiency can generally tolerate yogurt, a milk product. Yogurt contains lactase that catalyzes the degradation of lactose to glucose and galactose. ◀

GLYCOLYTIC PATHWAY

The identification of the precursors and products of each metabolic pathway is essential in the understanding of a biochemical process. The stoichiometry of the **Embden-Myerhof** glycolytic pathway, a cytosolic process, is expressed by equation 7.3.

$$\text{Glucose} + 2\,\text{ADP} + 2\,\text{P}_i + 2\,\text{NAD}^+ \rightarrow \quad (7.3)$$
$$2\,\text{pyruvate} + 2\,\text{ATP} + 2\,\text{H}_2\text{O}$$
$$+ 2\,\text{NADH} + 2\,\text{H}^+$$

Conversion of glucose into two molecules of pyruvate occurs with the generation of two molecules each of ATP and NADH. Although catabolic reactions capture chemical energy as ATP, two molecules of ATP are required to phosphorylate (1) glucose and (2) fructose 6-phosphate before ATP is generated. The phosphorylation reactions and the cleavage of the hexose bisphosphate into triose phosphates make up the first phase of the pathway; the generation of ATP and NADH occurs during the second phase (Figure 7–8).

First Phase of Glycolysis

Hexokinase or **glucokinase** catalyzes the reaction between ATP and glucose (Figure 6–7), yielding ADP and glucose 6-phosphate according to equation 7.4.

$$\text{ATP } (2\sim) + \text{glucose } (0\sim) \rightarrow \text{ADP } (1\sim)$$
$$+ \text{ glucose 6-phosphate } (0\sim) \quad (7.4)$$

There are two high-energy bonds in ATP, a reactant, and there is one high-energy bond in the products. Based on the decrease in the number of high-energy bonds, the reaction is exergonic, and the formation of products is favored (PRINCIPLE 2 OF BIOENERGETICS). Moreover, this reaction is one of the

three irreversible steps in the glycolytic pathway (Figure 7–9).

Hexokinase occurs in all cells including liver. **Glucokinase** occurs in liver. Hexokinase has a low K_m for glucose (about 30 μM) and is inhibited allosterically by glucose 6-phosphate. Glucokinase has a higher K_m for glucose (about 10 mM) and is not inhibited by glucose 6-phosphate. The concentration of glucose in the hepatic portal vein postprandially is about 10 mM, and hexokinase is saturated, but glucokinase is not saturated nor is it inhibited by intracellular glucose 6-phosphate. Because of these special properties of glucokinase, the liver has a high capacity for glucose metabolism.

Phosphoglucose isomerase catalyzes the conversion of glucose 6-phosphate to fructose 6-phosphate (Figure 7–9). There is no thermodynamic barrier for the interconversion of an aldehyde (glucose) and the ketone (fructose), and the isomerization reaction is functionally isoergonic.

Phosphofructokinase catalyzes the transfer of the γ-phosphoryl group from ATP to fructose 6-phosphate. The bioenergetics of the phosphofructokinase reaction parallels that of the hexokinase reaction. The reaction is exergonic and unidirectional.

Aldolase (fructose 1,6-bisphosphate aldolase) catalyzes the cleavage of fructose 1,6-bisphosphate to two triose phosphates (glyceraldehyde 3-phosphate and dihydroxyacetone phosphate). This is not a transferase reaction, and our use of group transfer potentials does not aid in the analysis of this reaction. The standard free energy change for this process is + 24 kJ/mol, indicating that formation of the triose phosphates is unfavorable under standard conditions. However, the free energy change under physiological concentrations of substrates and products is minimal (Table 7–2), and the aldolase reaction is bidirectional.

Triose phosphate isomerase mediates the conversion of a ketone (dihydroxyacetone phosphate) to an aldehyde (glyceraldehyde 3-phosphate). The structures and properties of the reactants and products are similar, and this isomerization is functionally isoergonic.

Second Phase of Glycolysis

Glyceraldehyde-3-phosphate dehydrogenase catalyses an oxidation-reduction reaction with the concomitant formation of a high-energy phosphate bond (an acyl~phosphate). The oxidation of glyceraldehyde 3-phosphate to phosphoglycerate by a pyridine nucleotide is thermodynamically very favorable (Table 5–3). In the glyceraldehyde-3-phosphate dehydrogenase reaction, this oxidation-reduction is accompanied by the formation of the acyl~phosphate linkage and much of the energy of the oxidation-reduction reaction is thereby conserved. This example illustrates one mechanism for

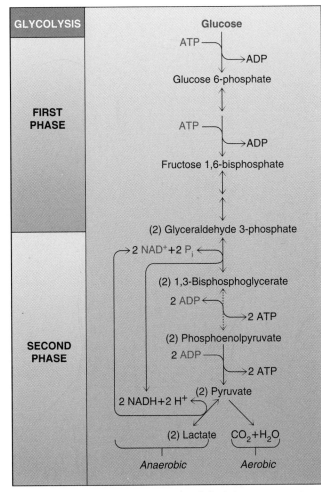

FIGURE 7–8. Overview of glycolysis.

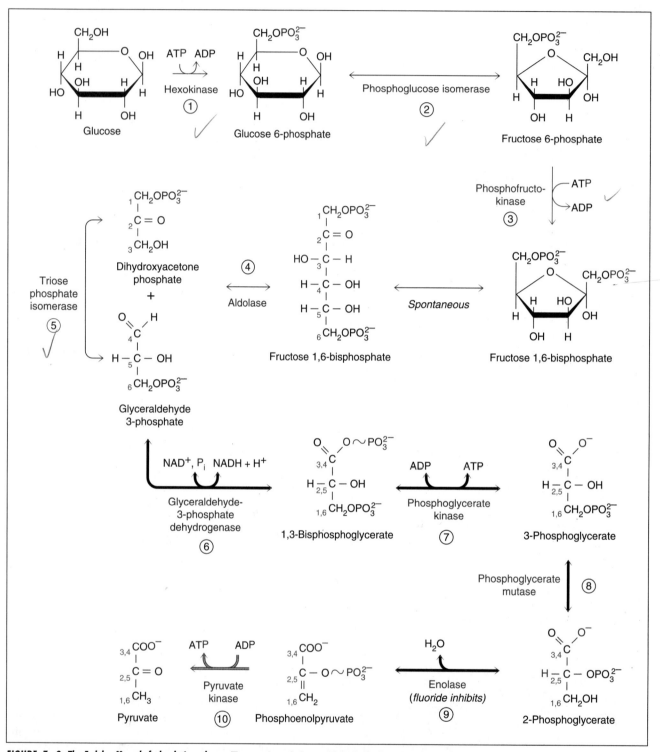

FIGURE 7–9. The Embden-Meyerhof glycolytic pathway. *Two moles of glyceraldehyde 3-phosphate are converted to two moles of pyruvate for each mole of glucose. This stoichiometry is indicated by the double arrows. The numbers on the trioses refer to their precursor atoms in glucose. Note that each of the phosphates of fructose 1,6-bisphosphate becomes the 3-phosphate of glyceraldehyde 3-phosphate, and C³ and C⁴ of the hexose molecule become C¹ of the triose molecule.*

TABLE 7–2.   Reactions and Bioenergetics of Glycolysis (25°C and pH 7)*

Reaction or Enzyme	Equation	$\Delta G^{\circ\prime}$ kJ mol^{-1}	$\Delta G'$ kJ mol^{-1}
Hexokinase (glucokinase)	Glucose + ATP → glucose 6-phosphate + ADP	− 16.6	− 33.5
Phosphoglucose isomerase	Glucose 6-phosphate ⇌ fructose 6-phosphate	2.09	− 0.28
Phosphofructokinase	ATP + fructose 6-phosphate → ADP + fructose 1,6-bisphosphate	− 14.2	− 26.8
Aldolase (fructose 1,6-bisphosphate aldolase)	Fructose 1,6-bisphosphate ⇌ glyceraldehyde 3-phosphate + dihydroxyacetone phosphate	21.8	− 0.15
Triose phosphate isomerase	Dihydroxyacetone phosphate ⇌ glyceraldehyde 3-phosphate	7.66	5.94
Glyceraldehyde-3-phosphate dehydrogenase	2 × (Glyceraldehyde 3-phosphate + NAD$^+$ + P$_i$ ⇌ 1,3-bisphosphoglycerate + NADH + H$^+$)	2 × (6.3)	2 × (1.4)
Phosphoglycerate kinase	2 × (1,3-Bisphosphoglycerate + ADP ⇌ 3-phosphoglycerate + ATP)	2 × (− 24.1)	2 × (− 15.3)
Phosphoglycerate mutase	2 × (3-Phosphoglycerate ⇌ 2-phosphoglycerate)	2 × (4.44)	2 × (− 1.3)
Enolase	2 × (2-Phosphoglycerate ⇌ phosphoenolpyruvate)	2 × (1.84)	2 × (− 4.76)
Pyruvate kinase	2 × (Phosphoenolpyruvate + ADP → pyruvate + ATP)	2 × (− 31.5)	2 × (− 21.8)
		− 85.3	− 138

*Standard free energy changes adapted from J.A. Bassham and G.H. Krause. Free energy changes and metabolic regulation in steady state photosynthetic carbon reduction. Biochimica et Biophysica Acta 189:207–221, 1969. Free energy changes from resting skeletal muscle calculated from the data of D.K. Srivastava and S.A. Bernhard. Enzyme-enzyme interactions and the regulation of metabolic reaction pathways. Current Topics in Cellular Regulation 28:1–68, 1986.

the conversion of oxidation-reduction energy to phosphate-bond energy.

Phosphoglycerate kinase catalyzes the conversion of ADP and 1,3-bisphosphoglycerate to ATP and 3-phosphoglycerate (Figure 7–9). The substrates (ADP, 1~; 1,3-bisphosphoglycerate, 1~) each contain one high-energy bond for a total of two, and the products (ATP, 2~; 3-phosphoglycerate, 0~) also contain two high-energy bonds. This reaction is functionally isoergonic (PRINCIPLE 1 OF BIOENERGETICS). *The phosphoglycerate kinase reaction is the only bidirectional kinase reaction in the glycolytic pathway.* The three other ATP-requiring kinase reactions (hexokinase, phosphofructokinase, and pyruvate kinase) are unidirectional. Since one mole of hexose yields two moles of triose, the phosphoglycerate kinase step accounts for the synthesis of two moles of ATP per mole of glucose.

Phosphoglycerate mutase mediates the transfer of the phosphoryl group from the alcohol on C^3 to that of C^2. Both 3-phosphoglycerate and 2-phosphoglycerate are low-energy oxygen esters of phosphate. This reaction is therefore functionally isoergonic (PRINCIPLE 4 OF BIOENERGETICS).

Enolase, in the next reaction of the glycolytic pathway, catalyzes the elimination of water from 2-phosphoglycerate to produce phosphoenolpyruvate. This reaction is a lyase reaction, and we cannot use the group transfer potentials in its analysis. Hydration-dehydration reactions such as this, however, lack an appreciable thermodynamic barrier, and these reactions are functionally isoergonic.

It is notable that the phosphate bond in 2-phosphoglycerate exhibits a low free energy of hydrolysis, whereas the phosphate bond in phosphoenolpyruvate exhibits a very large negative free energy of hydrolysis. Yet the reaction interconverting 2-phosphoglycerate and phosphoenolpyruvate is functionally isoergonic. How do we explain this apparent paradox? Free energy changes refer to the reactants relative to the products. With 2-phosphoglycerate, the hydrolysis product is glycerate (containing one carboxylate and two alcohol groups). With phosphoenolpyruvate, the hydrolysis product is pyruvate (containing a carboxylate and keto group). Phosphoenolpyruvate is energy rich when compared with its hydrolysis products, and 2-phosphoglycerate is energy poor when compared with its hydrolysis products. This analysis explains the apparent paradox.

Pyruvate kinase catalyzes the conversion of phosphoenolpyruvate and ADP to pyruvate and ATP. Two moles of ATP per mole of hexose are formed during this reaction. Although the number of high-energy bonds in the reactants and products is identical, we noted that this is the only situation where ATP is unable to phosphorylate its cognate substrate (equation 6.10). Consequently the pyruvate kinase step is the third unidirectional reaction of the glycolytic pathway (Table 7–3). Note that the free energy changes ($\Delta G'$) of these three irreversible reactions are the most negative (most favorable in the forward direction of glycolysis) of all of the reactions in the glycolytic pathway (Table 7–2).

Metabolism of 2,3-Bisphosphoglycerate

2,3-Bisphosphoglycerate (2,3-BPG) is an allosteric effector of hemoglobin. This effector, formerly

TABLE 7–3.   The Three Irreversible Enzyme-catalyzed Reactions of Glycolysis

1. Hexokinase (or glucokinase)
2. Phosphofructokinase
3. Pyruvate kinase

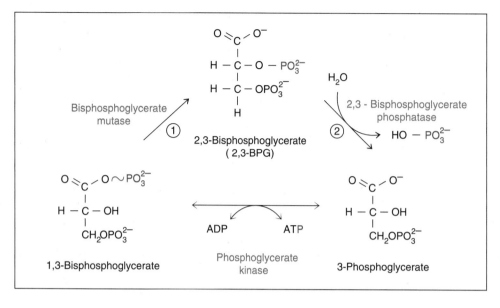

FIGURE 7-10. The 2,3-bisphosphoglycerate shunt.

called 2,3-diphosphoglycerate (2,3-DPG), is present in red blood cells. 2,3-BPG promotes the release of oxygen from hemoglobin (2,3-BPG makes hemoglobin dump oxygen). Erythrocytes synthesize and degrade 2,3-bisphosphoglycerate by a shunt from the glycolytic pathway. Both reactions are unidirectional (Figure 7-10). About 20% of glucose metabolized by erythrocytes is through 2,3-bisphosphoglycerate. Note that the bypass decreases the ATP yield by one mole per triose or by two moles per mole of hexose.

ATP Yield of Glycolysis

Let us consider additional aspects of the bioenergetics of the glycolytic pathway. We saw that two molecules of ATP are expended during the first phase of glycolysis. One ATP is required in the hexokinase reaction and the second in the phosphofructokinase reaction (Figure 7-9). Two molecules of ATP are generated in the phosphoglycerate kinase reaction, and two are formed by the pyruvate kinase reaction. That is, a total of four molecules of ATP are produced per hexose. It is noteworthy that the *net* yield of ATP in the glycolytic pathway is two (four minus two) per hexose. The standard free energy changes and the estimated cellular free energy changes of each reaction of glycolysis are given for general reference in Table 7-2. The free energy changes show that the three unidirectional reactions are accompanied by substantial decreases in free energy. The qualitative assessment of the bioenergetics of the glycolytic pathway (counting high-energy bonds) goes a long way toward explaining the metabolic strategy of glycolysis.

Regulation of Glycolysis

The main regulatory enzyme of the glycolytic pathway is phosphofructokinase. Other enzymes of the pathway can exhibit regulatory behavior (dispersive control of metabolism). What characteristics of the pathway favor a regulatory role for phosphofructokinase? This enzyme catalyzes a physiologically irreversible reaction, and this enzyme-catalyzed reaction represents the committed step in the pathway. These are two attributes that are important in metabolic control. In animals and in bacteria such as *Escherichia coli,* glucose 6-phosphate can be converted into glycogen, pentose phosphates, and pyruvate. Glucose 6-phosphate represents a metabolic branch point. Therefore, it would not be possible to increase glycolysis by increasing the transport or phosphorylation of glucose without altering the flux of metabolites through other pathways.

Phosphofructokinase activity is regulated by several allosteric effectors. Under conditions in which the levels of ATP are decreased, there is a concomitant increase in ADP and AMP. Under these physiological conditions, **AMP** serves as an allosteric activator of phosphofructokinase. Activation of phosphofructokinase promotes glycolysis and the generation of ATP. The formation of ATP occurs with a concomitant decrease in [AMP] that, in turn, decreases the allosteric activation of phosphofructokinase. **ATP** is both a substrate and an allosteric inhibitor of the phosphofructokinase reaction. When ATP concentrations are high, there is no need to accelerate glucose catabolism. This description indicates how the energy charge of ATP (Chapter 6) plays a role in metabolic control. Regulation by AMP is important in exercising skeletal muscle but probably is not important in other cells.

Citrate, another negative effector, accumulates in extrahepatic cells under conditions when fatty acids serve as a major source of metabolic fuel. Fatty acids are preferentially used during fasting, starvation, or intervals of low carbohydrate intake. Accumulated citrate acts as a negative allosteric effector of phosphofructokinase and inhibits further glucose degradation (Table 25-1).

TABLE 7–4. Allosteric Regulation of Phosphofructokinase-1 (PFK-1)

Activators	Inhibitors
AMP	ATP
Fructose 2,6-bisphosphate	Citrate

Fructose 2,6-bisphosphate activates phosphofructokinase allosterically. Current evidence indicates, moreover, that fructose 2,6-bisphosphate is the most important allosteric regulator of glycolysis (Table 7–4). Fructose 2,6-bisphosphate is formed from fructose 6-phosphate during a reaction catalyzed by 6-phosphofructose-2-kinase (Figure 7–11). Fructose 2,6-bisphosphate is degraded to fructose 6-phosphate in a reaction catalyzed by fructose 2,6-bisphosphate-2-phosphatase. A single protein contains the kinase and phosphatase activities that catalyze the formation and degradation of fructose 2,6-bisphosphate. This protein is often denoted in abbreviated form as kinase/phosphatase.

In liver, the phosphorylation of the kinase/phosphatase by protein kinase A decreases 6-phosphofructose-2-kinase activity and increases phosphatase activity (Table 25–2). Kinase/phosphatase phosphorylation occurs with a high glucagon-to-insulin ratio. Agents that elevate [cAMP] in the liver, such as glucagon, inhibit glycolysis by decreasing [fructose 2,6-bisphosphate]. In liver, elevated cyclic AMP produces an indirect (by protein phosphorylation) decrease in fructose 6-phosphate-2-kinase activity and an increase in fructose-2,6-bisphosphatase activity; these altered activities in turn produce a decrease in [fructose 2,6-bisphosphate] that decreases 6-phosphofructose-1-kinase (PFK) activity and the rate of glycolysis. The cAMP second messenger system is considered in more detail in the discussions of glycogen metabolism (Chapter 10) and signal transduction (Chapters 19 and 20).

Requirement for Regenerating NAD⁺, P_i, and ADP

The overall reaction for the conversion of glucose to two moles of pyruvate is given by the following equation:

$$\begin{matrix} \text{Glucose} & 2\text{ pyruvate} \\ + & + \\ 2\text{ ATP} & 4\text{ ATP} \\ + & + \\ 2\text{ NAD}^+ \rightleftharpoons & 2\text{ H}_2\text{O} \\ + & + \\ 2\text{ P}_i & 2\text{ NADH} + 2\text{ H}^+ \\ + & \\ 2\text{ ADP} & \end{matrix} \tag{7.5}$$

$$\Delta G^{\circ\prime} = -85\text{ kJ/mol}$$

Some of the decrease in free energy accompanying the conversion of glucose to pyruvate is captured as ATP, the common currency of energy exchange. Note that molecular oxygen is *not* involved in the process described by equation 7.5.

We can learn a considerable amount about biochemical operations by examining the stoichiometry given in a chemical equation such as equation 7.5. Besides the ATP required for the priming reactions in the first phase of glycolysis, a continual supply of ADP and P_i is necessary for continued glycolysis. ATP provides the energy for chemical work (biosynthesis), osmotic work, and mechanical work (motility) resulting in the continuous generation of ADP and P_i or of AMP and PP_i. A continual supply of NAD⁺ is also required to maintain glycolysis. NADH can be oxidized by pyruvate under anaerobic conditions or by an electron transport chain with oxygen as electron acceptor under aerobic conditions. Transport of electrons from cytosolic NADH to the electron transport chain occurs indirectly as described in Chapter 9.

FIGURE 7–11. Metabolism of fructose 2,6-bisphosphate.

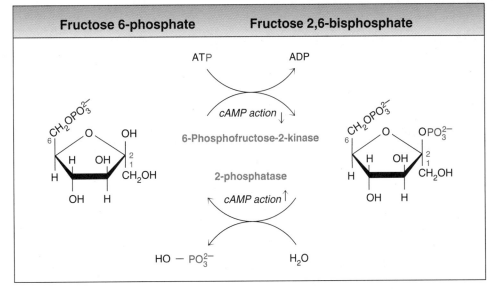

Lactate Dehydrogenase Reaction

Glucose is converted into two molecules of pyruvate by glycolysis. To regenerate NAD^+ under anaerobic conditions, NADH is oxidized by pyruvate in a reaction catalyzed by lactate dehydrogenase, a cytosolic enzyme (equation 7.6).

$$\text{Pyruvate} + \text{NADH} + H^+ \rightleftharpoons \text{lactate} + NAD^+ \quad (7.6)$$

The standard free energy of this reaction is -25.1 kJ/mol, and the equilibrium is far in the direction of products. This is a simple oxidation-reduction reaction, however, and the reaction is bidirectional (PRINCIPLE 7 OF BIOENERGETICS). Pyruvate metabolism is complicated. In contrast, lactate metabolism is simple. Lactate is formed from and converted to pyruvate.

The lactate dehydrogenase reaction plays an important role in human metabolism even though NADH can be oxidized by aerobic processes. Anaerobic glycolysis is the only form of energy production used by the erythrocyte owing to its lack of mitochondria. Anaerobic glycolysis also occurs in skeletal muscle. During a 100-meter sprint, for example, oxidative metabolism will not keep up with energy needs and lactate is generated.

Anaerobic glycolysis is also important during parturition. Parturition is accompanied by fetal anoxia. In uncomplicated deliveries, the fetus suffers no ill effects from anoxia. Prolonged anoxia, however, is postulated to produce nervous system deficits. Although the retina surrounding the fovea is highly aerobic, the fovea is quite active in anaerobic glycolysis. This portion of the retina relies on glycolysis to eliminate the need for colored mitochondrial pigments (cytochromes) required for aerobic respiration. Such pigments in this most sensitive area of the retina would decrease the response of photoreceptor cells and thereby decrease visual acuity.

Clinical Aspects of Glycolysis

▶ Acute and transient lactic acidosis and chronic lactic acidosis are common clinical problems. Circulatory failure, shock, coronary thrombosis, and asphyxia are conditions that impair the delivery of oxygen to tissues. These ailments curtail the production of ATP by oxidative phosphorylation (Chapter 9). 5′-AMP and inorganic phosphate trigger the rapid degradation of cellular glycogen, and the resulting glucose 1-phosphate is converted to lactate. There is an increase in the ratio of circulating lactate/pyruvate, indicating an increased cellular ratio of $NADH/NAD^+$ that prevails during hypoxia.

Mature erythrocytes lack mitochondria and require glycolysis for the generation of ATP. **Pyruvate kinase deficiency** in red cells is a rare inborn error of metabolism that results in hemolytic anemia. Immature red cells that contain mitochondria have normal ATP levels. Circulating lactate and pyruvate provide the fuel for oxidative metabolism and ATP production in these immature red cells. Maturation of the reticulocytes results in a loss of mitochondria, impaired ATP production, and hemolysis of red cells that contain inadequate pyruvate kinase.

Streptococcus mutans is a gram-positive, anaerobic bacterium (Table 1–2) that inhabits the mouth and derives all its energy from glycolysis. It produces dental caries by converting glucose to lactic acid, the cariogenic agent. As a result, the pH of the saliva decreases from about 6.8 to 5 or less, and lactic acid dissolves enamel.

The inhibition of enolase by **fluoride** played an important role in the elucidation of the glycolytic pathway. Glucose metabolism is inhibited by fluoride, and the accumulated product was identified as 3-phosphoglycerate. This inhibition requires millimolar concentrations of fluoride. Whether fluoride inhibition has any clinically important effects is unclear. It has been hypothesized that part of the anticariogenic action of fluoride is due to the inhibition of glycolysis in *Streptococcus mutans.* Physiological fluoride concentrations seem considerably less than millimolar. The content of fluoride in dental enamel is relatively high, however, and the question of fluoride action in bacteria is not resolved. Fluoride is incorporated into hydroxyapatite to produce harder fluorapatite, explaining, in part, the anticariogenic effect of fluoride (Chapter 2). ◀

PENTOSE PHOSPHATE PATHWAY

Another important scheme for glucose catabolism is the oxidative **Warburg-Dickens** pentose phosphate pathway. This pathway is responsible for the biosynthesis of five-carbon sugars found in nucleotides (ATP, NAD^+, $NADP^+$, coenzyme A, FAD), RNA, and DNA. Another important characteristic of the pathway is that it generates NADPH + H^+. The NADPH generated can be used in fatty acid (Chapter 11) and cholesterol (Chapter 12) biosynthesis. Erythrocytes also contain the enzymes of the pathway because, in these oxygen-carrying cells, NADPH plays a protective role against oxygen toxicity.

The pentose phosphate pathway contains an oxidative segment, which generates NADPH + H^+ and a nonoxidative segment. The nonoxidative segment involves the interconversion of many sugar phosphates including those with three-, four-, five-, six-, and seven-carbon atoms. Key enzymes in the nonoxidative segment of the pathway include transaldolase and transketolase. **Transaldolase** catalyzes the transfer of a three-carbon fragment and **transketolase,** a two-carbon fragment.

Oxidative Segment of the Pentose Phosphate Pathway

Glucose 6-phosphate represents the starting point for the oxidative reactions of the pentose phosphate pathway (Figure 7–12). Glucose-6-phosphate dehydrogenase catalyzes a reaction of substrate with $NADP^+$, yielding 6-phosphogluconate δ-lactone and $NADPH + H^+$. A hemiacetal (glucose 6-phosphate) is converted to a carboxylate ester. This is a simple oxidation-reduction reaction and is bidirectional (PRINCIPLE 7 OF BIOENERGETICS). **6-Phosphogluconate lactonase** then catalyzes the hydrolysis of the ester to produce 6-phosphogluconate. Hydrolysis of both low-energy and high-energy bonds (PRINCIPLE 5 OF BIOENERGETICS) is exergonic. Hydrolysis of the lactone makes the oxidative portion of the pathway unidirectional. Next, **6-phosphogluconate dehydrogenase** catalyzes an oxidative decarboxylation forming ribulose 5-phosphate (a pentose), $NADPH + H^+$, and carbon dioxide. At physiological concentrations of metabolites, the reaction proceeds in the direction of ribulose 5-phosphate. Each mole of glucose 6-phosphate yields two moles of $NADPH + H^+$ and one mole each of pentose phosphate and carbon dioxide.

Nonoxidative Segment of the Pentose Phosphate Pathway

This segment of the pathway is more intricate than the oxidative segment. Four enzymes of the pentose phosphate pathway catalyze the interconversion of three-, four-, five-, six-, and seven-carbon phosphate esters. Using a simple stoichiometry, we will illustrate how three pentose phosphates, derived from three molecules of glucose 6-phosphate, can be converted to two hexose phosphates (fructose 6-phosphate) and one triose phosphate (glyceraldehyde 3-phosphate). These reactions are summarized in equation 7.7.

Ribose 5-phosphate + 2 xylulose 5-phosphate ⇌

2 fructose 6-phosphate

+ glyceraldehyde 3-phosphate   (7.7)

Ribulose 5-phosphate is the pentose formed by the oxidative phase of the pentose phosphate pathway. Ribose 5-phosphate and xylulose 5-phosphate are derived from ribulose 5-phosphate through the action of an **isomerase** and an **epimerase** (Figure 7–12). In view of the similar chemical characteristics of reactants and products, both reactions are functionally isoergonic.

Transketolase mediates the transfer of a two-carbon fragment from xylulose 5-phosphate to ribose 5-phosphate to form sedoheptulose 7-phosphate and glyceraldehyde 3-phosphate (Figure 7–12). *Thiamine pyrophosphate is the cofactor for transketolase* (Table 2–3). ▶ Alcoholism is often associated with thiamine deficiency, and the transketolase reaction has been studied in individuals with this condition to gain an understanding of the pathophysiology of this disorder. ◀

Transaldolase operates on glyceraldehyde 3-phosphate and sedoheptulose 7-phosphate to produce fructose 6-phosphate and erythrose 4-phosphate. Transketolase catalyzes a reaction between erythrose 4-phosphate and a second molecule of xylulose 5-phosphate, yielding fructose 6-phosphate and glyceraldehyde 3-phosphate (Figure 7–12). All the reactions of the nonoxidative portion of the pentose phosphate pathway are isoergonic and bidirectional.

▶ The pathological lysis of red blood cells is called hemolysis. Hemolytic anemias can be produced by a variety of mechanisms. A common hereditary disorder is that of **glucose-6-phosphate dehydrogenase deficiency** in the red blood cell. This is one of the most common enzyme deficiencies. The administration of antimalarial drugs such as chloroquine or primaquine and of many other commonly used drugs including sulfonamides, antipyretics, and analgesics to individuals lacking glucose-6-phosphate dehydrogenase can produce hemolytic anemia. These drugs oxidize hemoglobin; disulfide bonds are formed from cysteine residues (Figure 3–5). Under normal circumstances, these disulfide bonds are reduced by glutathione, a tripeptide containing cysteine (Figure 4–12). Without NADPH generation, the reduction of glutathione is impaired, and the glutathione-mediated reduction of hemoglobin is thereby diminished. The oxidized form of hemoglobin precipitates and leads to hemolysis. Glucose-6-phosphate dehydrogenase deficiency is an X-linked (Table 16–5) recessive disorder that occurs in all races and ethnic groups. ◀

The oxidative segment of this pathway converts each mole of glucose 6-phosphate to a mole of ribulose 5-phosphate (a pentose phosphate) with the concomitant formation of two moles of NADPH. More NADPH than pentose phosphate is required in cells active in fatty acid and steroid biosynthesis. The NADPH is used in the reductive steps in these biosynthetic pathways.

The nonoxidative stage of the pathway converts the pentose phosphates to fructose 6-phosphate and glyceraldehyde 3-phosphate, avoiding the wasteful loss of carbon metabolites (Figure 7–12). Beginning with three molecules of glucose 6-phosphate (18C), three molecules of pentose phosphate (15C) and three molecules of carbon dioxide (3C) are produced. The pentose phosphates (15C) are converted into two molecules of fructose 6-phosphate (12C) and one molecule of glyceraldehyde 3-phosphate (3C). The order of the enzyme-catalyzed reactions is transketolase, transaldolase, and finally transketolase as illustrated in Figure 7–12.

The conversion of glucose 6-phosphate to ribulose 5-phosphate and carbon dioxide is exergonic and is made unidirectional by the hydrolysis reaction catalyzed by lactonase. The reactions in the nonoxidative segment are all freely reversible. The

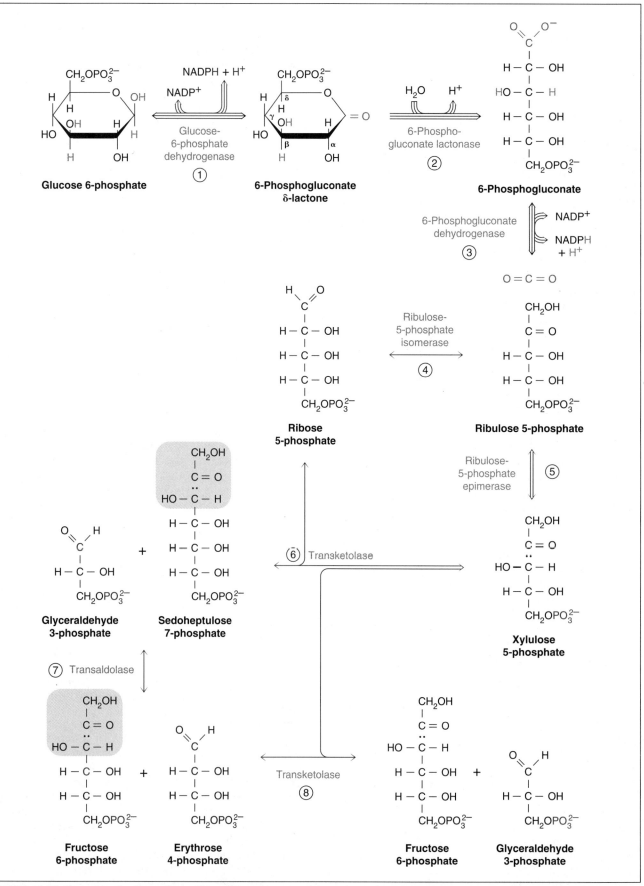

FIGURE 7–12. The pentose phosphate pathway. *The oxidative segment of the pathway (reactions 1 through 3) is accompanied by the formation of two moles of NADPH per mole of glucose. The number of lines in an arrow represents the number of reacting moles necessary to convert three moles of glucose 6-phosphate to two moles of fructose 6-phosphate, one mole of glyceraldehyde 3-phosphate, and three moles of carbon dioxide.*

nonoxidative portion can be thought of as providing great flexibility in the interconversion of a variety of sugar phosphates. The flux of these compounds will be governed by metabolic need. In contrast to glycolysis, note that ATP *per se* is not generated by the pentose phosphate pathway. In contrast to glycolysis, little is known about the regulation of the pentose phosphate pathway.

METABOLISM OF MANNOSE, FRUCTOSE, AND GALACTOSE

Monosaccharide Metabolism

We now consider the metabolism of mannose (from plants), fructose (from fruit), and galactose (from milk). The first step in the metabolism of carbohydrates is their phosphorylation. The conversion of **mannose** to a glycolytic intermediate requires only two steps. First, **hexokinase** catalyzes the exergonic phosphorylation of mannose to form mannose 6-phosphate (Figure 7–13). Second, **phosphomannose isomerase** catalyzes the isoergonic conversion of mannose 6-phosphate to fructose 6-phosphate, a familiar glycolytic metabolite (Figure 7–9). Mannose is not prevalent in human diets.

Fructose (fruit sugar) is derived from fruit, and it is also produced by the digestion of sucrose, or table sugar. Fructose may furnish from 30% to 60% of dietary carbohydrate, and daily intakes of 100 g are typical. Fructose can be phosphorylated during an exergonic process catalyzed by hexokinase to form fructose 6-phosphate (Figure 7–14), a glycolytic intermediate.

Besides hexokinase, the liver contains a special **fructokinase** that catalyzes the phosphorylation of fructose by ATP to yield **fructose 1-phosphate** in an exergonic and unidirectional process. This is not a usual glycolytic intermediate, and further reactions are required for metabolism. The product, fructose 1-phosphate, is cleaved in a reaction catalyzed by fructose-1-phosphate aldolase activity to form glyceraldehyde and dihydroxyacetone phosphate. Fructose 1,6-bisphosphate aldolase B (but not A or C) possesses fructose 1-phosphate aldo-

lase activity. **Glyceraldehyde kinase** mediates the phosphorylation of glyceraldehyde to yield glyceraldehyde 3-phosphate (Figure 7–14); this kinase reaction is exergonic and unidirectional. The triose phosphates produced during fructose metabolism are metabolized by glycolysis.

▶ **Essential fructosuria** is a benign metabolic anomaly that is caused by the absence of fructokinase. That 90% of ingested fructose is retained and only 10% is excreted in the urine of affected individuals indicates that hexokinase can substitute adequately for fructokinase. These individuals are asymptomatic. **Hereditary fructose intolerance** is caused by a deficiency of aldolase B in liver, kidney cortex, and small intestine. There is a buildup of fructose 1-phosphate in the affected cells. The affected individuals exhibit hepatomegaly, jaundice, hemorrhage, and renal disease. Both disorders are rare autosomal recessive diseases. Avoidance of fructose and sucrose in the diet relieves the symptoms. ◀

The catabolism of **galactose** is more complex than that of mannose and fructose. Galactose (Figure 7–3A) is derived from the disaccharide lactose found in milk (Latin *lac*). Lactose is hydrolyzed by a digestive enzyme (lactase); the sugars are absorbed by the gut and transported to the liver. In the liver, galactose is phosphorylated by ATP in a reaction catalyzed by **galactokinase** to yield ADP and galactose 1-phosphate (Figure 7–15). *Galactose is the only common aldohexose that is not a substrate for hexokinase.* Although liver has a large capacity to metabolize galactose, galactokinase and the other enzymes for galactose metabolism occur in many cell types including fibroblasts, red and white blood cells, and placenta.

Galactose 1-phosphate reacts with uridine diphosphoglucose (UDP-glucose) to yield UDP-galactose and glucose 1-phosphate. The isoergonic reaction is catalyzed by a **galactose-1-phosphate uridyltransferase** (Figure 7–15). Glucose 1-phosphate is converted to glucose 6-phosphate by **phosphoglucomutase** in an isoergonic reaction. Glucose 6-phosphate can be metabolized by glycolysis or by the pentose phosphate pathway. Glucose 1-phosphate can be converted to glycogen (Chapter 10).

FIGURE 7–13. Mannose metabolism.

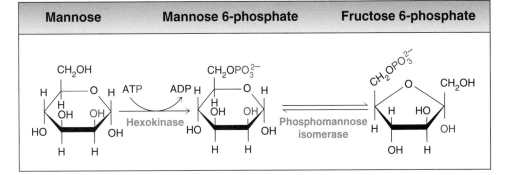

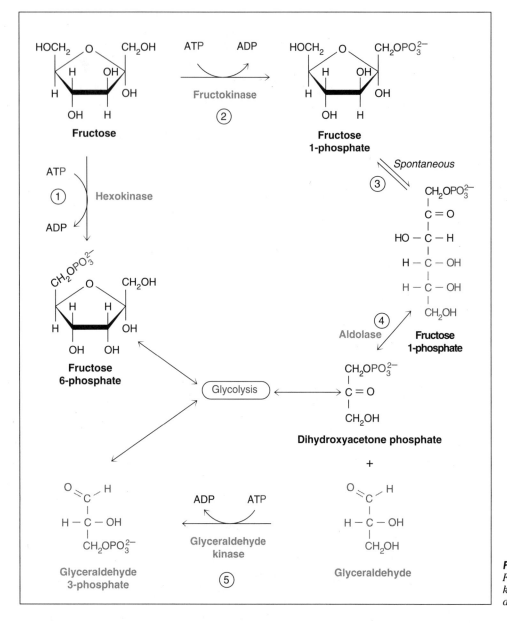

FIGURE 7-14. Fructose metabolism. *Fructokinase and glyceraldehyde kinase are hepatic enzymes that are unique to this pathway.*

UDP-galactose must be converted to UDP-glucose to regenerate the initial reactant. This reaction is catalyzed by an epimerase that converts the hydroxyl on C^4 to a ketone and then reduces it to give the hydroxyl of the alternative configuration (UDP-glucose) shown in Figure 7–15. The epimerase contains tightly bound NAD^+ as a prosthetic cofactor. UDP-glucose can now react with a second molecule of galactose 1-phosphate to yield glucose 1-phosphate and UDP-galactose. The UDP nucleotide is thus used repeatedly in a cyclic fashion to mediate the conversion of considerable galactose 1-phosphate to glucose 1-phosphate. UDP-glucose functions catalytically; UDP-glucose is regenerated after every reaction and is called the regenerating substrate. Galactose 1-phosphate, which is consumed by the process, is called the stoichiometric substrate. Metabolic cycles are discussed in more detail in Chapter 8.

Galactosemia

▶ The human disease of **galactosemia** is due to a deficiency of **galactose-1-phosphate uridyltransferase.** Excessive galactose 1-phosphate accumulates in cells with consequent deleterious effects. Affected infants exhibit vomiting, diarrhea, failure to thrive, and deranged hepatic function (jaundice and hepatomegaly), mental retardation, and increased susceptibility to sepsis by *E. coli.* Treatment consists of a diet lacking milk and milk products (specifically lactose). Galactose forms an essential component of many carbohydrate-containing glycoproteins. Withholding galactose is not harmful because the epimerase can catalyze the formation of UDP-galactose from UDP-glucose as necessary. A milder form of galactosemia is due to a hereditary deficiency of **galactokinase.** The second type of galactosemia is less severe than classi-

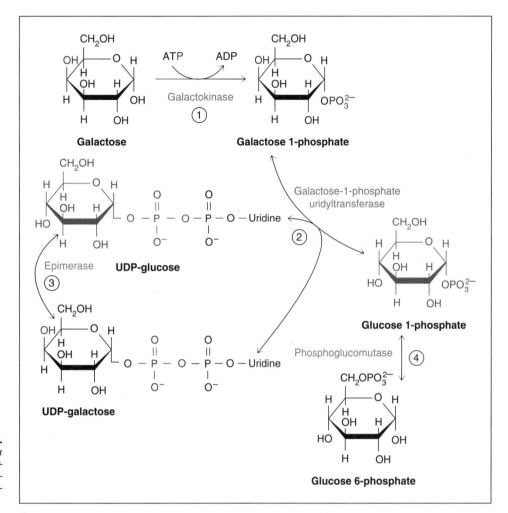

FIGURE 7–15. Galactose metabolism. *Classic galactosemia is due to a deficiency of the uridyltransferase. A variant form of galactosemia is due to a deficiency of galactokinase.*

cal galactosemia because there is not an accumulation of charged intracellular metabolites.

Both forms of galactosemia are transmitted as autosomal recessive diseases. The incidence of classical galactosemia (uridyltransferase deficiency) is about 1 in 70,000. The uridyltransferase gene is located on chromosome 9p13, and the galactokinase gene is located on chromosome 17q21–22 (Table 16–5). ◄

SUMMARY

The glycolytic pathway is the predominant pathway for glucose degradation in nature. There are two stages in the glycolytic pathway. During the first stage, two moles of ATP are consumed and one mole of glucose is converted into two moles of triose phosphate. In the second stage of glycolysis, two moles of triose phosphate are converted into two moles of pyruvate with the concomitant generation of four moles of ATP. The net yield of ATP per mole of glucose in the glycolytic pathway is two.

The three irreversible steps of the glycolytic pathway are catalyzed by hexokinase, phosphofructokinase, and pyruvate kinase. The hexokinase-catalyzed and phosphofructokinase-catalyzed reactions proceed with the loss of one high-energy bond. The pyruvate kinase reaction does not proceed with the loss of a high-energy bond, but phosphoenolpyruvate is exceptionally energy rich and this reaction is unidirectional.

The NADH produced by glycolysis must be regenerated to permit further glucose degradation. Under anaerobic conditions, NADH is oxidized by pyruvate to produce NAD^+ and lactate. Phosphofructokinase is the rate-limiting step of the glycolytic pathway. Phosphofructokinase is activated allosterically by fructose 2,6-bisphosphate and 5'-AMP; it is inhibited allosterically by citrate and ATP. Fructose 2,6-bisphosphate is the most important allosteric regulator of glycolysis.

The pentose phosphate pathway generates two moles of NADPH per mole of glucose. Glucose-6-phosphate dehydrogenase and 6-phosphogluconate dehydrogenase catalyze the formation of NADPH. The hydrolysis of 6-phosphogluconolactone is an exergonic process that ensures that the oxidative branch proceeds in the direction of pentose phosphates. Transaldolase, which transfers three-carbon units, and transketolase, which transfers two-carbon units, are key enzymes in the nonoxidative segment of the pentose phosphate pathway. Thiamine pyrophosphate is a prosthetic group for transketolase. All reactions of the nonoxidative branch are reversible and provide great metabolic flexibility.

Fructokinase and glyceraldehyde kinase are two hepatic enzymes that participate in fructose metabolism. Galactokinase is required for galactose metabolism. These kinase reactions proceed with the loss of a high-energy bond and are exergonic. Galactose-1-phosphate uridyltransferase and UDP-galactose epimerase are required for the conversion of galactose 1-phosphate to glucose 1-phosphate. Galactose-1-phosphate uridyltransferase is deficient in classical galactosemia.

SELECTED READINGS

DeFronzo, R.A., and E. Ferrannini. Regulation of hepatic glucose metabolism in humans. Diabetes/Metabolism Reviews 3:415–459, 1987.

Grant, J.P. Malabsorption syndromes. *In* D.C. Sabiston, Jr. (ed.). *Textbook of Surgery,* 14th ed. Philadelphia, W.B. Saunders Company, 1991, pp. 873–880.

Pilkis, S.J., and T.H. Claus. Hepatic gluconeogenesis/glycolysis: Regulation and structure/function relationships of substrate cycle enzymes. Annual Review of Nutrition 11:465–515, 1991.

Segal, S. Disorders of galactose metabolism. *In* C.R. Scriver, A.L. Beaudet, W.S. Sly, and D. Valle (eds.). *The Metabolic Basis of Inherited Disease,* 6th ed. New York, McGraw-Hill Book Company, 1989, pp. 453–480.

Semenza, G., and S. Auricchio. Small-intestinal disaccharidases. *In* C.R. Scriver, A.L. Beaudet, W.S. Sly, and D. Valle (eds.). *The Metabolic Basis of Inherited Disease,* 6th ed. New York, McGraw-Hill Book Company, 1989, pp. 2975–2997.

Unger, R.H., and D.W. Foster. Diabetes mellitus. *In* J.D. Wilson and D.W. Foster (eds.). *Williams Textbook of Endocrinology,* 8th ed. Philadelphia, W.B. Saunders Company, 1992, pp. 1255–1333.

Wood, T. *Pentose Phosphate Pathway.* New York, Academic Press, 1985.

CHAPTER EIGHT

The Krebs Cycle

Real research of a fundamental character requires a tremendous amount of time.

—HANS A. KREBS

A scientist must have the courage to attack the great unsolved problems of his time, and solutions usually have to be forced by carrying out innumerable experiments without much critical hesitation.

—OTTO WARBURG

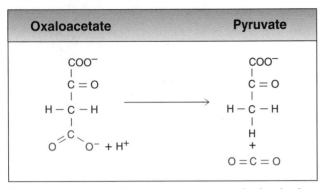

FIGURE 8–1. *Conversion of oxaloacetate to pyruvate and carbon dioxide, a simple decarboxylation.*

The aerobic metabolism of glucose to carbon dioxide and water provides much more energy than is liberated during anaerobic glycolysis. Following the conversion of glucose to pyruvate, pyruvate is converted to acetyl-CoA by oxidative decarboxylation before entering the Krebs cycle. The Krebs cycle is the final common pathway for the oxidation of carbohydrates, fatty acids, and amino acids (Figure 1–3). Oxidative decarboxylation reactions play a major role in metabolism. The Krebs cycle, which occurs in mitochondria (Table 1–1), is also called the **citric acid cycle** or the **tricarboxylic acid cycle.**

BIOENERGETICS OF DECARBOXYLATION REACTIONS

Decarboxylation reactions are common, and an understanding of their bioenergetics simplifies the study of biochemistry. There are two types of decarboxylation processes based on the presence or absence of an accompanying oxidation-reduction reaction: simple decarboxylation and oxidative decarboxylation.

A **simple decarboxylation** reaction is one occurring without a reduction of NAD^+ or $NADP^+$. The conversion of oxaloacetate to carbon dioxide and pyruvate provides an example of a simple decarboxylation reaction (Figure 8–1). The standard free energy change of this reaction is about -30 kJ/mol (equivalent to the hydrolysis of a high-energy bond). This process is exergonic and greatly favors formation of products. This example typifies all simple decarboxylation reactions, and knowing that decarboxylations are markedly exergonic will help us understand many aspects of metabolism.

Oxidative decarboxylation reactions include both oxidation-reduction and decarboxylation. This process involves decarboxylation coupled to the reduction of NAD^+, $NADP^+$, or another oxidizing agent. The oxidation of pyruvate to acetyl-CoA and carbon dioxide is an example of an oxidative decarboxylation reaction (Figure 8–2). The carbonyl group derived from C^2 of pyruvate is converted to the carboxylate level of oxidation. The standard free energy change for the reaction is appreciable (-34.9 kJ/mol), and the reaction is unidirectional.

Thiamine pyrophosphate and pyridoxal phosphate are the two major cofactors for decarboxylation reactions. Thiamine pyrophosphate (Figure 2–11) participates in (1) simple and (2) oxidative decarboxylation reactions. Pyridoxal phosphate (Figure 2–15) participates in simple decarboxylation reactions.

PRINCIPLE 6 OF BIOENERGETICS states that *decarboxylation reactions are exergonic.* This principle will aid our analysis of biochemical reactions and pathways. That decarboxylation reactions are markedly exergonic means that the products are especially stable when compared with the reactants. Carbon dioxide is the stable product that is generated, and this stability accounts for the exergonic nature of decarboxylation reactions. Moreover, the formation of more product molecules than of reactant molecules represents the formation of a less organized or more random state.

CONVERSION OF PYRUVATE TO ACETYL-CoA

Two molecules of pyruvate are formed from glucose during glycolysis. Prior to the Krebs cycle, we consider the pyruvate dehydrogenase reaction. The oxidative decarboxylation of pyruvate yields acetyl-CoA in a reaction catalyzed by the pyruvate dehydrogenase multienzyme complex (Figure 8–2). A multienzyme complex is a physical aggregate of enzymes that catalyze a series of interrelated reactions. This reaction, moreover, is physiologically irreversible. The unidirectional nature of the reaction is related to (1) the exergonic decarboxylation and (2) the exergonic oxidation of an α-keto car-

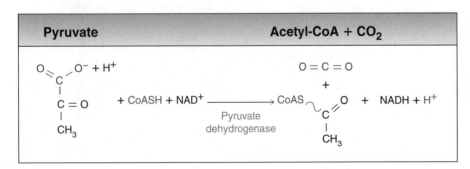

FIGURE 8–2. *Oxidative decarboxylation of pyruvate to carbon dioxide and acetyl-CoA.*

TABLE 8–1. Pyruvate Dehydrogenase Multienzyme Complex and Its Five Cofactors

Enzyme	Enzyme Designation	Prosthetic Cosubstrate	Soluble Substrate
Pyruvate decarboxylase	E_1	Thiamine pyrophosphate	—
Dihydrolipoyl transacetylase	E_2	Lipoamide	Coenzyme A
Dihydrolipoyl dehydrogenase	E_3	FAD	NAD^+

bonyl group by NAD^+ to form a carboxylate (Table 5–3).

The pyruvate dehydrogenase reaction requires the participation of three distinct enzyme activities (E_1, E_2, and E_3) and five different cofactors (Table 8–1). The advantage of multienzyme complexes is that the intermediates do not have to diffuse from enzyme to enzyme for the reaction to occur. All the reactions occur in close proximity in a multicomponent system.

The bioenergetics of the pyruvate dehydrogenase reaction aids in our understanding of this intricate process. First, the decarboxylation is exergonic. Second, a high-energy acetyl thioester forms during a reaction with lipoate (Figure 8–3). Third, acetyl-CoA, a product, forms by an isoergonic transthiolation. The effort that is required to decipher the intricacy of pyruvate dehydrogenase will pay multiple dividends because α-ketoglutarate dehydrogenase, α-ketobutyrate dehydrogenase, and branched-chain keto acid dehydrogenase use the same mechanism with three enzymes and five cofactors. Note that four of the five cofactors are vitamin derivatives (thiamine, pantothenate, riboflavin, and niacin).

OVERVIEW OF THE KREBS CYCLE

Acetyl-CoA is the source of the two-carbon fragments that are oxidized by the Krebs cycle. The structure of **coenzyme A** is shown in Figure 2–14. Acetyl-CoA results from the catabolism of carbohydrates, lipids, and amino acids (Figure 1–3).

A reaction between acetyl-CoA and oxaloacetate to form the six-carbon citrate initiates the cyclic process (Figure 8–4). Following an isomerization, a six-carbon compound undergoes oxidative decarboxylation to yield a five-carbon dicarboxylate. This five-carbon compound undergoes oxidative decarboxylation to form succinyl-CoA, a four-carbon derivative. The high-energy thioester of succinyl-CoA is conserved in a reaction that yields GTP from GDP and P_i by substrate level phosphorylation. Succinate is converted to oxaloacetate in three steps. The Krebs cycle pathway involves (1) a condensation and hydrolysis reaction, (2) two decarboxylation reactions, and (3) regeneration of oxaloacetate. The citrate synthase and α-ketoglutarate dehydrogenase reactions make the cycle function unidirectionally.

The Krebs cycle is catalytic in nature. The term catalytic in this context does not refer to the enzymes that catalyze the reactions. A catalyst is an agent that mediates a process and that is unchanged or regenerated at its completion. In the Krebs cycle, one molecule of oxaloacetate will mediate the oxidation of many molecules of acetyl-CoA because oxaloacetate is regenerated at the end of each oxidative sequence. One starts and ends with oxaloacetate, so in this sense the Krebs cycle functions catalytically. (The concept of the catalytic nature of the Krebs cycle is often difficult to grasp at first reading.)

In contrast to oxaloacetate, which can be reutilized, the acetyl group is formally consumed during each reaction cycle. The participation of acetyl-CoA is termed stoichiometric in contrast to catalytic. Stoichiometric is a chemical term indicating that the substrate is quantitatively consumed. A steady supply of acetyl-CoA must be available, since one molecule is destroyed during each turn of the cycle. Oxaloacetate is the **regenerating substrate,** and acetyl-CoA is the **stoichiometric substrate.**

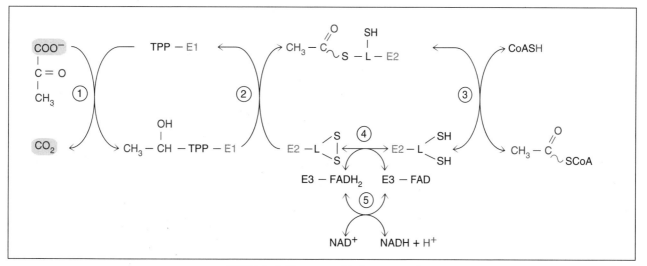

FIGURE 8–3. The pyruvate dehydrogenase reaction.

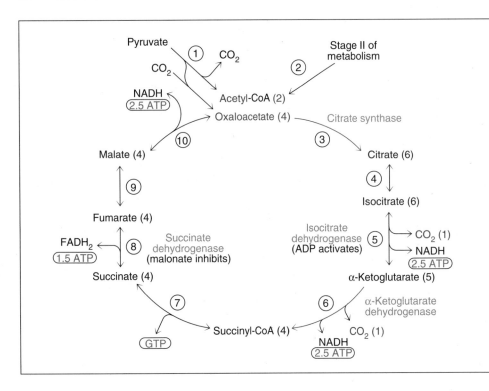

FIGURE 8–4. Overview of the Krebs cycle. *Acetyl-CoA (the stoichiometric substrate) reacts with oxaloacetate (the regenerating substrate) to initiate the cycle. The number of carbon atoms in each intermediate is shown. The two physiologically irreversible steps (catalyzed by citrate synthase and α-ketoglutarate dehydrogenase) are indicated by one-way arrows. The amount of ATP formed by oxidative phosphorylation is indicated.*

The net reaction of one turn of the Krebs cycle is given in equation 8.1:

$$
\begin{array}{ccc}
\text{Acetyl-CoA} & & 2\ CO_2 & \quad (8.1)\\
+ & & +\\
3\ NAD^+ & & 3\ NADH + 3\ H^+\\
+ & & +\\
FAD & \rightarrow & FADH_2\\
+ & & +\\
GDP + P_i & & GTP\\
+ & & +\\
2\ H_2O & & CoA
\end{array}
$$

Acetyl-CoA is oxidized by the reactions of the cycle. The standard free energy change for one turn of the Krebs cycle is about −47 kJ/mol (Table 8–2). NADH and FADH₂, reduced products of the process, will donate their reducing equivalents to the electron transport chain. Considerable energy is conserved when energy-producing exergonic reactions of electron transport are coupled to the endergonic formation of ATP (Chapter 9).

REACTIONS OF THE KREBS CYCLE

Initiation of the Cycle

Citrate synthase starts the Krebs cycle sequence by catalyzing the reaction of acetyl-CoA (the stoi-

TABLE 8–2. Reactions of the Krebs Cycle

Reaction	Enzyme	$\Delta G^{\circ\prime}$ per mole* (kJ)	Comments
1. Acetyl-CoA + oxaloacetate^{-2} + H$_2$O → citrate^{-3} + CoASH + H$^+$	Citrate synthase (condensing enzyme)	− 38.0	Irreversible
2. Citrate^{-3} ⇌ isocitrate^{-3}	Aconitase	6.66	
3. Isocitrate^{-3} + NAD$^+$ ⇌ α-ketoglutarate^{-2} + CO$_2$ + NADH	Isocitrate dehydrogenase	− 7.11	Regulatory enzyme
4. α-Ketoglutarate^{-2} + CoASH + NAD$^+$ → succinyl-CoA^{-1} + CO$_2$ + NADH	α-Ketoglutarate dehydrogenase	− 24.0†	Irreversible
5. Succinyl-CoA^{-1} + GDP^{-3} + P$_i^{-2}$ ⇌ succinate^{-2} + CoASH + GTP^{-4}	Succinyl CoA-synthetase (succinate thiokinase)	− 8.96‡	Substrate level phosphorylation
6. Succinate^{-2} + (FAD) ⇌ fumarate^{-2} + (FADH$_2$)	Succinate dehydrogenase	0.0	Inhibited by malonate
7. Fumarate^{-2} + H$_2$O ⇌ malate^{-2}	Fumarase	− 3.68	
8. Malate^{-2} + NAD$^+$ ⇌ oxaloacetate^{-2} + NADH + H$^+$	Malate dehydrogenase	28.0	
		− 47.09 *total*	

*Based on the data of M.J. Johnson at 25°C, pH 7.0. *In* P.D. Boyer, H. Lardy, and K. Myrbäck (eds.). *The Enzymes,* 2nd ed. New York, Academic Press, 1960, vol. 3, p. 407.

†Based on data in Tables 5–3 and 6–3.

‡Based on data in Table 6–3.

chiometric substrate), oxaloacetate (the regenerating substrate), and water to form citrate and coenzyme A. Note that this reaction of acetyl-CoA is not an acyl transfer reaction (Figure 8–5). Rather, the α-carbon of the acetyl group combines with the carbonyl group of oxaloacetate in a condensation reaction. A nonsystematic name for citrate synthase is condensing enzyme. Besides activating the acyl group for transfer reactions, formation of coenzyme A thioesters allows the acyl α-carbon to form a carbanion readily. The carbanion reacts with the electrophilic carbonyl group of oxaloacetate to form a new carbon-carbon bond (Figure 8–5). Following condensation, the hydrolysis of the thioester provides the major source of energy in driving the reaction from reactants toward products. The hydrolysis of both low- and high-energy linkages favors product formation (PRINCIPLE 5 OF BIOENERGETICS), and *the citrate synthase reaction is physiologically irreversible.*

Conversion of Citrate to Succinate

Aconitase catalyzes the elimination of water from citrate to produce *cis*-aconitate. Water combines with *cis*-aconitate to produce isocitrate. The isomerization is isoergonic and reversible. **Isocitrate dehydrogenase** catalyzes the decarboxylation that produces the first molecule of carbon dioxide. This is an oxidative decarboxylation coupled to the conversion of NAD^+ to $NADH + H^+$. The oxidation of an alcohol to a ketone by NAD^+ is endergonic, as exemplified by the lactate dehydrogenase reaction. Decarboxylations are exergonic (PRINCIPLE 6 OF BIOENERGETICS), and the decarboxylation provides a source of free energy to promote the overall reaction. Although the reaction is reversible *in vitro*, the forward reaction is favored under physiological conditions.

It is a paradox that the liberated carbon dioxide is not immediately derived from the acetyl group that condensed with oxaloacetate. Radiolabeling experiments show that the liberated carbon dioxide is derived originally from oxaloacetate. Although citrate lacks a chiral carbon atom, citrate is prochiral and the carboxyl groups are distinguishable. **Prochiral molecules** contain a carbon atom with three different substituents, and prochiral molecules can react stereospecifically with an enzyme's active site. Aconitase is the enzyme that distinguishes between the two different $-CH_2COO^-$ groups in citrate.

α-**Ketoglutarate dehydrogenase** catalyzes the second oxidative decarboxylation in the Krebs cycle. *The α-ketoglutarate dehydrogenase reaction is an exergonic oxidative decarboxylation and is unidirectional.* Carbon dioxide is liberated, NAD^+ is reduced, and succinyl-CoA is formed. Both decarboxylation and oxidation of a carbonyl group by NAD^+ are exergonic. This reaction is chemically analogous to the pyruvate dehydrogenase reaction. The reaction is mediated by a multienzyme complex composed of three different proteins and the same five cofactors used by pyruvate dehydrogenase (Table 8–1).

Succinate thiokinase catalyzes a reaction involving succinyl-CoA, GDP, and P_i to form succinate and GTP. Succinyl-CoA contains an energy-rich thioester linkage. The conservation of the energy-rich thioester of succinyl-CoA as a high-energy bond of phosphate is significant. The number of high-energy bonds in the reactants and products is the same (two), and the reaction is functionally isoergonic. This reaction is an example of substrate level phosphorylation; an energy-rich nucleoside triphosphate is formed by a process that does not involve the electron transport chain and oxygen.

Conversion of Succinate to Oxaloacetate

Succinate dehydrogenase catalyzes the oxidation of succinate to fumarate. The enzyme is located in the inner mitochondrial membrane. The reduced, enzyme-bound $FADH_2$ donates its electrons to coenzyme Q of the electron transport chain, and this initiates the synthesis of 1.5 moles of ATP per mole of $FADH_2$ (Chapter 9). (The oxidation of 1 mole of NADH initiates the synthesis of 2.5 moles of ATP.) The succinate dehydrogenase reaction is a simple oxidation-reduction reaction and is bidirectional (PRINCIPLE 7 OF BIOENERGETICS). Succinate dehydrogenase possesses two additional noteworthy properties. First, succinate dehydrogenase is inhibited by malonate ($^-OOC-CH_2-COO^-$), a three-carbon analogue of succinate. This property aided Krebs in the elucidation of this pathway by blocking the conversion of succinate to oxaloacetate. Second, succinate dehydrogenase is an integral inner mitochondrial membrane protein. Succinate dehydrogenase is the only Krebs cycle enzyme that is embedded within the inner mitochondrial membrane; all the other Krebs cycle enzymes occur in the mitochondrial matrix.

Fumarase catalyzes the hydration of fumarate to form malate in a reversible reaction. This reaction is an isoergonic lyase reaction. **Malate dehydrogenase** catalyzes the oxidation of malate by NAD^+ to produce oxaloacetate and NADH. The bioenergetics are similar to that of lactate dehydrogenase, and the equilibrium favors malate and not oxaloacetate. This is a simple oxidation-reduction reaction, however, and is bidirectional. Oxaloacetate can be reutilized in the oxidation of a second molecule of acetyl-CoA. This entire process of coupled reactions can then recur many times owing to the continuous regeneration of oxaloacetate.

ATP YIELD FOR KREBS CYCLE AND OXIDATIVE PHOSPHORYLATION REACTIONS

The standard free energy changes in the Krebs cycle are given in Table 8–2. Note that the stan-

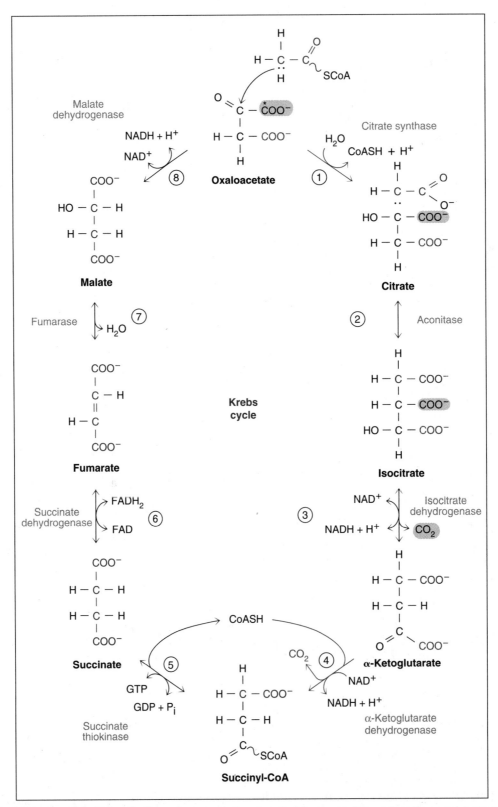

FIGURE 8–5. The eight reactions of the Krebs cycle. *The carbon atoms of carbon dioxide are not derived from the acetyl group added during this round of the catalytic cycle. Following the conversion of succinyl-CoA to succinate (reaction 5), the internal and external carbon atoms become equivalent.*

dard free energy change for the synthesis of citrate is equivalent to that of the hydrolysis of a thioester (Table 6–3). This hydrolysis drives the reaction toward the formation of citrate and makes the reaction physiologically irreversible. The standard free energy change of the isocitrate dehydrogenase reaction is -7 kJ/mol, but the forward reaction is greatly favored under physiological conditions. The free energy change of the isocitrate dehydrogenase reaction under physiological conditions is sufficient to allow this reaction to play the main regulatory role in the cycle. The next reaction (catalyzed by α-ketoglutarate dehydrogenase) is physiologically irreversible. *The irreversible α-ketoglutarate dehydrogenase reaction compels the cycle to function unidirectionally.*

We consider one ATP as equivalent to one high-energy bond for historical reasons. The reactants are ADP and P_i, and they form one new energy-rich linkage. This corresponds to the net formation of one energy-rich bond but disregards the high-energy bond present in ADP. Oxidative phosphorylation and the formation of ATP from ADP and P_i was discovered more than a decade before the conversion of ATP to AMP and PP_i. Because of historical precedence, the synthesis of one high-energy bond was equated with the conversion of ADP to ATP, and this convention continues. *An ATP equivalent is usually considered as one high-energy bond.* When ATP is converted to AMP and $2 P_i$, this represents the utilization of two high-energy bonds and is considered, by convention, two ATP equivalents even though a single ATP is involved. These conventions are followed throughout this book. This subtle point is sometimes difficult to grasp at first reading but should become second nature with repeated exposure and usage. Again, the conversion of ATP to ADP and P_i represents one high-energy bond or one ATP equivalent (easy to comprehend), and the conversion of 1 ATP to AMP and $2 P_i$ represents two high-energy bonds (easy) or *two* ATP equivalents (difficult).

One turn of the Krebs cycle produces one molecule of GTP by substrate level phosphorylation, three molecules of NADH, and one molecule of $FADH_2$. The oxidation of these reductants by the respiratory chain will lead to the production of ATP as described in Chapter 9. The oxidation of one mole of NADH will sustain the net formation of 2.5 moles of ATP, and the oxidation of a mole of succinate via $FADH_2$ will sustain the net formation of 1.5 moles of ATP. We can now calculate the yield of ATP from the complete oxidation of acetyl-CoA as shown in Table 8–3. We obtain a value of 10 moles of ATP per mole of acetyl-CoA. The conversion of pyruvate to acetyl-CoA results in the formation of one mole of intramitochondrial NADH. One mole of pyruvate yields 12.5 moles of ATP (10 ATP per acetyl-CoA and 2.5 from 1 NADH). How fractional values are obtained is considered in Chapter 9.

BIOENERGETICS OF DEHYDROGENASE REACTIONS

Simple oxidation-reduction reactions are reversible (PRINCIPLE 7 OF BIOENERGETICS). Simple oxidation-reduction reactions are defined as those (1) not involving a decarboxylation and (2) not directly involving molecular oxygen. Some oxidation-reduction reactions associated with decarboxylation are reversible, and others are not. Under physiological conditions, low carbon dioxide concentrations (millimolar) and high $NAD(P)^+/NAD(P)H$ ratios favor a unidirectional reaction in the direction of decarboxylation. We consider reactions involving oxygen in Chapter 9 and find that the reduction of molecular oxygen to water, R–OH, or R=O is physiologically irreversible. Since most oxidation-reduction reactions of metabolism are classified as simple, PRINCIPLE 7 OF BIOENERGETICS has broad applicability and provides considerable help and insight in the study of biochemistry.

AMPHIBOLIC NATURE OF THE KREBS CYCLE

As important as the Krebs cycle is in the oxidation of acetyl-CoA to carbon dioxide, with the concomitant formation of reducing equivalents and nucleoside triphosphate, this is but one facet of its overall usefulness. The intermediates in the cycle also serve as precursors for a variety of biosynthetic reactions. Krebs cycle participation in catabolic and anabolic reactions has prompted the use of the term **amphibolic** to describe the function of the tricarboxylate cycle in intermediary metabolism.

TABLE 8–3. ATP Yield from the Oxidation of Acetyl-CoA and Pyruvate by the Krebs Citric Acid Cycle and Oxidative Phosphorylation in Mitochondria*

Substrate	ATP Formed
NADH	2.5
$FADH_2$	1.5
Acetyl-CoA	
Isocitrate dehydrogenase (NADH)	2.5
α-Ketoglutarate dehydrogenase (NADH)	2.5
Succinate thiokinase (GTP)	1
Succinate dehydrogenase ($FADH_2$)	1.5
Malate dehydrogenase (NADH)	2.5
Yield from the oxidation of acetyl-CoA	10 *total*
Pyruvate	
Pyruvate dehydrogenase (NADH)	2.5
Acetyl-CoA	10
Yield from the oxidation of pyruvate	12.5 *total*

*ATP yield based on the values given by Hinkle and coworkers for animal mitochondria. (The yield for prokaryotes is generally less than the values given here.) Data from P.C. Hinkle, A. Kumar, A. Resetar, and D.L. Harris. Mechanistic stoichiometry of mitochondrial oxidative phosphorylation. Biochemistry 30:3576–3582, 1991.

Pyruvate Carboxylase Reaction

Let us consider the formation of Krebs cycle intermediates. These reactions are called **anaplerotic** (Greek "to fill up"). The generation of oxaloacetate from pyruvate and carbon dioxide is an important anaplerotic reaction. The carboxylation of pyruvate to oxaloacetate is endergonic, and chemical energy is required to sustain this reaction. **Pyruvate carboxylase** catalyzes an ATP-dependent carboxylation that yields oxaloacetate from bicarbonate and pyruvate (Figure 8–6). The standard free energy change for the ATP-dependent pyruvate carboxylase reaction is -3.2 kJ/mol. Under physiological conditions with a high [ATP]/[ADP] ratio, the reaction functions in the direction of oxaloacetate biosynthesis. Let us examine the bioenergetics of the component parts of the reaction:

$$\Delta G^{\circ\prime} \text{ (kJ/mol)}$$

			$\Delta G^{\circ\prime}$ (kJ/mol)	
Pyruvate$^-$ + HCO$_3^-$	$\rightleftharpoons$	oxaloacetate^{2-} + H$_2$O	$+27.2$	(8.2)
ATP + H$_2$O	$\rightleftharpoons$	ADP + P$_i$	-30.4	(8.3)
Pyruvate$^-$ + HCO$_3^-$ + ATP	$\rightleftharpoons$	oxaloacetate^{2-} + ADP + P$_i$	-3.2	(8.4)

The carboxylation of pyruvate is endergonic, but the conversion of ATP to ADP and P$_i$ is exergonic. The cleavage of ATP thus provides the chemical energy to promote the carboxylation reaction.

Let us examine the mechanism of this carboxylation reaction. Biotin serves as an intermediate carrier of activated carbon dioxide. Biotin is covalently attached to a lysyl residue of pyruvate carboxylase. Biotin and the lysyl side chain form a long mobile carrier of about 1.3 nm that is capable of accepting bicarbonate at one active site of the enzyme and transferring it to another active site of the same enzyme for further reaction.

The intermediate steps in the biotinyl transfer reaction most likely occur as illustrated in Figure 8–7. Although ATP is cleaved to ADP and P$_i$ during this process, the hydrolysis occurs indirectly. The oxygen of bicarbonate becomes covalently attached to the γ-phosphoryl group as ADP is displaced. Inorganic phosphate is released as the carboxyl group becomes attached to the biotinyl group. As noted in Chapter 6, the hydrolysis of ATP *per se* results in heat. To perform chemical work, the formation of activated intermediates during the cleavage of ATP is necessary as described for the pyruvate carboxylase reaction. The pyruvate carboxylase reaction exemplifies the concept of active intermediates being produced during ATP utilization.

The carboxy-biotinyl bond represents an activated carboxyl group. Its standard free energy of hydrolysis is -19.7 kJ mol^{-1}. This standard free energy of hydrolysis is less than that of other groups, but nonetheless this represents a respectable group transfer potential. *It is noteworthy that acetyl-CoA serves as an allosteric activator in the pyruvate carboxylase reaction* (Table 25–1). The activity of pyruvate carboxylase is nil in the absence of acetyl-CoA.

Malic Enzyme Reaction

Another specialized process that leads to the carboxylation of pyruvate is catalyzed by malic enzyme or malate dehydrogenase (decarboxylating; NADP), shown in Figure 8–8. The carboxylation part of the reaction is endergonic (PRINCIPLE 6 OF BIOENERGETICS). The reduction of a ketone to an alcohol by NADPH is exergonic (as for lactate dehydrogenase). The net standard free energy change is -2.6 kJ/mol. The conversion of products to reactants is an example of an oxidative decarboxylation. The reaction is reversible, and the direction in which the reaction proceeds depends upon the physiological requirements. Malic enzyme is important in the generation of NADPH, and this role is probably more important than the generation of malate.

REGULATORY STEPS IN THE OXIDATION OF PYRUVATE AND ACETYL-CoA

Pyruvate dehydrogenase and isocitrate dehydrogenase are the two main regulatory enzymes of mitochondrial oxidation reactions. The regulation of pyruvate dehydrogenase is intricate. **Pyruvate dehydrogenase** activity is regulated by phosphorylation-dephosphorylation reactions. The phosphorylated dehydrogenase is less active than the

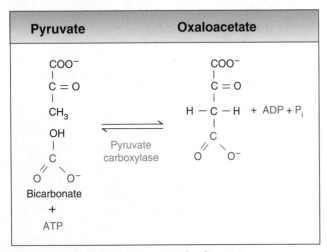

FIGURE 8–6. Pyruvate carboxylase reaction.

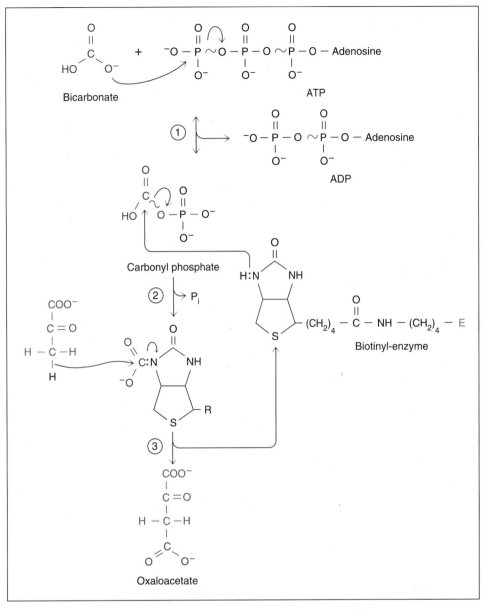

FIGURE 8–7. Role of biotin in the pyruvate carboxylase reaction. *(1) Bicarbonate reacts with ATP to form an energy-rich carbonyl ~phosphate, a mixed-acid anhydride, and ADP. (2) Biotin, the prosthetic group of pyruvate carboxylase, reacts with carbonyl ~phosphate to displace phosphate and form a carboxybiotin intermediate. (3) Pyruvate reacts with carboxybiotin to form oxaloacetate, and the enzyme is regenerated.*

unphosphorylated enzyme (Table 25–2). This observation and the metabolic logic of the cell can be used to deduce the effects of allosteric regulators of **pyruvate dehydrogenase kinase,** the enzyme that catalyzes the phosphorylation reaction (Figure 8–9).

Pyruvate dehydrogenase kinase is activated by acetyl-CoA and NADH. Activation of pyruvate dehydrogenase kinase by these compounds, which indicate a high-energy charge, mediates a decrease in pyruvate dehydrogenase activity by enzyme phosphorylation. Because of diminished pyruvate dehydrogenase activity as a result of phosphorylation, less acetyl-CoA, NADH, and ATP are generated.

Isocitrate dehydrogenase activity is regulated directly by ADP, which is stimulatory, and indirectly by energy charge (Table 25–1). When ATP levels fall, ADP is generated. This serves as a signal that additional Krebs cycle activity is required to re-

generate ATP, thus following the metabolic logic of the cell. Why is isocitrate dehydrogenase a regulatory enzyme? Why would considerable citrate synthesis occur at all when the catabolism of acetyl-CoA to carbon dioxide is not advantageous? The explanation for this apparent paradox is that the reactions of the Krebs cycle produce citrate for anabolic fatty acid biosynthesis. The oxidation of pyruvate to acetyl-CoA occurs within the mitochondrion. Acetyl-CoA serves as the precursor for fatty acid biosynthesis *de novo* in the cytosol. Acetyl groups are not transported across the inner mitochondrial membrane directly. To export two-carbon fragments, condensation with oxaloacetate to yield citrate is required. Citrate is then transported across the membrane to the cytosol, where it is converted to acetyl-CoA (Figure 11–14).

Citrate synthesis must exceed citrate degradation in the mitochondrion during fatty acid biosyn-

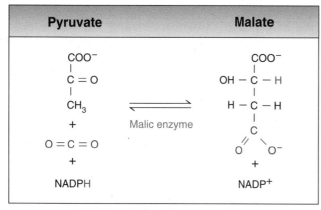

Pyruvate	Malate

$$
\begin{array}{ccc}
COO^- & & COO^- \\
| & & | \\
C = O & & OH - C - H \\
| & & | \\
CH_3 & \xrightleftharpoons{\text{Malic enzyme}} & H - C - H \\
+ & & | \\
 & & C \\
O = C = O & & O \quad O^- \\
+ & & + \\
NADPH & & NADP^+
\end{array}
$$

FIGURE 8–8. The malic enzyme reaction.

thesis from carbohydrates. The cell must, therefore, allow citrate synthesis to occur and to control its degradation. The first **exergonic** reaction in citrate catabolism is not catalyzed by aconitase but by isocitrate dehydrogenase, and this explains the importance of isocitrate dehydrogenase in the control of Krebs cycle metabolism.

CLINICAL ASPECTS OF OXIDATIVE METABOLISM

Pyruvate Dehydrogenase Deficiency

▶ The essential nature of pyruvate dehydrogenase and the Krebs cycle in human metabolism suggests that deficiencies in any of these activities would be incompatible with life. This supposition is substantiated by a paucity of cases of inborn errors of metabolism of enzymes in this pathway. The reported number of cases of pyruvate dehydrogenase deficiency is less than 100. If pyruvate cannot be metabolized by pyruvate dehydrogenase or subsequent reactions, pyruvate is converted to lactic acid. These disorders produce lactic acidosis, and affected individuals generally succumb early to their illness. These individuals frequently exhibit severe neurological deficits. ◀

Hepatic Encephalopathy

▶ In contrast to the rare **inborn errors of metabolism** involving pyruvate dehydrogenase or the Krebs cycle enzymes, hepatic encephalopathy is common. In Chapter 13, we consider the metabolism and disposal of ammonium ion by the urea cycle in liver. During severe liver disease that can result from cirrhosis or hepatitis, liver metabolism is compromised and blood ammonium levels increase. The encephalopathy that occurs during hepatic failure is characterized by confusion, stupor, coma, and sometimes death.

The precise mechanism for the encephalopathy is unclear, and there are probably several contributing factors. Many studies have shown that oxygen consumption in brain is markedly decreased (by 50%) during this condition. This finding shows that the brain's oxidative activity is decreased, but it does not pinpoint the mechanism. Three of the favored hypotheses for this encephalopathy involve derangements in Krebs cycle activity.

One hypothesis is that there is a decrease in

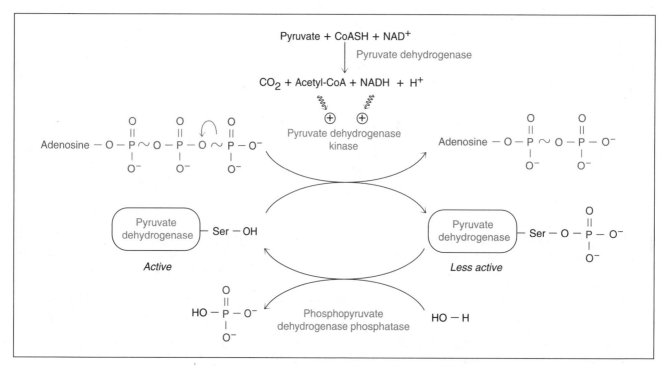

FIGURE 8–9. Phosphorylation and dephosphorylation of pyruvate dehydrogenase.

Krebs cycle intermediates as they are converted to glutamate from ammonium ion and α-ketoglutarate in an NAD(P)H-dependent reduction catalyzed by glutamate dehydrogenase. Because of this process, Krebs cycle intermediates are lost and Krebs cycle activity is diminished. A second hypothesis is that there is a decrease of pyruvate and α-ketoglutarate dehydrogenase activity during hepatic coma. This is postulated to be a direct effect of ammonium ion. A third hypothesis is that a shuttle for transporting reducing equivalents into brain mitochondria (Chapter 9) is inhibited during hepatic encephalopathy.

GABA (γ-aminobutyric acid), illustrated in Figure 19–20, is the chief inhibitory neurotransmitter in brain. The number of GABA receptors is increased during hepatic encephalopathy. Brain cells may be more sensitive to GABA, and increased sensitivity to an inhibitory neurotransmitter may lead to decreased neuronal activity and encephalopathy. More work is required before a complete explanation of hepatic encephalopathy is available. ◄

SUMMARY

The exergonic nature of decarboxylation reactions provides an explanation for the metabolism of pyruvate and acetyl-CoA. The conversion of pyruvate to acetyl-CoA involves a decarboxylation, and the metabolism of acetyl-CoA by the Krebs cycle involves two decarboxylation reactions.

Pyruvate dehydrogenase is a multienzyme complex that catalyzes the conversion of pyruvate to acetyl-CoA and carbon dioxide. The complex consists of three enzyme activities (E_1, E_2, and E_3), four vitamin derivatives (thiamine pyrophosphate, coenzyme A, FAD, and NAD^+), and lipoate. This reaction provides acetyl-CoA, the stoichiometric substrate, for the Krebs cycle. Pyruvate dehydrogenase is inhibited by the phosphorylation that is catalyzed by pyruvate dehydrogenase kinase. ATP, NADH, and acetyl-CoA inhibit pyruvate dehydrogenase, and this regulation thus follows the molecular logic of the cell. These three agents, which result from the activity of pyruvate dehydrogenase, activate the kinase and thereby inhibit pyruvate dehydrogenase indirectly. A phosphatase catalyzes the formation of unphosphorylated pyruvate dehydrogenase from the phosphorylated form during an exergonic hydrolysis reaction.

The Krebs cycle is initiated by a reaction between acetyl-CoA and oxaloacetate. This formation of citrate is unidirectional because of the exergonic hydrolysis of coenzyme A following the condensation reaction. Acetyl-CoA is consumed (the stoichiometric substrate) by the metabolic cycle; oxaloacetate is regenerated (the regenerating substrate). Isocitrate dehydrogenase, which catalyzes the first decarboxylation of the cycle, is activated allosterically by ADP. α-Ketoglutarate dehydrogenase, which catalyzes the second decarboxylation, catalyzes the second unidirectional reaction of the cycle. There are three NADH-generating reactions and one FADH$_2$-generating reaction (succinate dehydrogenase) in the Krebs cycle. GTP is formed during the action of the cycle by substrate level phosphorylation involving succinate thiokinase. The molar yield of ATP from oxidative phosphorylation in mitochondria is 1.5 per mole of $FADH_2$ and 2.5 per mole of NADH. The net yield of ATP in mitochondria from the oxidation of one mole of acetyl-CoA to carbon dioxide and water via the Krebs cycle and oxidative phosphorylation is 1 (substrate level phosphorylation) + 3 × 2.5 (for 3 NADH) + 1.5 (for 1 $FADH_2$) for a total of 10 moles of ATP. Since the conversion of pyruvate to acetyl-CoA generates 1 NADH, the net yield of ATP resulting from the complete oxidation of one mole of pyruvate is 10 + 2.5, or 12.5, moles.

Pyruvate carboxylase catalyzes an ATP-dependent carboxylation of pyruvate to form oxaloacetate. Biotin is a common cofactor for ATP-dependent carboxylation reactions. A carboxybiotin intermediate, an active carbon dioxide, participates in the reaction. It is noteworthy that acetyl-CoA is required by pyruvate carboxylase for expression of its activity. The Krebs cycle is the final common pathway of aerobic metabolism.

SELECTED READINGS

Krebs, H.A. The history of the tricarboxylic acid cycle. Perspectives in Biology and Medicine 14:154–170, 1970.

Krebs, H.A. *Reminiscences and Reflections.* London, Clarendon Press, 1981.

Krebs, H.A. The tricarboxylic acid cycle. *In* D.M. Greenberg (ed.). *Chemical Pathways of Metabolism.* New York, Academic Press, 1954, vol. 1, pp. 109–171.

Krebs, H.A., and W.A. Johnson. The role of citric acid in the intermediate metabolism in animal tissues. Enzymologia 4:148–156, 1937.

Robinson, B.H. Lactic acidemia. *In* C.R. Scriver, A.L. Beaudet, W.S. Sly, and D. Valle (eds.). *The Metabolic Basis of Inherited Disease,* 6th ed. New York, McGraw-Hill Book Company, 1989, pp. 869–888.

Sherlock, S. Fulminant hepatic failure. Advances in Internal Medicine 38:245–267, 1993.

Wiegand, G., and S.J. Remington. Citrate synthase: Structure, control and mechanism. Annual Review of Biophysics and Biophysical Chemistry 15:97–117, 1986.

OXIDATIVE

PHOSPHORYLATION

*If you accept the statement that only uninhibited investigators use inhibitors, you will soon find out
what kind of people work in the field of oxidative phosphorylation.*

—EFRAM RACKER

GENERATION OF ATP

The combined action of the Krebs cycle and oxidative phosphorylation is responsible for most of the ATP generated in humans. The exergonic transfer of electrons from NADH or $FADH_2$ to oxygen sustains the endergonic synthesis of ATP from ADP and P_i by **oxidative phosphorylation.** Oxidative phosphorylation, but not substrate level phosphorylation, requires an electron transport chain, molecular oxygen, and an ATP synthase.

The **chemiosmotic theory** combines the characteristics of (1) chemical reactions and (2) vectorial ion gradients (osmotic gradients). The chemiosmotic theory has broad applicability and is one of the most important unifying concepts in bioenergetics (PRINCIPLE 12 OF BIOCHEMISTRY). The chemiosmotic, or Mitchell, theory provides the conceptual framework for understanding the mechanism of oxidative phosphorylation. *The exergonic reactions of electron transport generate a proton gradient across a membrane that sustains ATP formation.*

The complete oxidation of organic fuel molecules to carbon dioxide and water liberates much more energy than can be obtained without oxygen utilization. The standard free energy changes during the conversion of glucose to (1) lactate, anaerobically, or (2) carbon dioxide and water, aerobically, are given by the following two equations:

$$
\begin{array}{llll}
 & & \Delta G^{\circ\prime} & \\
 & & \text{(kJ/mol)} & \\
\text{Glucose} & \rightarrow \quad 2 \text{ lactate}^{-1} & -196 & (9.1) \\
 & \qquad\quad + & & \\
 & \qquad\quad 2 \text{ H}^+ & & \\
\text{Glucose} & \rightarrow \quad 6 \text{ CO}_2 & -2870 & (9.2) \\
\quad + & \qquad\quad + & & \\
6 \text{ O}_2 & \qquad\quad 6 \text{ H}_2\text{O} & &
\end{array}
$$

In the reactions of the Krebs cycle, carbon dioxide, NADH, and $FADH_2$ are produced. NADH and $FADH_2$ donate electrons to the electron transport chain that passes them sequentially to O_2 to generate chemical energy and to form water. The generation of ATP from ADP and P_i ($\Delta G^{\circ\prime}$ positive) is coupled to a series of electron-transfer reactions ($\Delta G^{\circ\prime}$ negative) from reductants (NADH, $FADH_2$) to oxygen.

MITOCHONDRIAL STRUCTURE

Oxidative phosphorylation, which has an absolute requirement for a membrane, occurs in the mitochondrion, the powerhouse of the cell (Table 1–1). The inner mitochondrial membrane (Figure 9–1) contains the **electron transport chain** and the **ATP synthase** that mediates ATP formation. **Succinate dehydrogenase** of the Krebs cycle, which forms part of the electron transport chain, is an integral inner mitochondrial membrane protein. The remainder of the Krebs cycle enzymes are located in the matrix. The mitochondrion also con-

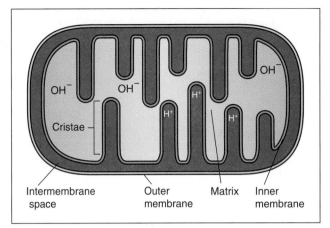

FIGURE 9–1. The mitochondrion. *Mitochondria are about 2 μm in length. Cristae, infoldings of the inner membrane, increase surface area and biochemical capacity. Electron transport generates a proton gradient, acid outside.*

tains the enzymes responsible for the β-oxidation of fatty acids. The reducing equivalents (NADH, $FADH_2$) formed during β-oxidation and during Krebs cycle activity are intramitochondrial. These reductants are generated at a location where they can readily react with the electron transport chain.

Electron transport from reductants to oxygen provides the energy to translocate protons from the interior to the exterior of the inner membrane, thereby establishing a proton-motive force. Exergonic proton transport from the exterior to the interior sustains ATP generation. Most oxygen consumed by humans is metabolized within the mitochondrion, and a typical cell such as a hepatocyte contains about 800 mitochondria.

The inner mitochondrial membrane, in contrast to the outer membrane, is impermeable to metabolites such as ATP, ADP, P_i, H^+, fatty acids, and small proteins. The inner membrane separates cytosolic metabolites from intramitochondrial substances. During metabolism, it is necessary to export considerable ATP from the mitochondrion to the cytosol before use. ATP is a charged, polar metabolite that cannot diffuse through lipid bilayers. The inner membrane contains several transport proteins, or **translocases,** one of which exchanges intramitochondrial ATP for extramitochondrial ADP. The ATP-ADP exchange protein is inhibited by a plant toxin called **atractyloside.**

Antiport describes the movement of metabolites across a membrane in opposite directions and is exemplified by the exchange of ATP for ADP. **Symport** involves the cotransport of two substances across a membrane in the same direction and is exemplified by pyruvate transport into the mitochondrion (Table 9–1). The transport of phosphate requires the formal cotransport of a proton. With phosphate transport, however, a proton is not involved. Rather, phosphate transport involves antiport of negatively charged hydroxide ion. The antiport of hydroxide is formally and bioenergetically equivalent to the symport of a proton.

TABLE 9–1. Mitochondrial Translocases*

Transporter	Function
Adenine nucleotides	$ADP^{-3} \rightleftarrows ATP^{-4}$
Phosphate	$P_i^- \rightleftarrows OH^-$
α-Ketoglutarate	Malate $\rightleftarrows$ α-Ketoglutarate
Glutamate-aspartate	Glu $\rightleftarrows$ Asp
Pyruvate	Pyruvate$^-$ H$^+$ $\rightleftarrows$
Fatty acid	Acylcarnitine $\rightleftarrows$ Carnitine
Dicarboxylate	Malate $\rightleftarrows$ P_i
Tricarboxylate	Citrate $\rightleftarrows$ Malate

*These proteins are located within the inner mitochondrial membrane. These transport processes involve symport (movement of metabolites in the same direction) or antiport (movement of metabolites in the opposite direction).

Some important compounds are not transported through the inner mitochondrial membrane, including NAD+/NADH, NADP+/NADPH, coenzyme A and its derivatives, and oxaloacetate. The lack of a transport system for oxaloacetate prevents its depletion from the mitochondrion. Transport of reducing equivalents across the inner mitochondrial membrane is mediated by the malate-aspartate shuttle and the glycerol phosphate shuttle. A given cell contains predominantly one or the other of these two systems.

Malate-Aspartate Shuttle

The **malate-aspartate shuttle** is intricate, requiring translocases that exchange (1) malate for α-ketoglutarate and (2) aspartate for glutamate (Table 9–1). Two sets of enzymes (intramitochondrial and extramitochondrial) are also required. These include (1) malate dehydrogenase and (2) aspartate aminotransferase (Figure 9–2). The malate-aspartate shuttle can transfer reducing equivalents from NADH into or out of the mitochondrion, depending upon the metabolic need. *The eventual yield of ATP is 2.5 moles per mole of cytosolic NADH that is oxidized using this shuttle.* The malate-aspartate shuttle system is located in liver and heart cells.

Glycerol Phosphate Shuttle

The glycerol phosphate shuttle is a second system for the transport of cytosolic reducing equivalents to the mitochondrial electron transport chain. This shuttle involves separate cytosolic and mitochondrial glycerol phosphate dehydrogenase enzymes (Figure 9–3). *The eventual yield of ATP is 1.5 moles per mole of cytosolic NADH oxidized.* Unlike the malate-aspartate shuttle, the glycerol phosphate shuttle is unable to transport mitochondrial reducing equivalents to the cytosol. The glycerol phosphate shuttle system is located in brain and muscle cells.

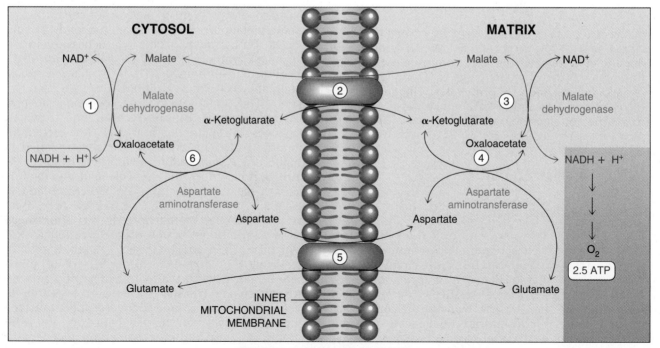

FIGURE 9–2. The malate-aspartate shuttle.

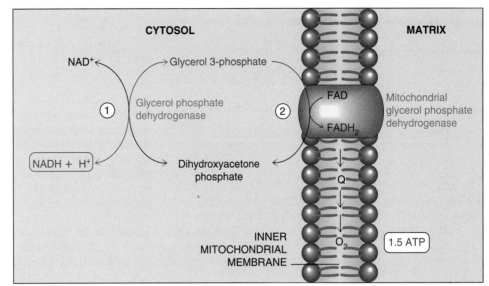

FIGURE 9–3. *The glycerol phosphate shuttle.*

COMPONENTS OF THE ELECTRON TRANSPORT CHAIN

Before considering the pathway for electron transport in mitochondria, we first consider the chemical nature of the four classes of components involved in electron transport. These constituents of electron transport include (1) flavoproteins (containing flavin mononucleotide, or FMN, and flavin adenine dinucleotide, or FAD), (2) coenzyme Q, (3) iron-sulfur proteins, and (4) cytochromes.

FMN and **FAD** undergo reversible oxidation-reduction reactions (Figure 2–12). FMN is bound firmly to complex I of the respiratory chain and does not function as a diffusible cosubstrate. FAD is tightly linked to complex II or succinate dehydrogenase. The flavins are derivatives of the vitamin riboflavin.

Coenzyme Q, in contrast to the flavin nucleotides, is diffusible and can move from donor to acceptor molecules during electron transport. The name coenzyme Q was initially given to a *q*uinone. It was also named ubiquinone because of its *u*biquitous or widespread distribution. Coenzyme Q is a benzoquinone with an unsaturated isoprenoid side chain (Figure 9–4A). The names coenzyme Q and ubiquinone and the abbreviations CoQ and UQ are used interchangeably. A subscript indicates the number of isoprenoid (five-carbon) units attached to the quinone ring, for example, CoQ_6 or CoQ_{10}. CoQ_{10} is the homologue that occurs in humans.

Iron-sulfur centers, like flavin nucleotides, are tightly bound to their proteins. The number of iron atoms in iron-sulfur centers varies from protein to protein. One, two, four, or more iron atoms are found. The structures of representative iron-sulfur

FIGURE 9–4. A. *Coenzyme Q.* *Coenzyme Q, a quinone, is a two-electron carrier. Quinones are aromatic dioxo compounds.* B. ***Representative iron-sulfur centers.*** *Iron-sulfur centers are one-electron carriers.*

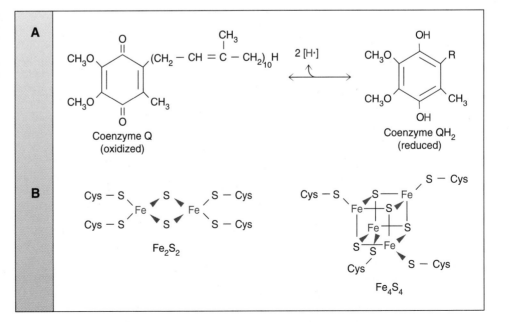

TABLE 9-2. Heme Components Found in Specific Cytochromes and Oxygen-Binding Proteins

Heme Group	Associated Protein
Heme a	Cytochrome a, a_3
Heme b	Hemoglobin, myoglobin, cytochrome b
Heme c	Cytochrome c
Protoheme	Cytochrome P-450

centers are illustrated in Figure 9-4B. The iron is linked to elemental sulfur (sulfide) and to cysteine thiol (-SH) groups contributed by the protein. Although several iron atoms may occur in a single center, iron-sulfur centers participate in one-electron transfer reactions.

Cytochromes are the final classes of components that participate in electron transport. They are so named because they are colored cellular components (cyto "cell," chrome "color"). The cytochromes are heme proteins. **Heme** is the iron-porphyrin that occurs in hemoglobin and myoglobin. The main varieties of cytochromes in mitochondria are the a, b, and c types of cytochromes. This classification of cytochromes is based on spectroscopic analysis. The cytochrome families are subclassified in terms of the historical order of their discovery (b_1, b_2, b_3 . . .) or the wavelength (nm) of a characteristic spectral absorption peak (b_{562}, b_{566}). Cytochromes are composed of specific proteins and hemes. The types of cytochrome are listed in Table 9-2, and the structures of three major varieties of heme are illustrated in Figure 9-5. Iron in cytochromes, but not hemoglobin, undergoes physiological oxidation-reduction between the ferrous (+2) and ferric (+3) states. Heme b in hemoglobin functions in the ferrous state.

PATHWAY OF MITOCHONDRIAL ELECTRON TRANSPORT

Complexes I, II, III, and IV

The components of the respiratory electron transport chain are found in the inner mitochondrial membrane. The electron transport chain consists of four independent complexes (I, II, III, and IV). Coenzyme Q and cytochrome c transport electrons between the complexes. Coenzyme Q transports electrons from complexes I and II to complex III; cytochrome c transports electrons from complex III to complex IV (Figure 9-6A). The order of the components that transport electrons approximates the increase in standard reduction potential, and this reaction sequence for transport is thermodynamically favored (Table 5-3). *The transfer of electrons from reductant to oxidant is exergonic; electron transfer proceeds with a decrease in free energy.* Part of the free energy of electron transport

is used to sustain ATP synthesis by oxidative phosphorylation.

The pathway for electron transport in mitochondria is shown in Figure 9-6B. NADH donates its electrons to complex I. Proton translocation reactions at site 1 provide energy for the synthesis of one mole of ATP per mole of NADH. ATP synthesis does not occur at site 1 *per se*; rather, ATP synthesis occurs on a protein called **ATP synthase.** Electrons are transferred from complex I to coenzyme Q to produce coenzyme QH_2. The flavin dehydrogenases such as succinate dehydrogenase (complex II) transport electrons to coenzyme Q without providing energy for proton translocation or ATP formation. Coenzyme QH_2, in turn, donates its electrons to complex III. Proton translocation at site 2 provides energy for the synthesis of 0.5 moles of ATP per mole of NADH or $FADH_2$.

Cytochrome c carries an electron from complex III to complex IV (cytochrome oxidase). Cytochrome c is a small (10 kDa), well-characterized protein. *Cytochrome c is, moreover, the only cytochrome of the mitochondrial electron transport chain that is hydrophilic* and resolvable from membranes without detergent. All the other cytochromes are integral inner mitochondrial membrane proteins and are lipophilic.

Cytochrome a,a_3 can be isolated as cytochrome oxidase or complex IV. The cytochrome oxidase reaction accounts for more than 95% of all oxygen consumed by humans. The reduction of oxygen by cytochrome oxidase accounts for the production of about 300 mL of water per day; this water is called metabolic water (Table 2-7). Besides cytochromes a and a_3, the oxidase complex contains two copper ions, each of which undergoes repetitive reduction (+1) and oxidation (+2). Proton translocation in complex IV provides the energy for the synthesis of one mole of ATP per mole of NADH or $FADH_2$.

Reactions of Molecular Oxygen

The cytochrome oxidase complex is the only member of the mitochondrial electron transport chain that reacts with oxygen physiologically. Oxygen radicals are natural by-products of oxidative phosphorylation, and they account for about 1% of total oxygen uptake. The major sources of radical generation are between complex I and CoQ and between CoQ and complex III. Reduced flavins and quinones react with oxygen to yield various oxygen radicals at these sites. Superoxide, peroxide, and hydroxyl free radicals react with proteins and nucleic acids and are toxic to the cell (Figure 5-5). Moreover, mitochondrial DNA is 15 times more sensitive to oxidative damage than is nuclear DNA (Chapter 17).

Let us consider the number of electrons transferred by various components of the electron transport chain and the stoichiometry of ATP formation. NADH transfers a pair of electrons as the hydride ion ($H:^-$), and $FMNH_2$, $FADH_2$, and coen-

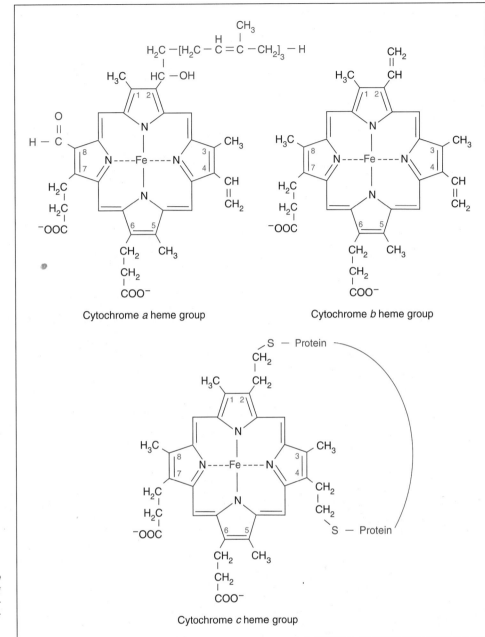

Cytochrome *a* heme group

Cytochrome *b* heme group

Cytochrome *c* heme group

FIGURE 9–5. Representative heme groups. *Hemes are iron-containing tetrapyrrole derivatives. The numbering system of the parent tetrapyrrole, called protoporphyrin IX, is illustrated.*

zyme QH_2 transfer two electrons and two protons. In contrast, iron-sulfur proteins and cytochromes transfer electrons one at a time. ATP yields are based historically upon electron pairs originating from NADH or succinate. A mole of NADH, whose electrons enter the respiratory chain at complex I, provides reducing equivalents that will sustain the synthesis of 2.5 moles of ATP. A mole of reduced $FADH_2$, whose electrons bypass complex I, provides reducing equivalents that will sustain the synthesis of 1.5 moles of ATP. Each electron pair reduces one atom of oxygen, or $\frac{1}{2}$ O_2. In nature, one entire molecule of oxygen (and not a half molecule) is the reactive species, and the cytochrome oxidase reaction involves molecular oxygen, 4 e^-, and 4 H^+. Because of these requirements, the cytochrome oxidase reaction is intricate.

The reactions of the electron transport chain, except for the reaction involving molecular oxygen, are simple oxidation-reduction reactions and are reversible (PRINCIPLE 7 OF BIOENERGETICS). The formation of water following the reduction of oxygen is exergonic and physiologically irreversible (PRINCIPLE 8 OF BIOENERGETICS).

INHIBITORS AND UNCOUPLERS OF OXIDATIVE PHOSPHORYLATION

Site-Specific Inhibitors and 2,4-Dinitrophenol

Site-specific inhibitors of oxidative phosphorylation, whose structures are illustrated in Table 9–3), block electron transport along the respiratory

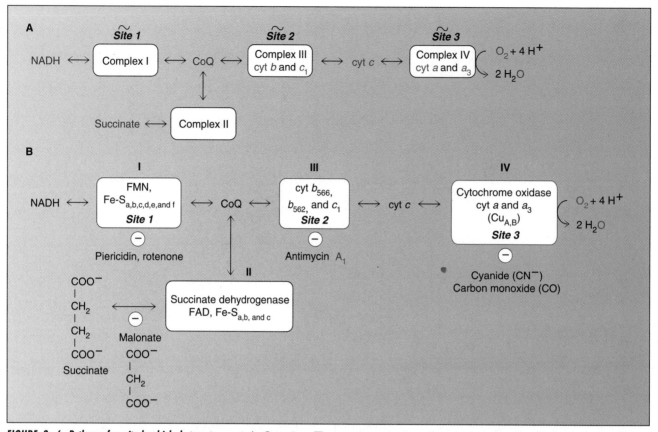

FIGURE 9-6. Pathway for mitochondrial electron transport. A. *Overview. The ~ represents sites of proton translocation. B. Components of each complex. Fe-S, iron-sulfur centers. Malonate is an inhibitor of succinate dehydrogenase. The loci of action of site specific inhibitors are indicated.*

chain (Figure 9-6B). This action inhibits oxygen consumption and secondarily abolishes the synthesis of ATP from ADP and P_i. **Uncouplers** of oxidative phosphorylation differ in their action from site-specific inhibitors. Electron transport from NADH and $FADH_2$ to oxygen proceeds, but the uncouplers indirectly abolish the conversion of ADP and P_i to ATP and H_2O. Because these agents separate the metabolically linked oxidation-reduction reactions of the electron transport chain from phosphorylation of ADP, they are called uncouplers of oxidative phosphorylation. 2,4-Dinitrophenol is an example of this class of compound (Figure 9-7). The action of 2,4-dinitrophenol and related compounds shows that ATP production relies on a continuously generated proton gradient, as described later.

Oligomycin, an antibiotic, represents another class of reagent that was used to determine the mechanism of oxidative phosphorylation (Figure 9-8). Oligomycin inhibits ATP synthase activity. The mechanism of action of oligomycin involves an oligomycin sensitivity conferring protein (OSCP).

At the time when the sites of action of the electron transport inhibitors were established in the 1950s, it was thought that the biosynthesis of ATP occurred at these sites. It was hypothesized that an energy-rich intermediate was formed and that the intermediate led to the generation of ATP by a process resembling substrate level phosphory-

lation. Even today, illustrations of the electron transport chain show ATP synthesis occurring at sites 1, 2, and 3. This should be regarded in a figurative and not a literal sense. Early workers surmised that uncouplers of oxidative phosphorylation destabilized the energy-rich intermediate that allowed electron transport and oxygen consumption to occur without ATP formation. The failure to identify an energy-rich intermediate in spite of exhaustive efforts by many investigators for more than a decade argued against the possibility of such a mechanism. With the advent of the chemiosmotic theory, the sites are now conceived to be responsible for proton translocation.

P/O Ratios

One important method of studying oxidative phosphorylation is to measure oxygen consumption under a variety of experimental conditions. A central property of oxidative phosphorylation is the P/O ratio. The P/O ratio refers to the number of ATP molecules formed from ADP and P_i per electron pair transported to an atom of oxygen (O or $\frac{1}{2} O_2$) to form water. With NADH as electron donor, the P/O ratio is between 2 and 3. With succinate as electron donor, the P/O ratio is between 1 and 2. Before the advent of the chemiosmotic theory, investigators thought that the P/O ratio

TABLE 9–3. Site-Specific Inhibitors of Electron Transport

Site	Inhibitor	Structure

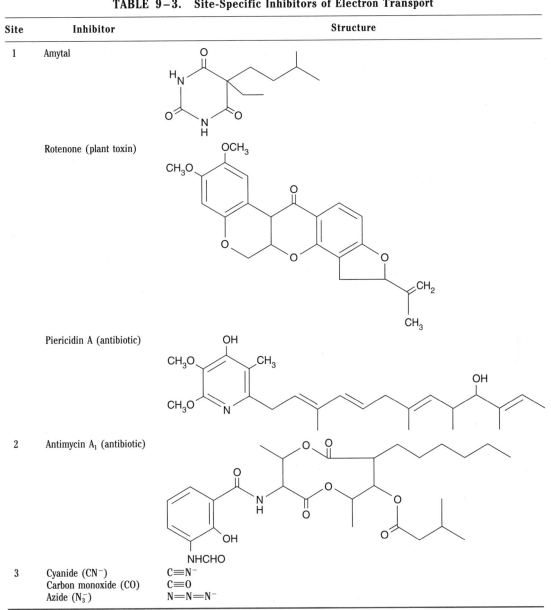

Site	Inhibitor	Structure
1	Amytal	
	Rotenone (plant toxin)	
	Piericidin A (antibiotic)	
2	Antimycin A₁ (antibiotic)	
3	Cyanide (CN⁻)	$C{\equiv}N^-$
	Carbon monoxide (CO)	$C{\equiv}O$
	Azide (N₃⁻)	$N{=}N{=}N^-$

would have to be an integral number. When mitochondriologists (whimsically called mitochondriacs) obtained nonintegral values, they rounded them off to an integral number. With the formulation of the chemiosmotic hypothesis, it became apparent that nonintegral P/O ratios are possible. Current data suggest that electron transport from a mole of NADH to oxygen sustains the synthesis of 2.5 moles of ATP, and from a mole of succinate to oxygen, 1.5 moles of ATP.

ROLE OF PROTON TRANSLOCATION IN OXIDATIVE PHOSPHORYLATION

We now address the mechanism by which the energy-yielding exergonic reactions of electron transport of the respiratory chain are coupled to the energy-requiring endergonic reaction of ATP formation from ADP and P_i. *The exergonic reactions of electron transport provide energy for the translocation of protons (H^+) from the mitochondrial matrix through the inner mitochondrial membrane to the exterior.* Electron transport generates and maintains an electrochemical proton gradient. The movement of charged protons from the mitochondrial matrix establishes both a concentration gradient and an electrical potential. The resulting proton-motive force consists of two components: an electrical potential (positive outside the mitochondrion) and a concentration gradient (acid outside the mitochondrion). An analogous situation occurs in bacteria, where protons are translocated from the interior to the exterior of the plasma membrane. The proton gradient serves as a source of energy as protons moving into mitochondria drive

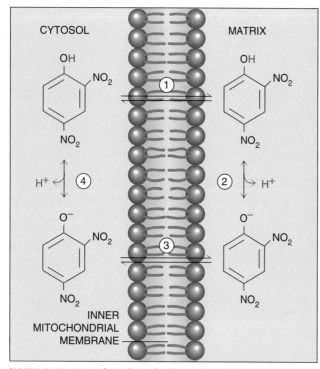

FIGURE 9–7. Action of 2,4-dinitrophenol as an uncoupler of oxidative phosphorylation. *Both the protonated and unprotonated forms of 2,4-dinitrophenol readily diffuse across the mitochondrial membrane. (1) The protonated (uncharged) form carries a proton from the side of higher to lower proton concentration. (3) The unprotonated (charged) species moves from the side of lower to higher proton concentration.*

ATP synthesis via an F_oF_1 ATP synthase. The three elements of the initial chemiosmotic theory (a membrane, an oxidation-reduction driven proton translocase, and a proton driven ATP synthase) are illustrated in Figure 9–9.

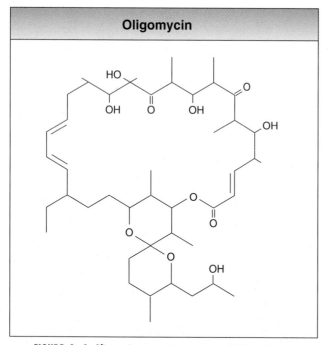

Oligomycin

FIGURE 9–8. Oligomycin, *an inhibitor of the ATP synthase.*

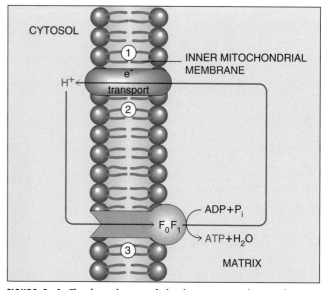

FIGURE 9–9. The three elements of the chemiosmotic mechanism of energy transduction. *(1) A membrane. (2) Exergonic electron transport generates a proton gradient across a membrane. (3) The proton gradient furnishes the energy for endergonic ATP production as catalyzed by ATP synthase.*

Let us consider possible mechanisms of proton translocation energized by electron transport. Peter Mitchell, the originator of the chemiosmotic theory, postulated the existence of oxidation-reduction loops to account for proton translocation. The concept is that protons and electrons are transported from the mitochondrial interior and protons are released at the exterior surface. Electrons are transported back (looped) to the internal aspect of the membrane for subsequent reaction. In the example illustrated in Figure 9–10, electrons and protons combine with FMN to yield $FMNH_2$. The reaction occurs on the matrix side of the mitochondrion. Two protons are discharged on the exterior of the mitochondrion and two electrons are transported via components within the membrane. The overall process of electron transport and proton translocation is exergonic.

Another hypothesis for proton translocation is that components of the electron transport chain

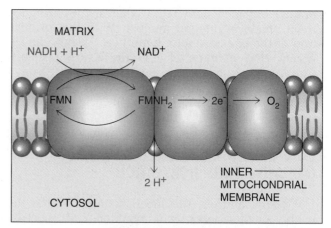

FIGURE 9–10. Redox loop.

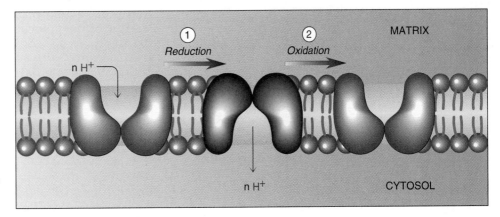

FIGURE 9–11. The proton pump mechanism for generating a proton gradient.

function as **proton pumps.** One scheme to account for proton pumping is that one or more protons bind to the internal face of a membrane protein and, following a conformational change energized by electron transport, protons are released from the pump on the exterior face (Figure 9–11).

A summary scheme showing the stoichiometry of proton translocation in animal mitochondria is shown in Figure 9–12. The number of protons translocated at sites 1 (4), 2 (2), and 3 (4) is noted in parentheses. There are suggestions that a proton pump participates in transport at sites 1 and 3 and a redox loop at site 2.

F_oF_1 ATP SYNTHASE

Protons moving down their electrochemical gradient in a bioenergetically favorable direction provide the energy for ATP biosynthesis. Peter Mitchell, the originator of this concept, referred to this source of energy as proticity (in analogy with electricity). The chemiosmotic theory for ATP formation by oxidative phosphorylation involves two distinct operations. First, electron transport generates a proton gradient across an impermeable membrane. Second, protons move down their electrochemical gradient from the outside to the inside of the mitochondrion (or from the outside to the inside of a bacterial cell) to energize ATP formation by ATP synthase. The ATP synthase uses the proton current to support the biosynthesis of ATP from ADP and P_i.

Structure

ATP synthase is an aggregate of polypeptides that form a mushroom-shaped molecule on the inner aspect of the inner mitochondrial membrane. The enzyme is called the F_oF_1 ATPase (Table 9–4). The F_o (o for oligomycin-sensitive, not zero) is embedded in the membrane (Figure 9–13). The F_1 portion is composed of several polypeptide chains designated α, β, γ, δ, and ϵ; F_1 forms the mushroom top. When separated from the membrane, F_1 possesses ATPase activity. Its predominant func-

tion in the physiological situation, however, is ATP synthesis, and the name ATP synthase more accurately describes this function. The composition of the mammalian mitochondrial enzyme is $\alpha_3\beta_3\gamma\delta\epsilon_{1-2}$. This intricate enzyme contains nine or ten subunits. The triplet of $\alpha\beta$ subunits provides three ATP binding sites per molecule.

ATP synthases isolated from the mitochondria of animals, plants, and protozoa, from plant chloroplasts (site of photophosphorylation), and from bacteria are homologous. The F_1 subunit can be resolved from the F_o subunit. Following the separation of F_o from F_1, the membrane containing F_o is permeable to protons. After reconstituting the F_1 with the F_o component, the membrane becomes proton impermeable. Oligomycin interacts with OSCP (oligomycin sensitivity conferring protein) of F_o to inhibit proton translocation through the ATP synthase.

ATP Synthesis

How ATP synthesis might occur is illustrated in Figure 9–14. In this scheme, protons are not involved directly in catalysis. Protons bind to the face of the F_1 complex toward the cytosol, and after promoting the formation of an energized conformation that sustains ATP synthesis, protons are then released on the matrix face of the F_1 complex. Another conformational transition occurs to produce the initial state.

SUCCESSES OF THE CHEMIOSMOTIC THEORY

The chemiosmotic theory provides the explanation for the following phenomena. First, ATP synthesis by oxidative phosphorylation requires a membrane. Second, respiring mitochondria generate a proton gradient. Third, uncoupling agents such as 2,4-dinitrophenol abolish ATP synthesis without inhibiting electron transport from NADH or succinate to oxygen. 2,4-Dinitrophenol dissipates proton gradients (Figure 9–7), and this property explains its action as an uncoupler of oxidative phosphorylation. Without a proton gradient and a

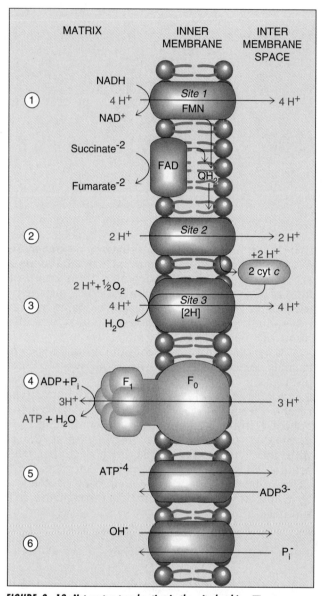

FIGURE 9–12. Net proton translocation in the mitochondrion. *The transport of two electrons through sites 1, 2, and 3 from NADH to oxygen provides the energy for proton translocation. The number of protons translocated at these sites is noted. A total of 10 protons are transported per electron pair corresponding to one molecule of NADH or one gram atom of oxygen.*

transport of phosphate from the exterior to the interior of the mitochondrion (this is equivalent to the transport of hydroxide ion from the interior to the exterior of the mitochondrion). The exchange of intramitochondrial ATP for extramitochondrial ADP does not require proton movement.

ATP YIELD FROM THE COMPLETE OXIDATION OF GLUCOSE

We can now calculate the amount of ATP produced from ADP and P_i when one mole of glucose is completely oxidized to carbon dioxide and water. We noted before that the net yield of ATP is two during the conversion of glucose to pyruvate by glycolysis. Two moles of GTP are formed during the succinate thiokinase reaction of the Krebs cycle from two moles of glucose-derived acetyl-CoA. The energy content of GTP is equivalent to that of ATP. The four ATP equivalents produced during glycolysis and directly by the Krebs cycle (succinate thiokinase reaction) are examples of substrate level phosphorylation.

Although measurements of the number of ATP molecules formed during electron transport phosphorylation have been performed over a 50-year period, variation has been observed. When fractional values for the P/O ratio (ATP formed per gram atom of oxygen) were obtained, the values were assumed initially to correspond to whole numbers and were accordingly rounded off to an integer. Chemiosmotic theory, however, provides a basis for the existence of fractional values because protons are the coupling currency, and *the number of protons transported by a coupling site need not be a multiple of the protons needed to synthesize ATP from ADP and P_i*. In mitochondria, ATP efflux and

corresponding counterforce against physiological proton translocation, the rate of electron transport (and oxygen consumption) is more rapid than that of normal mitochondria.

Let us now consider the size of the proton-motive force and compare it with the energy required for ATP synthesis. The standard free energy of formation of ATP and H_2O from ADP and P_i is +30.4 kJ mol⁻¹. However, the actual free energy of ATP formation from ADP and P_i under physiological conditions, the phosphorylation potential (ΔG_p), is about +50 kJ/mol. Thermodynamic calculations and experiments suggest that three protons per molecule of ATP are required. In mitochondria, moreover, a fourth proton is required for the

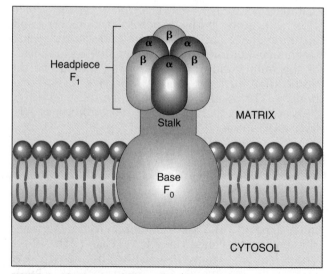

FIGURE 9–13. Structure of ATP synthase. *The base (F_0 domain) spans the membrane, and the headpiece (F_1 domain) occurs in the matrix. Each pair of α and β-subunits forms a dimer that binds ADP and P_i or ATP.*

TABLE 9–4.   Components of the Mitochondrial ATP Synthase (F$_o$F$_1$ ATPase)

Component	Subunit Composition	Function
F$_o$	Several types of subunit including 10 copies of DCCD-binding proteolipid	DCCD-binding proteolipid forms proton channel
F$_1$	$\alpha_3\beta_3\gamma\delta\epsilon$	$\alpha\beta$-dimer binds ATP
Stalk	One copy each of OSCP and F$_6$	Required to bind F$_o$ to F$_1$

DCCD, dicyclohexylcarbodiimide; OSCP, oligomycin sensitivity–conferring protein.

ADP and P$_i$ influx must occur. The influx of P$_i$ into the mitochondrion requires an exchange with hydroxide. The exchange of hydroxide ion is equivalent to the cotransport of P$_i$ with a proton. Current research indicates that a total of four protons are required for ATP synthesis in mitochondria: three for the ATP synthase reaction and one for P$_i$ transport.

Hinkle and coworkers reported that the "ideal" mechanistic stoichiometries for ATP formation are close to 1 at sites 1 and 3, and close to 0.5 at site 2, in rat liver mitochondria. The yield of ATP is 2.5 per mole of NADH and 1.5 per mole of FADH$_2$. The yield of ATP from glucose metabolism depends upon the nature of the shuttle system used to transport reducing equivalents from the cytosol into the mitochondrion. The gross yield from the oxidation of glucose corresponds to 30 ATP molecules per mole of glucose if the glycerol phosphate shuttle is used, and 32 ATP molecules if the malate-aspartate shuttle is used. These values are based upon the number of ATP, NADH, and FADH$_2$ molecules formed during glycolysis and Krebs cycle function, as shown in Table 9–5.

Textbooks published before 1992 report different values for the ATP yield from NADH and succinate than are used in this book. Before that time, the yield was reported as three ATP molecules per NADH and two ATP molecules for succinate (FADH$_2$). Because current books contain different values, the yield of ATP from the metabolism of glucose will probably be eliminated from standardized examinations for several years. Moreover, future work may prompt additional changes in the values for the ATP yield.

REGULATION OF GLYCOLYSIS, THE KREBS CYCLE, AND OXIDATIVE PHOSPHORYLATION BY ADENINE NUCLEOTIDES

The main function of glycolysis, the Krebs cycle, and oxidative phosphorylation is to mediate ATP

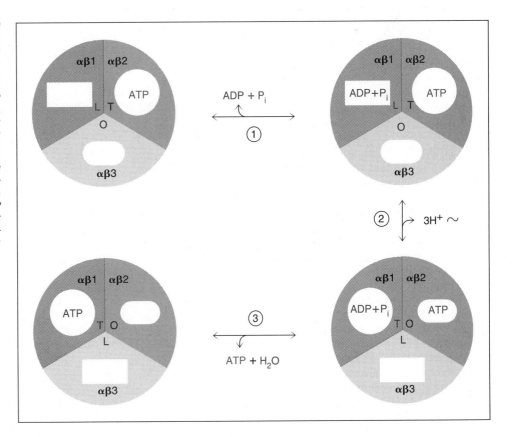

FIGURE 9–14. Mechanism of ATP synthase. Each nucleotide-binding domain is made of an $\alpha\beta$ subunit dimer. Each ATP synthase contains three binding sites with loose (L), tight (T), and little (open, or O) affinity. (1) ADP and P$_i$ bind to an L site. (2) The energy of a proton current changes the nature of the binding sites: an L site is converted to a T site, a T site is converted to an O site, and an O site is converted to an L site. (3) The ATP that was synthesized during the previous cycle is released. ADP and P$_i$ are converted to ATP that remains tightly bound to the enzyme and is released during the next cycle.

TABLE 9–5. ATP Yield from the Complete Oxidation of Glucose

	ATP produced
Glycolysis *per se*	2
2 NADH from glycolysis	3 or 5 (glycerol phosphate or malate-aspartate shuttles, respectively)
Pyruvate dehydrogenase (2 NADH)	5
Isocitrate dehydrogenase (2 NADH)	5
α-Ketoglutarate dehydrogenase (2 NADH)	5
Succinate thiokinase (2 GTP or 2 ATP)	2
Succinate dehydrogenase (2 FADH$_2$)	3
Malate dehydrogenase (2 NADH)	5
	30 or 32

1 Glucose → 30 ATP (glycerol phosphate shuttle) or 32 ATP (malate-aspartate shuttle)
1 Acetyl-CoA → 10 ATP
1 Pyruvate → 12.5 ATP

Based on the values of P.C. Hinkle, M.A. Kumar, A. Resetar, and D.L. Harris. Mechanistic stoichiometry of mitochondrial oxidative phosphorylation. Biochemistry 30:3576–3582, 1991.

formation. ATP and its metabolites play an important role in the regulation of these activities. ATP plays an inhibitory role, and ADP or AMP plays a stimulatory role. Let us consider the reactions that the energy charge of adenine nucleotides regulates.

Phosphofructokinase is the rate-limiting and regulatory enzyme of glycolysis (Chapter 7). That ATP is an inhibitor makes physiological sense in that ATP will decrease the rate of glucose metabolism and ATP production. ATP inhibits phosphofructokinase allosterically (Figure 4–2). AMP increases the rate of glycolysis and stimulates ATP formation. AMP performs this function by activating phosphofructokinase allosterically. The concentration of AMP generally is low. Only when ATP is degraded does the AMP concentration increase. These are just the conditions needed to activate the glycolytic pathway. Regulation by adenine nucleotides is important in active skeletal muscle but not in aerobic cells such as heart or brain.

Pyruvate dehydrogenase is regulated indirectly by adenine nucleotides. ATP activates pyruvate dehydrogenase kinase, and phosphorylated pyruvate dehydrogenase is inhibited (Table 25–2). Acetyl-CoA and NADH also activate pyruvate dehydrogenase kinase. ATP, acetyl-CoA, and NADH are substances that signify ample energy and serve as a signal to decrease the activity of a pivotal regulatory enzyme. This strategy follows the metabolic logic of the cell.

Isocitrate dehydrogenase is the main regulatory enzyme of the Krebs cycle (Table 25–1). ADP activates isocitrate dehydrogenase. When ADP is converted to ATP, ADP's concentration is low and it is a less effective activator. Regulation of isocitrate dehydrogenase in mitochondria permits synthesis of citrate, a precursor of cytosolic acetyl-CoA and malonyl-CoA for fatty acid biosynthesis in liver, and appropriately limits isocitrate degradation.

Oxidative phosphorylation is regulated by the levels of ADP. Under most physiological conditions, electron transport is tightly coupled to ATP formation from ADP and P$_i$. The requirements for oxidative phosphorylation include ADP, P$_i$, O$_2$, and reducing equivalents (NADH or FADH$_2$). ADP availability stimulates the rate of oxidative phosphorylation by providing substrate for the ATP synthase reaction. Phosphate is generally present in excess and does not limit the rate of ATP synthesis. When ADP is converted to ATP, the lack of ADP availability naturally decreases the rate of ADP phosphorylation. A low rate of ATP formation via ATP synthase allows the proton-motive force to reach a summit (electropositive and acidic outside). When the ADP concentration is low and the rate of ATP synthesis is slow, the proton gradient *per se* retards additional proton translocation from the matrix to the intermembrane space. Only when ADP and P$_i$ are bound to ATP synthase is proton transport down its electrochemical gradient permitted, thereby accounting for control by ADP levels. Diminished ability to translocate protons against the proton-motive force results in a simultaneous decrease in electron transport from reductants (NADH and FADH$_2$). The rate of electron transport is thereby diminished.

The time course of the response of electron transport, proton translocation, and ATP synthesis to ADP availability is very rapid (on the order of milliseconds.) During vigorous muscular activity, the supply of oxygen becomes limiting. Under these conditions, ATP is supplied by anaerobic glycolysis (Chapter 7) and by the creatine phosphokinase reaction (Figure 4–13). Allosteric activation and regulation of metabolism makes biochemical and physiological sense (the molecular logic of the cell).

MITOCHONDRIAL DYSFUNCTION

▶ Mitochondrial function is essential for health and well-being. Primary defects in the electron transport chain are rare. Individuals with aberrations in each of the four complexes of oxidative phosphorylation have been reported. Individuals with complex I, III, and IV defects have lactic acidosis just as those with pyruvate dehydrogenase and Krebs cycle enzyme defects do. Some individuals with reported defects in the complexes of the respiratory chain have survived into adulthood.

Mitochondrial function may be altered in pathological states. Under anoxic conditions secondary to vascular occlusion, cells lack oxygen and oxidative phosphorylation is impaired because of the absence of substrate (oxygen). If excessive or prolonged, anoxia leads to cellular and tissue death. Mitochondrial oxidative phosphorylation in heart may be diminished in disorders such as diabetes mellitus, hypertension, and various heart diseases. Arterial occlusion followed by reperfusion results in the generation of toxic superoxide, peroxides, and hydroxyl free radicals (Figure 5–5). These deleterious processes occur commonly in the clinical setting. The defect in oxidative phosphorylation is secondary to the illness.

Cyanide is one of the most toxic and rapidly acting poisons known, and individuals can die within a few minutes of exposure. Hydrogen cyanide, a volatile substance, is currently used in gas chambers for the execution of criminals. Cyanide binds tightly to ferric ($+3$) iron. Cyanide's role as a site 3 specific inhibitor explains its mechanism of toxicity. Cyanide reacts with ferric iron of cytochrome oxidase and inhibits electron transport. Since oxygen consumption is blocked, venous blood is as red as arterial blood. Treatment of cyanide poisoning is based on converting the ferrous iron of hemoglobin to the ferric form, which then binds to cyanide. Amyl nitrate injection promotes this oxidation.

Rhodanese, a liver mitochondrial enzyme, catalyzes the conversion of cyanide to the nontoxic thiocyanate. Cyanide reacts with thiosulfate to form thiocyanate and sulfite, as shown in equation 9.3.

$$CN^- + {}^-S\text{--}SO_3^- \rightarrow SCN^- + SO_3^{2-} \qquad (9.3)$$

Intravenous injections of sodium thiosulfate and amyl nitrate are used for the treatment of cyanide poisoning. ◄

SUMMARY

There are three fundamental tenets of the chemiosmotic theory. First, a membrane is required. Second, exergonic reactions of the electron transport chain generate a proton gradient across a proton-impermeable membrane. Third, proton translocation down its electrochemical gradient provides ATP synthase with the energy to drive ATP synthesis.

The respiratory chain is made up of several different classes of substances. Components of the respiratory chain include (1) flavins, (2) iron-sulfur proteins, (3) coenzyme Q, and (4) cytochromes. Coenzyme Q shuttles electrons from complexes I and II to complex III. Cytochrome c shuttles electrons from complex III to complex IV. Sites 1, 2, and 3 of the respiratory chain refer to sites of proton translocation. Electron transport inhibitors block oxidation-reduction reactions at specific locations along the electron transport chain. As a result of the action of the site specific inhibitors, electrons cannot be transferred from substrates to oxygen. Rotenone is a site 1 specific inhibitor, antimycin is a site 2 specific inhibitor, and cyanide and carbon monoxide are site 3 specific inhibitors.

Uncouplers of oxidative phosphorylation such as 2,4-dinitrophenol permit oxidation-reduction and oxygen consumption, but they abolish ATP formation. Uncouplers exert this effect by dissipating the proton gradient across the membrane. Oligomycin is an antibiotic that inhibits ATP synthase.

The proton-motive force is made up of an electrical potential gradient and a pH gradient. The stoichiometry for ATP synthesis by the ATP synthase is three protons per molecule of ATP. In mitochondria, an additional proton is required for the transport of P_i into the mitochondrion from the cytosol. A total of four protons is required for the synthesis of ATP that is used in the cytosol. The transport of reducing equivalents into mitochondria requires intricate and indirect transport systems. These transport systems include the malate-aspartate shuttle and the glycerol phosphate shuttle.

With one mole of NADH as donor, 2.5 moles of ATP per mole of reductant are formed by oxidative phosphorylation. This corresponds to one mole of ATP at site 1, 0.5 mole at site 2, and one mole at site 3. With one mole of succinate ($FADH_2$) as reductant, 1.5 moles of ATP are formed. The metabolism of one mole of acetyl-CoA by the Krebs cycle and oxidative phosphorylation results in the formation of 10 moles of ATP; one mole of pyruvate yields 12.5 moles of ATP. The metabolism of one mole of glucose yields 30 moles of ATP using the glycerol phosphate shuttle, and 32 moles of ATP using the malate-aspartate shuttle. These shuttle systems transport reducing equivalents formed during glycolysis into the mitochondrion. The relative proportion of the two shuttle systems varies from cell to cell. The malate-aspartate shuttle is more important in liver and heart, and the glycerol phosphate shuttle is more important in muscle and brain.

SELECTED READINGS

Boyer, P.D., B. Chance, L. Ernster, P. Mitchell, E. Racker, and E.C. Slater. Oxidative phosphorylation and photophosphorylation. Annual Review of Biochemistry 46:955–1026, 1977.

Corral-Debrinski, M., G. Stepien, J.M. Shoffner, M.T. Lott, K. Kanter, and D.C. Wallace. Hypoxemia is associated with mitochondrial DNA damage and gene induction: Implications for cardiac disease. Journal of the American Medical Association 266:1812–1816, 1991.

Hatefi, Y. The mitochondrial electron transport chain and oxidative phosphorylation system. Annual Review of Biochemistry 54:1015–1069, 1985.

Hinkle, P.C., and R.E. McCarty. How cells make ATP. Scientific American 238(3):104–123, 1978.

Hinkle, P.C., M.A. Kumar, A. Resetar, and D.L. Harris. Mechanistic stoichiometry of mitochondrial oxidative phosphorylation. Biochemistry 30:3576–3582, 1991.

Mitchell, P. Vectorial chemistry and the molecular mechanics of chemiosmotic coupling: Power transmission by proticity. Biochemical Society Transactions 4:399–430, 1976.

Pedersen, P.L., and L.M. Amzel. ATP synthases. Journal of Biological Chemistry 268:9937–9940, 1993.

CHAPTER TEN

CARBOHYDRATE

METABOLISM

The most powerful way devised by civilization for finding new facts is the experimental method.

—LUIS F. LELOIR

In von Gierke's disease, an almost complete deficiency of one enzyme, glucose-6-phosphatase, offers a satisfactory explanation for the accumulation of glycogen in the liver and kidney.

—GERTY T. CORI

PRINCIPLES OF BIOSYNTHESIS

Life depends on the continual provision and deployment of ATP. The chemical energy of ATP provides the chemical energy for biosynthetic pathways. Part of the necessity for this strategy lies in the tenets of bioenergetics. The deployment of energy for biosynthetic reactions follows a general theme—to make the overall process exergonic. Moreover, pathways for both synthesis and degradation are exergonic and proceed with the liberation of free energy (PRINCIPLE 19 OF BIOCHEMISTRY). It is not possible for a single pathway, however, to be simultaneously exergonic in both directions.

A consideration of the pathways for glucose degradation and biosynthesis (gluconeogenesis) illustrates these ideas. The standard free energy change for glycolysis is about -85 kJ per mole of glucose and results in the formation of two moles of ATP (Table 7–2). The standard free energy change for gluconeogenesis is about -21 kJ per mole of glucose but occurs at a cost of four moles of ATP and two moles of GTP. Both pathways are exergonic. Moreover, separate pathways for biosynthesis and degradation permit differential regulation of both processes. With different pathways, it is possible to accelerate one and inhibit the other. Coordinate regulation of opposing and parallel pathways of metabolism is widespread in nature.

GLUCONEOGENESIS

Gluconeogenesis is the synthesis of glucose from noncarbohydrate sources. The following substances can be used to produce net increases of glucose: pyruvate, lactate, glycerol, Krebs cycle intermediates via oxaloacetate, and amino acids that are catabolized to pyruvate and Krebs cycle intermediates. It is noteworthy that humans are *unable* to use fatty acids with an even number of carbon atoms to produce net increases of glucose. It is also noteworthy that gluconeogenesis occurs in liver and kidney. An overview of gluconeogenesis is given in Figure 10–1.

Pyruvate Kinase Bypass Reactions

There are three irreversible steps in glycolysis (Table 10–1), one of which is catalyzed by pyruvate kinase. Pyruvate cannot be phosphorylated directly by ATP in humans. We noted in Table 6–3 that the standard group transfer potential of phosphoenolpyruvate is very high (≈ 60 kJ/mol) compared with that of ATP (≈ 30 kJ/mol). The phosphorylation of pyruvate by ATP does not occur in part because of the unfavorable thermodynamic barrier.

Nature has evolved a two-step sequence for phosphoenolpyruvate (PEP) formation that in-

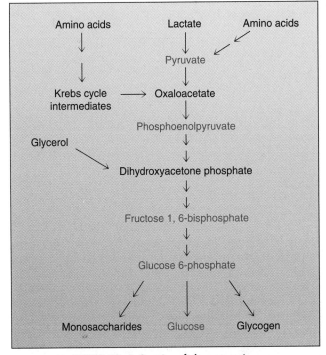

FIGURE 10–1. Overview of gluconeogenesis.

volves **pyruvate carboxylase** and **phosphoenolpyruvate carboxykinase** (Figure 10–2). The bioenergetics of phosphoenolpyruvate formation involves an ATP-dependent carboxylation reaction. The free energy of carboxylation is nearly equal to that of the hydrolysis of ATP. The carboxylation reaction energizes pyruvate in preparation for the next reaction. The decarboxylation of oxaloacetate provides an additional driving force for the formation of phosphoenolpyruvate with GTP as the phosphoryl donor. High ratios of ATP/ADP and GTP/GDP promote PEP synthesis. The following are noteworthy properties of these two reactions. First, pyruvate carboxylase is a biotin-containing enzyme. Second, pyruvate carboxylase requires acetyl-CoA as an allosteric activator. Third, GTP serves as the phosphorylating agent in the phosphoenolpyruvate carboxykinase reaction.

The conversion of pyruvate into glucose requires the mitochondrial and cytosolic compartments. There are two pathways for this process in humans, and each is important. The first pathway begins with pyruvate or alanine, and the second begins with lactate, which is more reduced. Ala-

TABLE 10–1.   Reactions Unique to Glycolysis and Gluconeogenesis

Glycolysis	Gluconeogenesis
Hexokinase	Glucose-6-phosphatase
Phosphofructokinase	Fructose-1,6-bisphosphatase
Pyruvate kinase	Pyruvate carboxylase
	Phosphoenolpyruvate carboxykinase (GTP-requiring)

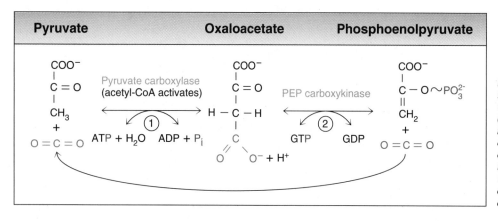

FIGURE 10–2. The two-step conversion of pyruvate to phosphoenolpyruvate. *Two high-energy bonds (ATP and GTP) energize the synthesis of energy-rich phosphoenolpyruvate (PEP). Note that carbon dioxide acts catalytically in the two-step process. Reaction 1 occurs in mitochondria, and reaction 2 occurs in mitochondria and the cytosol.*

nine is converted to pyruvate by transamination, and pyruvate enters the mitochondrion by symport with a proton and is converted to oxaloacetate. Oxaloacetate *per se* cannot be transported through the inner mitochondrial membrane. Oxaloacetate is reduced by NADH to form malate as catalyzed by **malate dehydrogenase.** Malate is translocated into the cytosol via the dicarboxylate carrier and is oxidized by NAD^+ to reform oxaloacetate (Figure 10–3). Oxaloacetate is then converted into phosphoenolpyruvate in a GTP-dependent reaction catalyzed by **cytosolic phosphoenolpyruvate carboxykinase.** In the pathway initiated by alanine or pyruvate, reducing equivalents for gluconeogenesis are transported from the mitochondrion to the cytosol as malate.

In the second pathway, lactate is converted to pyruvate, generating NADH, before entering the mitochondrion. Pyruvate is first converted to oxaloacetate and subsequently to phosphoenolpyruvate by **mitochondrial phosphoenolpyruvate carboxykinase.** Phosphoenolpyruvate is then translocated into the cytosol via the tricarboxylate carrier. Both pathways generate one cytosolic NADH per triose that is required for further reactions of gluconeogenesis.

Phosphofructokinase Bypass Reaction

Phosphoenolpyruvate is converted to fructose 1,6-bisphosphate by a reversal of glycolysis (Figure 10–4). The biochemical strategy used to bypass the phosphofructokinase reaction is conceptually easier to understand than the pyruvate phosphorylation sequence. Fructose 1,6-bisphosphate is hydrolyzed to form fructose 6-phosphate in a reaction catalyzed by **fructose-1,6-bisphosphatase.** This hydrolysis reaction is exergonic and unidirectional (PRINCIPLE 5 OF BIOENERGETICS). Fructose 6-phosphate is converted into glucose 6-phosphate by the phosphoglucose isomerase reaction.

Hexokinase Bypass Reaction

To bypass the hexokinase reaction in liver, intestine, and kidney cells, glucose 6-phosphate is hydrolyzed and released into the bloodstream. Glucose 6-phosphate is transported into the endoplasmic reticulum via a transport protein called GLUT7, and exergonic hydrolysis is catalyzed by **glucose-6-phosphatase.** Glucose liberated in the endoplasmic reticulum is released from the cell.

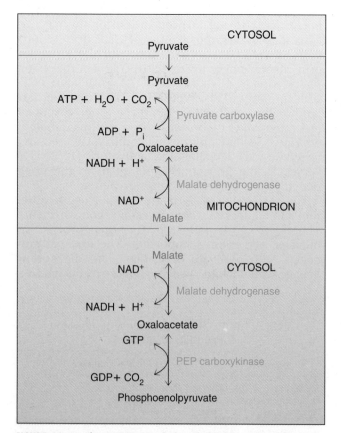

FIGURE 10–3. The participation of the mitochondrion and cytosol in the conversion of pyruvate to phosphoenolpyruvate.

Regulation

Fructose 2,6-bisphosphate regulates glycolysis and gluconeogenesis in a reciprocal fashion. In

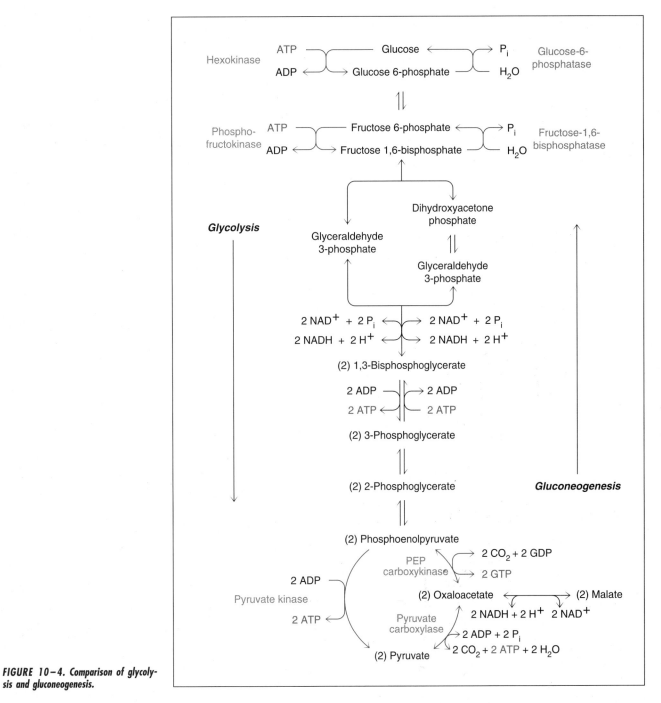

FIGURE 10–4. Comparison of glycolysis and gluconeogenesis.

Chapter 7, we noted that fructose 2,6-bisphosphate is the most important regulator of glycolysis; fructose 2,6-bisphosphate is a potent allosteric activator of phosphofructokinase and hence of glycolysis. Fructose 2,6-bisphosphate is also an inhibitor of fructose-1,6-bisphosphatase and thereby functions as an inhibitor of gluconeogenesis. We also noted that high plasma glucagon elevates hepatic cyclic AMP concentrations.

The phosphorylation of fructose-6-phosphate-2–kinase/phosphatase in liver by protein kinase A increases phosphatase activity and decreases fructose-6-phosphate-2-kinase activity (Table 25–2). In liver, elevated cyclic AMP action produces an increase in fructose-2,6-bisphosphatase activity and a decrease in kinase activity; these two changes produce a decrease in [fructose 2,6-bisphosphate]. This process removes an inhibitor of fructose-1, 6-bisphosphatase activity and thereby promotes gluconeogenesis. A decrease in [fructose 2,6-bisphosphate] removes an activator of fructose-6-phosphate-1-kinase (phosphofructokinase) activity and thereby decreases the rate of glycolysis (Table 25–1). This provides an example of the reciprocal regulation of anabolic and catabolic pathways. Pyruvate carboxylase requires **acetyl-CoA** for the expression of activity. *The second enzyme of gluconeogenesis, phosphoenolpyruvate carboxykinase, is the rate-limiting enzyme for the pathway.* Its activity is regulated by enzyme induction. Pyruvate kinase is inhibited by ATP and alanine. **Alanine** is a favored gluconeogenic precursor that is released from muscle and serves as a signal to inhibit glycolysis. Liver pyruvate kinase is also inhibited by phosphorylation by protein kinase A.

Bioenergetics

The overall stoichiometry for the conversion of two moles of pyruvate into one mole of glucose using pyruvate carboxylase and phosphoenolpyruvate carboxykinase is given in equation 10.1.

$$
\begin{array}{ccc}
2\ \text{Pyruvate}^- & & \text{Glucose} \qquad (10.1) \\
+ & & + \\
6\ \text{NTP}^{-4} & & 6\ \text{NDP}^{-3} \\
+ & \rightarrow & + \\
2\ \text{NADH} & & 6\ \text{P}_i \\
+ & & + \\
6\ \text{H}_2\text{O} & & 2\ \text{NADH} + 2\ \text{H}^+
\end{array}
$$

The six moles of nucleoside triphosphate (NTP) correspond to two moles of GTP (for the conversion of two moles of oxaloacetate to two moles of phosphoenolpyruvate) and four moles of ATP (two each in the pyruvate carboxylase reaction and in the phosphoglycerate kinase reaction as shown in Figure 10–4). NADH is the reducing agent, and two moles are required per mole of glucose.

The standard free energy change for the conversion of two moles of pyruvate into glucose is $+148$ kJ. The terminal high-energy bond of nucleoside triphosphates is equivalent to that of ATP at -30.4 kJ mol^{-1} (Table 6–3). The exergonic utilization of six high-energy phosphate bonds corresponds to -182.4 kJ. The net standard free energy change for the process in equation 10.1 is -34.4 kJ mol^{-1}, and the overall gluconeogenic process is exergonic. The free energy for the conversion of glucose to two moles of pyruvate by the glycolytic pathway is about -85 kJ mol^{-1} (Table 7–2). Thus, both glycolysis and gluconeogenesis are exergonic. These values illustrate PRINCIPLE 18 OF BIOCHEMISTRY, stating that biochemical processes proceed with the liberation of free energy. The conversion of pyruvate to glucose is made possible by means of the phosphorylating potential of ATP and GTP and the exergonic hydrolytic reactions following these phosphorylation reactions.

Diabetes Mellitus

Gluconeogenesis is important in normal glucose homeostasis. The liver of a normal 70-kg adult produces about 100 g of glucose from the time of an evening meal until breakfast the next morning. ▶ Understanding the role of gluconeogenesis in the hyperglycemia of diabetes is also an important reason for emphasizing gluconeogenesis and its hormonal and biochemical regulation. Diabetes mellitus is characterized by a high glucagon-to-insulin ratio (as noted in Chapters 3 and 25). The hyperglycemia of diabetes is due to (1) a lack of

transport of glucose into cells owing to insulin deficiency and (2) a high rate of gluconeogenesis because the action of glucagon is not restrained by insulin (Table 25–6).

Glucagon activates the cyclic AMP second messenger system that leads to the phosphorylation of fructose-6-phosphate-2-kinase/phosphatase (as noted in Chapter 7). Following enzyme phosphorylation, the concentration of cellular fructose 2,6-bisphosphate decreases. This removes an inhibitor of fructose-1,6-bisphosphatase and an activator of phosphofructokinase (fructose-6-phosphate-1-kinase). The net result is an increase in gluconeogenesis or in the rate of conversion of pyruvate to glucose. The elevated glucagon-to-insulin ratio in diabetes contributes to the hyperglycemia of diabetes by this mechanism. Glucagon also induces the enzymes of gluconeogenesis (Table 25–1).

The normal value for a fasting serum glucose concentration is less than 6.7 mM, or 120 mg/dL. A fasting serum glucose 7.8 mM (140 mg/dL) or greater on at least two occasions is an often-cited standard for the diagnosis of diabetes mellitus. When diabetes is suspected but when the fasting serum glucose levels are less than 7.8 mM, oral glucose tolerance tests may reveal a diabetic state. The usefulness of oral **glucose tolerance tests** is diminished by the influence of many factors other than diabetes. For example, age, diet, gastrointestinal function, medication, and stress can confound the issue. Oral glucose tolerance tests should be performed only on well persons who have been consuming a normal diet with adequate carbohydrate (>150 g/d) for at least 3 days. The test is performed following an overnight fast. After a serum sample is drawn, individuals are given 100 g of glucose by mouth, and serum samples are taken at 60, 90, and 120 minutes. Ranges of values for normal and diabetic individuals are given in Table 10–2. Individuals with limited carbohydrate intake (because of starvation or illness) have decreased carbohydrate tolerance (high serum glucose in response to a glucose load) but may not have diabetes. It is for this reason that the tested individual should have been on a regular diet for at least 3 days before the test. ◀

LACTOSE BIOSYNTHESIS

We will consider lactose biosynthesis as a prototype in understanding the energetics of biosynthetic processes. Lactose is a disaccharide consisting of galactose covalently bonded to glucose (Figure 10–5). We can formally describe the generation of lactose as a condensation reaction involving galactose and glucose as shown in the following chemical equation.

$$\text{Galactose} + \text{glucose} \rightarrow \text{lactose} + \text{H}_2\text{O} \qquad (10.2)$$

A **condensation reaction** involves the joining of two molecules together with the liberation of a

TABLE 10-2. Serum Glucose Concentrations for Oral Glucose Tolerance Tests

Time	Values, mM (mg/dL)	
	Normal	Diabetic
Fasting	3.9–5.8 (70–105)	≥ 7.8 (≥ 140)
60 min	6.7–9.4 (120–170)	≥ 11 (≥ 200)
90 min	5.6–7.8 (100–140)	≥ 11 (≥ 200)
120 min	3.9–6.7 (70–120)	≥ 7.8 (≥ 140)

small molecule such as water. The standard free energy of reaction 10.2 is about + 15 kJ/mol. The equilibrium constant is small, and the generation of product from these reactants does not occur physiologically by this process.

The lactose synthase reaction serves as a prototype for the condensation reactions involved in the biosynthesis of glycogen, triglyceride, proteins, DNA, and RNA. The biosynthesis of these compounds does not proceed as the reverse of a hydrolysis reaction. Rather, biochemically activated precursors are used. The activated precursors are characteristically energy-rich compounds. An energy-rich compound and a substrate react to form a product and a leaving group. In lactose synthesis, for example, the activated precursor is UDP~galactose, the acceptor is glucose, and UDP is the leaving group. **Lactose synthase** catalyzes the biosynthesis of lactose according to the following chemical equation.

UDP-galactose + glucose → lactose + UDP   (10.3)

Let us consider this process using the principles of bioenergetics (counting high-energy bonds) developed in Chapter 6. The reactants contain a total of two energy-rich linkages (Figure 10–6). UDP-galactose contains two high-energy bonds (the galactosyl~phosphate is one energy-rich bond, and the pyrophosphate acid anhydride linkage is the second). The products contain a single energy-rich bond. UDP contains one high-energy bond (the pyrophosphate acid anhydride bond); lactose contains a low-energy glycosidic bond. The reaction proceeds with the loss of a high-energy bond and is exergonic (PRINCIPLE 2 OF BIOENERGETICS). Moreover, the reaction is unidirectional.

The role of UDP-galactose in the condensation reaction to produce lactose illustrates the tenet of **group activation.** In subsequent chapters, we will consider the manner of activation of fatty acids, amino acids, deoxyribonucleotides, and ribonucleotides. In all these situations, the activated precursor is attached to a leaving group by a high-energy bond. These energy-rich bonds require ATP directly or indirectly for their synthesis, as stated by Lipmann's law.

BIOENERGETICS AND METABOLISM OF GLYCOSIDIC DIPHOSPHATES

Glucose 6-phosphate is a pivotal metabolite in carbohydrate metabolism. Glucose 6-phosphate is converted to glucose 1-phosphate in a reaction catalyzed by phosphoglucomutase (Figure 10–7). Both compounds contain a low-energy bond, and their facile interconversion is consistent with the lack of an appreciable thermodynamic barrier for the reaction (PRINCIPLE 4 OF BIOENERGETICS). The group transfer potential of the glycosyl group of glucose 1-phosphate is increased after the reaction with UTP.

In the UDP-glucose pyrophosphorylase step (Figure 10–7), the reactants have two high-energy bonds, both in UTP. The products have three high-energy bonds (UDP-glucose contains the energy-rich phosphoric acid anhydride and the energy-rich glycosidic-diphosphate bond; PP$_i$ contains the energy-rich simple acid anhydride linkage). Under standard conditions, the reaction proceeds from products to reactants (PRINCIPLE 3 OF BIOENERGETICS). The standard free energy change for the reaction is + 6.9 kJ/mol, and the reaction is bidirectional. This is an unusual example in a biosynthetic pathway because the products have more high-energy bonds than the reactants.

The standard free energy of hydrolysis of inorganic pyrophosphate is − 33.4 kJ/mol (Table 6–3). This reaction is catalyzed by pyrophosphatase. The hydrolysis serves to pull the reaction in the direction of UDP-glucose formation. The sum of these two reactions is given as follows.

			$\Delta G^{\circ\prime}$ (kJ/mol)	
UTP + glucose 1-phosphate	⇌	UDP-glucose + PP$_i$	+ 6.9	(10.4)
PP$_i$ + H$_2$O	→	2 P$_i$	− 33.4	(10.5)
UTP + glucose 1-phosphate + H$_2$O	→	UDP-glucose + 2 P$_i$	− 25.6	(10.6)

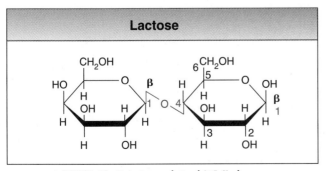

Lactose

FIGURE 10–5. Lactose, galactosyl (β1,4) glucose.

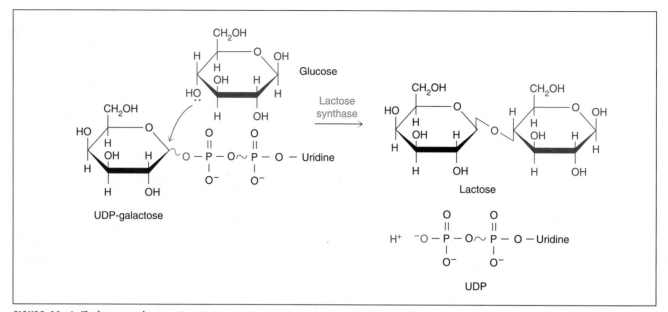

FIGURE 10–6. The lactose synthase reaction. *UDP-galactose represents activated galactose. The ~ denotes the location of the high-energy bonds.*

Reactions 10.4 and 10.5 have a common component—pyrophosphate. The example illustrates the utility of pyrophosphate cleavage. The hydrolysis of pyrophosphate converts an unfavorable reaction into a very favorable process.

ATP serves as the common currency of energy exchange (Lipmann's law). The energy of ATP is used for carbohydrate biosynthesis in the following fashion. An appropriate leaving group such as UDP must be reconverted into the nucleoside triphosphate before it can participate in the activation of another sugar. This reconversion is described in equation 10.7.

$$UDP + ATP \rightleftharpoons UTP + ADP; \Delta G°' \cong 0 \quad (10.7)$$

ATP is then regenerated by substrate level phosphorylation or by oxidative phosphorylation. The enzyme that catalyzes the isoergonic reaction in Equation 10.7 is nucleoside diphosphate kinase and is described in Chapter 6.

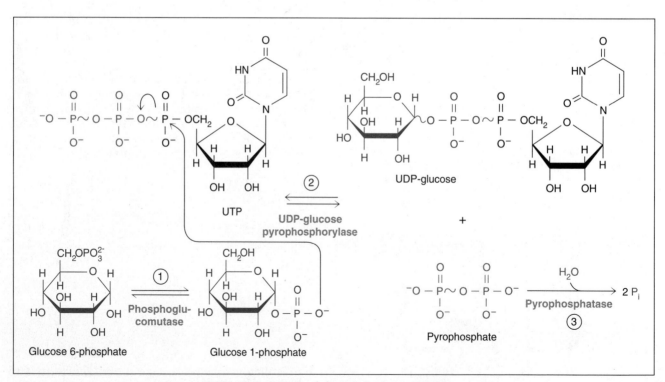

FIGURE 10–7. Conversion of glucose 6-phosphate to UDP-glucose.

GLYCOGEN METABOLISM

Glycogen is the storage form of carbohydrate and occurs in all nucleated animal cells. Glycogen is a branched polymer of glucosyl residues. α-1,4-Glycosidic bonds form linear chains, and α-1,6-glycosidic bonds form branches (Figure 7–6). Glycogen chains are 10–14 residues long, and each molecule contains about 4000 of these chains. Glycogen metabolism is particularly important in liver (the organ responsible for maintaining blood glucose) and muscle (the tissue responsible for movement).

The study of glycogen biosynthesis (**glycogenesis**) and degradation (**glycogenolysis**) was the prototype that led to the establishment of the principle that the pathway for biosynthesis differs from that for degradation (PRINCIPLE 19 OF BIOCHEMISTRY). Both glycogen biosynthesis and degradation are exergonic.

Two enzyme activities are required for glycogen biosynthesis. One enzyme catalyzes the addition of glucosyl residues forming the α-1,4 linkages (**glycogen synthase**), and a second enzyme mediates the formation of the α-1,6 branches (**branching enzyme**). Two different enzyme activities are required for glycogenolysis. These involve the cleavage of the straight chain α-1,4-glucosyl residues by phosphorolysis (the enzyme is **glycogen phosphorylase**) and α-1,6-hydrolysis activity (**debranching enzyme**). These processes are outlined in Figure 10–8.

Glycogenesis

Glycogen synthase catalyzes the reaction between glycogen containing n glucosyl residues (glycogen$_n$) with UDP-glucose to form a new α-1,4-glycosidic linkage (glycogen$_{n+1}$) and UDP (Figure 10–9). This transferase reaction proceeds with a loss of one high-energy bond and is exergonic. This process is repeated until a chain extending 12–16 glucosyl groups from a branch point is formed. **Branching enzyme (amylo-1,4-1,6-transglycosylase)** catalyzes the formation of an α-1,6 branch on the proximal portion of the donor chain (Figure 10–10). The branching enzyme reaction does not require the input of further chemical energy.

The glycogen synthase reaction requires a primer to which the glucosyl groups are added. The initial synthesis of each glycogen molecule requires the participation of a protein called **glycogenin** that functions as a primer. Glycogenin reacts with UDP-glucose to form a glycosylated protein in an autocatalytic process. The glucose residue is attached to a tyrosyl hydroxyl group. After the addition of about eight glucosyl residues, the oligosaccharide-protein complex functions as a primer to which additional glucosyl residues can be added to form the glycogen macromolecule as catalyzed by glycogen synthase.

From a bioenergetics viewpoint, the branching enzyme reaction is isoergonic because reactants and products contain only low-energy bonds (PRINCIPLE 4 OF BIOENERGETICS). The reaction, however, is not reversible as is the case for most isoergonic reactions. The evidence for the irreversible nature of the reaction is based on the existence in humans of an inborn error of metabolism (type III glycogen storage disease) in which the biochemical defect is inadequate debranching enzyme activity. If the branching enzyme reaction were reversible, one enzyme could catalyze both formation and elimination of the branches. The production of a severe metabolic disease by the deficiency of brancher activity underscores the importance of

FIGURE 10–8. *Overview of glucose 6-phosphate and glycogen metabolism.*

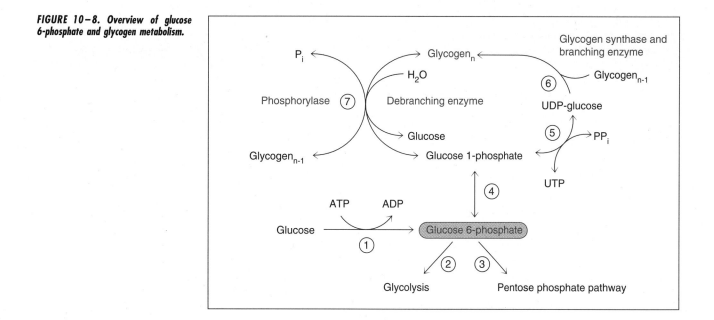

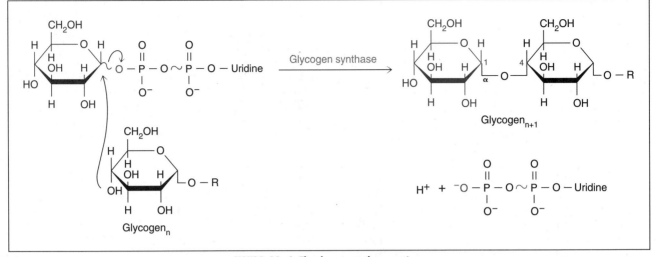

FIGURE 10–9. *The glycogen synthase reaction.*

the reaction in humans and indicates that reversal of brancher activity (which is debrancher activity) does not occur physiologically. There is, moreover, another glycogen storage disease (type IV) produced by deficient branching enzyme activity. Both disorders result in inappropriate accumulation of glycogen and are examples of **glycogen storage diseases;** these are discussed later in this chapter.

Glycogenolysis

Two enzymes are necessary for glycogenolysis (the degradation or lysis of glycogen). **Glycogen phosphorylase** (usually called phosphorylase) catalyzes a reaction between phosphate and glycogen to yield glucose 1-phosphate and glycogen$_{n-1}$ (Figure 10–11). Note that this is a phosphorolysis and not a hydrolysis reaction. This phosphorolysis (lysis by phosphate) reaction occurs at α-1,4-glycosidic bonds. Phosphorylase contains pyridoxal phosphate as a covalently bound prosthetic group. The Schiff base of pyridoxal phosphate does not participate in catalysis; rather, the phosphate group acts as a proton donor. This function of pyridoxal phosphate represents an unusual and noteworthy situation. The number of low-energy bonds in the reactants and products is the same, and the reaction is functionally isoergonic. The reaction proceeds in the direction of products at physiological metabolite concentrations.

Phosphorylase reactions occur until a glucosyl unit about four residues from a branch point is reached. Then a single protein with two enzymatic activities, called **debranching enzyme,** eliminates the branch by a two-step process (Figure 10–12). Transglycosylase activity of debranching enzyme transfers a triglucosyl fragment to the end of a chain. This reaction, which is isoergonic, does not require any additional energy. The α-1,6 hydrolysis reaction is exergonic, and the reaction is unidirectional (PRINCIPLE 5 OF BIOENERGETICS). Most of the glucosyl residues from glycogen are released as phosphate esters by the phosphorylase reaction. The resulting glucose 1-phosphate is converted into glucose 6-phosphate as catalyzed by phosphoglucomutase. About 10% of the residues are hydrolytically released as free glucose by the debranching reaction.

REGULATION OF GLYCOGENESIS AND GLYCOGENOLYSIS

The regulation of glycogenesis and glycogenolysis is intricate. The regulated enzymes include **glycogen synthase** and **glycogen phosphorylase.** (Branching and debranching enzymes do not play a regulatory role.) Both glycogen synthase and phosphorylase are regulated allosterically and by protein phosphorylation.

FIGURE 10–10. *Schematic diagram depicting the action of branching enzyme in glycogen biosynthesis.*

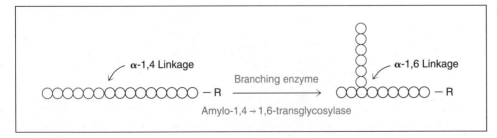

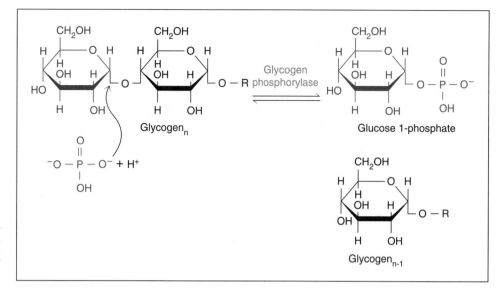

FIGURE 10–11. The glycogen phosphorylase reaction. *The α-1,4-glycosidic bond is cleaved by phosphate in a reaction called phosphorolysis.*

Many extracellular signaling molecules mediate their physiological responses through the cyclic AMP–second messenger system. The hormone, neurotransmitter, adhesion molecule, or local mediator is the first messenger, and cyclic AMP is one of several second messengers. The first messenger is extracellular, and the second messenger is intracellular. The process whereby an extracellular molecule affects intracellular function is called **signal**

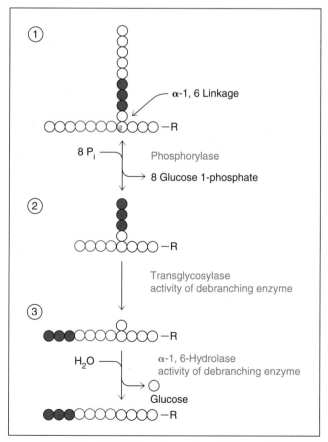

FIGURE 10–12. The debranching reactions of glycogenolysis.

transduction. Because the process is so prevalent, we will consider the second messenger scheme in detail. The regulation of glycogen metabolism by protein kinases was the first process shown to be regulated by the cyclic AMP second messenger system. The regulation is labyrinthine and intricate. After one understands this scheme, however, it is much easier to understand other phosphorylation-dephosphorylation processes that are encountered in biochemistry.

We consider the process step-by-step to facilitate understanding. We first identify the changes in activity of key enzymes that occur in response to protein phosphorylation. We then consider the overall change in glycogen metabolism that results from the activation of the cyclic AMP second messenger system and the accompanying protein phosphorylation reactions. We finally consider the reversal of the overall process by dephosphorylation.

Glucagon and Hyperglycemia

An early observation that led to the discovery of protein kinase A and the glycogen cascade of regulatory reactions was that glucagon (a hormone) leads to prompt hyperglycemia (elevation of serum glucose levels). The chief organ responsible for maintenance of blood glucose is the liver. *Liver cells contain glucose-6-phosphatase and can release free glucose into the bloodstream.* Muscle and nearly all other tissues lack glucose-6-phosphatase and are unable to release glucose into the bloodstream. Glucagon promotes glycogenolysis (the breakdown of glycogen) in liver. Glucagon leads to an increase in the rate of glycogenolysis by activating glycogen phosphorylase. Glucagon also leads to the inhibition of glycogen synthase. Our objective is to learn how the changes in the activity of phosphorylase and glycogen synthase arise in response to the action of glucagon.

Several aspects contribute to the intricacy of the glycogen regulatory scheme. First, control of glycogen metabolism involves a cascade. A **cascade** is a serial system in which one enzyme catalyzes the modification of a second enzyme, which in turn, catalyzes the modification of a third enzyme. The cascade can involve additional steps. Cascades can result in amplification of a response. If the first enzyme of a cascade catalyzes the modification of 100 molecules of a second enzyme, and the second enzyme catalyzes the modification of 100 molecules of a third protein, the end result is that the primary enzyme alters the activity of 100^2, or 10,000, molecules. A small amount of the first enzyme can therefore alter the activity of many target molecules.

The second difficulty with the glycogen cascade is not the biochemistry but the nomenclature. Protein kinases catalyze phosphorylation reactions, i.e., the formation of an ester bond between a phosphate and the hydroxyl group of a serine, threonine, or tyrosine residue. One important enzyme in glycogen metabolism catalyzes the breakdown of glycogen by a phosphorylase reaction (cleavage of glycogen by phosphate). The hindrance comes when we consider the phosphorylation (the chemical modification) of phosphorylase (the enzyme that cleaves with phosphate). Another challenge in the glycogen regulatory scheme is the inconsistent terminology used in naming the phosphorylated and the unphosphorylated proteins. Still another predicament is that the phosphorylation of some proteins enhances their activity, and the phosphorylation of others inhibits their activity. That the overall result follows the molecular logic of the cell serves, however, as an aid in understanding metabolic regulation.

Let us consider the physiological response to glucagon in more detail. Glucagon interacts with its receptor on the plasma membrane of the liver cell, producing conformational changes that result in activation of the plasma membrane–associated adenylyl cyclase. Adenylyl cyclase is activated by glucagon receptors by a mobile trimeric **G-protein** that catalyzes the hydrolysis of GTP. G_s stimulates adenylyl cyclase. G_i, activated by other extracellular signals, inhibits adenylyl cyclase. Active G-proteins contain GTP; inactive G-proteins contain GDP that was produced by the hydrolysis of GTP catalyzed by the G-protein.

Cyclic AMP, formed from ATP in the cytosol by stimulated adenylyl cyclase, specifically activates protein kinase A (Figure 10–13). This protein kinase is a tetramer consisting of two different subunits: R (regulatory) and C (catalytic). The R_2C_2 complex is inactive. Cyclic AMP binds to the complex to dissociate the R subunits from the C subunits. The free C subunits are active. Each R subunit has two cyclic AMP-binding sites. Protein kinase A, which exhibits broad substrate specificity, has three actions in the glycogen cascade: (1) activation of phosphorylase kinase (which, in turn, activates the glycogen-cleaving phosphorylase), (2) inhibition of glycogen synthase, and (3) actions that result in inhibition of phosphoprotein phosphatase–1 (Figure 10–14).

The free catalytic subunit of protein kinase A, generated by the action of cyclic AMP, catalyzes the phosphorylation of specific serine residues of phosphorylase kinase. Following phosphorylation, phosphorylase kinase is *activated*. Phosphorylase kinase is an intricate enzyme consisting of a tetramer of the four different subunits $(\alpha\beta\gamma\delta)_4$. The serine residues of phosphorylase kinase that are phosphorylated in the reaction catalyzed by protein kinase A are in the four α- and four β-subunits. In contrast to protein kinase A, phosphorylase kinase is a protein kinase with restricted substrate specificity; it catalyzes the phosphorylation of the enzyme called (glycogen) phosphorylase. Phosphorylase kinase remains active until the phosphoryl groups added by protein kinase A are hydrolytically removed by phosphoprotein phosphatase–1.

Phosphorylase kinase catalyzes the reaction of ATP with serine 14 of phosphorylase, and phosphorylase becomes *activated*. The historical and still current terms describing phosphorylase are **phosphorylase a** (the active and phosphorylated enzyme) and **phosphorylase b** (the less active, nonphosphorylated enzyme). Phosphorylase exists as a dimer, and each subunit can accept phosphate at serine 14. Phosphorylase a catalyzes the breakdown of glycogen to glucose 1-phosphate, and phosphoglucomutase mediates the conversion of glucose 1-phosphate to glucose 6-phosphate (Figure 10–4). Glucose-6-phosphatase catalyzes the exergonic hydrolysis of its substrate to form free glucose that is released into the bloodstream. This biochemical mechanism accounts for glucagon mediated hyperglycemia. Phosphorylase continues to cleave glycogen until inactivated by the hydrolytic removal of the phosphoryl group at serine 14 as catalyzed by phosphoprotein phosphatase–1.

Reactions Leading to Inhibition of Glycogen Synthase

Protein kinase A also catalyzes the phosphorylation glycogen synthase (Figure 10–14). Following phosphorylation, however, glycogen synthase and glycogen synthesis become *inhibited*. Phosphorylated glycogen synthase is called the **D** form. Its activity was thought to be *d*ependent on an allosteric effector, glucose 6-phosphate. Unphosphorylated glycogen synthase is called the **I** form. Its activity is *i*ndependent of the allosteric effector, glucose 6-phosphate. The nomenclature designating the D- and I-forms is set by precedent. The concentrations of glucose 6-phosphate required for activation, however, may not be achieved physiologically. The phosphorylated glycogen synthase remains inactive until the phosphoryl group

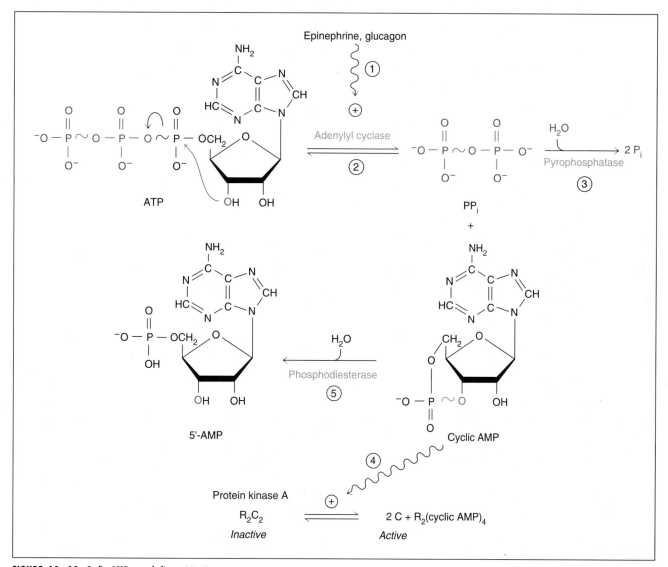

FIGURE 10–13. Cyclic AMP metabolism. *(1) Epinephrine and glucagon (and other hormones) stimulate adenylyl cyclase activity via plasma membrane receptors through G-proteins. (2) Adenylyl cyclase catalyzes the isoergonic conversion of ATP to cyclic AMP. (3) Pyrophosphatase catalyzes the exergonic hydrolysis of substrate to pull reaction 2 forward. (4) Cyclic AMP activates protein kinase A by forming a noncovalent complex with the regulatory, or R, subunits and dissociating them from the catalytic, or C, subunits. (5) Phosphodiesterase catalyzes the exergonic hydrolysis of cyclic AMP to 5'-AMP.*

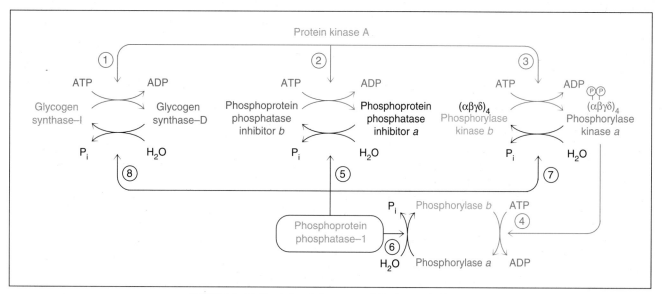

FIGURE 10–14. Regulation of glycogen metabolism by protein kinases.

145

is hydrolytically removed by phosphoprotein phosphatase–1.

Reactions Leading to Inhibition of Phosphoprotein Phosphatase–1

There is a family of phosphoprotein phosphatases designated 1, 2A, 2B, and 2C whose function is to remove phosphoryl groups added by protein kinases (Table 20–7); we need only consider the first enzyme for the glycogen cascade. Phosphoprotein phosphatase–1 is inhibited by a protein that is a substrate for protein kinase A. The native or unphosphorylated form of phosphatase-1 inhibitor does not inhibit protein phosphatase–1. The phosphorylated form of phosphatase-1 inhibitor, generated by the action of protein kinase A, binds to phosphatase-1 and inhibits phosphatase–1 activity. When the inhibitor is bound to protein phosphatase–1, the enzyme is inactive toward other substrates. The phosphorylated form of phosphatase inhibitor is dephosphorylated by protein phosphatase–1 or other phosphatases. Not only does the action of cyclic AMP lead to the activation of protein kinases, activation of protein kinase A leads to the inhibition of phosphoprotein phosphatase–1 (Figure 10–14). These are the responses that occur during the glycogenolytic and hyperglycemic phase of metabolism produced by glucagon.

Other protein kinases catalyze the phosphorylation of glycogen synthase (glycogen synthase kinase–3 and casein kinase–2) at serines that differ from those phosphorylated by protein kinase A. These other phosphoryl groups are also removed by the action of phosphatase-1. Inhibition of phosphatase-1 by the cyclic AMP–dependent reaction inhibits the removal of the phosphoryl groups added by the action of glycogen synthase kinase–3 and casein kinase–2, and phosphorylation mediated by these two kinases may be responsible for the inhibition of glycogen synthase. Whatever the mechanism, however, the important point is that phosphorylation of glycogen synthase is inhibitory.

Dephosphorylation Reactions

Let us consider the biochemistry for removing the phosphoryl groups from the acceptor proteins that lead to the decline of the glycogenolytic response. When the concentration of glucagon in the blood decreases, glucagon dissociates from its receptor in the liver cell plasma membrane. The G_s protein, which functions as an intermediary between the receptor and adenylyl cyclase, catalyzes the hydrolysis of GTP to form GDP and P_i, and the G protein no longer stimulates adenylyl cyclase. Adenylyl cyclase returns to its less active form, and cyclic AMP is no longer generated. Cyclic AMP

phosphodiesterase catalyzes the exergonic hydrolysis of cyclic AMP to 5'-AMP (Figure 10–13). Cyclic AMP levels fall, and cyclic AMP dissociates from the regulatory subunits of protein kinase A. Inactive protein kinase A holoenzyme forms from the regulatory and catalytic subunits. The phosphorylation of glycogen synthase, phosphoprotein phosphatase inhibitor–1, and phosphorylase kinase ceases.

Dephosphorylation of phosphatase inhibitor allows phosphoprotein phosphatase–1 to become active. Phosphoprotein phosphatase–1 catalyzes the hydrolysis of phosphate from serine 14 of phosphorylase a to produce the less active phosphorylase b. Phosphoprotein phosphatase–1 catalyzes the hydrolysis of phosphate from the α- and β-subunits of phosphorylase kinase to produce the less active enzyme. The dephosphorylation of both phosphorylase kinase and phosphorylase decreases the rate of glycogenolysis. Phosphoprotein phosphatase–1 catalyzes the hydrolysis of glycogen synthase–D to produce the more active unphosphorylated glycogen synthase–I. All components are now in their initial state (Figure 10–14).

The bioenergetics of these phosphorylation-dephosphorylation processes is straightforward. The phosphorylation reactions catalyzed by these protein kinases involve the formation of low-energy protein phosphoserine residues, and these reactions proceed with the loss of a high-energy bond and are exergonic (PRINCIPLE 2 OF BIOENERGETICS). Moreover, the hydrolysis reactions that remove phosphate from proteins are exergonic (PRINCIPLE 5 OF BIOENERGETICS). Both kinase and phosphatase reactions do not occur simultaneously, however, because they are differentially regulated.

Allosteric Regulation of Glycogen Metabolism

As complex as this scheme is, the physiological situation is even more elaborate. Glycogen phosphorylase, phosphorylase kinase, and glycogen synthase are all regulated by noncovalent allosteric effectors. Phosphorylase, for example, is activated by 5'-AMP. 5'-AMP serves as a signal that the energy charge and ATP levels are low. Since glycogen is a fuel whose metabolism leads to ATP generation, both aerobically and anaerobically, activation of glycogenolysis follows the molecular logic of the cell. ATP and glucose 6-phosphate are allosteric inhibitors of phosphorylase. The inhibition by ATP is reciprocal to the effect described for 5'-AMP. When ATP levels are high, there is no need to degrade glycogen for energy production. When glucose 6-phosphate levels are high, this serves as a signal that glucose should be stored. Hence, the inhibition of phosphorylase and the activation of glycogen synthase (Table 25–1).

Phosphorylase kinase is activated by calcium. The δ-subunit of phosphorylase kinase is the calcium-binding protein called **calmodulin.** The activation of muscle phosphorylase kinase by calcium plays an important role in the activation of phosphorylase kinase and the downstream processes of phosphorylase activation. The depolarization of muscle by acetylcholine mobilizes cytosolic calcium to trigger muscle contraction. Calcium also activates phosphorylase kinase, promoting glycogenolysis. Glycogenolysis is activated during periods of muscle contraction.

Differential Regulation of Glycogenesis and Glycogenolysis

The advantage of separate pathways for the synthesis and degradation of a compound is that the pathways can be differentially regulated. Besides the activation of phosphorylase, the cyclic AMP–second messenger system mediates the inactivation of glycogen synthase. The inhibition of glycogen synthase does not involve a cascade (the phosphorylation of one enzyme that catalyzes the phosphorylation of a second protein). Rather, protein kinase A catalyzes the direct reaction of glycogen synthase and ATP to form phosphorylated glycogen synthase and ADP (Figure 10–14).

This mechanism for the regulation of glycogenesis and glycogenolysis (Table 25–2) occurs in all nucleated cells. The hormones or neurotransmitters that activate adenylyl cyclase to initiate the process may differ from cell to cell. The action of cyclic AMP in muscle, produced in response to epinephrine but not glucagon, is to promote glycogenolysis. Muscle and other cells lacking glucose-6-phosphatase use the liberated metabolites (glucose 1-phosphate and glucose) for glycolysis and ATP production.

GLYCOGEN STORAGE DISEASES

▶ Several rare inborn errors in glycogen metabolism have been described, and these are listed numerically in Table 10–3 along with the corresponding enzyme defects. When the liver is the chief organ affected, as in types I, III, and VI, the signs include hypoglycemia and hepatomegaly. The hypoglycemia is associated with hypoinsulinemia and hyperglucagonemia, and this hormonal profile serves to distinguish these disorders from other causes of hypoglycemia. When muscle is affected, as in types III, V, and VII, the symptoms are related to the inability of metabolism to provide energy for muscle contraction. The inheritance of these disorders is autosomal recessive except for one form of type VI that is X-linked.

It is noteworthy that the type I glycogen storage disease **(von Gierke disease)** is due to a deficiency of glucose-6-phosphatase. Besides hepatomegaly, the kidneys of affected individuals are usually twice the normal size. Hypoglycemia, lactic acidemia, and elevated blood triglycerides are hallmarks of the disorder. These individuals fail to increase blood glucose following galactose or fructose ingestion or glucagon injection as does a normal individual. As a result of the inability to release glucose into the bloodstream because of a deficiency of glucose-6-phosphatase, glucose is converted to lactate, which is released into the bloodstream. The liver also synthesizes lactate from glycogen, galactose, fructose, and glycerol, substances ordinarily converted to glucose. Treatment is symptomatic, and the prognosis is guarded.

Type II glycogen storage disease **(Pompe disease)** involves the heart, skeletal muscle, and nervous system. It is due to a deficiency of acid α-glu-

TABLE 10–3.   Glycogen Storage Diseases

Type*	Defective Enzyme	Organ Affected	Glycogen in the Affected Organ	Clinical Features
I Von Gierke disease	Glucose-6-phosphatase	Liver and kidney	Increased amount; normal structure	Massive enlargement of the liver. Failure to thrive. Severe hypoglycemia, ketosis, hyperlipemia
II Pompe disease	α-1,4-Glucosidase (lysosomal)	All organs	Massive increase in amount; normal structure	Cardiorespiratory failure causes death, usually before age 2
III Cori disease	Amylo-1,6-glucosidase (debranching enzyme)	Muscle and liver	Increased amount; short outer branches	Similar to type I, but milder course
IV Anderson disease	Branching enzyme (α-1,4 → α-1,6)	Liver and spleen	Normal amount; very long outer branches	Progressive cirrhosis of the liver. Liver failure causes death, usually before age 2
V McArdle disease	Phosphorylase	Muscle	Moderately increased amount; normal structure	Limited ability to perform strenuous exercise because of painful muscle cramps
VI Hers disease	Phosphorylase	Liver	Increased amount	Similar to type I, but milder course
VII Tarui disease	Phosphofructokinase	Muscle	Increased amount; normal structure	Similar to type V
VIII	Phosphorylase kinase	Liver	Increased amount; normal structure	Mild liver enlargement. Mild hypoglycemia

* Some of the type VI disorders are X-linked; otherwise, the glycogen storage diseases are autosomal recessive.

cosidase, a lysosomal enzyme whose gene is on chromosome 17 (Table 16–5). Because of this defect, there is an accumulation of glycogen particles in vacuoles. This malady, in contrast to von Gierke disease, is not associated with hypoglycemia. α-Glucosidase was not mentioned in our consideration of the normal catabolism of glycogen, but the failure of affected individuals to survive for more than 1–2 years indicates that it is an important enzyme in the degradation of glycogen.

Type V glycogen storage disease **(McArdle disease)** is due to a deficiency of muscle phosphorylase. Fatigue with exercise and muscle cramps appear in the second or third decade of life. Unlike in normal individuals, there is no increase in venous lactate following exercise. Liver glycogen metabolism is normal, and hypoglycemia is absent. ◄

BACTERIAL GLYCAN METABOLISM AND DENTAL CARIES

Glycans are extracellular polymers of glucose produced by bacteria. *Streptococcus mutans,* the microbe that is responsible for the initiation of dental caries, produces a glycan polymer containing α-1,6 and α-1,3 linkages. The polymer is named **mutan,** after the bacteria. Mutan is formed from sucrose in reactions catalyzed by extracellular glucosyl transferases:

$$\text{Sucrose} + \text{mutan}_n \rightarrow \text{mutan}_{n+1} + \text{fructose} \quad (10.8)$$

The glycosidic bond of sucrose is a high-energy bond with a standard free energy of hydrolysis of -30 kJ/mol. The product contains a low-energy glycosidic bond, and the overall reaction is exergonic. Note that ATP and nucleotide derivatives cannot participate in glycan formation because they are intracellular metabolites, and glycan formation occurs extracellularly.

► Sucrose is the most cariogenic sugar in the diet, and its role in mutan formation explains this phenomenon. The α-1,3 linkages confer insolubility and promote bacterial colonization on enamel, and these substances are more important for producing caries than glycans containing α-1,6 linkages, which are soluble. Salivary glycoproteins bind to the surfaces of teeth to form a pellicle. Bacteria bind to the glycoprotein in the pellicle to form plaque. Calcified pellicle forms calculus (Latin "stone"). The formation of mutan promotes adhesion and colonization of *S. mutans* to plaque. Fructans, which are polymers of fructose containing β-1,2-furanoside bonds, are an extracellular energy storage form of carbohydrate for bacteria in plaque and are only secondarily involved in cariogenesis. They are synthesized by a reaction analogous to that for glycans with sucrose as the extracellular fructosyl donor.

S. mutans is a gram-positive, anaerobic bacterium that inhabits dental plaque and derives all its energy by glycolysis. These bacteria produce dental caries by converting sugars to lactic acid, the cariogenic agent. As a result, plaque pH decreases from about 6.8 to 5 or less, and lactic acid dissolves enamel. A carbohydrate-containing meal, especially one with simple sugars (monosaccharides and disaccharides), produces a prompt and brisk decrease in plaque pH. Compounds that are fermented by *S. mutans* include all the common dietary sugars (glucose, fructose, sucrose, lactose, and maltose), sorbitol, and mannitol. The sugars are taken up by a phosphoenolpyruvate-dependent phosphotransferase system, resulting in the formation of a sugar phosphate that can be metabolized by the Embden-Meyerhof glycolytic pathway. The bacteria also possess hexokinase to initiate hexose degradation, as required. Fluoride is anticariogenic and bacteriostatic, and this is postulated to be due to inhibition of *S. mutans* enolase. The bacterial phosphoglyceromutase and proton-translocating ATPase (the F_oF_1 ATP synthase operating in the reverse direction) may also be inhibited by low concentrations (≈ 0.25 mM) of fluoride.

Buffers in saliva counteract the decrease in plaque pH produced by bacteria. The pH of saliva increases with increased flow, and this is protective. Caries is common in conditions associated with decreased salivary flow (xerostomia). Dry mouth can result from irradiation of salivary glands and administration of anticholinergic medication. Sjögren syndrome is a chronic inflammatory and autoimmune disorder in which the salivary and lacrimal glands undergo progressive destruction by white blood cells with decreased production of saliva (xerostomia) and tears. Primary Sjögren syndrome involves these symptoms alone; secondary Sjögren syndrome involves this diad and rheumatoid arthritis. ◄

SUMMARY

The pathway for the biosynthesis of a compound differs from that of its degradation. This principle allows both synthesis and degradation to be exergonic, and this biochemical strategy permits independent and interdependent regulation. This principle applies to glycolysis and gluconeogenesis, glycogenolysis and glycogenesis, and other pathways of metabolism.

Gluconeogenesis uses four ATP, two GTP and two NADH molecules during the conversion of two pyruvate to one glucose molecule. Pyruvate carboxylase (a biotin-containing enzyme) and phosphoenolpyruvate carboxykinase (a GTP-requiring enzyme) bypass the pyruvate kinase reaction. Fructose-1,6-bisphosphatase bypasses the phosphofructokinase reaction. Glucose-6-phosphatase bypasses the hexokinase reaction. Glycolysis occurs in all cells; gluconeogenesis is important in liver and kidney.

Phosphofructokinase is the chief regulatory enzyme of glycolysis and fructose-1,6-bisphosphatase is an important regulatory step in gluconeogenesis. These enzymes are reciprocally regulated. Fructose 2,6-bisphosphate is the main regulatory molecule. Fructose 2,6-bisphosphate activates phosphofructokinase and inhibits fructose-1,6-bisphosphatase. High glucagon-to-insulin ratios activate gluconeogenesis. This situation promotes cyclic AMP production and activates protein kinase A. The phosphorylation of fructose-6-phosphate-2-kinase/phosphatase activates fructose-2,6-bisphosphatase activity. The destruction of fructose 2,6-bisphosphate leads to an increase in fructose-1,6-bisphosphatase activity and increased gluconeogenesis. Pyruvate carboxylase requires acetyl-CoA for the expression of activity.

The reaction responsible for lactose biosynthesis serves as a prototype for carbohydrate condensation reactions. UDP-galactose ($2\sim$) reacts with glucose to produce lactose ($0\sim$) and UDP ($1\sim$). The reaction proceeds with the loss of one high-energy bond and is exergonic. The synthesis of glycogen exhibits similar bioenergetics.

Two enzymes involved in glycogen biosynthesis are glycogen synthase and branching enzyme. Glycogen synthase transfers activated glucose to a carbohydrate primer to form an α-1,4-glycosidic bond in an exergonic process. Branching reactions involve the transfer of a block of glycosyl residues to the C^6 hydroxyl group of an acceptor residue with the concomitant formation of an α-1,6-glycosidic branch. Two enzymes are required for glycogenolysis: glycogen phosphorylase and debranching enzyme. The first enzyme catalyzes the phosphorolytic cleavage of α-1,4-glycosidic bonds to yield glucose 1-phosphate and glycogen containing one less glucose residue. This reaction is exergonic under physiological conditions. About 90% of the glycogen is cleaved by the phosphorylase reaction. The second enzyme, a debranching enzyme, has two activities. Debranching enzyme moves a triglucosyl chain from a branch to the straight chain, forming a new α-1,4-bond. Debranching enzyme then catalyzes the hydrolysis of an α-1,6 bond to yield free glucose and a glycogen with one fewer glucose residue. This reaction is exergonic and unidirectional.

The protein kinase cascade that participates in the regulation of glycogen metabolism has been well characterized. The activation of phosphorylase requires two serial protein kinase steps—a cascade. The first enzyme is protein kinase A. This enzyme catalyzes the phosphorylation and activation of phosphorylase kinase. The second enzyme, phosphorylase kinase, catalyzes the phosphorylation and activation of phosphorylase (converting the *b* form to the *a* form). Protein kinase A also catalyzes the phosphorylation and inactivation of glycogen synthase (converting the I form to the D form). Protein kinase A holoenzyme is made up of R_2C_2 subunits (inactive) and is dissociated following the binding of cyclic AMP to the regulatory subunits. Free C subunits are active. These protein kinase reactions occur in the cytosol. Protein kinase A is the only protein kinase that dissociates during activation. Other protein kinase activities are altered by conformational changes.

Von Gierke disease is caused by a deficiency of glucose-6-phosphatase, a hepatic enzyme. Pompe disease is a lysosomal disease that is caused by a deficiency of α-1,4-glucosidase, which occurs in all nucleated cells. McArdle disease is caused by a deficiency of muscle phosphorylase.

SELECTED READINGS

Cori, G.T. Glycogen structure and enzyme deficiencies in glycogen storage disease. Harvey Lectures 48:145–171, 1952–1953.

DeFronzo, R.A., and E. Ferrannini. Regulation of hepatic glucose metabolism in humans. Diabetes/Metabolism Reviews 3:415–459, 1987.

Hardie, D.G. *Biochemical Messengers: Hormones, Neurotransmitters, and Growth Factors.* London, Chapman & Hall, 1991.

Hers, H.G., F. Van Hoof, and T. de Barsy. Glycogen Storage Diseases. *In* C.R. Scriver, A.L. Beaudet, W.S. Sly, and D. Valle (eds.). *Metabolic Basis of Inherited Disease,* 6th ed. New York, McGraw-Hill Book Company, 1989, pp. 425–452.

Larner, J. Insulin and the stimulation of glycogen synthesis. Advances in Enzymology 63:173–231, 1990.

Olefsky, J.M. Diabetes Mellitus. *In* J.B. Wyngaarden, L.H. Smith, Jr., and J.C. Bennett (eds.). *Cecil Textbook of Medicine,* 19th ed. Philadelphia, W.B. Saunders Company, 1291–1310, 1992.

CHAPTER ELEVEN

FATTY ACID AND

TRIGLYCERIDE

METABOLISM

Vitalism had a strong influence on biological thinking and for all we know, it will raise its Hydra-head again, because the idea that life processes can be entirely explained by known laws of physics and chemistry is hard to accept by some.

—Carl F. Cori

Lipids are defined operationally as biomolecules that are soluble in organic solvents such as chloroform/methanol. As a corollary, lipids are poorly soluble in water. Lipids, particularly triglycerides (triacylglycerols), are a source of concentrated chemical energy, and lipids represent an important food. Membranes are lipid bilayers that contain proteins (Figure 1–4); phospholipids and cholesterol are important components of eukaryotic membranes. The diverse chemical classes of lipids are given in Table 11–1.

FATTY ACIDS

Nomenclature

Fatty acids are represented by the formula R—COOH, where R is an alkyl group. Fatty acids are divided into short- (2 to 4 carbon atoms), medium- (6 to 10 carbon atoms), and long- (12 to 26 or more carbon atoms) chain classes. Most fatty acids present in human cells are of the long-chain variety. Almost all fatty acids in nature contain an even number of carbon atoms (Table 11–2).

Like amino acids, fatty acids exist at physiological pH as the anionic carboxylate:

$$R—COOH \rightleftharpoons RCOO^- + H^+ \qquad (11.1)$$

The hydrophobic alkyl chain and the hydrophilic carboxyl group give fatty acids detergent properties. The alkyl side chain seeks a nonpolar environment, and the carboxylate seeks an aqueous environment. The concentration of fatty acid in the circulation is 0.5 to 0.7 mM, and most of this fatty acid is bound to albumin. Free fatty acids are not found as structural constituents of membranes.

TABLE 11–1.   Classification of Lipids

Lipid	Function
Fatty acids	Metabolic fuel; component of several other classes of lipids
Triglycerides	Main storage form of fatty acids and chemical energy
Phospholipids	Component of membranes; source of arachidonic acid, inositol triphosphate, and diglyceride for signal transduction
Sphingolipids	Component of membranes
Cholesterol	Component of membranes; precursor of bile salts and steroid hormones
Bile salts	Lipid digestion and absorption; main product of cholesterol metabolism
Steroid hormones	Intercellular signals that regulate gene expression in target cells
Eicosanoids	Regulators of physiological functions
Vitamins	Vision; calcium metabolism; antioxidants; blood coagulation
Ketone bodies	Metabolic fuel

Unsaturated Fatty Acids

Double bonds in naturally occurring unsaturated fatty acids have the *cis* configuration. Those with one double bond are **monounsaturated fatty acids,** and those with two or more double bonds are **polyunsaturated fatty acids.** Plant and fish fats contain more polyunsaturated fatty acids than those of mammals or fowl (Table 11–3). Human cells contain at least twice as many unsaturated as saturated fatty acid derivatives.

The carbon atoms of fatty acids are designated by numbers or letters. The lettering system describes C^2 (starting from the carboxylate as C^1) as the α-carbon, C^3 as the β-carbon, and the methyl group at the end of the chain as the ω-carbon (Figure 11–1). β-Oxidation refers to the oxidation of the β-carbon atom.

TABLE 11–2.   Some Naturally Occurring Fatty Acids

Common Name	Systematic Name	Carbon Atoms	Double Bonds	Position of Double Bonds	Unsaturated Fatty Acid Class
Saturated fatty acids					
Formate	—	1	0	—	—
Acetate	Ethanoate	2	0	—	—
Propionate	Propanoate	3	0	—	—
n-Butyrate	Butanoate	4	0	—	—
Laurate	Dodecanoate	12	0	—	—
Myristate	Tetradecanoate	14	0	—	—
Palmitate	Hexadecanoate	16	0	—	—
Stearate	Octadecanoate	18	0	—	—
Arachidate	Eicosanoate	20	0	—	—
Unsaturated fatty acids					
Palmitoleate	*cis*-9-Hexadecenoate	16	1	9	ω-7
Oleate	*cis*-9-Octadecenoate	18	1	9	ω-9
Linoleate	*cis,cis*-9,12-Octadecadienoate	18	2	9,12	ω-6
Linolenate	*cis,cis,cis*-9,12,15-Octadecatrienoate	18	3	9,12,15	ω-3
γ-Linolenate	*cis,cis,cis*-6,9,12-Octadecatrienoate	18	3	6,9,12	ω-6
Arachidonate	*cis,cis,cis,cis*-5,8,11,14-Eicosatetraenoate	20	4	5,8,11,14	ω-6
EPA	Eicosapentaenoate	20	5	5,8,11,14,17	ω-3
DHA	Docosahexaenoate	22	6	4,7,10,13,16,19	ω-3

TABLE 11–3. Fatty Acid Composition of Some Fats of Animal and Plant Origin

	Saturated (%)	Monounsaturated (%)	Polyunsaturated (%)
Animal Fats			
Fish	28	29	43
Chicken	40	38	22
Pork	40	46	14
Beef	54	44	2
Butter	59	37	4
Vegetable Oils			
Safflower	11	11	78
Sunflower	12	18	70
Corn	14	26	60
Sesame	14	43	43
Soybean	15	27	58
Peanut	20	45	35
Margarine	20	48	32
Cottonseed	29	19	52
Coconut	86	12	2

Two systems are used to designate the position of double bonds. In the Δ (delta) system, the carboxylate is considered as C^1, and the position of the double bond is denoted by the carbon atom of the double bond closest to the carboxylate. Palmitoleic acid, for example, is denoted as 16:1Δ9. The compound contains 16 carbon atoms and one *cis*-double bond, and the position of the double bond is between C^9 and C^{10} (Figure 11–1).

In the n or ω-system, palmitoleic acid is denoted as 16:1n-7 or 16:1ω-7. The position of the double bond is between C^9 (16 − 7 = 9) and C^{10}. Linoleic acid, an essential fatty acid for humans that must be derived from the diet, can be denoted as 18:2Δ9,12, 18:2ω-6, or 18:2n-6. This corresponds to an 18-carbon compound with two double bonds beginning at C^9 and at C^{12}. The double bond nearest the end of the alkyl chain occurs at the ω-6

position (Figure 11–1). The Δ system is unambiguous. The ω or n system assumes that the double bonds are separated by three carbon atoms.

Unsaturated fatty acids are divided into four classes based upon the position of the double bond relative to the ω-end of the molecule (Table 11–4). Each class makes up a family of fatty acids, and all the members of that family can be synthesized from the parent fatty acid. For example, arachidonic acid (20:4ω-6) is synthesized from linoleic acid (18:2ω-6 or 18:2Δ9,12). No member of the oleic acid class (ω-9) in humans can be converted to the ω-6 class. Moreover, no member of the ω-6 class can be converted to the ω-3 class.

Cis and Trans Isomerism

A double bond in an alkyl side chain can occur in the *cis* or *trans* configuration (Figure 2–7). Nearly all double bonds in naturally occurring fatty acids in humans, other animals, plants, and bacteria are of the *cis* configuration. *Trans* double bonds, however, are formed during the catalytic hydrogenation of vegetable oils to make margarine. *Trans* fatty acid derivatives are found in many commercially made cookies, candies, and fried foods. The purpose of hydrogenation is to change the physical properties of oils into solid products, which are easier to manipulate. The greater the number of double bonds, the lower is the melting point. Fats containing several unsaturated bonds exist as oils or liquids at room temperature, and those containing few unsaturated bonds exist as solids. When ingested by humans, fatty acids with *trans* double bonds can be oxidized or incorporated into structural lipids. *Trans* fatty acids do not accumulate in human tissues, and cells contain enzyme activities required to completely oxidize such nutrients.

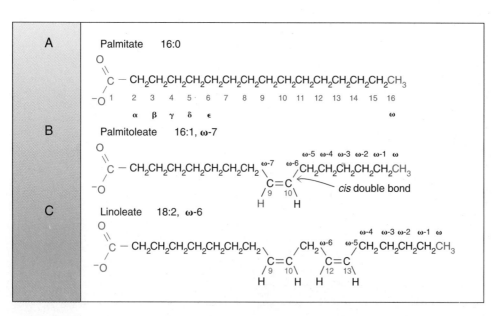

FIGURE 11–1. Fatty acids. A. *Palmitate, the conjugate base of the 16-carbon saturated fatty acid. The carbon atoms are numbered 1 through 16 beginning from the carboxylate. The α-carbon is attached to the carboxylate. B. Palmitoleate. The ω-carbon is at the end of the alkyl chain. The double bond nearest the methyl end of the alkyl chain occurs at the ω-7 position. C. Linoleate, an essential fatty acid.*

TABLE 11–4. Fatty Acid Nomenclature

Descriptive Name	Numeric	Δ	n	ω
		Abbreviation System		
Palmitate	16:0			
Palmitoleate	9–16:1	16:1Δ9	16:1n-7	16:1ω-7
Linoleate	9,12–18:2	18:2Δ9,12	18:2n-6	18:2ω-6
Linolenate	9,12,15–18:3	18:3Δ9,12,15	18:3n-3	18:3ω-3

Composition of Dietary Fats

Lipids in the diet are composed of a mixture of fatty acid derivatives. Because of the perceived health consequences of fats in the diet, the composition of saturated, monounsaturated, and polyunsaturated fatty acids in human diets has been a topic for medical investigation. Fats derived from animal sources contain more saturated fatty acids than those from plant sources. An exception is coconut oil, which contains about 86% saturated fatty acid (see Table 11–3). The polyunsaturated fatty acids in the common plant oils are in the ω-6 class. Certain fish oils contain between a quarter and a third of fatty acids of the ω-3 class.

▶ Saturated fatty acids raise both "good" cholesterol (HDL) and "bad" cholesterol (LDL; see Chapter 12). Monounsaturated fatty acids raise HDL and lower LDL, and polyunsaturated fatty acids maintain HDL but lower LDL. *Trans* fatty acids lower HDL and raise LDL. Diets that contain monounsaturated and polyunsaturated fatty acids are used therapeutically for the treatment of hypercholesterolemia (elevated blood cholesterol). The ω-3 class of polyunsaturated fatty acids is produced by plants that grow in cold sea water. Fish such as salmon that feed on this vegetation (directly or indirectly) contain large amounts of the ω-3 class of fatty acids. These fatty acids are effective in lowering the levels of plasma triglycerides, and they may protect against thrombosis. ◀

Essential Fatty Acids

Those fatty acids that are required for optimal health and cannot be synthesized are called essential fatty acids (Table 2–4) and must be obtained from the diet. The parent fatty acids of the ω-6 class (**linoleate**) and the ω-3 class (**linolenate**) are the two essential fatty acids (Figure 2–25). Linoleic acid is a precursor of prostaglandins and other eicosanoids. The role of linolenic acid in metabolism is unclear.

ESTERS

Triglycerides

Triglycerides are compounds that contain glycerol to which three fatty acids or three acyl groups are attached (Figure 11–2). Glycerol is a compound with three carbon atoms each of which contains an alcohol side chain. C^2 is a prochiral carbon atom and can become asymmetrical when different groups are bound to the alcohol groups of C^1 and C^3; naturally occurring glycerol derivatives correspond to L-glyceraldehyde and exist in the L-configuration. Bonds that link a fatty acid to an alcohol are esters (Table 2–2), and these are low-energy bonds (Table 6–1). Ester linkages are prevalent in lipids. The three fatty acids that occur in each triglyceride usually differ. Moreover, the fatty acyl group at C^2 is usually unsaturated. Butter and margarine consist predominantly of triglyceride.

Cholesterol and Cholesteryl Esters

Cholesterol, an alcohol, contains 27 carbon atoms and one double bond (Figure 11–3). Cholesterol is a steroid, and steroids are characterized by a cyclopentane ring attached to a saturated three-membered phenanthrene ring system. Cholesterol contains methyl groups at positions 18 and 19, and an eight-membered alkyl side chain. When the alcohol group of cholesterol is attached to an acyl group, the resulting cholesteryl ester is apolar. Cholesterol occurs in membranes, but cholesteryl esters do not.

PHOSPHOLIPIDS

Glycerolipids

Glycerolipids, which contain glycerol, are derived from phosphatidate (Figure 11–4). Phospha-

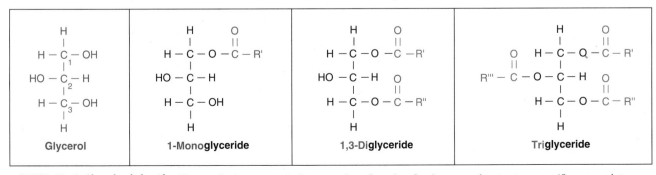

FIGURE 11–2. Glycerol and glycerides. *The numbering system indicates* sn-1, sn-2, *and* sn-3, *where* sn *refers to stereospecific nomenclature.*

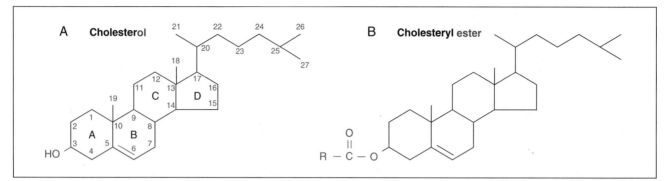

FIGURE 11–3. Cholesterol and cholesteryl ester. A. *Cholesterol. The four rings of the steroid are labeled A, B, C, and D. The methyl groups labeled 18 and 19 are called angular methyl groups. Note the double bond between carbon atoms 5 and 6 and the alcohol at carbon 3.* B. *Cholesteryl ester. An acyl group is attached to the alcohol via a low-energy ester bond.*

tidate is not a storage form of lipid but is a key metabolic intermediate in lipid metabolism. The phosphate of complex lipids is bonded as a low-energy ester to glycerol and a second alcohol to form a phosphodiester (Figure 11–5). These compounds are important constituents of membranes. Moreover, phosphatidylinositol phosphate derivatives play a role in the generation of intracellular regulatory compounds. Removal of the *sn*-2 acyl group from phosphatidylcholine results in lysophosphatidylcholine. These compounds lyse membranes; hence, the *lyso* prefix.

Sphingolipids

Sphingolipids are derivatives of **sphingosine,** an amino alcohol (Figure 11–6). The acylation of the amino group produces **ceramide.** Attachment of choline phosphate to C^1 results in **sphingomyelin.** Attachment of a monosaccharide to C^1 results in a **cerebroside,** and attachment of an oligosaccharide results in a **ganglioside.** These sphingolipids were isolated from nervous tissue, thereby accounting for their names. The sphingolipids occur in all human tissues, however, and are important components of membranes.

DIGESTION AND ABSORPTION OF LIPIDS

Human adults ingest between 60 and 150 grams of fat, on the average, per day. To aid in the digestion and absorption of lipid, the liver secretes bile that contains bile salts and phosphatidylcholine, which function as detergents to solubilize dietary fat. Solubilization facilitates digestion and absorption of dietary fat.

Digestive Enzymes

The stomach produces gastric lipase that is stable and active at the low pH found in the stomach. **Gastric lipase** initiates lipid digestion, which is completed in the small intestine by pancreatic lipase. **Pancreatic lipase** digests triglyceride to produce a mixture of 2-monoglycerides and fatty acids. **Colipase** is a low-molecular-mass protein (12 kDa) produced by the pancreas that is required for pancreatic lipase activity. Pancreatic juice also contains an **esterase** that acts on monoglycerides, cholesterol esters, and esters of vitamin A. The pancreas also secretes a **phospholipase** that catalyzes the hydrolytic removal of the 2-acyl group of phospholipids.

Bile Salts

Bile salts, which are oxidation products of cholesterol (Figure 11–7), form micelles consisting of colloidal particles with a polar exterior exposed to water and a nonpolar interior. The hydrophobic portion of bile salts points to the interior, and the carboxylate and alcohol groups point to the exterior. Besides providing the vehicle for the transport of lipids from the intestinal lumen to epithelial cells where absorption occurs, micelles participate in the absorption of free fatty acids, monoglycerides, cholesterol, and fat-soluble vitamins.

Absorption

After fatty acids and 2-monoglycerides are taken up by the intestinal epithelium and are converted

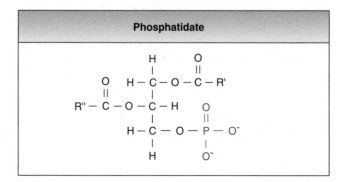

FIGURE 11–4. Phosphatidate. *Acyl groups are attached in ester linkage at* sn-1 *and* sn-2, *and phosphate is attached in ester linkage at* sn-3. *Each of these three bonds is of the low-energy variety.*

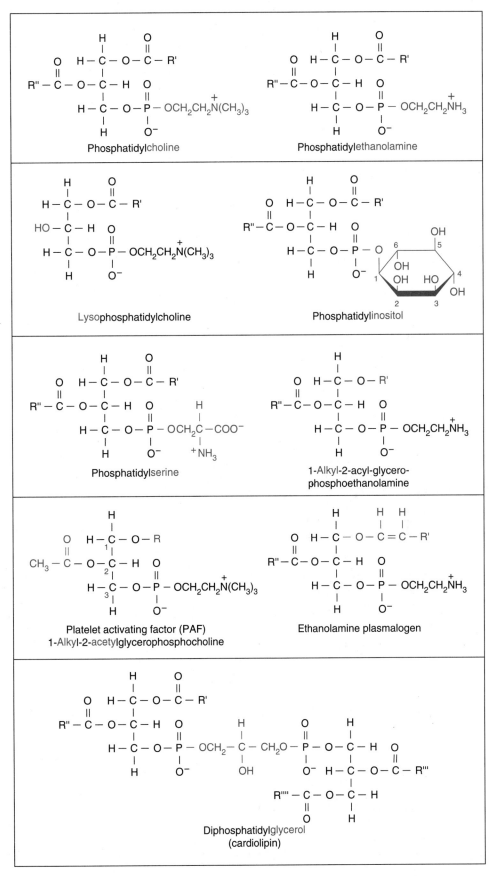

FIGURE 11–5. Representative glycerolipids. *A nonsystematic name for phosphatidylcholine is lecithin. The 1-alkyl phospholipids and platelet activating factor contain an alkyl group attached via an ether bond to the sn-1 carbon atom. The other compounds contain an acyl group attached to alcohol at sn-1.*

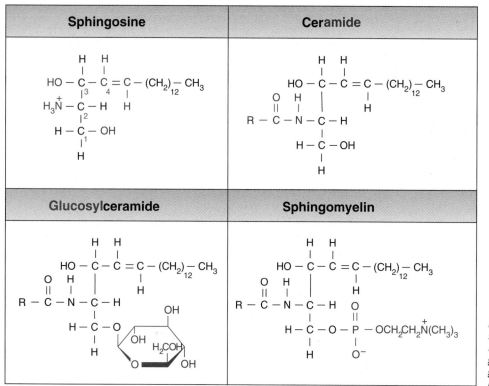

FIGURE 11–6. Sphingosine and representative sphingolipids. Sphingosine is a C_{18} compound with hydroxyl groups on C^1 and C^3, an amino group on C^2, and a trans double bond at C^4.

to triglyceride by the mucosal cells, dietary lipid is released into the lymph from the intestine as **chylomicrons.** Chylomicrons, which are made up of lipid and protein, represent one form of circulating lipoprotein. The contents of the chylomicrons are delivered to tissues as described in Chapter 12. Short- and medium-chain fatty acids, which are present in food in only small amounts, are absorbed into the portal blood and delivered to the liver as free fatty acids. Short- and medium-chain fatty acids bypass the lipoprotein pathway for intestinal absorption, and this property can be used to advantage in human therapeutics.

β-OXIDATION OF FATTY ACIDS

The first step in the complete oxidation of fatty acids involves the formation of fatty acyl coenzyme A, which undergoes a succession of reactions to produce acetyl-CoA and a fatty acyl-CoA shortened by two carbon atoms. β-Oxidation continues sequentially until acetoacetyl-CoA is degraded into two acetyl-CoA molecules. The acetyl-CoA produced by β-oxidation is metabolized by the Krebs cycle, the final common pathway of metabolism. During β-oxidation, the fatty acyl–CoA is first oxidized to yield $FADH_2$, and then a subsequent reaction yields NADH. These reduced coenzymes transfer their electrons to the respiratory chain as described in Chapter 9.

Comparison of β-Oxidation and Krebs Cycle Reactions

The reactions of β-oxidation are given in abbreviated form in equation 11.2.

$$\text{Fatty acyl–CoA} \xrightarrow[\text{FAD} \quad \text{FADH}_2]{} \text{trans-}\Delta^2\text{-enoyl-CoA} \xrightarrow[\text{H}_2\text{O}]{}$$

$$\text{L-3-hydroxyacyl-CoA} \xrightarrow[\text{NAD}^+ \quad \text{NADH} + \text{H}^+]{} \text{3-keto fatty acyl–CoA} \quad (11.2)$$

The reactions are analogous to three reactions of the Krebs cycle (those given in equation 11.3). The first oxidation involves a saturated hydrocarbon chain and FAD. The second reaction is a hydration. The third reaction involves the oxidation of a hydroxyl group by NAD^+.

$$\text{Succinate} \xrightarrow[\text{FAD} \quad \text{FADH}_2 \quad \text{H}_2\text{O}]{} \text{fumarate} \xrightarrow{}$$

$$\text{malate} \xrightarrow[\text{NAD}^+ \quad \text{NADH} + \text{H}^+]{} \text{oxaloacetate} \quad (11.3)$$

β-Oxidation of fatty acyl–CoA occurs within the mitochondrion, whereas the biosynthesis of fatty acids occurs within the cytosol (Table 1–1). This separation permits independent regulation of the two pathways.

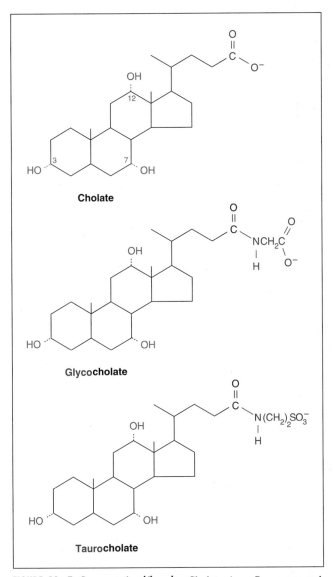

FIGURE 11-7. Representative bile salts. *Cholate is a* C_{24} *compound with three hydroxyl groups and a carboxylate. Glycocholate contains glycine linked to cholate, and taurocholate contains taurine linked to cholate. The amide bonds are of the low-energy variety.*

Acyl-CoA and Fatty Acylcarnitine

The conversion of a free fatty acid into fatty acyl–coenzyme A was the first reaction in biochemistry found to yield pyrophosphate following the cleavage of ATP (Figure 6–8). The product is fatty acyl–CoA with an energy-rich thioester bond. This priming reaction occurs in the cytosol. There are at least four acyl-CoA synthetases that differ in the size of the substrate and their intracellular location (Table 11–5). The chemistry and bioenergetics of each of the enzyme-catalyzed reactions for the biosynthesis of variable length acyl-CoA molecules are the same.

The inner mitochondrial membrane lacks a translocase to mediate the transport of acyl–coenzyme A or coenzyme A. Instead, fatty acylcar-

TABLE 11-5.   Substrate Specificity of the Fatty Acyl–CoA Synthetases

Fatty Acid Substrate Chain Length	Location
Short: 2–3 carbon atoms	Mitochondrion
Medium: 4–10 carbon atoms	Mitochondrion
Long: 12 or more carbon atoms	Endoplasmic reticulum
Arachidonate-specific (20:4ω-6)	Endoplasmic reticulum

nitine is used to transport fatty acyl molecules into the mitochondrion. Before transfer through the inner mitochondrial membrane, the fatty acyl group is transferred to carnitine.

$$
\begin{array}{ccc}
\text{Fatty acylcarnitine} & & \text{fatty acyl-CoA} \\
+ & \xrightleftharpoons{\text{Carnitine}} & + \\
\text{CoA} & \text{acyltransferase} & \text{carnitine} \\
& \text{I and II} &
\end{array}
\qquad (11.4)
$$

Recall that acylcarnitine derivatives are high-energy oxygen esters (Table 6–2). The number of high-energy bonds on each side of equation 11.4 is the same. According to PRINCIPLE 1 OF BIOENERGETICS, reaction 11.4 is isoergonic and can proceed in either direction depending upon physiological need. Following the formation of fatty acylcarnitine in the cytosol as catalyzed by carnitine acyltransferase I, fatty acylcarnitine is transported into the mitochondrion by a translocase in exchange for free carnitine (Figure 11–8). Once inside the mitochondrion, carnitine acyltransferase II catalyzes the conversion of the fatty acylcarnitine to fatty acyl–

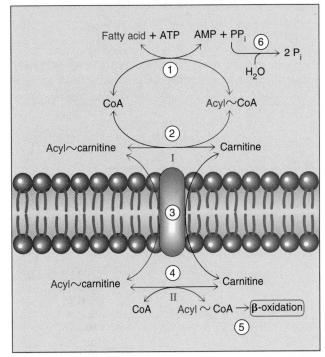

FIGURE 11-8. Transport of fatty acids from the cytosol into the mitochondrion. *The hydrolysis of pyrophosphate, reaction 6, ensures that the formation of acyl-CoA is unidirectional.*

CoA. The reactions of β-oxidation are now able to proceed. Because of the high-energy nature of the special oxygen ester (fatty acylcarnitine), additional chemical energy is not required to convert fatty acylcarnitine to fatty acyl–CoA.

A GTP-linked mitochondrial matrix enzyme catalyzes the synthesis of fatty acyl–CoA from any free fatty acid that may be present. The chemistry and bioenergetics of this process differ from that of the ATP-dependent enzymes. Products of the reaction include fatty acyl–CoA, GDP, and P_i. This is not a mainstream enzyme, but it is important in salvaging fatty acids in the mitochondrion.

The First Spiral

The pathway for β-oxidation is shown in Figure 11–9. **Acyl-CoA dehydrogenase** is a flavoprotein, and it transfers electrons to the respiratory chain at the level of coenzyme Q. Acyl-CoA dehydrogenase, similar to succinate dehydrogenase, is an FAD-requiring enzyme. Acyl-CoA dehydrogenase donates its electrons to an **electron-transferring protein**, also containing FAD, that donates electrons to coenzyme Q within the inner mitochondrial membrane. The hydration of enoyl-CoA corresponds to the hydration of fumarate (to form malate) in the Krebs cycle. The oxidation of L-β-hydroxyacyl-CoA by NAD⁺ corresponds to the oxidation of malate (to form oxaloacetate) in the Krebs cycle. The reaction catalyzed by **thiolase**, a thiolytic cleavage, produces acetyl-CoA and fatty acyl–CoA. The exergonic metabolism of acetyl-CoA by the Krebs cycle also helps pull β-oxidation forward.

Repeating Spirals

The process of oxidation, hydration, oxidation, and thiolysis is repeated sequentially until the car-bon chain is too short (two or three carbon atoms) for subsequent β-oxidation. In the usual case, with an even number of carbon atoms, two molecules of acetyl-CoA are formed during the final thiolytic reaction. With an odd number of carbon atoms, acetyl-CoA and propionyl-CoA are produced. The metabolic fate of propionyl-CoA is considered later in this chapter.

Rate-Limiting Step

The rate-limiting step in the β-oxidation pathway is the formation of fatty acylcarnitine as catalyzed by carnitine acyltransferase I. The biosynthesis of fatty acids occurs in the cytosol, and the source of most of the carbon atoms for fatty acid synthesis is malonyl-CoA. Malonyl-CoA inhibits the synthesis of fatty acylcarnitine, and fatty acyl groups cannot be translocated into the mitochondrion for fatty acid oxidation. Carnitine acyltransferase I, which occurs at the crossroads of fatty acid biosynthesis and fatty acid oxidation, plays a central regulatory role (Table 25–1).

ATP Yield During the β-Oxidation of Fatty Acids

Let us calculate the net yield of ATP from the complete oxidation of one mole of palmitate to carbon dioxide and water mediated by β-oxidation, the Krebs cycle, and oxidative phosphorylation. Each spiral of β-oxidation generates $FADH_2$ (leading to 1.5 ATP) and NADH (leading to 2.5 ATP). The 16-carbon fatty acid undergoes seven spirals of β-oxidation to produce eight molecules of acetyl-CoA. During the seventh spiral, acetoacetyl-CoA is cleaved by coenzyme A to yield two molecules of acetyl coenzyme A. The yield of ATP from seven

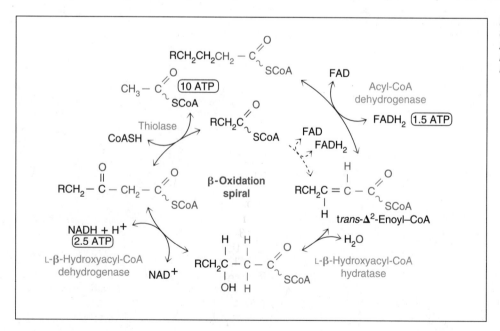

FIGURE 11–9. β-Oxidation of fatty acyl–CoA. *Each spiral generates $FADH_2$, NADH, acetyl-CoA, and a fatty acyl–CoA that is shortened by two carbon atoms.*

TABLE 11–6. ATP Yield from the β-Oxidation of Palmitate in Mitochondria*

	ATP Yield
Seven β-oxidation spirals	
7 NADH $\times$ 2.5	17.5
7 FADH$_2$ $\times$ 1.5	10.5
Eight acetyl-CoA $\times$ 10 ATP	80
−2 ATP equivalents for fatty acid activation	−2
Net	106 moles of ATP per mole of palmitate

* Values used for ATP yields are from P.C. Hinkle, A. Kumar, A. Resetar, and D.L. Harris. Mechanistic stoichiometry of mitochondrial oxidative phosphorylation. Biochemistry 30:3576–3582, 1991.

moles of FADH$_2$, seven moles of NADH, and eight moles of acetyl-CoA is 108 moles of ATP. Recall, however, that palmitate must first be converted into palmitoyl-CoA before β-oxidation, and this reaction requires one molecule of ATP and the expenditure of two high-energy bonds. By convention, we denote the conversion of an ATP to AMP as two ATP equivalents. One ATP is required for the conversion of AMP to ADP, and a second ATP equivalent is required for the conversion of ADP and P$_i$ to ATP by substrate level or oxidative phosphorylation. The net ATP yield from the complete oxidation of one mole of palmitate is 108 − 2, or 106, moles of ATP (Table 11–6).

OXIDATION OF UNSATURATED FATTY ACIDS

The oxidation of unsaturated fatty acids is more intricate than the oxidation of saturated fatty acids. When an unsaturated fatty acid undergoes β-oxidation, an NADPH-dependent reduction is required for each double bond in the fatty acid. This reduces the molar ATP yield by 2.5 for each double bond when compared with the corresponding saturated fatty acid. The presence of the two unsaturated bonds in linoleic acid (18:2Δ9,12), for example, decreases the net ATP yield by five moles of ATP (2.5 for each double bond) when compared with the corresponding saturated fatty acid (18:0).

Let us consider the complete oxidation of linoleoyl-CoA. Linoleic acid is *cis,cis*-9,12-octadecadienoic acid. It contains a double bond after a carbon with an even number (12) and after a carbon with an odd number (9). The metabolism of fatty acids with unsaturation at these two different locations (even and odd) differs; metabolism with unsaturation at an odd-numbered carbon atom is more intricate than that with an unsaturation at an even-numbered carbon atom.

Following two spirals of β-oxidation of linoleoyl-CoA, a Δ^5-*cis*, Δ^8-*cis*-tetradecadienoyl-CoA results (Figure 11–10). A Δ^2-*trans* double bond forms during a reaction catalyzed by acyl-CoA dehydrogenase. **Enoyl-CoA isomerase** catalyzes the conversion of the Δ^2-*trans* bond to a Δ^3-*trans* double bond. **3,5-Dienoyl-CoA isomerase** then converts the Δ^3-*trans*, Δ^5-*cis* double bonds to Δ^2-*trans*, Δ^4-*trans* double bonds.

The 2,4-dienoyl derivative undergoes an **NADPH-dependent reduction**, catalyzed by **2,4-dienoyl-CoA reductase,** to form a *trans*-Δ^3 fatty acyl–CoA, which is converted to a Δ^2-*trans* compound, catalyzed by enoyl-CoA isomerase. The Δ^2-*trans* fatty acyl–CoA is a normal β-oxidation intermediate. The compound undergoes two spirals of β-oxidation that results in the formation of a Δ^4-*cis* fatty acyl–CoA (Figure 11–10), which undergoes the first step of β-oxidation. The Δ^2-*trans*-Δ^4-*cis* compound is a substrate for 2,4-dienoyl-CoA reductase. The product contains a Δ^3-*trans*-double bond and it undergoes an isomerization catalyzed by enoyl-CoA isomerase to form the Δ^2-*trans*-acyl-CoA, a normal substrate for β-oxidation.

The metabolism of fatty acids with double bonds beginning at even-numbered carbon atoms, such as the Δ^{12} position of linoleate, requires only two additional enzyme activities not required for saturated fatty acid metabolism: 2,4-dienoyl-CoA reductase and enoyl-CoA isomerase. The metabolism of fatty acids with double bonds beginning at odd-numbered carbon atoms, such as the Δ^9 position of linoleate, requires another enzyme, 3,5-dienoyl-CoA isomerase. *For each double bond, the ATP yield is decreased by 2.5 when compared with the saturated fatty acid.*

α-, β-, AND ω-FATTY ACID OXIDATION

α- and β-Oxidation in Peroxisomes

α-Oxidation, which occurs in peroxisomes, involves NADPH, molecular oxygen, cytochromes, free fatty acid (not the CoA derivative), an α-hydroxylase, and an α-oxidase. The precise mechanism of α-oxidation has not been established. An α-hydroxy fatty acid is an intermediate, and carbon dioxide is a product. The metabolism of **phytanate,** a degradation product of the phytol side chain of chlorophyll, requires the α-oxidation pathway (Figure 11–11). β-Oxidation of phytanate is not possible because the methyl group on the β-carbon prohibits it. The α-oxidation step, however, generates a substrate for the β-oxidation pathway.

▶ A rare inborn error of lipid metabolism, **Refsum disease,** or **phytanate storage disease,** results from a defect in the α-hydroxylase step of α-oxida-

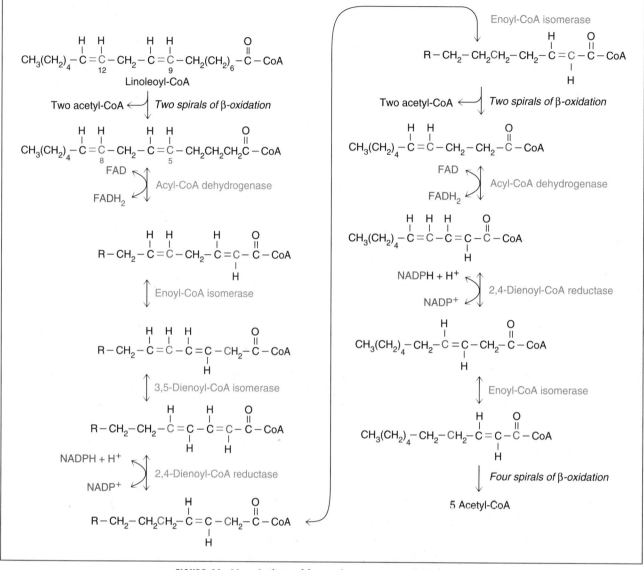

FIGURE 11–10. β-Oxidation of fatty acyl–CoA containing double bonds.

tion. This autosomal recessive disease is characterized by retinitis pigmentosa, peripheral neuropathy, nerve deafness, and cerebellar ataxia. Phytanate is not an endogenous substance but is of dietary origin. Phytanate occurs in dairy products and ruminant fats, where it is derived from the metabolism of chlorophyll. Treatment consists of a diet that is low in phytanate. ◄

Peroxisomes also possess a pathway for β-oxidation. There are differences in the peroxisomal and mitochondrial processes of β-oxidation. Of great importance, peroxisomes can initiate the oxidation of fatty acids that are longer than 18 carbon atoms, but mitochondria cannot. Moreover, carnitine is required for the translocation of fatty acids into mitochondria but not into peroxisomes. Translocation of the long-chain fatty acids into peroxisomes occurs by simple diffusion. Both mitochondrial and peroxisomal β-oxidation require acyl-CoA synthe-

tases that use ATP and generate AMP, PP_i, and acyl-CoA. The first oxidation step in the peroxisomal pathway, which differs from that of the mitochondrial pathway, uses oxygen as the oxidant. Products include the *trans* α, β-unsaturated fatty acyl–CoA and hydrogen peroxide. Recall that peroxisomes are organelles where hydrogen peroxide is generated (Table 1–1). Hydrogen peroxide is degraded to oxygen and water in a reaction mediated by catalase.

The unsaturated fatty acyl–CoA in peroxisomes is metabolized by the familiar steps of β-oxidation. In contrast to the mitochondrial system, however, fatty acyl–CoA hydratase and hydroxyacyl-CoA dehydrogenase activities in peroxisomes reside on a single polypeptide chain. The peroxisome is required for the initial stages of oxidation of fatty acids with carbon chains longer than 18. The process is initiated within the peroxisome, and the

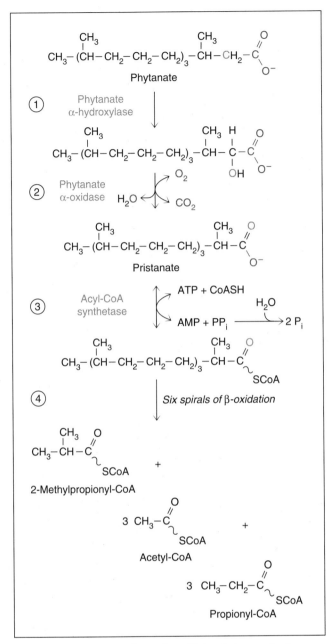

FIGURE 11–11. Overview of α- and β-oxidation of phytanate by the peroxisome.

fatty acyl molecules are eventually translocated to the mitochondrion as carnitine derivatives. The yield of ATP for β-oxidation by the peroxisomal pathway is uncertain.

Zellweger Syndrome

▶ That the peroxisomal pathway for the β-oxidation of long-chain fatty acids is physiologically important is illustrated by a rare group of hereditary peroxisomal disorders typified by Zellweger syndrome. These disorders are due to a defect in peroxisome biosynthesis. Long-chain fatty acids, such as hexacosanoate (26:0), accumulate in the blood. The gene for this disorder is located on chromosome 7 (Table 16–5), but the nature of the biochemical defect is unknown. The peroxisome is required for the initial stages of oxidation of acyl groups that are longer than 18 carbon atoms. The mitochondrion will operate on fatty acids that are 18 carbon atoms and shorter. The accumulation of long-chain fatty acids in Zellweger syndrome demonstrates that the peroxisome plays an important role in the degradation of long-chain fatty acids. ◀

ω-Oxidation by the Endoplasmic Reticulum

This process involves NADPH, oxygen, and cytochrome P-450. The substrates include medium- and long-chain free fatty acids (and not the thioesters). The ω-methyl group is first hydroxylated and then oxidized to a carboxylate; the product of ω-oxidation is a dicarboxylate. Either of the two carboxylates forms a thioester with coenzyme A, and the product is metabolized by β-oxidation.

METABOLISM OF PROPIONYL–COENZYME A

Vitamin B_{12} in the Conversion of Propionate to Succinyl-CoA

Only a small proportion of fatty acids in nature contain an odd number of carbon atoms. These fatty acids are metabolized by the β-oxidation pathway. The final thiolytic cleavage, however, yields acetyl-CoA and propionyl-CoA. The metabolism of phytanate also produces propionyl-CoA (Figure 11–11). Propionyl-CoA is converted into succinyl-CoA by three reactions. In the first step, **propionyl-CoA carboxylase** catalyzes an ATP-dependent carboxylation. Carboxylation reactions are generally endergonic, and ATP serves as the source of chemical energy that sustains this process. The bioenergetics of the propionyl-CoA carboxylase reaction is analogous to that of the pyruvate carboxylase reaction (Figure 8–6). D-Methylmalonyl-CoA undergoes an isoergonic isomerization to yield the L-isomer (Figure 11–12).

Methylmalonyl-CoA mutase, which uses **5′-deoxyadenosylcobalamin** as coenzyme (Figure 2–1), catalyzes the transfer of the CoA-carbonyl group to the adjacent methyl-carbon atom to yield succinyl-CoA. This is one of two reactions in human metabolism that requires the participation of vitamin B_{12} and is noteworthy because of this characteristic (Table 2–3). The other involves the reaction of methyltetrahydrofolate with homocysteine to form tetrahydrofolate and methionine (Chapter 13).

▶ Pernicious anemia results from a deficiency of vitamin B_{12}. The role that intrinsic factor plays in the absorption of B_{12} is discussed in Chapter 2. One sign of pernicious anemia and B_{12} deficiency is the excretion of methylmalonate in the urine. Since

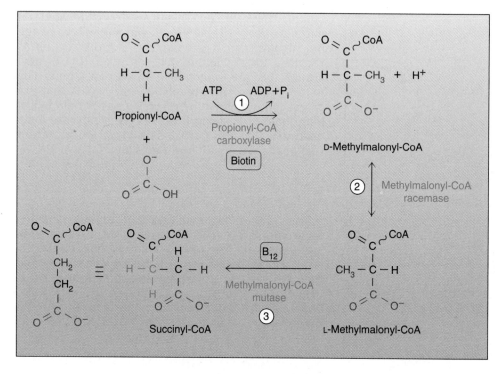

FIGURE 11–12. Conversion of propionyl-CoA to succinyl-CoA. *Propionyl-CoA carboxylase uses biotin as prosthetic group, and methylmalonyl-CoA mutase uses 5′-deoxyadenosylcobalamin (a vitamin B_{12} derivative) as coenzyme. This B_{12}-requiring reaction should be mastered.*

methylmalonyl-CoA cannot be metabolized by the mutase pathway, the compound is degraded by hydrolases (the precise natures of which are unknown), and the resulting four-carbon acid is excreted in the urine. ◀

Oxidation of Succinyl-CoA

Succinyl-CoA is a Krebs cycle metabolite. The complete oxidation of succinyl-CoA or other Krebs cycle metabolites is not as trivial as one might imagine. The reaction of oxaloacetate, a four-carbon metabolite of succinyl-CoA, with acetyl-CoA will not account for the oxidative metabolism of succinate because the Krebs cycle regenerates four-carbon metabolites during one turn of the cycle. *To oxidize any intermediate of the cycle, the metabolite must first be converted to pyruvate and then to acetyl-CoA (equation 8.1).* To oxidize succinyl-CoA completely, therefore, it must first be converted to malate by the customary reactions of the Krebs cycle (Figure 11–13).

Malate undergoes an oxidative decarboxylation reaction, which is catalyzed by one of three malic enzymes, to form pyruvate, carbon dioxide, and reduced NAD(P)H. The mitochondrial matrix contains two different enzymes that catalyze the conversion of malate to pyruvate. One is specific for NADP$^+$, and the second uses either NAD$^+$ or NADP$^+$ as oxidant. Alternatively, malate can be transported into the cytosol and converted into pyruvate by the cytosolic malic enzyme, an NADP$^+$-dependent process. Pyruvate, a product of

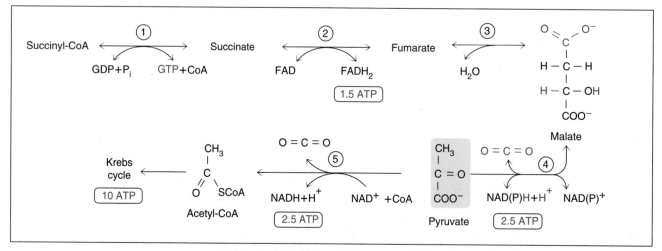

FIGURE 11–13. Oxidative metabolism of succinyl-CoA.

the malic enzyme reaction, is metabolized by the mitochondrial pyruvate dehydrogenase reaction to form acetyl-CoA, the stoichiometric substrate of the Krebs cycle.

The net ATP yield for the metabolism of succinyl-CoA by the mitochondrial pathway is calculated as follows, where the ATP yield is shown in parentheses: succinyl-CoA to succinate and GTP (1); succinate to fumarate and FADH$_2$ (1.5); malate to pyruvate, carbon dioxide, and NAD(P)H (2.5); and pyruvate to its usual products (12.5). The net yield is therefore 17.5 moles of ATP per mole of succinyl-CoA by the mitochondrial pathway (Figure 11–13). The yield is the same for the pathway involving cytosolic malic enzyme, assuming that the malate-aspartate shuttle (Figure 9–2) is used for the transfer of reducing equivalents into the mitochondrion.

FATTY ACID AND LIPID BIOSYNTHESIS

Acetyl-CoA, an energy-rich thioester, is required for fatty acid biosynthesis. Acetyl-CoA serves as a primer for fatty acid biosynthesis and as a precursor of malonyl-CoA. Malonyl-CoA is a three-carbon precursor of the two-carbon fragments that are incorporated stepwise during fatty acid biosynthesis. We consider the biosynthesis of malonyl-CoA and the bioenergetics of its condensation reactions in fatty acid biosynthesis in the next section.

One tenet of biochemistry considered in Chapter 10 is that the pathway for the biosynthesis of a compound differs from that of its degradation. Synthesis and degradation of fatty acids and complex lipids follow this unifying principle. We note that NADPH is the major reductant for biosynthetic reactions (PRINCIPLE 16 OF BIOCHEMISTRY). Accordingly, NADPH is essential for the biosynthesis of fatty acids.

Fatty Acid Synthase as a Multienzyme Complex

Biosynthesis of fatty acids is catalyzed by a polyprotein called **fatty acid synthase.** A polyprotein is a single protein with more than one activity, and fatty acid synthase is formed from two chains of this polyprotein. The biosynthetic intermediates do not diffuse away from the polyprotein but are passed from one enzyme active site to the next active site by acyl carrier protein as noted below. Such channeling of biosynthetic intermediates is characteristic of a unit of metabolism, called a **metabolon.**

Chemical Equation for Palmitate Biosynthesis

The stoichiometry for the formation of palmitate (16 carbon atoms) beginning from one mole of ace-

tyl-CoA and seven moles of malonyl-CoA is given by equation 11.5.

$$\text{Acetyl-CoA} + 7 \text{ malonyl-CoA}^- + 7 \text{ H}^+ \\ + 14 \text{ NADPH} + 14 \text{ H}^+ \quad (11.5)$$

$$\downarrow$$

$$\text{CH}_3(\text{CH}_2)_{14}\text{COO}^- + \text{H}^+ + 7 \text{ CO}_2 + 8 \text{ CoA} \\ + 14 \text{ NADP}^+ + 6 \text{ H}_2\text{O}$$

In equation 11.5, one water molecule is required to hydrolyze palmitoyl-CoA to palmitate and CoA to account for the stoichiometry of six (and not seven) water molecules in the products. Acetyl-CoA serves as the primer for biosynthesis; acetyl-CoA furnishes the two carbon atoms farthest from the carboxyl group (Figure 11–1). The other carbon atoms are derived from malonyl-CoA; two carbon atoms are incorporated into the chain, and carbon dioxide is expelled for each malonyl-CoA reactant. All carbon atoms of fatty acids, however, are derived from acetyl-CoA because the same carbon atom of carbon dioxide that carboxylates acetyl-CoA to form malonyl-CoA is discharged as carbon dioxide during biosynthesis. The decarboxylation reaction provides free energy to make fatty acid biosynthesis exergonic. Besides acetyl-CoA and malonyl-CoA, NADPH is required for fatty acid biosynthesis.

Formation of Malonyl-CoA from Acetyl-CoA

Genesis of Acetyl-CoA

Malonyl-CoA, derived from acetyl-CoA, is required for fatty acid biosynthesis. Mitochondria furnish the acetyl groups used for malonyl-CoA and fatty acid biosynthesis. Most of the acetyl-CoA is derived from carbohydrate, but a portion is derived from amino acids. When carbohydrates serve as progenitors of fatty acids, pyruvate (derived from glycolysis) is transported into the mitochondrion and is converted to acetyl-CoA by the pyruvate dehydrogenase reaction (Figure 8–3). Because CoA derivatives are unable to cross the inner mitochondrial membrane, acetyl-CoA condenses with oxaloacetate to form citrate. Citrate is then exported from the mitochondrion by means of an antiport system located in the inner mitochondrial membrane (Figure 11–14).

Fate of Cytosolic Oxaloacetate

Following translocation from the mitochondrion, citrate is converted to acetyl-CoA and oxaloacetate in a reaction catalyzed by **ATP-citrate lyase** (Figure 11–15), a cytosolic enzyme. Let us consider the fate of the oxaloacetate generated in the cytosol as a result of the ATP-citrate lyase reaction. Recall that oxaloacetate per se cannot be transported across the inner mitochondrial membrane. How-

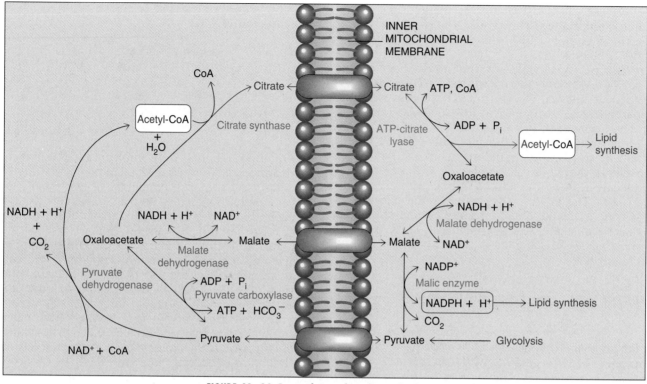

FIGURE 11–14. Export of citrate from the mitochondrion.

ever, cytosolic oxaloacetate can be reduced by NADH to malate as catalyzed by malate dehydrogenase, and malate can then be transported into the mitochondrion (Figure 11–14). After oxidation to oxaloacetate within the mitochondrion, the four-carbon compound can serve again as a carrier of an acetyl group to the cytosol. A second route for cytosolic malate involves its oxidative decarboxylation to form pyruvate, carbon dioxide, and NADPH as catalyzed by **malic enzyme** (NADP-requiring) as shown in Figure 11–14. (Malic enzyme refers to the malic acid [malate] substrate.) The malic enzyme reaction generates cytosolic NADPH that can be used in lipid biosynthesis. This reaction is an oxidative decarboxylation that is modestly endergonic under standard conditions but readily proceeds under physiological concentrations of metabolites in the direction of NADPH. The oxidation of an alcohol (malate) to a ketone (pyruvate) by $NAD(P)^+$ is an endergonic process analo-

gous to that of the lactate dehydrogenase reaction (equation 5.25). However, the decarboxylation yielding pyruvate and carbon dioxide is exergonic, and the decarboxylation provides sufficient free energy to drive the reaction forward. Pyruvate, following its translocation into the mitochondrion, can be converted to acetyl-CoA or oxaloacetate, depending upon metabolic need.

The Acetyl-CoA Carboxylase Reaction

Acetyl-CoA carboxylase catalyzes the synthesis of malonyl-CoA, a crucial intermediate in fatty acid biosynthesis, according to equation 11.6.

$$\text{Acetyl-CoA} + \text{ATP} + \text{HCO}_3^- \rightarrow$$
$$\text{malonyl-CoA} + \text{ADP} + \text{P}_i \quad (11.6)$$

The reactants exhibit three high-energy bonds (one in acetyl-CoA and two in ATP) and the products exhibit two high-energy bonds (one each in ma-

Citrate		Acetyl-CoA	Oxaloacetate

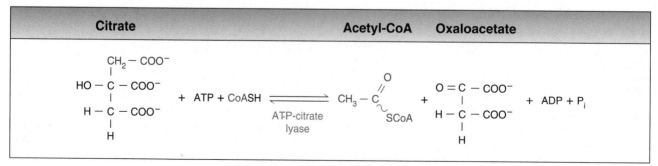

FIGURE 11–15. The ATP-citrate lyase reaction.

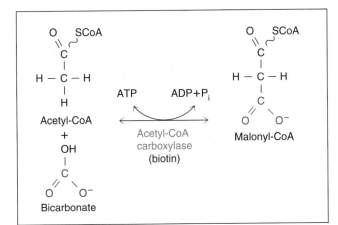

FIGURE 11–16. The acetyl-CoA carboxylase reaction.

lonyl-CoA and ADP). The reaction is functionally isoergonic, however, because the carboxylation is endergonic and requires energy (Figure 11–16). Acetyl-CoA carboxylase contains covalently bound biotin, and the mechanism and bioenergetics of this reaction parallel the example of pyruvate carboxylase illustrated in Figure 8–8. *The acetyl-CoA carboxylase reaction is the rate-limiting reaction in fatty acid biosynthesis* (Table 25–1). As an example of the reciprocal regulation of metabolism, malonyl-CoA (the product of the acetyl-CoA carboxylase reaction) inhibits the rate-limiting step of fatty acid oxidation by blocking the synthesis of fatty acylcarnitine, thereby inhibiting fatty acid transport into the mitochondrion.

The stoichiometry for the biosynthesis of palmitate from acetyl-CoA, bicarbonate, and ATP is summarized in equation 11.7.

$$8 \text{ Acetyl-CoA} + 7 \text{ ATP}^{4-} + 7 \text{ HCO}_3^- + 14 \text{ NADPH} \\ + 14 \text{ H}^+$$

$$\downarrow$$

$$CH_3(CH_2)_{14}COO^- + H^+ + 7 \text{ CO}_2 + 8 \text{ CoA} + 6 \text{ H}_2O \\ + 7 \text{ ADP}^{3-} + 7 \text{ P}_i^{2-} + 14 \text{ NADP}^+ \quad (11.7)$$

Acetyl-CoA furnishes all the carbon atoms of palmitate. ATP and bicarbonate are required for further activation of acetyl-CoA, and NADPH serves as the reductant for biosynthesis.

Pathway for Fatty Acid Biosynthesis

The fatty acid synthase complex involves two types of thiol groups. One of these, called the **central thiol,** is made up of 4′-phosphopantetheine, a derivative of coenzyme A that is covalently linked by a phosphodiester bond to a serine residue of **acyl carrier protein,** or **ACP.** The 4′-phosphopantetheine can be regarded as protein-bound coenzyme A (Figure 2–14). The 4′-phosphopantetheine of the acyl carrier protein contains the thiol group upon which the fatty acid chain is built. ACP shut-

tles the growing chain from one enzyme active site to another as a mobile carrier. A second important thiol group, called the **peripheral thiol,** belongs to a cysteinyl residue on β-*k*etoacyl-ACP *synthase* (KSase). The growing fatty acyl group is transiently transferred to the peripheral sulfhydryl group before recurring condensation reactions of the fatty acid synthetic spiral.

The Condensation Reaction of Fatty Acid Elongation

To initiate biosynthesis, acetyl-CoA reacts with the central thiol to form a covalent thioester bond and CoA is displaced. The acetyl group is then transferred to the peripheral thiol, where it is also bound as a thioester (Figure 11–17). The high-energy nature of the thioester linkage is retained as the transfer occurs from coenzyme A to the central thiol and then to the peripheral thiol. Next, the malonyl group of malonyl-CoA is transferred to the central thiol (4′-phosphopantetheine) of ACP. Now the reactants are poised for the first condensation reaction. The α-carbon of malonyl-ACP attacks the carbonyl group covalently linked to the peripheral thiol (Figure 11–17). This reaction is driven by the concomitant decarboxylation, yielding acetoacetyl-ACP. The rare substitution of propionyl-CoA for acetyl-CoA during the initial step of fatty acid biosynthesis accounts for the unusual occurrence of fatty acids containing an odd number of carbon atoms.

The condensation reaction of fatty acid biosynthesis is catalyzed by β-**ketoacyl–ACP synthase.** *The decarboxylation reaction, which is very exergonic, and the displacement of the energy-rich thioester ensures that the equilibrium lies far to the right.* The *acetyl* group from *acetyl*-CoA forms the terminus of *aceto*acetyl-ACP (Figure 11–17). The initial acetyl group will form the last two carbon atoms at the ω-end of the fatty acid (Figure 11–1).

The Reduction Spiral

Acetoacetyl-ACP undergoes a reduction at the expense of NADPH + H$^+$, yielding D-β-hydroxybutyryl-ACP and NADP$^+$ in a reaction mediated by β-ketoacyl-ACP **reductase.** The next step involves a dehydration to 2,3-*trans*-butenoyl-ACP (crotonyl-ACP), catalyzed by β-hydroxyacyl–ACP **dehydratase.** The double bond is reduced by NADPH + H$^+$ in a reaction catalyzed by 2,3-*trans*-enoyl–ACP **reductase.** Two NADPH molecules are required for each two-carbon unit that is added during biosynthesis.

Preparation for the Second and Subsequent Condensation Reactions

The butyryl group, formed by the first reduction spiral, is transferred from the central thiol of ACP to the peripheral thiol group. The peripheral thiol was the location of the starting acetyl group. Ma-

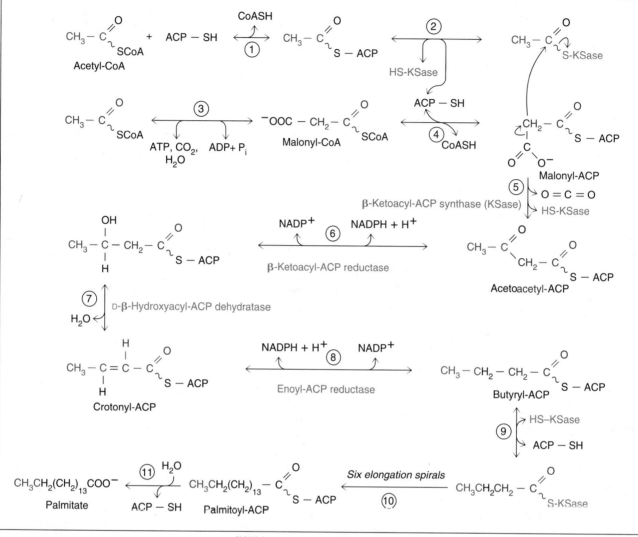

FIGURE 11–17. Fatty acid biosynthesis.

lonyl-CoA next combines with ACP. The α-carbon of malonyl-ACP attacks the carbonyl group of the butyryl group, and carbon dioxide is discharged. The 3-ketohexanoyl group resides on ACP. This group is reduced, dehydrated, reduced, and transferred to the peripheral thiol group as before. This process continues until the 16-carbon palmitoyl group is formed.

Palmitate is released from the fatty acid synthase complex by an exergonic hydrolysis reaction. That fatty acid synthesis by the multienzyme complex stops at palmitate is probably due to limitations in the size of an active site of fatty acid synthase. Biochemists have whimsically suggested that the fatty acid synthase complex counts to 16 carbon atoms and then liberates the fatty acid. The 16-carbon palmitate can undergo further reactions including elongation and desaturation.

Elongation Reactions

Stearic and oleic acids are major constituents of fatty acids found in human cells. Although the fatty acid synthase complex stops at 16 carbon atoms, human cells can extend the length of the fatty acid chain. Two-carbon units can be added to endogenously synthesized or dietary fatty acids by elongation reactions. The two-carbon donor for the endoplasmic reticulum pathway is malonyl-CoA, and that in the mitochondrion is acetyl-CoA. The endoplasmic reticulum pathway is quantitatively more important. This strategy agrees with the role of the mitochondrion functioning as a catabolic organelle.

The substrate for the elongation reactions is fatty acyl–CoA and not fatty acyl–ACP. The two-carbon units from malonyl-CoA are added at the carboxyl end of the molecule, and the reaction is analogous to the condensation reaction that occurs during conventional fatty acid biosynthesis. The endoplasmic reticulum contains the enzyme activities found in the fatty acid synthetase complex that successively reduce, dehydrate, and reduce the compound to produce fatty acyl–CoA containing two additional carbon atoms. The fatty acyl–CoA substrate for the elongation reaction can be saturated or unsaturated. More than one elongation reaction can occur, and fatty acids up to 26 carbon atoms can be synthesized. In contrast to the endoplasmic reticulum elongation process, acetyl-CoA and not malonyl-CoA donates the two-carbon units in the mitochondrion. The elongation process is the reversal of β-oxidation except that an NADPH reductase substitutes for the FAD-requiring enzyme-catalyzed reaction.

Bioenergetics of Fatty Acid Biosynthesis

One mole of ATP is required for the generation of each mole of acetyl-CoA from citrate; thus, eight moles of ATP are required for the eight 2-carbon fragments required for the synthesis of one mole of palmitate. Seven additional moles of ATP are required for the synthesis of seven moles of malonyl-CoA from acetyl-CoA and carbon dioxide. A total of 15 ATP equivalents are required for the synthesis of palmitate from citrate. Fourteen moles of NADPH are required for the biosynthesis of one mole of palmitate. If these reducing equivalents were employed to provide energy for oxidative phosphorylation, using identical yields of ATP for NADPH and NADH, 14 moles of NADPH would provide energy for the synthesis of 2.5×14, or 35, additional moles of ATP. Fatty acid biosynthesis is thus energetically expensive. Fatty acid biosynthesis, however, occurs when there is abundant precursor to provide both the mass and the energy to sustain the process.

Several steps of fatty acid biosynthesis are chemically similar those of β-oxidation (Table 11-7). Both include a β-keto acid, an unsaturated fatty acid, and a β-hydroxy acid; all chemical intermediates are thioesters. A high ratio of [NADPH] to [NADP⁺], which occurs physiologically, favors biosynthesis. A high ratio of [NAD⁺] to [NADH], also physiological, favors β-oxidation. Note, however, that NADPH is required for the catabolism of unsaturated fatty acids, and this is an unusual situation. The thermodynamic driving force for biosynthesis resides in the utilization of malonyl-CoA for the condensation reaction. Liberation of carbon dioxide provides energy (about −28 kJ/mol) that promotes biosynthesis.

Source of Reducing Equivalents

The origin of NADPH for fatty acid biosynthesis depends on the cell type. In liver, for example, NADPH is generated mainly from the two NADP⁺-requiring reactions of the pentose phosphate pathway. These two reactions are catalyzed by glucose-6-phosphate dehydrogenase and 6-phosphogluconate dehydrogenase. In adipose tissue, NADPH is generated by malic enzyme (Figure 11–14) and the pentose phosphate pathway (Figure 7–12). Fatty acid synthesis in humans is quantitatively more important in liver.

FATTY ACID DESATURATION

Fatty acid synthase catalyzes the formation of palmitate, a saturated fatty acid. Human cells possess the machinery for converting saturated to unsaturated fatty acids. This ability permits the generation of an appropriate balance of products to maintain physiological membrane fluidity.

Since fatty acid desaturation is more intricate than a simple oxidation-reduction reaction, we consider it in some detail. A variety of fatty acyl–CoA molecules can serve as substrate, and the location of the double bond that is formed is dependent upon which desaturase catalyzes the final step in the process. These include Δ4, Δ5, Δ6, and Δ9 desaturases. In saturated fatty acyl–CoA substrates, the double bond is produced at the Δ⁹ position. In unsaturated fatty acyl–CoA substrates, a *cis* double bond is constructed three carbon atoms from the most proximal double bond toward the α-carbon. The inability of humans to produce double bonds between the ω-terminus and the Δ⁹ position accounts for the lack of production of linoleic acid (18:2Δ9,12) and linolenic acid (18:3Δ9, 12,15), dietary essential fatty acids. One pathway in the metabolism of the ω-6 family is illustrated in Figure 11–18.

The following equation gives the stoichiometry for the general desaturation process.

$$R—CH_2CH_2\cdots CO{\sim}SCoA + O_2 + NADPH + H^+ \rightarrow$$
$$R—CH{=}CH\cdots CO{\sim}SCoA$$
$$+ 2 H_2O + NADP^+ \quad (11.8)$$

A simple oxidation-reduction reaction involving only NADP⁺ would be reversible. The reduction of oxygen to water is exergonic. The bioenergetics of the oxygen-dependent process makes the overall reaction very exergonic, and the reaction is physiologically irreversible (PRINCIPLE 8 OF BIOENERGETICS). The pathway for electron transport from NADPH is illustrated in Figure 11–19.

TABLE 11–7. Comparison of Fatty Acid Oxidation and Biosynthesis

Requirement	Oxidation	Synthesis *de novo*
Acetyl-CoA	+	+
Malonyl-CoA	−	+
NAD⁺	+	−
NADPH	+*	+
Coenzyme A	+	+
ACP	−	+
Mitochondria	+	−
Cytosol	−	+
Multienzyme complex	−	+
L-Hydroxyacyl intermediate	+	−
D-Hydroxyacyl intermediate	−	+

* 2,4-Dienoyl-CoA reductase.

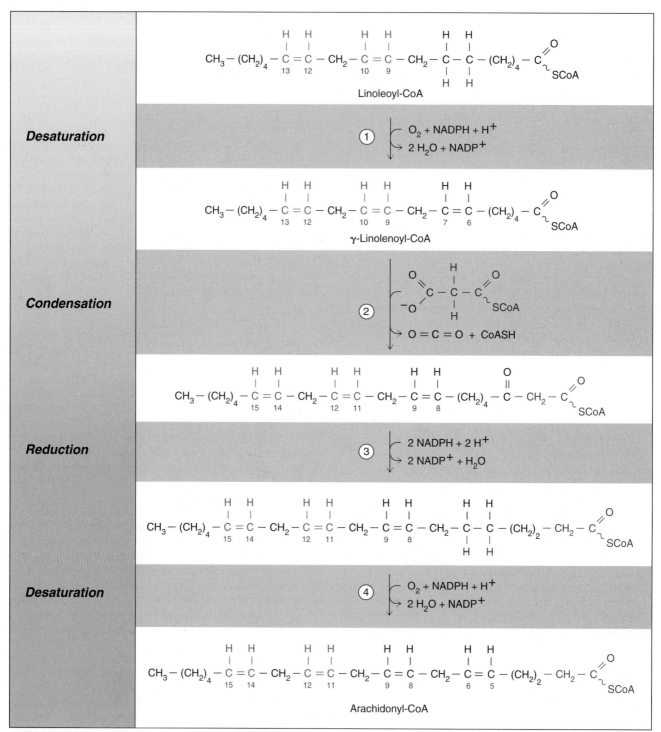

FIGURE 11–18. Conversion of linolenoyl-CoA to arachidonoyl-CoA. *Malonyl-CoA serves as the donor of C^1 and C^2 to form a 20-carbon metabolite.*

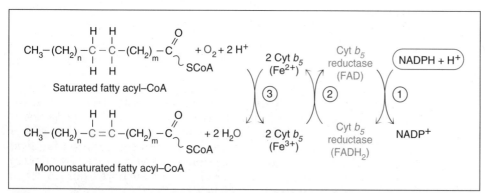

Saturated fatty acyl–CoA

Monounsaturated fatty acyl–CoA

FIGURE 11–19. Pathway for fatty acid desaturation. *Each desaturation is a four-electron process (two from NADPH and two from fatty acyl–CoA) that requires molecular oxygen.*

TRIGLYCERIDE BIOSYNTHESIS

Triglyceride ester bonds are low energy in nature. Acyl-CoA is a high-energy thioester, and acyl-CoA is the activated form of the acyl group that participates in biosynthetic condensation reactions. The reaction of acyl-CoA with an acceptor alcohol is illustrated by the following equation.

$$R—CO{\sim}SCoA + HO—R' \rightarrow$$
$$R—CO—OR' + HSCoA \quad (11.9)$$

This reaction proceeds with a decrease in the number of high-energy bonds and is exergonic (PRINCIPLE 2 OF BIOENERGETICS). This general principle provides the rationale for understanding nearly all acyl transfer reactions in lipid metabolism.

There are two pathways for triglyceride biosynthesis. The first is the **general pathway** and is operational in liver and other organs where fatty acid biosynthesis occurs. The second is the **intestinal pathway** and is responsible for the resynthesis of triglyceride following the digestion and absorption of dietary triglyceride (Figure 11–20). The precursor for the intestinal pathway is 2-monoglyceride, the end product of triglyceride digestion.

General Pathway

There are two major pathways for the formation of phosphatidate beginning from dihydroxyacetone phosphate, a glycolytic intermediate, or from glycerol 3-phosphate. Note that NADPH is the reductant (Figure 11–21) in accord with PRINCIPLE 16 OF BIOCHEMISTRY. Each acyltransferase reaction in these pathways is accompanied by the loss of a high-energy bond and is exergonic (PRINCIPLE 2 OF BIOENERGETICS). Hydrolysis reactions are also exergonic and unidirectional.

Intestinal Pathway

The biosynthesis of triglyceride from 2-monoglyceride occurs in the intestinal epithelium. An intestinal **monoglyceride acyltransferase** catalyzes the formation of *sn*-1,2-diglyceride, and **1,2-diglyceride acyltransferase** catalyzes the biosynthesis of triglyceride. The bioenergetics of the intestinal pathway of triglyceride biosynthesis is straightforward (Figure 11–20).

KETONE BODY METABOLISM

Lipids are the main storage form of chemical energy in humans, and lipids are the main fuel for ATP production during fasting and starvation. Ketone body is a nonsystematic term for **acetoacetate, β-hydroxybutyrate,** and **acetone.** Ketone bodies are produced by the liver during fasting,

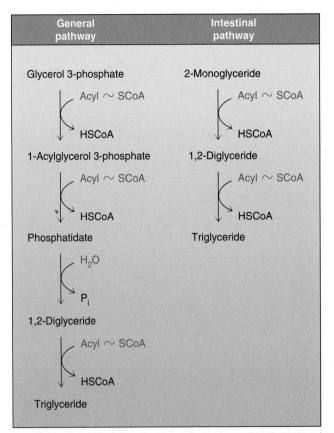

FIGURE 11–20. General and intestinal pathways for triglyceride synthesis. *The acyltransferase reactions and the hydrolysis reaction are exergonic and unidirectional.*

starvation, and diabetic ketoacidosis (Table 25–6). Ketone bodies are carried by the circulation to extrahepatic cells, where two of them are oxidized to produce energy. Although this is a contradiction in terms, ketone bodies can be considered as water-soluble lipids. Acetone is a metabolic dead end that is expired from the lungs or excreted in the urine; it cannot be oxidized to produce energy.

Ketone Body Synthesis

Ketone body synthesis occurs exclusively in liver mitochondria. Ketone bodies are synthesized from acetyl-CoA or acetoacetyl-CoA that is derived during the β-oxidation of fatty acids (Figure 11–22). Acetoacetyl-CoA is not the direct precursor of acetoacetate. Rather, acetoacetyl-CoA reacts with acetyl-CoA to form **HMG-CoA (β-hydroxyl-β-methylglutaryl–CoA).** Glutarate, the parent compound, is a five-carbon dicarboxylate. The synthesis of HMG-CoA involves a condensation and hydrolysis that resembles citrate synthesis (Figure 8–5). The HMG-CoA synthase reaction is exergonic and unidirectional.

HMG-CoA undergoes an aldol-lyase reaction to form acetoacetate and acetyl-CoA. Acetoacetate is the first ketone body formed. Acetoacetate can be reduced by NADH to form β-hydroxybutyrate. This

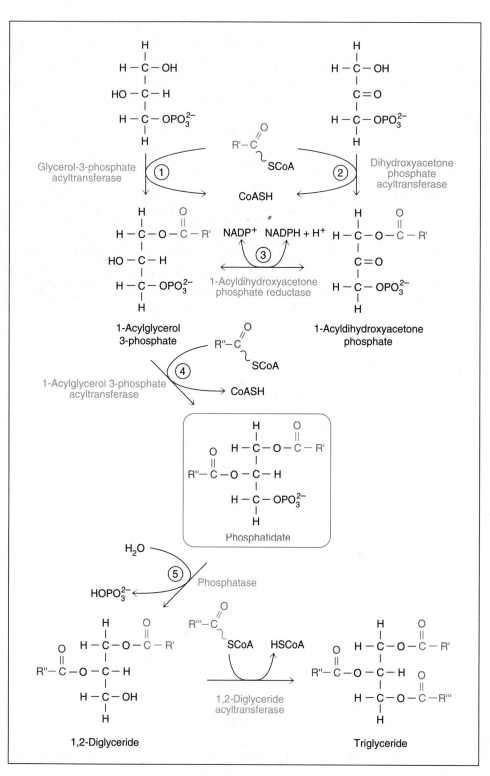

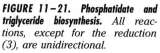

FIGURE 11–21. Phosphatidate and triglyceride biosynthesis. *All reactions, except for the reduction (3), are unidirectional.*

is a simple oxidation-reduction reaction and is bi-directional. Acetoacetate and β-hydroxybutyrate are the two important ketone bodies. Ketone bodies are also formed during the catabolism of a few amino acids, as noted in Chapter 13. A small fraction of acetoacetate undergoes nonenzymatic decarboxylation to form carbon dioxide and ace-tone. Decarboxylation reactions are exergonic, and this reaction does not occur to a greater extent because humans lack an enzyme for catalysis.

Ketone Body Oxidation

After their release from the liver into the circula-tion, ketone bodies are metabolized by mitochon-dria of extrahepatic cells. β-Hydroxybutyrate is ox-idized by NAD^+ to form acetoacetate and NADH. Now let us consider the key step in the catabolism of acetoacetate. This compound reacts with suc-cinyl-CoA, an intermediate of the Krebs cycle, to form acetoacetyl-CoA and succinate (Figure 11–

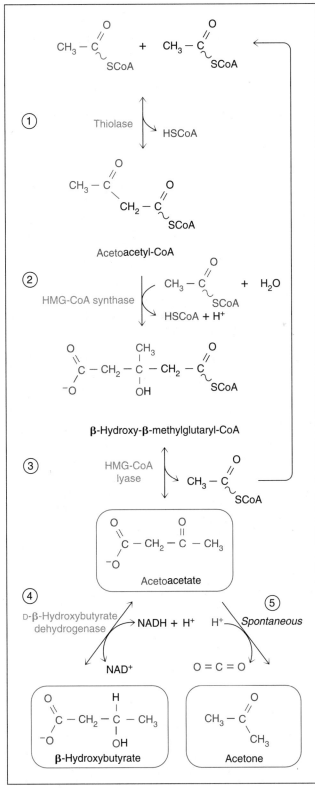

FIGURE 11–22. Ketone body synthesis in liver mitochondria.

Diabetic Ketoacidosis

▶ Ketone body metabolism is important in fasting, starvation, and diabetes mellitus. There is a high glucagon-to-insulin ratio in these three conditions. Glucagon promotes and insulin inhibits lipolysis in adipose cells. Fatty acids are liberated from adipose tissue and are transported to the liver as a complex with serum albumin. Once inside the liver cell, the fatty acyl group undergoes β-oxidation and produces ketone body precursors.

The production of inordinate amounts of ketone bodies in diabetes mellitus results in **diabetic ketoacidosis,** a metabolic acidosis. This is related to the generation of large amounts of acetoacetate and β-hydroxybutyrate. The excretion of ketones

23). Both compounds are high-energy thioesters, and the reaction is isoergonic. Acetoacetyl-CoA is a metabolic intermediate of β-oxidation. It is cleaved by CoASH in a reaction catalyzed by thiolase to form two moles of acetyl-CoA. Acetyl-CoA in the mitochondria is metabolized by the familiar reactions of the Krebs cycle.

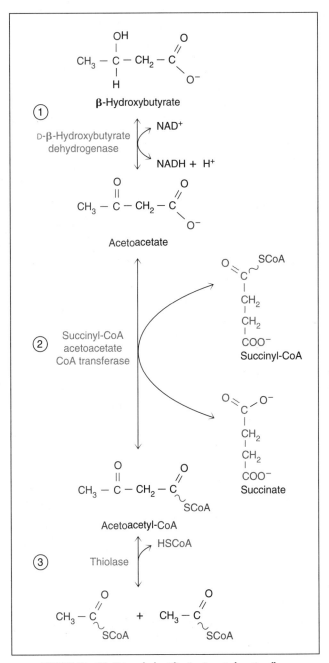

FIGURE 11–23. Ketone body utilization in extrahepatic cells.

in the urine is called ketonuria. Acetone is often detectable by smell on the breath of an individual with diabetic ketoacidosis. Its odor is reminiscent of fruity chewing gum. ◄

REGULATION OF FATTY ACID OXIDATION AND BIOSYNTHESIS

The reaction catalyzed by acetyl-CoA carboxylase is the chief regulatory step in fatty acid biosynthesis in eukaryotes (Table 25–1). This enzyme is activated by citrate (the precursor of the acetyl-CoA building blocks for biosynthesis) and is inhibited by palmitoyl-CoA (one of the products). Citrate promotes the conversion of less active monomeric enzymes to more active polymeric aggregates that take the shape of filaments. Increased cytosolic citrate serves as a signal that fuel molecules are abundant, and this signal promotes the formation of fatty acid.

Two mitochondrial reactions participate in fatty acid biosynthesis from carbohydrate: pyruvate dehydrogenase and citrate synthase. The participation of these mitochondrial reactions in fatty acid biosynthesis also explains why isocitrate dehydrogenase, a reaction distal to citrate formation, is a key regulatory step in the Krebs cycle (Table 25–1). Citrate is formed in the mitochondrion and is then exported to the cytosol. This can occur because isocitrate dehydrogenase is not maximally activated, thereby permitting the formation and transport of citrate from the mitochondrion.

Malonyl-CoA inhibits carnitine acyltransferase I, thus inhibiting fatty acid translocation into the mitochondrion. Conditions that favor fatty acid biosynthesis thereby produce an inhibitor of a step required before fatty acid oxidation. The synthesis of fatty acylcarnitine is the rate-limiting process in β-oxidation.

SUMMARY

Fatty acids in lipids represent a concentrated source of fuel for the generation of ATP. The first step in fatty acid metabolism involves the formation of fatty acyl–CoA. Coenzyme A and its derivatives are not translocated across the inner mitochondrial membrane. Fatty acylcarnitine is formed in an isoergonic reaction from fatty acyl–CoA, and the carnitine ester is then translocated into the mitochondrion in exchange for carnitine (an antiport system). Fatty acyl–CoA is re-formed and undergoes β-oxidation. The four steps in β-oxidation include an FAD-dependent oxidation, a hydration, an NAD⁺-dependent oxidation, and a thiolysis reaction involving coenzyme A. Acetyl-CoA and a fatty acyl–CoA with two fewer carbon atoms are produced. The steps and order of β-oxidation parallel four steps in the Krebs cycle (from succinate to oxaloacetate).

The oxidation of unsaturated fatty acids requires isomerases that catalyze the translocation of double bonds and 2,4-dienoyl reductase. The substrate for this reductase is NADPH. The metabolism of fatty acids that contain a double bond at an odd-numbered carbon atom involves three enzyme activities besides those of the β-oxidation spiral: 3,5-dienoyl-CoA isomerase, enoyl-CoA isomerase, and 2,4-dienoyl reductase. The metabolism of fatty acids that contain a double bond at an even-numbered carbon atom involves the latter two enzymes.

The oxidation of fatty acids with an odd number of carbon atoms yields acetyl-CoA and propionyl-CoA during the final thiolytic cleavage. Propionyl-CoA is converted to succinyl-CoA by a three-step pathway. The pathway involves (1) an ATP- and biotin-dependent carboxylation, (2) an isomerization, and (3) a vitamin B_{12}–dependent transfer reaction. In the last-mentioned, methylmalonyl-CoA is converted to succinyl-CoA. Succinyl-CoA must be converted to malate, pyruvate, and acetyl-CoA before its complete oxidation to carbon dioxide as mediated by Krebs cycle reactions.

A general principle of metabolism is that NADPH is the reductant for biosynthetic reactions. NADPH is the reductant for fatty acid and cholesterol biosynthesis. The requirement of NADPH for the catabolism of unsaturated fatty acids is atypical. Fatty acid biosynthesis has an unusual bioenergetic feature. The rate-limiting reaction in fatty acid biosynthesis is catalyzed by acetyl-CoA carboxylase. This enzyme catalyzes the conversion of acetyl-CoA to malonyl-CoA in an ATP-dependent and biotin-dependent reaction. The carboxylate on the α-carbon atom provides additional activation for the condensation reactions that generate palmitate. Decarboxylation reactions proceed with a decrease in free energy equivalent to that of the hydrolysis of the high-energy bonds of ATP.

Fatty acid biosynthesis occurs on a polyprotein. Fatty acid synthase has two important thiol groups that form thioester intermediates during synthesis. A peripheral thiol is contributed by an enzymatic cysteine on the ketoacyl-ACP synthase domain. The central thiol is contributed by 4′-phosphopantetheine, covalently linked to ACP. A malonyl group, bound to the central thiol as a thioester, reacts with the acetyl group, parked on the peripheral thiol. The peripheral thiol is displaced, the acetoacetyl group is attached to the central thiol, and carbon dioxide is liberated in an exergonic process. The ketone group of acetoacetyl-ACP is reduced, water is eliminated, and the resulting double bond is reduced during the first cycle. The four-carbon group is then transferred to the peripheral thiol. A second malonyl group becomes attached to the central thiol, and the second condensation reaction occurs. The reductive cycle commences. The process is repeated until the 16-carbon palmitate is synthesized.

Cytosolic acetyl-CoA is derived from mitochondrial citrate. The requirement to synthesize citrate in the mitochondrion for fatty acid biosynthesis accounts for regulation of the Krebs cycle at the isocitrate dehydrogenase and not citrate synthase step. ATP-citrate lyase converts citrate into acetyl-CoA and oxaloacetate.

Acyl-CoA is the energy-rich donor of fatty acids for biosynthesis of triglycerides and other esters. Low-energy esters are the products of such acyl-transfer reactions. Phosphatidate, which is derived from dihydroxyacetone phosphate or glycerol, is a key intermediate of lipid biosynthesis. Phosphate is cleaved from phosphatidate by exergonic hydrolysis. Triglyceride is formed from 1,2-diglyceride and acyl-CoA.

The three ketone bodies are acetoacetate, β-hydroxybutyrate, and acetone. Acetyl-CoA combines with acetoacetyl-CoA to form HMG-CoA. A hydrolysis reaction makes this process exergonic. HMG-CoA undergoes a lyase reaction to form acetoacetate and acetyl-CoA.

The synthesis of fatty acylcarnitine is rate-limiting in the β-oxidation of fatty acids. Carnitine acyl-transferase I is inhibited by malonyl-CoA, a key precursor of fatty acid biosynthesis. Acetyl-CoA carboxylase is the rate-limiting process in fatty acid biosynthesis. Citrate, a precursor of cytosolic acetyl-CoA that is used for fatty acid biosynthesis, activates acetyl-CoA carboxylase. This is an example of feed-forward activation.

SELECTED READINGS

Foster, D.W., and J.D. McGarry. Metabolic derangements and treatment of diabetic ketoacidosis. New England Journal of Medicine 309:159–169, 1977.

Smeland, T.E., M. Nada, D. Cuebas, and H. Schulz. NADPH-dependent β-oxidation of unsaturated fatty acids with double bonds extending from odd-numbered carbon atoms. Proceedings of the National Academy of Science USA 89:6673–6677, 1992.

Steinberg, D. Refsum disease. In C.R. Scriver, A.L. Beaudet, W.S. Sly, and D. Valle (eds.). The Metabolic Basis of Inherited Disease, 6th ed. New York, McGraw-Hill Book Company, 1989, pp. 1533–1550.

Vance, D.E., and J.E. Vance. Biochemistry of Lipids and Membranes. Menlo Park, Calif., Benjamin/Cummings, 1986.

CHAPTER TWELVE

COMPLEX LIPID

METABOLISM

The ways chosen by Nature for making organic compounds are easy enough to rationalize—by hindsight. Biochemistry remains, by and large, an empirical science and predicting the course of even the simplest biochemical reactions, on whatever grounds, remains a venture of risk.

—KONRAD BLOCH

Glycerolipids, which possess a glycerol backbone, and **sphingolipids,** which possess a sphingosine backbone, are two major categories of lipid. Members of both classes of lipid are important constituents of membranes. An important principle of bioenergetics facilitates understanding the reactions of complex lipid biosynthesis. *Compounds with a high group-transfer potential donate their activated groups to a substrate, yielding products with a low group-transfer potential.* Energy-rich donors in lipid metabolism include acyl-CoA and CDP-derivatives. The following two equations illustrate this principle:

$$\text{Acyl} \sim \text{SCoA} + \text{ROH} \rightarrow \text{Acyl} - \text{OR} + \text{CoASH} \quad (12.1)$$

$$\text{CMP} \sim \text{phosphocholine} + \text{ROH} \rightarrow \quad (12.2)$$
$$\text{RO} - \text{phosphocholine} + \text{CMP}$$

The products are low-energy oxygen esters (or amides) and phosphodiesters. The pathway for the biosynthesis of these phospholipids is readily understandable in terms of the fundamental tenets of bioenergetics.

GLYCEROLIPIDS

Biosynthesis of Glycerolipids

Phosphatidate, Phosphatidylinositol, Phosphatidylglycerol, and Cardiolipin

Phosphatidate and cytidine nucleotide derivatives are key metabolites in the biosynthesis of glycerolipids. Phosphatidate reacts with CTP to form CDP-diglyceride and PP$_i$ (Figure 12–1). **CDP-diglyceride** is the activated form of phosphatidate. CDP-diglyceride is an intermediate in the biosynthesis of phosphatidylinositol, phosphatidylglycerol, and cardiolipin (Figure 12–2). High-energy compounds are converted into low-energy products, and the hydrolysis of low-energy bonds provides the chemical energy to make the pathway exergonic.

Salvage and *De Novo* Pathways for Choline and Ethanolamine

CDP-ethanolamine and **CDP-choline** are activated phosphate esters that participate in the bio-

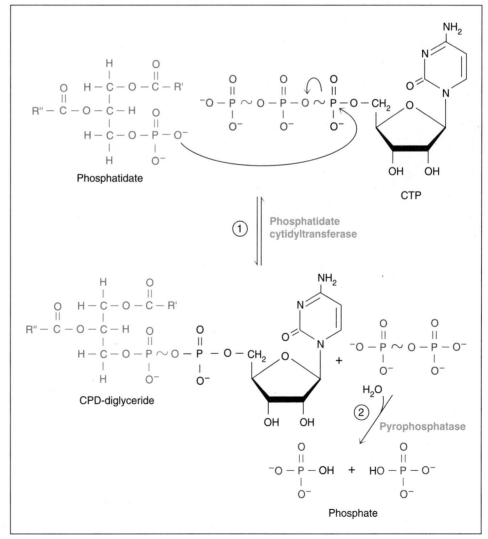

FIGURE 12–1. Synthesis of CDP-diglyceride. (1) The reactants and products of this isoergonic reaction both contain a total of two high-energy bonds. (2) The hydrolysis of PP$_i$ by an independent pyrophosphatase pulls reaction 1 forward.

Phosphatidate

CTP

① Phosphatidate cytidyltransferase

CPD-diglyceride

② Pyrophosphatase

Phosphate

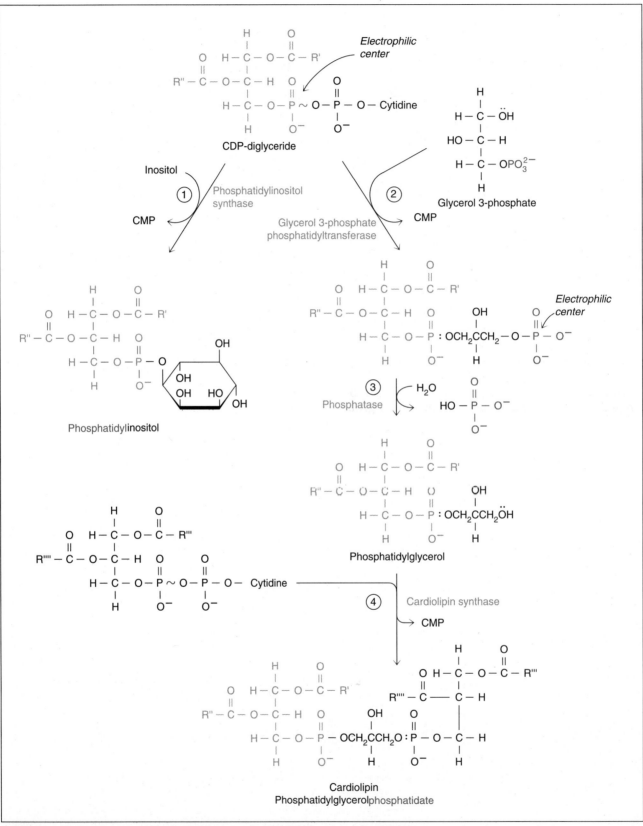

FIGURE 12–2. Biosynthesis of (1) phosphatidylinositol, (2, 3) phosphatidylglycerol, and (4) cardiolipin. *Each reaction in this figure is exergonic and unidirectional.*

synthesis of complex lipids; the simple acid anhydride between the two phosphates is energy rich (Figure 12–3). The biochemistry and bioenergetics of phosphatidylcholine and phosphatidylethanolamine synthesis are analogous. When phosphatidylethanolamine is derived from phosphatidylserine and when phosphatidylcholine is derived from phosphatidylethanolamine, new ethanolamine and choline moieties are formed from precursors, and the pathways are called *de novo* **pathways.** In the sequences outlined in Figure 12–3, however, ethanolamine and choline per se are the starting substances, and the processes are called **salvage pathways.** Choline and ethanolamine are not synthesized anew *(de novo);* rather, preformed choline and ethanolamine are reutilized or salvaged.

Metabolism of Ethanolamine, Choline, and Serine Derivatives

Phosphatidylserine is a minor constituent of membranes; however, it is an important precursor of phosphatidylethanolamine. Moreover, phosphatidylethanolamine can be converted to phosphatidylcholine (in liver) by three successive methylation reactions. The activated methyl donor is *S*-adenosylmethionine (AdoMet). This substance is synthesized from methionine and ATP, a type IV reaction of ATP (Figure 6–10). The amino group of phosphatidylethanolamine reacts in succession with three molecules of *S*-adenosylmethionine to form the monomethyl-, dimethyl-, and trimethyl derivatives (choline) as shown in Figure 12–4.

The formation of phosphatidylserine occurs by an exchange reaction involving phosphatidylethanolamine. An enzyme found in the endoplasmic reticulum catalyzes the exchange of esterified ethanolamine and serine (Figure 12–5). Phosphatidylserine can undergo a decarboxylation reaction to produce phosphatidylethanolamine. This decarboxylation reaction is exergonic as are most decarboxylation reactions (PRINCIPLE 6 OF BIOENERGETICS), and conversion to phosphatidylethanolamine is unidirectional.

Metabolism of Phosphatidylinositol Bisphosphate (PIP₂)

Even though phosphatidylinositol derivatives constitute only 5% of the phospholipid in plasma membranes, they play an important role in metabolic regulation and signal transduction. Signal transduction refers to the processes whereby extracellular substances (hormones, growth factors, neurotransmitters, adhesion molecules) influence intracellular metabolism. The hormones are called first messengers, and intracellular regulatory molecules are called second messengers. **Phosphatidylinositol 4,5-bisphosphate** is a key metabolite in signal transduction. It is converted into two second messengers through the action of phospholipase C; these second messengers are diglyceride and inositol 1,4,5-trisphosphate.

Physiological Actions of Diglyceride and Inositol 1,4,5-Trisphosphate

Phosphatidylinositol 4,5-bisphosphate (PIP₂) is a glycerolipid containing inositol 4,5-bisphosphate that is connected to a glycerol backbone via a phosphodiester (Figure 12–6). The compound undergoes an exergonic hydrolysis reaction catalyzed by phospholipase C to form two physiologically important regulatory second messengers: diglyceride and inositol 1,4,5-trisphosphate. Diglyceride is an activator of protein kinase C. **Protein kinase C is an enzyme** that catalyzes the phosphorylation of several proteins and thereby alters their activity to mediate a variety of physiological responses. Low concentrations of calcium are required for protein kinase C activity (C refers to calcium). Protein kinase C is also a prime target for phorbol esters such as phorbol myristoyl acetate, a tumor promoter (Figure 21–4). The other product of the phospholipase C reaction, inositol trisphosphate (IP₃), interacts with calcium storage sites (endoplasmic reticulum) within the cell and increases the intracellular *concentration* of calcium.

The Inositol Cycle of PIP₂ Metabolism

Phosphatidylinositol 4,5-bisphosphate is made and degraded in a cyclic fashion and thus undergoes continual turnover. This pathway can be divided into a lipid cycle, which involves the reactions of diglyceride, and an inositol phosphate cycle, which involves the reactions of the cyclic alcohol. Inositol 1,4,5-trisphosphate, one of the products of the phospholipase C reaction, undergoes three successive hydrolysis reactions to form inositol (Figure 12–7A). Ionic lithium (Li⁺), at therapeutic concentrations (low millimolar) in humans, is a potent inhibitor of the **inositol phosphate phosphatase.** ▶ Lithium is one of the substances that is used in the treatment of manic depression in humans, and inhibition of this phosphatase accounts for many of its effects on neuronal metabolism. ◀

The Lipid Cycle of PIP₂ Metabolism

Let us now consider the fate of diglyceride, the other product of the phospholipase C reaction. Diglyceride is converted to CDP-diglyceride in two reactions (Figure 12–7B). CDP-diglyceride reacts with inositol to form phosphatidylinositol and CMP (Figure 12–7C). Phosphatidylinositol undergoes two successive phosphorylation reactions with ATP as the phosphoryl donor to regenerate PIP₂ and complete the cycles.

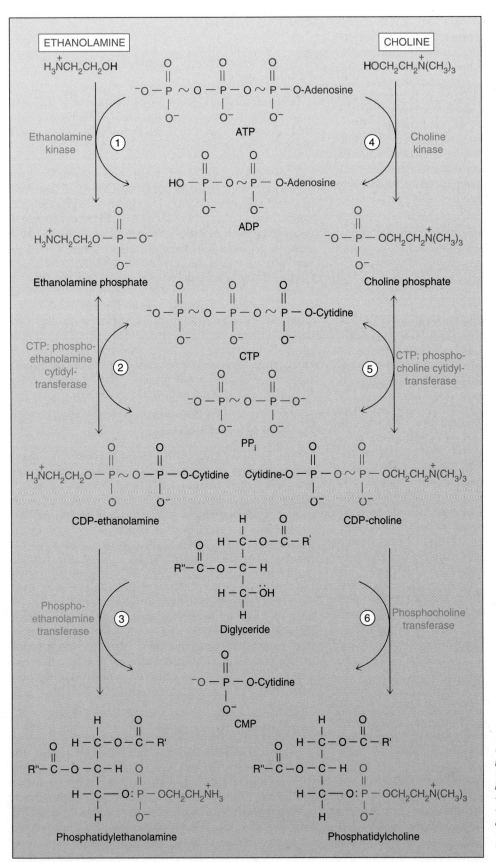

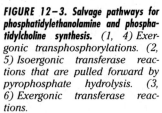

FIGURE 12–3. Salvage pathways for phosphatidylethanolamine and phosphatidylcholine synthesis. (1, 4) Exergonic transphosphorylations. (2, 5) Isoergonic transferase reactions that are pulled forward by pyrophosphate hydrolysis. (3, 6) Exergonic transferase reactions.

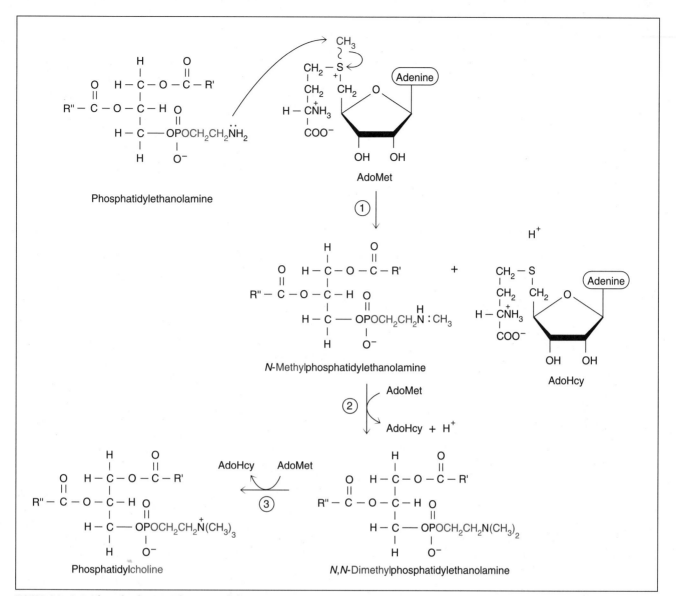

FIGURE 12–4. S-Adenosylmethionine (AdoMet) metabolism. *A single enzyme catalyzes each of the three exergonic methylation reactions (1–3).* *AdoHcy, S-adenosylhomocysteine.*

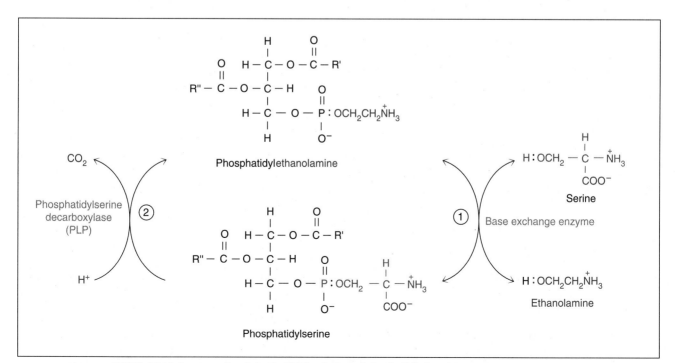

FIGURE 12–5. Interconversion of phosphatidylethanolamine and phosphatidylserine. *PLP, pyridoxal phosphate.*

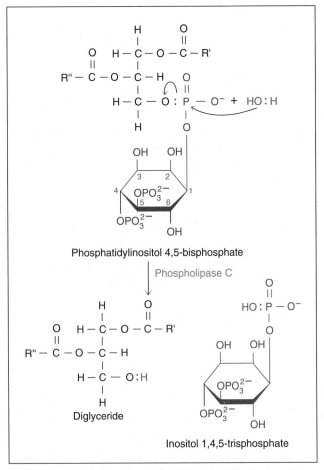

Phosphatidylinositol 4,5-bisphosphate

Phospholipase C

Diglyceride

Inositol 1,4,5-trisphosphate

FIGURE 12–6. Hydrolysis of phosphatidylinositol 4,5-bisphosphate. *Phospholipase C has a broad substrate specificity and is not restricted to phosphatidylinositol phosphate compounds.*

SPHINGOLIPIDS

Biosynthesis of Sphingolipids

Sphingolipids are derivatives of the amino alcohol **sphingosine.** There are three general classes of sphingolipids: sphingomyelin, cerebrosides, and gangliosides. These three classes differ with respect to the substituent attached to the C^1-hydroxyl group of sphingosine. **Sphingomyelin** contains phosphocholine, **cerebrosides** contain a monosaccharide, and **gangliosides** contain an oligosaccharide. An important intermediate in the formation of the three classes of sphingolipids is **ceramide** (N-acylsphingosine).

Conversion of Palmitoyl-CoA and Serine to Ceramide

Free sphingosine does not occur as an intermediate in ceramide biosynthesis. The carbon atoms that contribute to sphingosine (C_{18}) include palmitoyl-CoA (C_{16}) and two from serine. The first enzyme **(3-ketosphinganine synthase)** in the pathway contains pyridoxal phosphate as a cofactor. The conversion of precursors to 3-ketosphinganine is

accompanied by a decarboxylation of the seryl group and the displacement of coenzyme A (Figure 12–8). Both processes make the reaction highly exergonic.

3-Ketosphinganine, a ketone, is reduced by **NADPH** to form sphinganine, an alcohol (Figure 12–8). Sphinganine is converted to **dihydroceramide** in a reaction with acyl~SCoA. The reactant contains a high-energy thioester bond, and the product, a low-energy N-acyl bond. The reaction proceeds with the loss of a high-energy bond and is exergonic.

A double bond is introduced at C^4 by an oxidation reaction; the oxidant, denoted A, has not been identified. Based upon the succinate dehydrogenase and acyl-CoA dehydrogenase reactions, FAD would serve as an appropriate oxidant. Like the succinate and acyl-CoA dehydrogenase reactions, the product contains a *trans* double bond. Oxidation of AH_2 pulls the synthesis of ceramide forward.

Conversion of Ceramide to Sphingomyelin

Ceramide is an intermediate in the biosynthesis of the three major classes of sphingolipids (sphingomyelin, cerebrosides, gangliosides). The formation of sphingomyelin from ceramide is unusual in that a high-energy precursor is not involved. The phosphocholine donor in this exchange reaction is phosphatidylcholine (Figure 12–9). The reactants and products are low-energy compounds. The bioenergetic principle of this reaction corresponds to that of PRINCIPLE 4 OF BIOENERGETICS, and the process is functionally isoergonic. The metabolism of diglyceride, as illustrated in Figure 12–7, pulls the exchange reaction in the direction of sphingomyelin.

Conversion of Ceramide to Cerebroside and Several Gangliosides

The bioenergetics for the biosynthesis of cerebrosides and gangliosides is identical to that for lactose biosynthesis (Figure 10–6). Cerebrosides and gangliosides contain carbohydrate linked to the terminal alcohol group of ceramide via a low-energy glycosidic bond. The donors of the carbohydrates are the energy-rich uridine diphosphate sugars. The formation of cerebroside involves a reaction of ceramide with UDP-galactose. The reactants contain two high-energy bonds (bonds in UDP-galactose), and the products contain only one high-energy bond (in UDP). The reaction proceeds with the loss of one high-energy bond and is exergonic and unidirectional (Figure 12–10). The pathway for the biosynthesis of some gangliosides is illustrated in Figure 12–11. After the addition of the first sugar to ceramide, other activated sugars are transferred to the carbohydrate portion of intermediates in the pathway. Each of these exer-

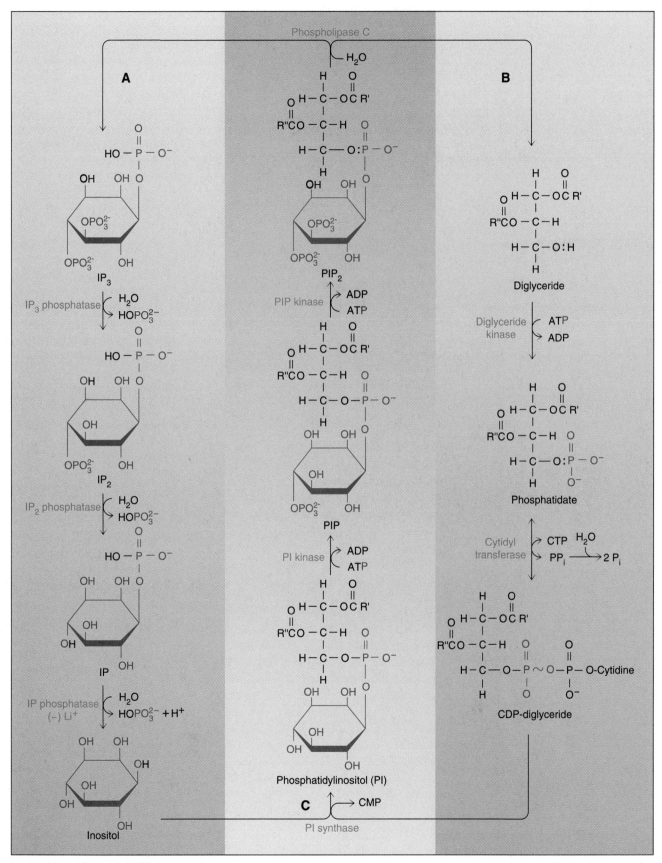

FIGURE 12–7. The phosphatidylinositol cycle. *The two parts of the cycle include* (A) *the inositol phosphate segment and* (B) *the lipid segment. All the reactions except for the cytidyltransferase reaction are unidirectional as indicated by the arrows.*

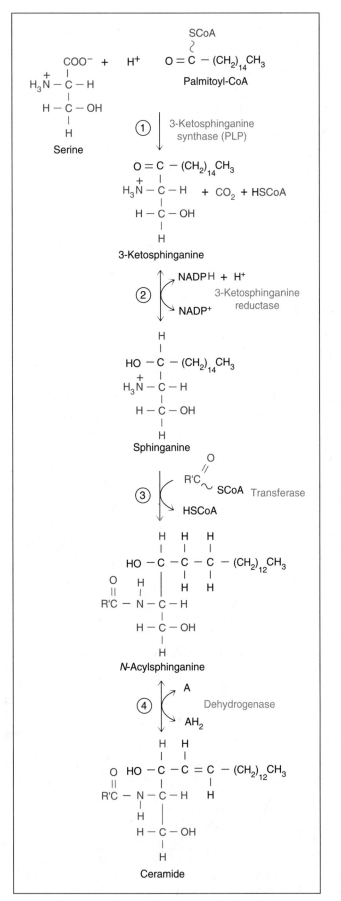

FIGURE 12–8. Ceramide biosynthesis. *Exergonic reactions are depicted with unidirectional arrows.*

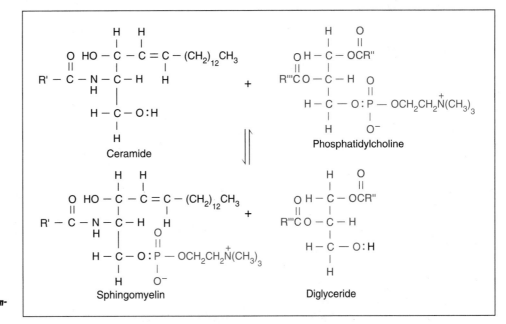

FIGURE 12–9. Sphingomyelin biosynthesis.

gonic reactions is catalyzed by an individual glycosyltransferase.

Phosphoadenosylphosphosulfate (PAPS): Active Sulfate

Sulfate esters (formed by the combination of an alcohol with sulfate) occur in sphingolipids. The donor of sulfate in biosynthetic reactions is **3′-phosphoadenosine-5′-phosphosulfate,** or **PAPS.** The standard free energy of hydrolysis of phosphoadenosylphosphosulfate to form 3′-phosphoadenosine monophosphate and sulfate is about −75 kJ/mol. Because of the extraordinary energy richness of this linkage, several steps are required

in the pathway for PAPS metabolism to ensure that the overall process is exergonic. Its intricacy is even more formidable than the pathway for synthesizing phosphoenolpyruvate from pyruvate.

In the first step of active sulfate metabolism, ATP reacts with sulfate to form adenosylphosphosulfate (APS). This substance contains a mixed acid-anhydride linkage between phosphate and sulfate (Figure 12–12). In Table 6–2, we noted that acid anhydrides are energy rich. Hydrolysis of pyrophosphate helps to pull the reaction forward. APS reacts with ATP to form PAPS and ADP in an exergonic kinase reaction. An important function of PAPS is to donate the sulfuryl group for the synthesis of sulfate esters. PAPS undergoes reactions with substrates that yield low-energy sulfate esters.

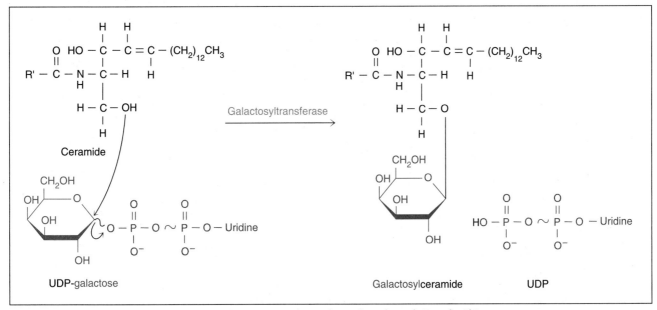

FIGURE 12–10. Conversion of ceramide to galactosylceramide (a cerebroside).

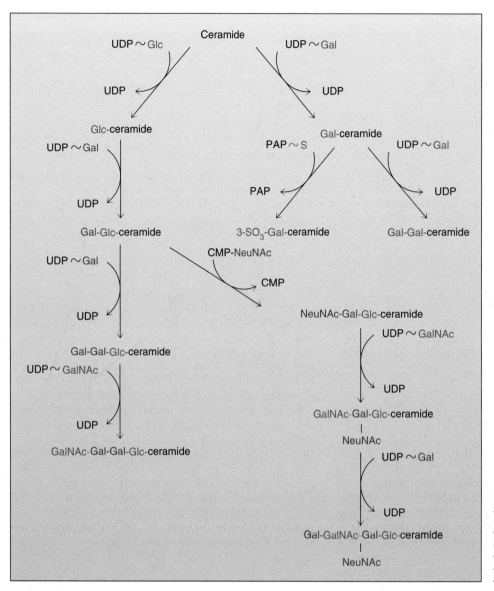

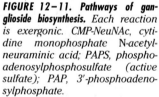

FIGURE 12–11. Pathways of ganglioside biosynthesis. *Each reaction is exergonic. CMP-NeuNAc, cytidine monophosphate N-acetylneuraminic acid; PAPS, phosphoadenosylphosphosulfate (active sulfate); PAP, 3'-phosphoadenosylphosphate.*

The loss of the high-energy bond makes these processes exergonic.

The product of the sulfuryl transfer reactions (3'-phosphoadenylate) undergoes an exergonic hydrolysis to give AMP. Adenylate kinase catalyzes the conversion of AMP to ADP, and a variety of processes (substrate level phosphorylation, oxidative phosphorylation) are responsible for the regeneration of ATP. A total of three high-energy bonds is required for each sulfation reaction (ATP → AMP + 2 P_i; ATP → ADP + P_i). The exceptional high energy of the P—O—S bond of PAPS explains the requirement for multiple steps in PAPS metabolism. The role of PAPS in the sulfation of sphingolipids is illustrated in Figure 12–13.

CMP-N-Acetylneuraminate Metabolism

N-Acetylneuraminate is an acetylated nine-carbon compound that occurs in several sphingolipids and glycoproteins. The donor is CMP-*N*-acetylneuraminate. The unusual nature of this compound is due to the attachment of the sugar to a nucleoside monophosphate (CMP), not to a nucleoside diphosphate.

The precursor for all *N*-acetylhexoses is **fructose 6-phosphate,** and the amido group of **glutamine** is the source of the amino groups that occur in sugars. The pathway for the conversion of fructose 6-phosphate to *N*-acetylmannosamine 6-phosphate is shown in Figure 12–14. Hexosamines occur mainly as the *N*-acetyl derivative, and the second step of the pathway is an acetylation reaction. Hydrolase, acetylase, and kinase reactions make the pathway exergonic.

Phosphoenolpyruvate provides three carbon atoms in a reaction with *N*-acetylmannosamine 6-phosphate to form *N*-acetylneuraminate 9-phosphate (Figure 12–15). CMP-*N*-acetylneuraminate donates its activated sugar to various sphingolipid acceptors to form the appropriate derivative. The

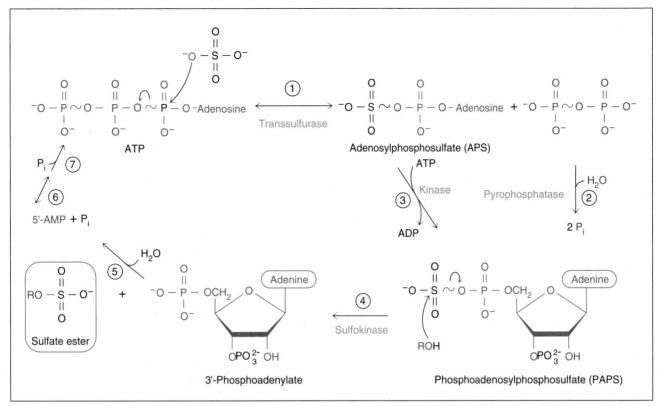

FIGURE 12–12. Phosphoadenosylphosphosulfate (PAPS) metabolism. *Bidirectional and unidirectional reactions are indicated by the corresponding arrows.*

FIGURE 12–13. Synthesis of galacto-cerebroside 3-sulfate from ceramide. *The C^3 hydroxyl group (a nucleophile) of the galactosyl residue of galactocerebroside reacts with the sulfur atom (an electrophile) of activated sulfate (PAPS) to form the low-energy sulfate ester.*

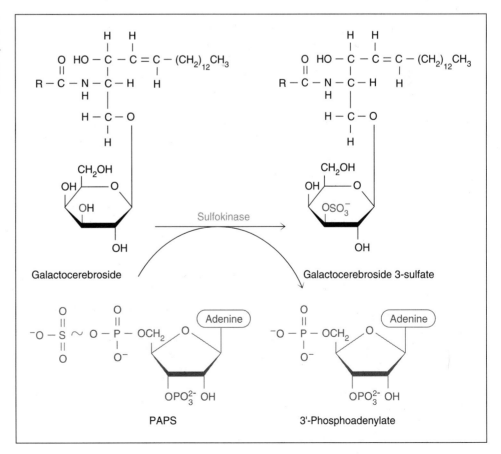

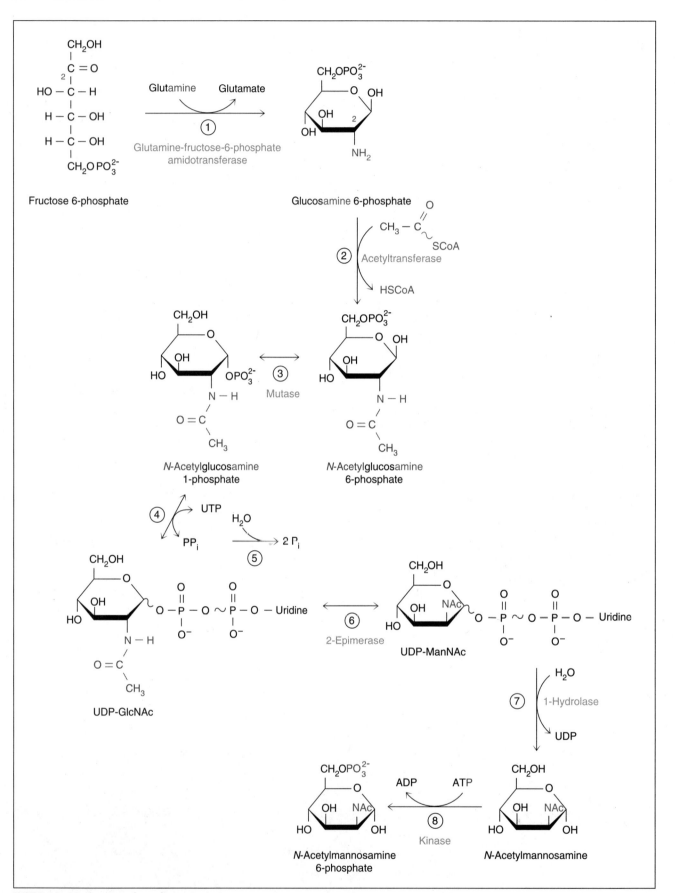

FIGURE 12–14. Hexosamine biosynthesis. *Glutamine donates its amido nitrogen to fructose 6-phosphate in the first and rate-limiting reaction of the pathway. Exergonic reactions are depicted with unidirectional arrows.*

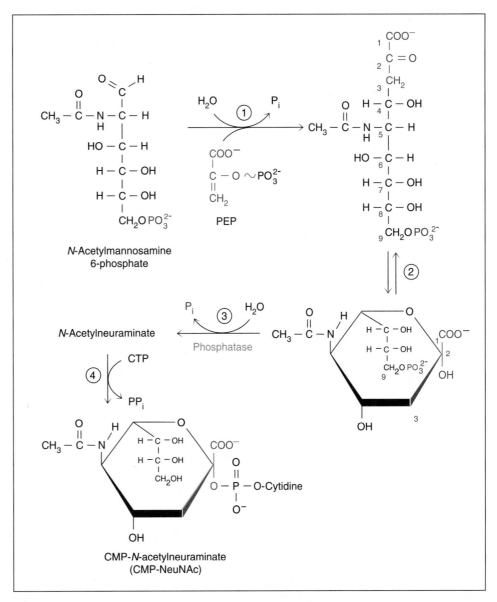

FIGURE 12–15. Biosynthesis of CMP-N-acetylneuraminate. *Formation of the six-membered ring is nonenzymatic. Exergonic reactions are depicted with unidirectional arrows.*

N-Acetylmannosamine 6-phosphate

PEP

N-Acetylneuraminate

Phosphatase

CTP

PP$_i$

CMP-N-acetylneuraminate (CMP-NeuNAc)

free energy of hydrolysis of the glycosidic linkage has not been determined. By comparison with other glycosidic bonds involving the hemiketal group, the standard free energy of hydrolysis is estimated to be about − 20 kJ/mol. Since CMP-N-acetylneuraminate is the universal donor of N-acetylneuraminate, its activation is sufficient to promote group transfer.

Sphingolipidoses

Gangliosides are complex lipids that are derivatives of sphingosine. The intricate pathways for the degradation of sphingolipids are illustrated in Figures 12–16 and 12–17. Each hydrolytic reaction in these pathways is catalyzed by a specific enzyme. Although the pathways are formidable, the bioenergetics is straightforward. ▶ The sphingolipidoses are celebrated lysosomal diseases, and the enzyme deficiencies are given for general reference in Table 12–1. Only experts know all these deficiencies by rote. Gaucher disease is due to a deficiency of **β-glucosidase.** Tay-Sachs disease is due to a deficiency of **hexosaminidase A** (Table 12–1). Tay-Sachs disease is generally fatal by age 3. The course of Gaucher disease is variable. ◀

CHOLESTEROL

Biosynthesis of Cholesterol

Cholesterol is the major sterol of animals, but it is not found in plants or in prokaryotes to any significant extent. It is a structural component of animal cell membranes, and animal cells cannot survive without it. Cholesterol (Figure 11–3) is the precursor of bile salts and steroid hormones. Cholesterol biosynthesis occurs in the cytosol of nu-

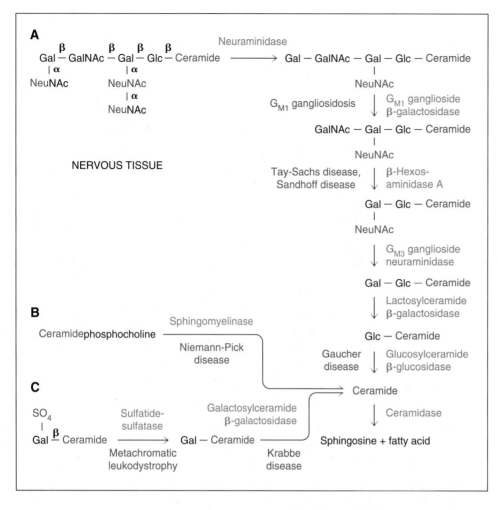

FIGURE 12–16. Pathway for the metabolism of sphingolipids in nerve cells. *Each reaction in this figure represents an exergonic hydrolysis. Water and the monomeric product are omitted for clarity. A. Ganglioside metabolism. B. Sphingomyelin metabolism. C. Sulfatide metabolism. A deficiency of enzyme activity leads to an accumulation of the corresponding substrate and the designated disease. (See also Table 12–1.)*

cleated cells. Cholesterol is formed entirely from acetyl-CoA. An overview of the biosynthesis of cholesterol is shown in Figure 12–18.

Formation of the Five-Carbon Isoprenoid Precursors of Cholesterol

Acetoacetyl-CoA forms in a reaction catalyzed by **thiolase,** an enzyme usually associated with degradation (Figure 12–19). The next reaction, which is

catalyzed by **HMG-CoA synthase,** is similar to the citrate synthase reaction of the Krebs cycle and is physiologically irreversible. *The rate-limiting reaction in cholesterol biosynthesis is catalyzed by HMG-CoA reductase* (Table 25–3). The carbonyl group is reduced to (1) a thiohemiacetal during the first reduction and then to (2) an alcohol during the second reduction by **NADPH.** The removal of CoASH makes the second reduction unidirectional. Note that NADPH is the favored reductant for biosynthetic reactions (PRINCIPLE 16 OF BIOCHEMISTRY), including cholesterol biosynthesis.

Mevalonate, formed by the HMG-CoA reductase reaction, undergoes two successive phosphorylation reactions involving ATP. The products include 5-phosphomevalonate and then 5-pyrophosphomevalonate and two ADP molecules (Figure 12–20). Note that the formation of 5-pyrophosphomevalonate does not involve a direct transfer of the pyrophosphate group from ATP as occurs in a type III reaction of ATP (Figures 6–6 and 6–9). The formation of 5-pyrophosphomevalonate requires two successive type I phosphorylation reactions; the first is exergonic, and the second is isoergonic. Isopentenyl pyrophosphate is formed during an exergonic decarboxylation reaction. The isomerase reaction that follows is functionally isoergonic and bidirectional.

TABLE 12–1. Enzyme Deficiencies in Selected Sphingolipidoses

Disease	Enzyme	CNS Involvement*	Visceral Involvement*
Fabry	α-Galactosidase	–	+
Farber	Ceramidase	±	–
GM₁ gangliosidosis	β-Galactosidase	+	+
Gaucher†	β-Glucosidase	±	+
Metachromatic leukodystrophy	Sulfatide sulfatase	+	–
Niemann-Pick	Sphingomyelinase	+	+
Tay-Sachs	Hexosaminidase A	+	–

* ± Designates variable.
† Most prevalent.

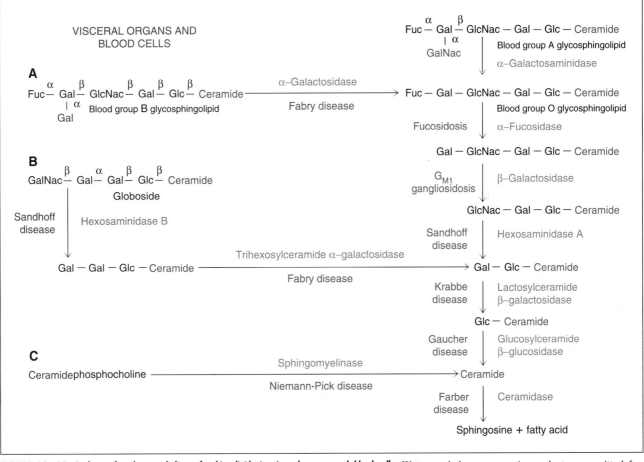

FIGURE 12–17. *Pathway for the metabolism of sphingolipids in visceral organs and blood cells. Water and the monomeric product are omitted for clarity. A. Blood group substance metabolism. B. Globoside metabolism. C. Sphingomyelin metabolism. A deficiency of enzyme activity leads to an accumulation of the corresponding substrate and the designated disease. (See also Table 12–1.)*

Condensation of Isoprenoid Precursors to Form Cholesterol

A molecule of **dimethylallyl pyrophosphate** condenses with **isopentenyl pyrophosphate** to yield **geranyl pyrophosphate** and pyrophosphate (Figure 12–21). Geranyl pyrophosphate condenses with a second molecule of isopentenyl pyrophosphate, yielding **farnesyl pyrophosphate** and pyrophosphate. Then two molecules of farnesyl pyrophosphate condense to form **squalene.** Squalene reacts with molecular oxygen and undergoes an epoxidation and subsequent ring closures, yielding **lanosterol.** Reactions of molecular oxygen with hydrocarbons, and the reduction of oxygen to form water are exergonic (PRINCIPLE 8 OF BIOENERGETICS). *Lanosterol is the first compound in the pathway containing the steroid nucleus.* Lanosterol is converted to **cholesterol** by removal of three methyl groups, reduction of a double bond, and isomerization involving double bond migration (Figure 12–21).

Three ATP molecules are required for the formation of each isoprenoid unit. Six isoprenoid units are required for the synthesis of cholesterol for a total of 18 molecules of ATP. In addition, molecular oxygen is involved in the formation of squalene epoxide and reduction to water. Exergonic kinase, pyrophosphatase, and oxidation reactions promote cholesterol formation.

Conversion of Cholesterol to Neutral Sterols and Bile Salts

Cholesterol is the precursor of steroid hormones, bile salts, and neutral sterols. Humans are unable to degrade completely the steroid ring to carbon dioxide and water. Although the complete oxidation of cholesterol or its derivatives is thermodynamically feasible, animals lack enzymes needed for catabolizing steroid rings. A result is that cholesterol cannot be degraded to produce metabolic energy, and the deposition of excess cholesterol in humans results in disease. We next consider the conversion of cholesterol to (1) neutral sterols by enteric bacteria and (2) bile salts by liver cells.

Neutral Sterols

Cholesterol, synthesized by the liver, is excreted into the gut in bile. Cholesterol, a polar lipid, aids

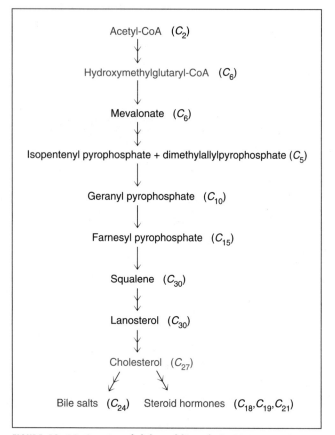

FIGURE 12–18. Overview of cholesterol biosynthesis. *Multiple arrows indicate that several steps are required to produce the designated metabolic transformation.*

in the emulsification of dietary fat. Some of the enteric cholesterol is converted to neutral sterols by intestinal bacteria. **Coprostanol** and **cholestanol,** neutral sterols, are stereoisomers that are formed by the bacterial reduction of the double bond of cholesterol. Coprostanol and cholestanol differ in the stereochemistry joining the A and B rings.

Primary and Secondary Bile Salts

Bile salts are divided into two classes: primary and secondary. **Primary bile salts** are synthesized by humans. **Secondary bile salts** result from the action of intestinal bacteria on the primary bile salts. The physical and physiological properties of the bile salts are similar.

The first and rate-limiting step in the conversion of cholesterol to bile salts is catalyzed by **cholesterol 7α-hydroxylase.** The α-positions are those under the steroid ring as viewed on the printed page (Figure 12–22). The reaction involves NADPH, molecular oxygen, and the cytochrome P-450 electron transport chain of the endoplasmic reticulum (Table 1–1). The reaction is exergonic and irreversible. Deoxycholate and lithocholate are secondary bile salts. They are derived from primary bile salts by the action of enteric bacteria. This conversion involves an exergonic hydrolysis of

conjugated glycine or taurine, and the reduction of the hydroxyl group at C^7 of the steroid ring.

Cholesterol cannot be oxidized to carbon dioxide and water. The only way to rid the body of excess cholesterol is via excretion of cholesterol, neutral sterols, and bile salts in the feces. Liver synthesizes about 500 mg of bile salts daily, and these and recirculating bile salts are excreted into the gut in bile. The liberation of bile salts by the liver, their transit to the ileum, and their absorption in the ileum and return to the liver is called **enterohepatic (gut-liver) circulation.** About 94% of the intestinal bile salts is reabsorbed, and 6% is lost in the feces. ▶ Oral administration of anion exchange resins captures a greater percentage of bile salts and increases their excretion in the feces. This is one therapy used in the treatment of hypercholesterolemia. ◀

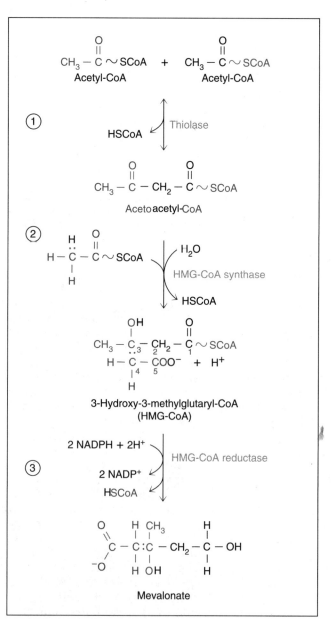

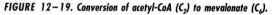

FIGURE 12–19. Conversion of acetyl-CoA (C_2) to mevalonate (C_6).

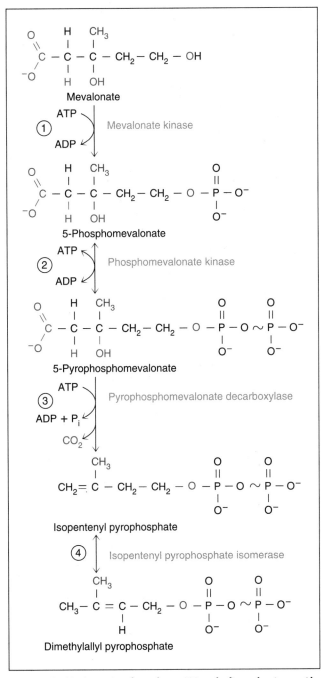

FIGURE 12–20. *Conversion of mevalonate (C₆) to the five-carbon isoprenoids: isopentenyl pyrophosphate and dimethylallyl pyrophosphate.*

LIPOPROTEINS

Lipoprotein Metabolism

The transport of hydrophobic cholesterol and triglyceride in the aqueous bloodstream requires an elaborate lipoprotein transport system. We consider this intricate system in detail because of the association of atherosclerosis, the leading cause of death in the Western world, with cholesterol and triglyceride metabolism. Lipoprotein densities are inversely related to their lipid content: the higher

the lipid content, the lower the density. The main components of lipoprotein transport and their properties are given for general reference in Table 12–2. Note that apo-**A** occurs in HDL with α-electromobility, and apo-**B** occurs in LDL with β-mobility.

The lipoprotein particles perform three major functions. One role is to transport dietary fat from the intestinal mucosa, where it is absorbed, to other tissues by **exogenous lipid transport.** A second function of the lipoprotein transport system is to transfer triglyceride and cholesterol from liver to other tissues by **endogenous lipid transport.** The third function is to transfer cholesterol from extrahepatic tissues to the liver by **reverse cholesterol transport** (Figure 12–23).

Enzymes

Lecithin is a nonsystematic name for phosphatidylcholine, and *lecithin-cholesterol acyltransferase* (**LCAT,** pronounced "el cat") catalyzes the transfer of the *sn*-2 fatty acyl group of phosphatidylcholine to cholesterol; the products include cholesteryl ester and lysolecithin. Note that this reaction converts the polar cholesterol molecule to the nonpolar ester (Figure 12–24). The polar hydroxyl group of cholesterol occurs at the surface of lipoprotein particles in contact with the aqueous environment, while the nonpolar cholesteryl ester occurs in the interior of lipoprotein particles.

Lipoprotein lipase catalyzes the hydrolysis of triglyceride in very low density lipoprotein (VLDL) and chylomicrons. This enzyme is located at the capillary surface throughout the body where it is bound to heparin. Lipoprotein lipase is responsible for generating fatty acids and glycerol at the tissue level where the fatty acid will be taken up by the surrounding cells. This enzyme is also known as **heparin-sensitive lipase.** Following the intravenous injection of heparin, lipase activity in the serum is elevated. This is not a physiological means of regulation but is caused by the displacement of the enzyme from its normal location by a competing ligand, namely, injected heparin.

Hepatic lipase catalyzes the hydrolysis of triglyceride and phospholipids in high-density lipoprotein (HDL) and intermediate-density lipoprotein (IDL). The enzyme is located in liver sinusoids and plays a role in the metabolic degradation of these two classes of lipoprotein. The fatty acids are taken up by the liver.

Acid lipase catalyzes the hydrolysis of triglyceride and cholesteryl ester in lysosomes. The pH optimum of all lysosomal enzymes is acidic. Acid lipase participates in the catabolism of lipoproteins that are taken up by receptor-mediated endocytosis. Of these four enzymes of lipoprotein metabolism, only acid lipase functions within cells.

Properties of Apolipoproteins

The apolipoproteins (apoproteins) are designated by letters, and members of a class are fur-

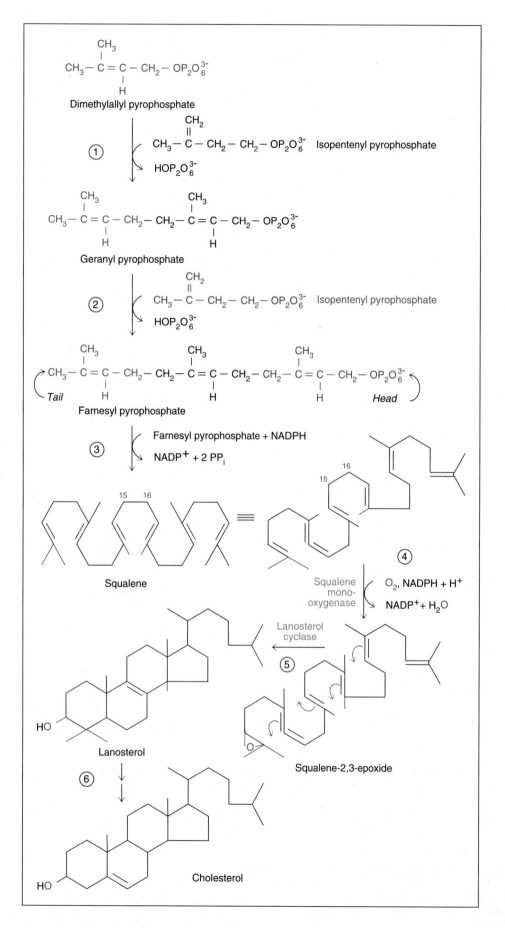

FIGURE 12–21. Cholesterol biosynthesis.

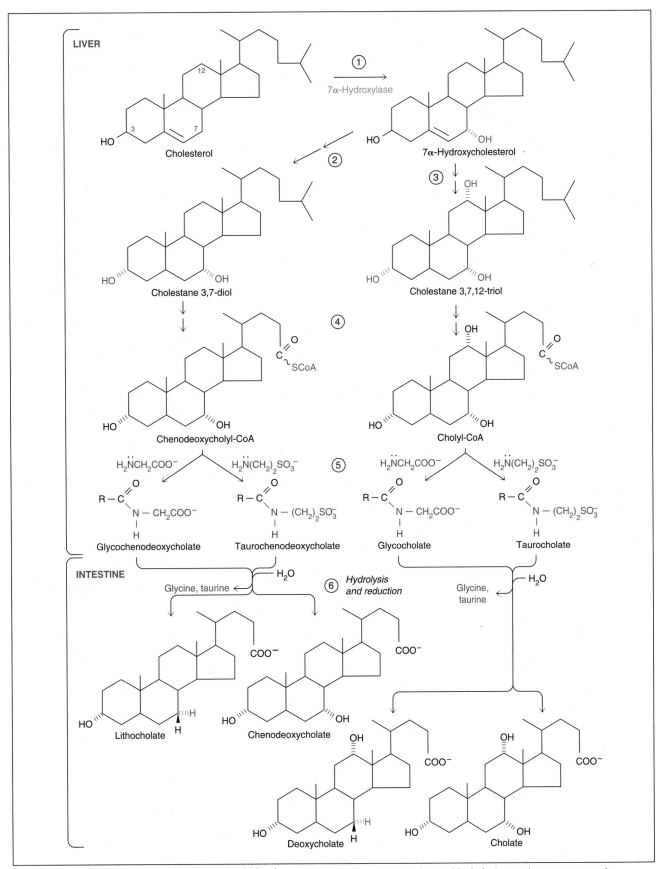

FIGURE 12–22. Overview of the biosynthesis of bile salts. *The hydroxylation, acyltransfer, and hydrolysis reactions are exergonic.*

TABLE 12-2. Properties of Plasma Lipoproteins

Lipoprotein	Major Lipid	Electrophoretic Mobility*	Major Apoproteins
Chylomicron	Triglyceride	None	B-48, A-I, IV
Very low density (VLDL)	Triglyceride	Pre-β	B-100, E, C-I, II, III
Intermediate density (IDL)	Triglyceride and cholesteryl esters	β	B-100, E
Low density (LDL)	Cholesteryl esters	β	B-100
High density (HDL)	Phospholipids and cholesterol	α_1	A-I, II

* Electrophoresis of plasma proteins resolves them into albumin and α, β, and γ-globulin fractions. These fractions, which contain a multitude of proteins, are heterogeneous.

ther distinguished by numbers. The lipoproteins were initially described by their electrophoretic mobility, and the apoprotein of the α-lipoprotein was initially named A, and the apolipoprotein of the β-lipoprotein was named B. With the discovery of other classes and subclasses of apoproteins, the complexity of this nomenclature increased. Apo-A-I is the main structural protein of HDL, the α-lipoprotein. HDL, however, contains lipoproteins from all classes except apo-B and apo-E.

The B apoproteins are designated B-48 and B-100; the numbers refer to their relative molecular masses, with B-48 having a molecular mass that is 48% of that of B-100 at 100%. These proteins form aggregates of higher molecular mass under physiological conditions. Apo-B-48 is synthesized by the intestine, and B-100 is synthesized by the liver. They correspond to the same gene, and the difference is due to variation in the metabolism of the RNA molecules that direct the biosynthesis of these two proteins (Chapter 16). Apo-B-48 is the main protein of the chylomicrons. Apo-B-100 is the predominant protein of VLDL, IDL, and LDL (low-density lipoprotein). Properties of these proteins are listed in Table 12-3 for general reference.

Exogenous Lipid Transport by Chylomicrons

Properties of Chylomicrons

Chylomicrons carry dietary fat (triglyceride and cholesterol) from the small intestine to other tis-

sues of the body. Triglycerides are synthesized from fatty acids and monoglycerides, products of triglyceride digestion, in the enterocytes. Apo-B-48, apo-A-I, and apo-A-IV are synthesized on ribosomes in the rough endoplasmic reticulum and combine with triglyceride, cholesterol, and phospholipid. The chylomicrons with their lipid cargo enter secretory vesicles, are released into the intercellular space, and pass into the lymph.

Chylomicrons contain chiefly triglyceride, and 98% of their mass is lipid. Chylomicrons are large complexes that refract light and give the plasma a milky appearance postprandially. Chylomicrons enter the blood from the lymphatics through the thoracic duct. Their main function is to transport dietary fat, primarily triglyceride. The triglyceride is hydrolyzed, and fatty acids are delivered to extrahepatic and hepatic cells. Capillary lipoprotein lipase plays a key role in the delivery of fatty acids to extrahepatic cells. Chylomicrons also transport cholesterol as cholesteryl ester from the enterocyte.

Metabolism of Chylomicrons

Chylomicrons interact with other plasma lipoproteins in an intricate fashion. Chylomicrons receive apo-C-II and apo-E from HDL (Figure 12-25). Lipoprotein lipase acts on chylomicrons to degrade triglyceride to fatty acids and glycerol, and apo-C-II functions as an activator in this process. As triglyceride is hydrolyzed at various tissues, the size

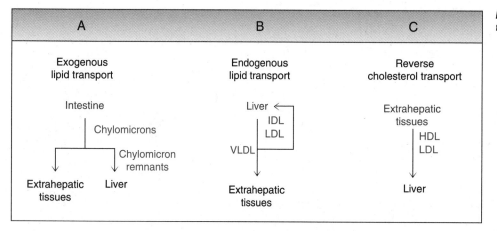

FIGURE 12-23. Overview of lipid transport.

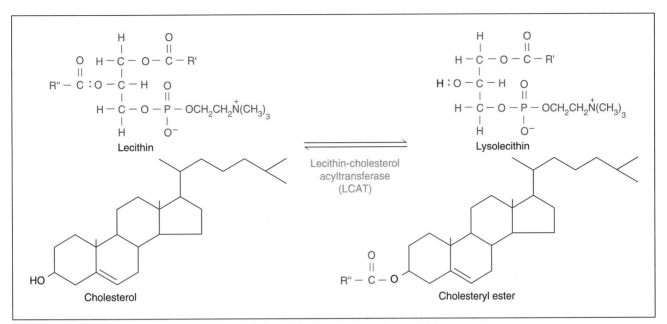

FIGURE 12–24. The lecithin-cholesterol acyltransferase (LCAT) reaction.

of the chylomicrons decreases, and chylomicron remnants result. Chylomicron remnants contain cholesterol, cholesteryl ester, apo-B-48, and apo-E. The metabolism of chylomicrons is expressed by equation 12.3.

$$\text{Chylomicrons} + 3n\ H_2O \xrightarrow[\text{(apo-C-II)}]{\substack{\text{Lipoprotein} \\ \text{lipase}}} \qquad (12.3)$$
$$\text{chylomicron remnants} + 3n\ \text{fatty acids}$$
$$+ n\ \text{glycerol}$$

The chylomicron remnants are removed from the circulation by the liver in a process that involves recognition of the remnant by a receptor that binds apo-E but is distinct from the LDL receptor. The chylomicron remnants are digested by lysosomal acid lipase in liver to yield cholesterol and fatty acids.

Chylomicrons transport triglyceride to adipocytes, muscle, and other tissues. By taking up the chylomicron remnant, liver acquires dietary cho-lesterol. Exogenous lipid transport involves both triglyceride and cholesterol. Glycerol liberated in the extracellular space can be metabolized in cells that contain glycerol kinase, such as liver and kidney. Adipocytes lack glycerol kinase.

Endogenous Lipid Transport by VLDL, IDL, and LDL

Biosynthesis of VLDL

VLDL synthesis occurs in the liver. The main function of VLDL is to transport triglyceride from the liver to other tissues. There are two sources of fatty acids that constitute hepatic triglyceride: fatty acids synthesized from dietary carbohydrate and fatty acids taken up by the liver. The two sources of the latter include free fatty acid transported as an albumin complex and the lipids contained in lipoproteins. The apoproteins (A, B-100, C, and E) combine with triglyceride, phospholipid, and cho-

TABLE 12–3. Apoproteins of the Plasma Lipoproteins

Apoprotein	Plasma Lipoprotein Containing an Appreciable Amount	Major Site of Synthesis	Function
A-I	HDL, chylomicrons	Intestine, liver	LCAT activation
A-II	HDL	Intestine, liver	Structural
A-IV	Chylomicrons	Intestine	Structural
B-100	LDL, VLDL, IDL	Liver	Recognition by LDL receptor
B-48	Chylomicrons, chylomicron remnants	Intestine	Chylomicron formation
C-I	VLDL, HDL	Intestine	Structural
C-II	VLDL, HDL	Liver	Lipoprotein lipase activation
C-III	VLDL, HDL	Liver	Inhibition of VLDL uptake by liver
D	HDL	?	Structural
E	VLDL, chylomicron remnants, IDL	Liver, macrophages	Recognition by LDL and chylomicron remnant receptors

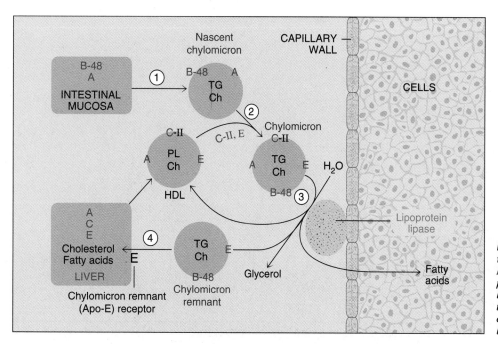

FIGURE 12–25. Exogenous lipid transport and chylomicron metabolism. *Not drawn to scale. The apolipoproteins are designated by their letters. A, apo-A-I and A-IV; TG, triglyceride; Ch, cholesterol and cholesteryl ester; PL, phospholipid.*

lesterol, and the resulting VLDL is released from hepatocytes. VLDL are about 60% triglyceride and 90% lipid. The VLDL interacts with HDL and receives additional apo-C and apo-E (Figure 12–26).

Metabolism of VLDL, IDL, and LDL

The delivery of fatty acids from VLDL resembles that from chylomicrons. The triglyceride within VLDL is digested by lipoprotein lipase, and fatty acids and glycerol are discharged. VLDL is converted to IDL. The amount of triglyceride and cholesterol in IDL is intermediate between that of VLDL and LDL. Some IDL is taken up by the liver, in a process that involves recognition by an apo-B-100/apo-E receptor, and the remaining IDL is converted to LDL. The conversion of IDL to LDL involves the discharge of more triglyceride as catalyzed by lipoprotein lipase. Most of the apo-C proteins are lost during the conversion of VLDL to

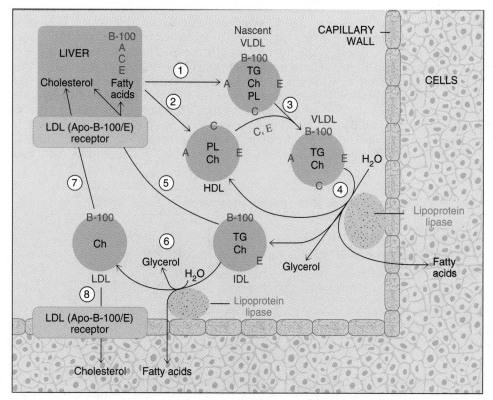

FIGURE 12–26. Endogenous lipid transport and VLDL metabolism. *Not drawn to scale. The apolipoproteins are designated by their letters. C, apo-C-I, C-II and C-III; TG, triglyceride; Ch, cholesterol and cholesteryl ester; PL, phospholipid.*

IDL, and apo-E is lost during the conversion of IDL to LDL. The LDL (apo-B-100/apo-E) receptor can still recognize and take up LDL containing only apo-B-100.

LDL contains most of the cholesterol in the plasma after an overnight fast, and 75% is in the form of cholesteryl ester. About half the LDL is taken up by the liver and the remainder by extrahepatic tissues. The uptake of LDL depends upon the recognition by an apo-B-100/apo-E receptor. Some LDL uptake occurs by nonreceptor-mediated uptake. By these processes, cholesteryl ester is delivered from LDL to the liver and to extrahepatic tissues. Some of the LDL cholesteryl ester is obtained from HDL. The function of this three-component system (VLDL, IDL, and LDL) is to transport large amounts of triglyceride and small but important amounts of cholesterol from the liver to extrahepatic tissues.

HDL and Reverse Cholesterol Transport

Biosynthesis of HDL

This class of lipoprotein particle is synthesized in both liver and intestine. HDL interacts with both chylomicrons and VLDL (Figures 12–25 and 12–26). Apo-A-I and apo-A-II are synthesized by ribo-somes on the rough endoplasmic reticulum. The proteins combine with phospholipids and are secreted into the extracellular space as disk-shaped (discoidal) particles and then enter the blood plasma as nascent HDL.

Metabolism of HDL

Discoidal HDL interacts with cells and HDL$_2$ and is converted into HDL$_3$. The subsequent conversion of HDL$_3$ to HDL$_2$ involves two different processes. First, HDL$_3$ receives free cholesterol that is released from cells and is converted to cholesteryl ester in a reaction catalyzed by LCAT (Figure 12–27). Second, some of the cholesteryl ester is transferred from HDL$_3$ to VLDL in exchange for triglyceride. This exchange is mediated by one or more plasma lipid transfer proteins. HDL$_2$ is larger and less dense than its precursor, HDL$_3$. HDL$_2$ metabolism involves two pathways: (4) HDL$_2$ is acted on by hepatic lipase and is converted back to HDL$_3$; (6) HDL$_2$ may also be taken up and degraded by the liver.

The transport of cholesterol from extrahepatic cells to the liver is called reverse cholesterol transport. The liver is the main organ for converting cholesterol to bile salts, and bile salts are the chief excretory metabolite of cholesterol. The movement of cholesterol from the plasma mem-

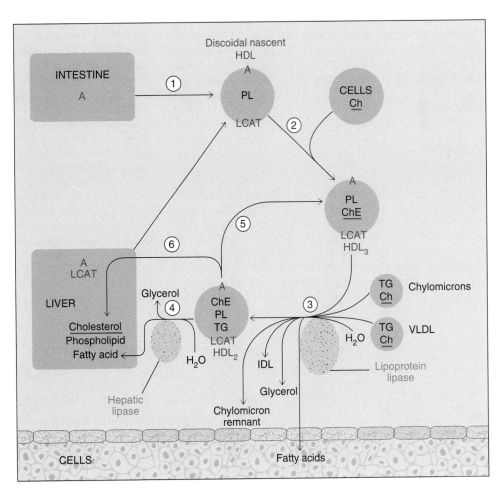

FIGURE 12–27. Reverse cholesterol transport and HDL metabolism. *Cholesterol is transported from extrahepatic cells to the liver. The apolipoproteins are designated by their letters. A, apo-A-I, A-II; TG, triglyceride; Ch, cholesterol; ChE, cholesteryl ester; PL, phospholipid.*

brane of cells to HDL involves diffusion. After the cholesterol becomes associated with HDL, LCAT catalyzes the conversion of cholesterol to cholesteryl ester. The nonpolar cholesteryl ester moves to the hydrophobic core of the HDL particle, or the cholesteryl ester can move to the hydrophobic core of VLDL.

Lipid Transfer Proteins

Lipid transfer proteins mediate the movement of cholesteryl esters, triglyceride, and phospholipids between lipoproteins. At least two separate lipid transfer proteins are present in human plasma. One transfers all three lipids noted, and the second mediates the transfer only of phospholipids. A lipid transfer protein facilitates the movement of cholesteryl ester from HDL to VLDL after synthesis that is catalyzed by the LCAT reaction. The transfer of triglyceride from VLDL to HDL may be mediated by the same transfer protein. A lipid transfer protein also mediates the translocation of phospholipid from chylomicrons and VLDL to HDL.

▶ People who have high HDL levels are resistant to the development of atherosclerosis. Premenopausal women have higher HDL levels than men or than postmenopausal women. The most widely held idea on the protection against atherosclerosis by HDL is that this system removes cholesterol from peripheral tissues and the cardiovascular system. For this reason, HDL is sometimes called "good" cholesterol. People with high LDL levels, on the other hand, are prone to the development of atherosclerosis. LDL is sometimes called "bad" cholesterol because it may serve as a source for the cholesterol that accumulates in atherosclerotic plaques. ◀

Lipoprotein Receptors

The LDL receptor, which is the best characterized of the lipoprotein receptors, recognizes both apo-B-100 and apo-E (Table 12–4). The LDL receptor, which occurs in many cell types, participates in the removal of LDL from the plasma based upon the recognition of apo-B-100. The LDL receptor also participates in the removal of IDL, which contains apo-B-100 and apo-E, from plasma. The LDL receptor does not take part in the uptake of VLDL even though this lipoprotein contains apo-B-100. Apo-C-III blocks the interaction of the LDL receptor with VLDL. Although chylomicron remnants contain apo-E, these particles are not acted upon by the LDL receptor. Modification of apo-B-100 by oxygen promotes the uptake of LDL by endothelial cells and macrophages (Table 12–4). This process may play a role in the pathogenesis of atherosclerosis.

The LDL Receptor

The LDL receptor gene encodes a glycoprotein with a molecular mass of about 160 kDa. The extracellular LDL binding region consists of 292 amino acids. These are cysteine-rich regions that contain seven 40–amino acid repeats (Figure 12–28). The receptor contains a region that is homologous to epidermal growth factor (Table 20–5). The receptor contains a single transmembrane domain and a cytoplasmic domain of about 50 amino acid residues. The LDL receptor gene is located on human chromosome 19 (Table 16–5).

The LDL receptor participates in the endocytosis of LDL and IDL particles. The receptor becomes located in coated pits within the plasma membrane; the coating is an internal meshwork of a protein called **clathrin.** Following the recognition and binding of the receptor with ligands on the lipoprotein particle, the coated pit is taken up by endocytosis to form a coated vesicle (Figure 12–29). The contents of the coated vesicles are delivered to lysosomes, and the receptor is recycled. The lysosomes catalyze the hydrolysis of cholesteryl ester to produce free cholesterol that is released to the cytosol. Cathepsins (Table 1–1) catalyze the hydrolysis of the proteins derived from the coated vesicles.

Intracellular cholesterol has a number of functions. Increased free intracellular cholesterol leads to decreased LDL receptor and HMG-CoA reductase biosynthesis. The result of this action is that cells synthesize less cholesterol (decreased HMG-CoA reductase activity), and they take up less cholesterol from the blood plasma (decreased LDL receptor). A decrease in the amount of receptor is called down regulation. The expression of the LDL receptor is regulated in accord with the metabolic logic of the cell. When the cell has adequate cholesterol, the LDL receptor is unnecessary, and it is not expressed. When the cell contains inadequate

TABLE 12–4. Lipoprotein Receptors

Receptor	Recognition	Lipoprotein	Tissue	Metabolic Role	Comment
Chylomicron remnant	Apo-E	Chylomicron remnants	Liver	Uptake of dietary fat by liver	Also called apo-E receptor
HDL	Unknown	HDL	Liver, possibly other tissues	HDL binding to cells	
LDL	Apo-B-100, apo-E	LDL, IDL	Liver, many other tissues	Removal of LDL, IDL, from circulation	Mediates delivery of cholesterol from liver to tissues
Scavenger	Chemically modified apo-B-100	Modified or damaged LDL	Endothelium, macrophages	Removal of chemically altered LDL	Poorly defined function

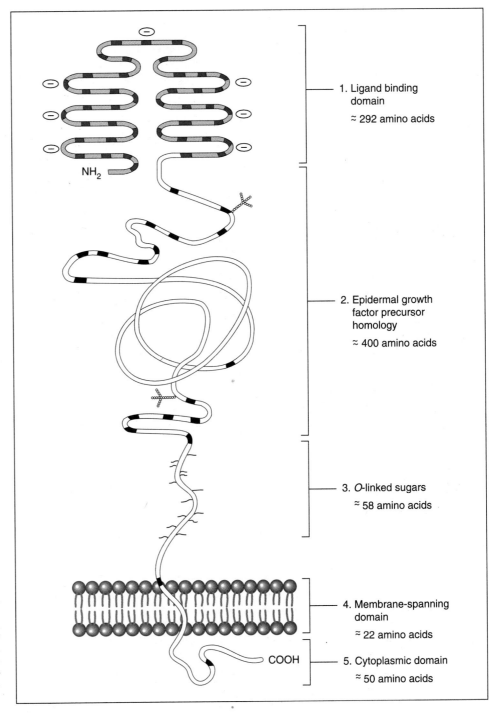

1. Ligand binding domain

≈ 292 amino acids

2. Epidermal growth factor precursor homology

≈ 400 amino acids

3. *O*-linked sugars

≈ 58 amino acids

4. Membrane-spanning domain

≈ 22 amino acids

5. Cytoplasmic domain

≈ 50 amino acids

NH₂

COOH

FIGURE 12–28. LDL receptor topology. *Adapted, with permission, from M.S. Brown and J.L. Goldstein. The LDL receptor and HMG-CoA reductase—two membrane molecules that regulate cholesterol homeostasis. Current Topics in Cellular Regulation 26:3–15, 1985.*

cholesterol, the LDL receptor expression is increased. This probably occurs in conjunction with increased HMG-CoA reductase expression.

An increase in free cholesterol increases the activity of acyl-CoA cholesterol acyltransferase (ACAT). This enzyme catalyzes the conversion of cholesterol to cholesteryl ester (Figure 12–30). The ester in the reactants is energy rich and in the products is energy poor, and the reaction is exergonic. The cholesteryl ester can be stored in droplets or micelles within the cell. Cholesterol hydrolase catalyzes the hydrolysis of the ester to form

free cholesterol. In liver, cholesterol can be converted to bile salts. Both cholesterol and bile salts are secreted with the bile, in which they participate in the digestion and absorption of dietary lipids.

The Chylomicron Remnant Receptor

The chylomicron remnant receptor, which is confined to the liver, recognizes apo-E. Although the LDL receptor also recognizes apo-E, the receptors differ. The chylomicron remnant pathway ac-

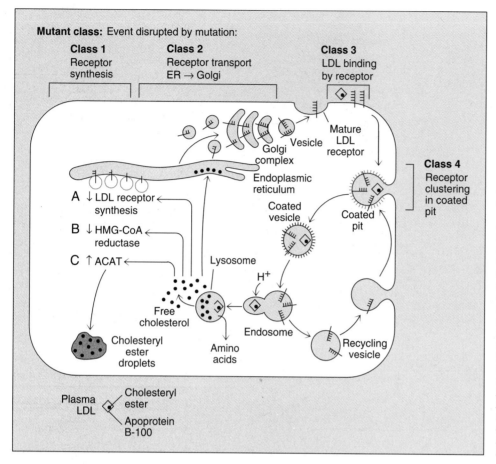

FIGURE 12–29. Function of the LDL receptor in the endocytosis of lipoproteins. The receptor is synthesized in the endoplasmic reticulum and transported to the cell surface via the Golgi. Plasma LDL binds to the receptors, which cluster to form coated pits. The receptor is taken up by endocytosis forming an endosome, a precursor of the lysosome. The lipid and protein components of LDL are hydrolyzed. The mutant classes refer to different defects in LDL receptor metabolism that lead to familial hypercholesterolemia. Modified, with permission, from M.S. Brown and J.L. Goldstein. The LDL receptor and HMG-CoA reductase—two membrane molecules that regulate cholesterol homeostasis. Current Topics in Cellular Regulation 26:3–15, 1985.

counts for the transport of dietary cholesterol and triglyceride to the liver.

Nonreceptor-Mediated Lipoprotein Uptake

There is modest uptake of cholesterol-containing lipoproteins by nonreceptor-linked pathways. Some of these pathways operate in macrophages and other scavenger cells. When the plasma concentration of lipoprotein particles rises, the rate of degradation by the nonreceptor-linked pathways in-creases. ▶ This is postulated to contribute to the deposition of cholesterol in macrophages of arterial walls to produce atherosclerotic plaques. The deposition of cholesterol in the macrophages of tendons and skin produces xanthomas. ◀

Hyperlipoproteinemias

▶ **Primary hyperlipoproteinemias** are due to defects in lipoprotein metabolism. **Familial hyper-**

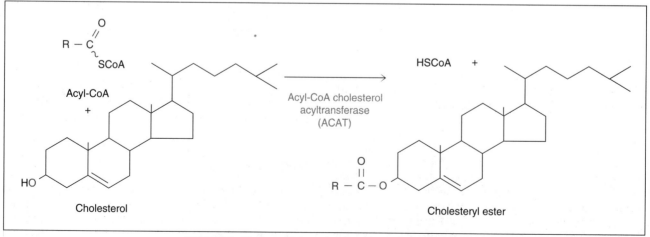

FIGURE 12–30. The acylcholesterol acyltransferase (ACAT) reaction.

TABLE 12-5. Major Secondary Forms of Hyperlipoproteinemia

Disorder	Plasma Lipoprotein Elevation	Proposed Mechanism
Alcoholic hyperlipidemia	VLDL (usually chylomicrons)	Increased secretion of VLDL in individuals genetically predisposed to hypertriglyceridemia
Diabetes mellitus	VLDL	Increased secretion and delayed catabolism of VLDL
Hypothyroidism	LDL	Decreased catabolism of LDL owing to suppressed LDL receptors
Nephrotic syndrome	VLDL and LDL	Increased secretion and decreased catabolism of VLDL and LDL
Uremia	VLDL	Decreased catabolism of VLDL

cholesterolemia is an autosomal dominant disease with an incidence of 1 in 500 live births. It is caused by defects in LDL receptor function (Figure 12-29). **Secondary hyperlipoproteinemias** result from other disorders such as diabetes mellitus and other causes that are listed in Table 12-5. Premature atherosclerosis is a common result of many hyperlipoproteinemias. ◄

STEROID HORMONES

Steroid Hormone Biosynthesis

Conversion of cholesterol to steroid hormones is essential for life. The main steroid hormones (Table 20-8) include cortisol (a glucocorticoid produced by the adrenal cortex), aldosterone (a mineralocorticoid produced by the adrenal cortex), estrogen (a sex hormone produced by the ovary), testosterone (a sex hormone produced by the testes), and progesterone (a progestational hormone produced by the ovary).

Conversion of Cholesterol to Pregnenolone

All steroid hormones are synthesized from **pregnenolone,** a C_{21} compound (Figure 12-31). This substance results from the action of the side-chain cleavage enzyme complex on 20,22-dihydroxycholesterol. The process requires NADPH, oxygen, mitochondrial cytochrome P-450, and **adrenodoxin**. Side-chain cleavage involves multiple hydroxylation reactions and the reduction of molecular oxygen to water. These oxidation reactions are exergonic (PRINCIPLE 8 OF BIOENERGETICS). *The conversion of cholesterol to pregnenolone is rate-limiting in steroid hormone biosynthesis.*

Conversion of Pregnenolone to Progesterone, Aldosterone, and Cortisol

The conversion of pregnenolone to **progesterone** requires two activities. A 3β-ol dehydrogenase catalyzes the NAD+-dependent oxidation of the alcohol to a ketone and double bond migration (Figure 12-31). The steroid hormone pathway in the corpus luteum of the ovary ends at progesterone. The conversion of progesterone to **aldosterone** requires four reactions. These are catalyzed by an endoplasmic reticulum 21-hydroxylase and mito-

chondrial 11β-hydroxylase, 18-hydroxylase, and 18-hydroxysteroid oxidase. All four reactions require NADPH, oxygen, and cytochrome P-450, and they are unidirectional. The metabolism of progesterone to **cortisol** requires three reactions. These are catalyzed by endoplasmic reticulum 17α- and 21-hydroxylases and a mitochondrial 11β-hydroxylase. These hydroxylations involve cytochrome P-450, are unidirectional, and are analogous to those described for aldosterone biosynthesis.

Conversion of Pregnenolone to Testosterone and Estradiol

The metabolism of pregnenolone to testosterone requires four endoplasmic reticulum enzymes: a 17α-hydroxylase, a $C_{17,20}$ side-chain cleavage enzyme, a 3β-hydroxysteroid dehydrogenase, and a 17β-hydroxysteroid dehydrogenase. The pathway, illustrated in Figure 12-31, ends at testosterone in the Leydig cells of the testes. Progesterone can also be converted to testosterone (not shown in Figure 12-31), and the pregnenolone (major) and progesterone (minor) pathways form an intricate network. Testosterone is reduced to dihydrotestosterone in target cells in a reaction catalyzed by 5α-reductase.

The metabolism of testosterone to **estradiol** involves the elimination of the C^{19} methyl group and conversion of ring A to an aromatic group. This process requires three NADPH molecules, three oxygen molecules, and cytochrome P-450. The hydroxylation and oxidation reactions of steroid hormone synthesis are exergonic and unidirectional (PRINCIPLE 8 OF BIOENERGETICS).

Structures of the Steroid Hormones

The following describes the salient features of the various classes of steroid hormones. Estradiol contains 18 carbon atoms and an aromatic A ring. Testosterone contains 19 carbon atoms. Progesterone, aldosterone, and cortisol contain 21 carbon atoms. Aldosterone is unique because it contains an aldehyde group on C^{18}. Glucocorticoids (and aldosterone) contain a hydroxyl group on C^{11} (Figure 12-31).

Congenital Adrenal Hyperplasia

► Congenital adrenal hyperplasia is a group of disorders arising from defects in enzymes of the

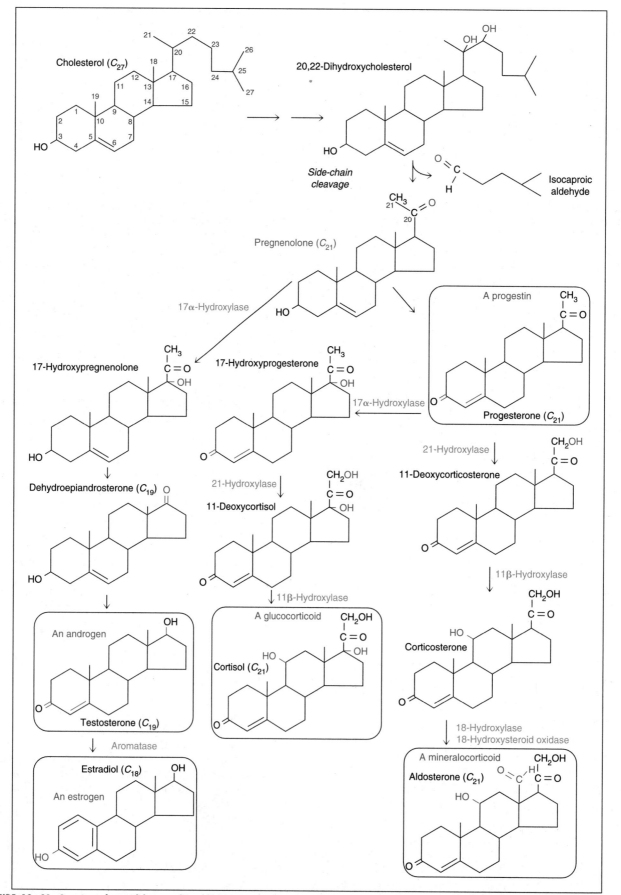

FIGURE 12–31. Overview of steroid hormone biosynthesis. *All the oxidation or hydroxylation reactions involve molecular oxygen, cytochrome P-450, and NADPH. The most common cause of congenital adrenal hyperplasia is a deficiency of progesterone 21-hydroxylase.*

adrenal cortex required for cortisol biosynthesis. The most common enzyme defect, which accounts for 90% of the cases, is due to a deficiency of **progesterone 21-hydroxylase,** which is required for glucocorticoid and mineralocorticoid synthesis (Figure 12–31). As a result, there is a deficiency of cortisol and aldosterone. The plasma levels of 17-hydroxyprogesterone are greatly elevated, and there is excessive production of dehydroepiandrosterone, an androgen. Excessive androgen production in females leads to genital ambiguity in the newborn, often requiring surgical correction. Salt wasting and hypotension are also commonly observed. Affected male infants have normal external genitalia, and the disorder may go unrecognized in early infancy. Androgen excess in both males and females leads to rapid growth and accelerated skeletal maturation.

The incidence of congenital adrenal hyperplasia, which is an autosomal recessive disease, is about 1 in 12,500 live births. The progesterone 21-hydroxylase gene is on the short arm of chromosome 6 (Table 16–5). Affected individuals are treated with synthetic glucocorticoids such as dexamethasone and synthetic mineralocorticoids such as fludrocortisone. These agents indirectly decrease the synthesis of pregnenolone and the formation of androgen. ◄

EICOSANOIDS

Physiological Actions

Almost all mammalian cells except erythrocytes produce one or more of the eicosanoids, 20-carbon compounds (Greek *eikosil,* "twenty"), that include prostaglandins (PGs), prostacyclins (PGIs), thromboxanes (TXs), and leukotrienes (LTs). The physiological responses to these lipid mediators are related to the production of pain and fever, alteration of blood platelet (thrombocyte) activity, and induction of labor. Their tremendous medical importance prompts their detailed consideration.

The eicosanoids are local mediators and are active near their site of formation and are not transported via the circulation to target cells as are hormones. Circulating eicosanoids are chiefly inactive metabolites. The eicosanoids are not stored in cells but are synthesized on demand. The eicosanoids are evanescent, with lifetimes of less than a minute. The chemistry of the eicosanoids is intricate. Only individuals who work with these substances regularly know their structures and metabolism by rote. Although the eicosanoids and steroid hormones are essential, their physiological concentrations are in the nanomolar range—they are not abundant compounds.

Chemical Structures

The prostaglandins and prostacyclins can be considered as derivatives of prostanoate, a compound that does not occur per se in nature. Prostanoate contains a cyclopentane ring with two side chains (Figure 12–32). The configuration is such that the aliphatic chain from C^8 extends below the plane of the cyclopentane ring, and the aliphatic chain linked to C^{12} projects above the plane of the ring. E, F, G, and H are primary prostaglandins. E received its name because it is soluble in ether. F received its name because it is soluble in phosphate buffer (Swedish *fosfat*). G and H represent cyclic endoperoxides (where —O—O— is a peroxide).

The eicosanoids are derived from unsaturated fatty acids. Eicosatrienoate (20:3Δ5,8,11) is the precursor to series 1 compounds containing one aliphatic double bond. Arachidonate (20:4Δ5,8,11,14) is the precursor of the series 2 compounds containing two aliphatic double bonds. Eicosapentaenoate (20:5Δ5,8,11,14,17) is the precursor to series 3 compounds containing three aliphatic double bonds. We concentrate on the series 2 compounds and arachidonate metabolites next.

There are two major divisions of the eicosanoids. These are (1) the **cyclic** prostaglandins and their derivatives (prostacyclins and thromboxanes) that contain the cyclopentane ring and (2) the **linear** leukotrienes (leuko, isolated originally from leukocytes; triene, three double bonds) and tetraenes. The cyclic and linear pathways for biosynthesis are depicted in Figure 12–33. The nomenclature for the *hydroperoxyeicosatetraenoates* is formidable, and the use of the abbreviation HPETE is convenient. HOO— represents hydroperoxy. Eicosa refers to the 20 carbon atoms, and tetraene refers to four double bonds. HPETE combines with glutathione, and the products are called leukotrienes.

The Cyclooxygenase Pathway

Generation of Arachidonate

The first step in the metabolism of the prostaglandins involves the generation of precursor polyunsaturated fatty acid from phospholipid. Most phospholipids contain polyunsaturated fatty acids linked to C^2. Phospholipase A_2 catalyzes the liberation of arachidonate from phospholipids (Figure 12–33). *Phospholipase A_2 catalyzes the rate-limiting reaction in the pathways of eicosanoid biosynthesis.* The hydrolysis catalyzed by phospholipase A_2 is exergonic and unidirectional. Arachidonate can enter the linear (lipoxygenase) or cyclic (cyclooxygenase; see below) eicosanoid pathway. The specificity of the various types of phospholipases is illustrated in Figure 12–34. We noted earlier in this chapter that phospholipase C catalyzes the hydrolysis of PIP_2 to form diglyceride and inositol 1,4,5-trisphosphate.

Biosynthesis of PGH$_2$, a Cyclic Eicosanoid

The second stage of prostaglandin biosynthesis involves the reaction of arachidonate with two

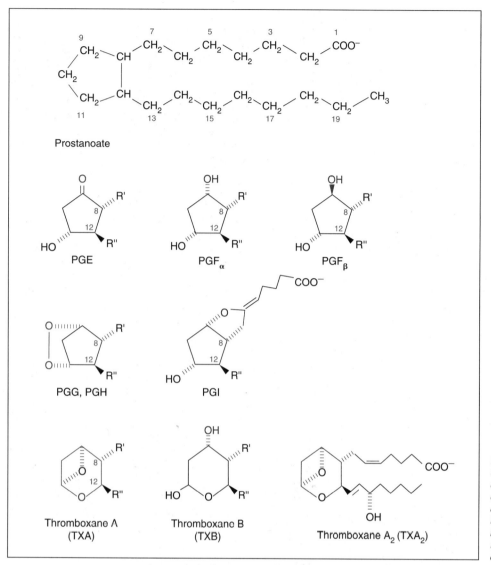

Prostanoate

PGE

PGF$_\alpha$

PGF$_\beta$

PGG, PGH

PGI

Thromboxane A (TXA)

Thromboxane B (TXB)

Thromboxane A$_2$ (TXA$_2$)

FIGURE 12–32. Structures of the eicosanoids. *Prostanoate is the parent compound of the eicosanoids containing a cyclopentane ring. A dashed line indicates that the bond projects below the plane of the paper, and a triangular line indicates that the bond projects above the plane of the paper.*

molecules of oxygen to form PGH$_2$, the precursor for the other prostaglandins, prostacyclins, and thromboxanes. The enzyme responsible for this reaction is **cyclooxygenase,** sometimes called **prostaglandin endoperoxide synthase.** The enzyme is bound to the membranes of the endoplasmic reticulum, and this is common for enzymes that catalyze reactions of long-chain fatty acids.

Prostaglandin endoperoxide synthase has two activities. The first is the **cyclooxygenase** activity that is responsible for the formation of the cyclopentane ring. The second is the **hydroperoxidase** activity that converts a hydroperoxide to an alcohol (Figure 12–33). ► That cyclooxygenase is inhibited irreversibly by aspirin is noteworthy. Aspirin acetylates an active-site serine residue (Figure 4–5). Inactivation of cyclooxygenase inhibits the biosynthesis of all three classes of compounds that are derived from PGH$_2$. Other nonsteroidal anti-inflammatory agents inhibit cyclooxygenase, but the inhibition is not covalent or irreversible as is the case with aspirin.

Low doses of aspirin, 325 mg every other day,

are reported to reduce the incidence of myocardial infarction and stroke. This effect is postulated to be the result of cyclooxygenase inhibition. There is not complete agreement on the use of this agent prophylactically for prevention of these cardiovascular diseases, and additional studies are needed to clarify this situation. ◄

Conversion of PGH$_2$ to Other Prostaglandins and to Prostacyclins and Thromboxanes

The conversion of PGH$_2$ to PGE$_2$ involves an isomerization reaction; the hydrogen linked to C^9 adds to the oxygen on C^{11} to form an alcohol, and the other oxygen of the peroxide forms a double bond with carbon, yielding a ketone (Figure 12–35). The formation of PGF$_{2\alpha}$ involves a reduction of the two peroxide oxygen atoms to two alcohol groups.

Arterial walls contain **prostacyclin synthase,** which catalyzes the conversion of PGH$_2$ to prostacyclin with a new five-membered oxygen-containing ring. This reaction involves the formation of an ether bond linking C^9 and C^6. PGI$_2$ can undergo a

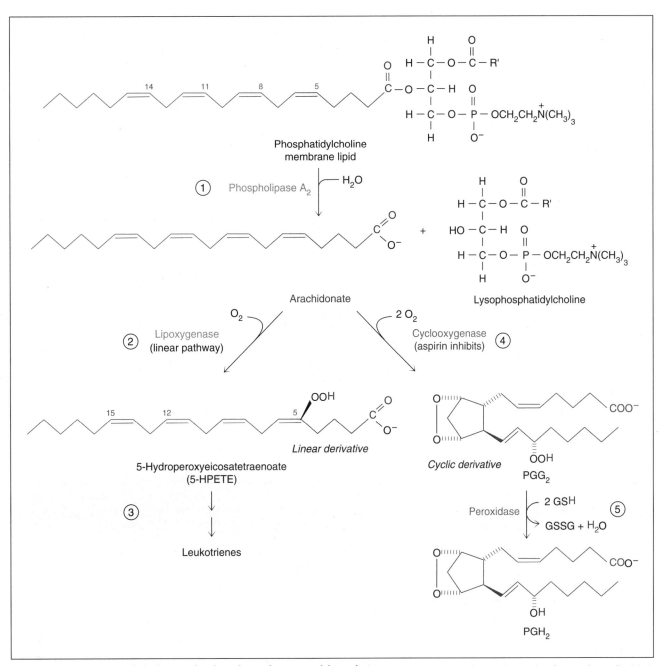

FIGURE 12–33. Overview of the linear and cyclic pathways for eicosanoid biosynthesis. *(1) Phospholipase A_2 catalyzes the first and rate-limiting reaction of the pathways. (2) Lipoxygenase catalyzes the committed step in the linear pathway to form HPETE. (3) 5-HPETE is converted into the linear leukotrienes. Cyclooxygenase catalyzes (4) the formation of the cyclopentane ring and 15-peroxide and (5) the conversion of the 15-peroxide to the 15-alcohol.*

hydrolysis to form a 6-keto compound (6-keto $PGF_{1\alpha}$). Blood platelets (thrombocytes) contain **thromboxane synthase.** This enzyme catalyzes the formation of the six-membered oxane ring of the thromboxanes. The 9,11-epoxide can undergo hydrolysis to form two alcohol groups (Figure 12–35).

The Linear Lipoxygenase Pathway

Lipoxygenases catalyze the insertion of oxygen in the 5, 12, or 15 position of the various eicosanoids. The products are *hydroperoxyeicosatetraen*-

oates, or HPETEs (Figure 12–33). We consider only the insertion of peroxide at C^5. 5-HPETE undergoes a dehydration reaction to form an epoxide named leukotriene A_4 (Figure 12–36). Next, the thiol group of glutathione, a tripeptide, reacts with C^6 to form a thioether (C—S—C) bond. This reaction converts an epoxide to an alcohol in leukotriene C_4. Leukotriene C_4 undergoes hydrolysis to form leukotriene D_4, a dipeptide derivative, and glutamate. Leukotriene D_4 undergoes hydrolysis to form leukotriene E_4 and glycine. The hydrolysis reactions are exergonic and unidirectional. These compounds are converted to more than a dozen metabolites.

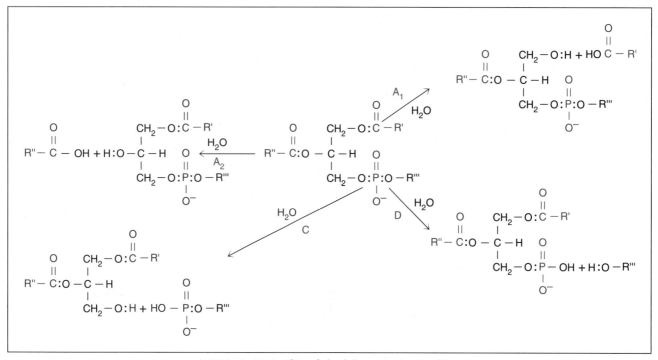

FIGURE 12-34. Specificity of phospholipases A₁, A₂, C, and D.

PLASMALOGENS AND PLATELET ACTIVATING FACTOR

Plasmalogens are phosphoglycerolipids that contain an ether bond at *sn*-1 (Figure 11-5) and phosphoethanolamine or phosphocholine at *sn*-3. These substances occur in the membranes of brain, heart, erythrocytes, and other tissues in variable amounts. Plasmalogens make up about 20% of the phospholipid in human nervous tissue but less than 1% of that in liver. The pathway for biosynthesis begins with the exergonic acylation of dihydroxyacetone phosphate (Figure 12-37). Long-chain fatty acid alcohols are derived from acyl-CoA by reduction by two molecules of NADPH.

$$\text{Acyl-SCoA} + 2\ \text{NADPH} + 2\ \text{H}^+ \rightleftharpoons \quad (12.4)$$

$$\text{Alcohol} + 2\ \text{NADP}^+ + \text{CoASH}$$

The alcohol displaces the acyl group from C^1 to form an ether. After four additional steps (3 through 6, Figure 12-37), the alkyl side chain is oxidized to produce a plasmalogen. The requirements for the desaturation include oxygen, a reductant (NADPH), and cytochrome b_5. The reduction of oxygen to water makes this desaturation reaction exergonic and unidirectional. These requirements are the same as those for the desaturation of acyl-CoA (Figure 11-19).

Platelet activating factor (PAF), an ether-containing phospholipid (Figure 11-5), was named because it causes platelet degranulation. PAF, however, acts on a variety of cells including muscle, liver, kidney, and brain. PAF is also released during inflammation and allergic responses. This lipid mediator is synthesized by a variety of cells including leukocytes, platelets, kidney, and vascular endothelium. PAF is unusual owing to the esterification of *sn*-2 to acetate and not a long-chain acyl group.

Platelet activating factor is derived from 1-alkyl-2-acylglycerol-3-phosphocholine. This substance is formed by a pathway analogous to that of the corresponding phosphoethanolamine derivative illustrated in Figure 12-37. PAF is synthesized on demand and is not stored in cells. The PAF cycle is illustrated in Figure 12-38. Phospholipase A₂ catalyzes the hydrolysis of 1-alkyl-2-acylglycerol-3-phosphocholine to generate lyso-PAF. Lyso-PAF undergoes an acetylation to form PAF. PAF is the active substance that mediates the physiologic responses. PAF is inactivated by hydrolysis forming lyso-PAF. This compound is reconverted to 1-alkyl-2-acylglycerol-3-phosphocholine during an acyltransfer reaction. Following an appropriate stimulus, the cycle is repeated. Each step in the PAF cycle is exergonic.

SUMMARY

Acyl-CoA molecules serve as energy-rich donors for lipid biosynthesis. Phosphatidate, a key intermediate in lipid metabolism, is converted to triglyceride or to phospholipids. CDP-diglyceride is activated diglyceride. CDP-diglyceride reacts with inositol to form phosphatidylinositol. CDP-choline and CDP-ethanolamine are activated intermediates in phosphatidylcholine and phosphatidylethanolamine formation.

Phosphatidylinositol 4,5-bisphosphate is an im-

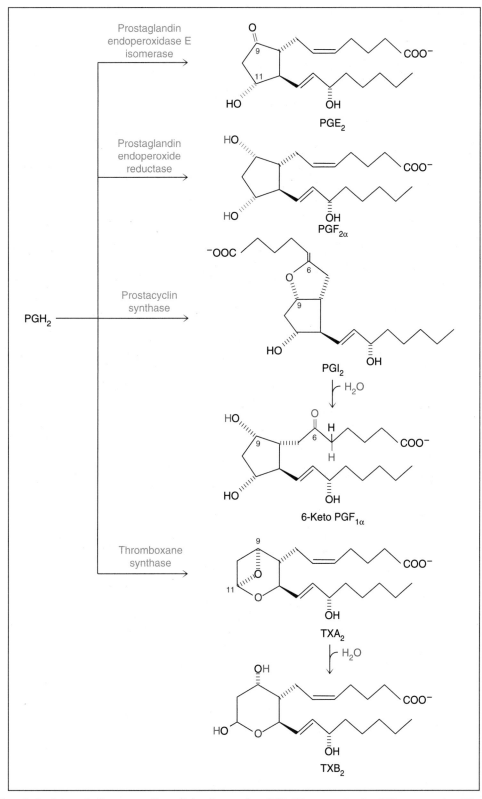

FIGURE 12-35. Biosynthesis of prostaglandins, prostacyclins, and thromboxanes from PGH₂. *PG, prostaglandin; PGI, prostacyclin; TX, thromboxane.*

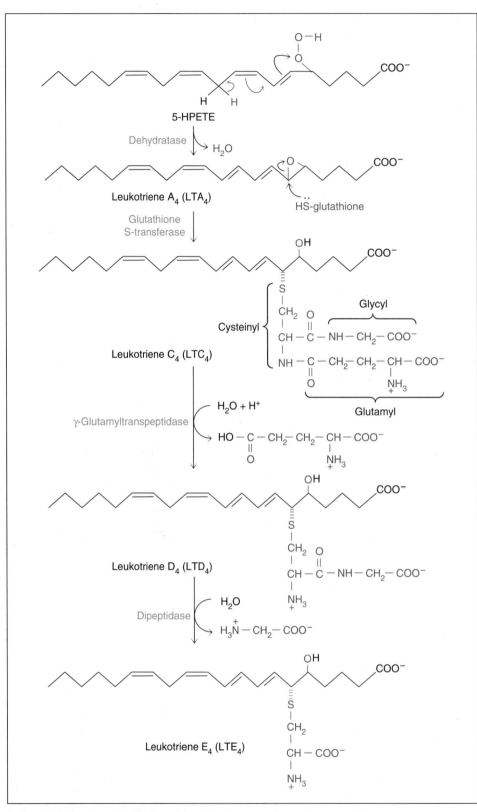

FIGURE 12–36. Leukotriene biosynthesis from 5-HPETE. *The formation of a thioether bond between leukotriene A_4 and glutathione is a distinctive feature of leukotriene metabolism.*

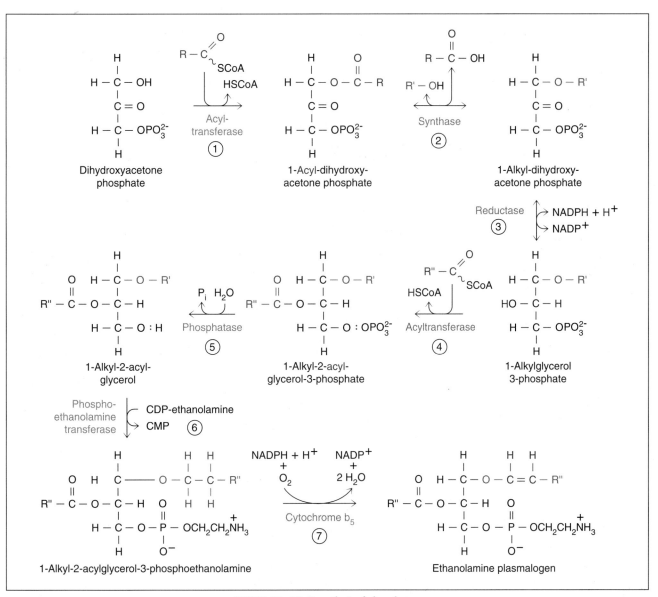

FIGURE 12–37. Biosynthesis of plasmalogen.

portant regulatory molecule. It is converted into two second messengers through the action of phospholipase C; these second messengers are diglyceride and inositol 1,4,5-trisphosphate. Sphingosine is a C_{18} alcohol derived from palmitate and serine. Acyl-CoA serves as a precursor for ceramide (*N*-acylsphingosine). UDP-sugars are activated sugars that are donated to ceramide during the formation of cerebrosides and gangliosides.

All 27 carbon atoms of cholesterol are derived from acetyl-CoA. Hydroxymethylglutaryl-CoA reductase catalyzes the rate-limiting reaction of cholesterol biosynthesis. This enzyme catalyzes the reduction of its substrate to mevalonate in a four-electron transfer reaction. Components of the cholesterol biosynthesis pathway include mevalonate (C_6), isopentenyl pyrophosphate (C_5), dimethylallyl pyrophosphate (C_5), geranyl pyrophosphate (C_{10}), farnesyl pyrophosphate (C_{15}), squalene (C_{30}),

lanosterol (C_{30}), and cholesterol (C_{27}). Reactions involving molecular oxygen required for the conversion of squalene to lanosterol are exergonic and unidirectional.

Cholesterol is absorbed from the intestine and is also synthesized in all nucleated cells. Cholesterol is an important component of plasma membranes. Cholesterol is converted to bile salts, quantitatively the most important pathway of cholesterol metabolism in humans. Chylomicrons transport dietary lipid (triglyceride and cholesterol) from the intestine to the tissues. VLDL transports triglyceride from the liver to extrahepatic cells. LDL ("bad" cholesterol) transports cholesterol from the liver to extrahepatic cells. HDL ("good" cholesterol) transports cholesterol from extrahepatic cells to the liver in a process called reverse cholesterol transport.

Apo-B-100 and apo-E are recognized by the LDL

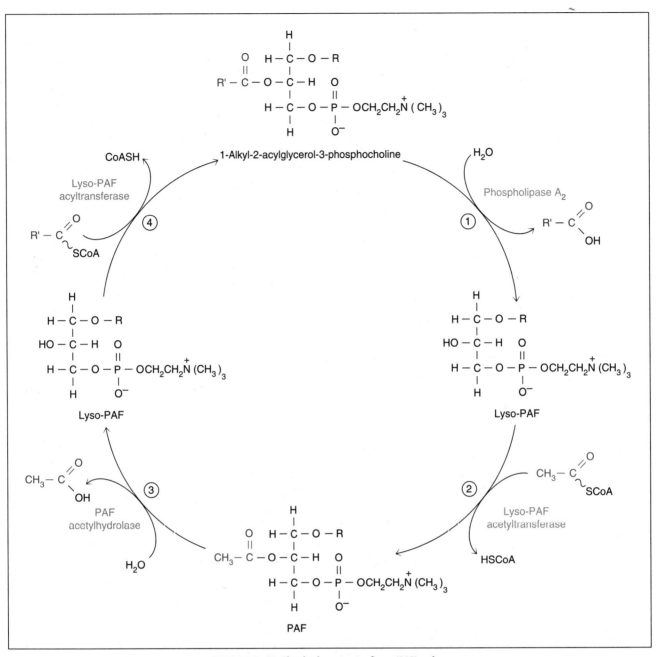

FIGURE 12–38. The platelet activating factor (PAF) cycle.

receptor. The LDL receptor mediates the cellular uptake of LDL and IDL. Familial hypercholesterolemia, a primary hyperlipoproteinemia, is an autosomal dominant disease that is caused by defects in LDL receptor function. Apo-E is recognized by the chylomicron remnant receptor on liver cells. Reverse cholesterol transport requires HDL and LCAT. LCAT is activated by apo-A-I. Lipoprotein lipase (heparin-sensitive lipase) is located in the capillary endothelia throughout the body and is activated by apo-C-II. Lipoprotein lipase operates on chylomicrons and VLDL to generate fatty acids from triglyceride for cellular metabolism.

Cholesterol is converted into steroid hormones by several oxidation reactions involving cyto-chrome P-450. Cholesterol is converted to pregnenolone, the precursor of the five classes of steroid hormone. Steroid hormones include progesterone (C_{21}), aldosterone (C_{21} with an aldehyde group at C^{18}), cortisol (C_{21} with a hydroxyl group at C^{11}), testosterone (C_{19}), and estradiol (C_{18} with an aromatic A ring).

Phospholipase A_2 catalyzes the rate-limiting step in the biosynthesis of the eicosanoids. Cyclooxygenase, which is inhibited by aspirin, catalyzes the biosynthesis of PGH_2. PGH_2 can be converted to PGE_2, $PGF_{2\alpha}$, and prostacyclin (PGI_2). PGH_2 is also converted to thromboxanes. The lipoxygenase pathway is responsible for the synthesis of linear leukotrienes. The fatty acid forms a thioether with the tripeptide glutathione. Glutamate and glycine are removed from the parent leukotrienes sequentially by hydrolysis. Plasmalogens contain an unsaturated alkyl-ether and platelet activating factor contains a saturated alkyl-ether attached to *sn*-1.

SELECTED READINGS

Bansal, V.S., and P.W. Majerus. Phosphatidylinositol-derived precursors and signals. Annual Review of Cell Biology 6:41–76, 1990.

Criqui, M.H., et al. Plasma triglyceride level and mortality from coronary heart disease. New England Journal of Medicine 328:1220–1225, 1993.

Goldstein, J.L., and M.S. Brown. Regulation of the mevalonate pathway. Nature 343:425–430, 1990.

Hunninghake, D.B., et al. The efficacy of intensive dietary therapy alone or combined with lovastatin in outpatients with hypercholesterolemia. New England Journal of Medicine 328:1213–1219, 1993.

Kikkawa, U., A. Kishimoto, and Y. Nishizuka. The protein kinase C family: Heterogeneity and its implications. Annual Review of Biochemistry 58:31–44, 1989.

Orth, D.N., W.J. Kovacs, and C.R. DeBold. The adrenal cortex. *In* J.D. Wilson and D.W. Foster (eds.). *Williams Textbook of Endocrinology,* 8th ed. Philadelphia, W.B. Saunders Company, 1992, pp. 489–619.

Parker, C.W. Lipid mediators produced through the lipoxygenase pathway. Annual Review of Immunology 5:65–84, 1987.

Ross, R. The pathogenesis of atherosclerosis: A perspective for the 1990s. Nature 362:801–809, 1993.

CHAPTER THIRTEEN

AMINO ACID

METABOLISM

A clean experiment is worth more than a few hundred dirty calculations.

—EFRAM RACKER

The principal use of amino acids is to provide the building blocks of proteins. Proteins are the main structural and functional molecules of all living organisms. Because the composition of dietary amino acids does not necessarily match the composition of proteins that are synthesized in human cells, numerous interconversions occur to produce an appropriate balance. The liver is an important organ for amino acid metabolism. Amino acids also participate in the metabolism of a variety of nonprotein compounds.

Amino acids are derived from the breakdown of dietary and body proteins. About 85% of the amino acids resulting from the hydrolysis of endogenous body proteins are reutilized for protein biosynthesis. Oxidation of the carbon skeletons of amino acids accounts for about 12–15% of the metabolic energy of humans. Since there are 20 genetically encoded amino acids, each amino acid provides a small amount of the total metabolic energy of humans.

PROTEIN DIGESTION

Proteases

Proteolytic enzymes can be injurious to cells. It is for this reason that proteolytic digestive enzymes are synthesized and stored as inactive precursors called **zymogens** (the Greek roots mean "to give rise to" enzymes). The conversion of zymogens to enzymes occurs in the digestive tract. That the intestine itself does not undergo autodigestion is astonishing. **Pepsinogen,** produced by the chief cells of the stomach, is the precursor of **pepsin.** Some peptide bonds are unstable in acid, and gastric acid catalyzes the conversion of a few pepsinogen molecules to active **pepsin,** which converts the remaining pepsinogen to pepsin. Pepsin exhibits a pH optimum of about 1.5. This optimum is unusual, but it reflects the physiological requirements for gastric digestion. Pepsin is an endopeptidase and catalyzes the hydrolysis of proteins into large polypeptides. The active site of pepsin contains **aspartate,** which reacts with carbonyl groups of peptide bonds via its carboxylate oxygen.

Trypsin, chymotrypsin, and **elastase** are endopeptidases that catalyze the hydrolysis of internal peptide bonds of proteins. Their substrate specificity is given in Table 4–2. Because their active sites contain serine, these enzymes are called **serine proteases.** Trypsinogen is converted to trypsin, the active enzyme, by the action of a peptidase named

enterokinase or **enteropeptidase.** Trypsin catalyzes the conversion of chymotrypsinogen, procarboxypeptidases A and B, and proelastase to their active enzyme forms. Carboxypeptidase A catalyzes the removal of most of the amino acid residues from the carboxyl end of a protein, one at a time, except for lysine, arginine, and proline. **Carboxypeptidase B** catalyzes the removal of only lysine and arginine.

Intestinal Peptidases

The intestinal mucosa produces di- and tripeptidases that catalyze the hydrolysis of small peptides to free amino acids during the final stages of digestion. The intestine and pancreas produce aminopeptidases. These enzymes are exopeptidases that catalyze the hydrolysis of amino acid residues from the amino terminus. A prominent enzyme in this class is called **leucine aminopeptidase.** It is named because of its preference for leucine as the amino terminal residue. The enzyme, however, has broader specificity than the name implies and will catalyze the hydrolytic removal of other residues. All the peptidases catalyze hydrolysis reactions, and all these reactions are exergonic and unidirectional.

Absorption of Amino Acids and Peptides

Intestinal cells take up free amino acids and some di- and tripeptides by special transport proteins. All of the peptides are hydrolyzed to free amino acids in enterocytes before their release into the hepatic portal vein. Newborn infants are able to take up some proteins without prior digestion. Immunoglobulins of the A type (IgA, Table 16–10) from colostrum of maternal milk are absorbed intact, providing the newborn with passive immunity. The newborn loses the ability to take up intact immunoglobulins about 2 days postpartum.

TRANSAMINATION REACTIONS

Amino acid metabolism consists of pathways for amino groups and for carbon skeletons. Transamination reactions are pivotal for both the degradation and biosynthesis of the majority of the standard amino acids. The structures of the reactants and products of aminotransferase reactions are quite similar, and this accounts for the isoergonic nature of these reactions (Figure 13–1).

FIGURE 13–1. A transamination reaction. The amino group of one amino acid is donated to a keto acid, forming new amino and keto acids.

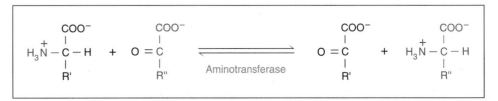

There are several enzymes that catalyze transamination reactions, and **pyridoxal phosphate** (a derivative of vitamin B_6, Figure 2–15) is the cofactor. Transaminases generally demonstrate a preference for one of the pairs of the amino group donor and acceptor and exhibit a varying latitude for the other cognate pair. The involvement of glutamate and α-ketoglutarate as substrates is prevalent and pivotal. The ability of most amino acids to donate their amino groups to α-ketoglutarate to form glutamate is responsible in part for the central role of glutamate in nitrogen metabolism. Glutamate is also a common amino group donor in the formation of many other amino acids. For example, glutamate reacts with oxaloacetate to form aspartate (Figure 4–10), and glutamate reacts with pyruvate to form alanine (Figure 4–11).

Transamination reactions are intricate, and the alanine aminotransferase reaction is representative. The aldehyde of pyridoxal phosphate forms an adduct with the amino group of a specific lysine residue of each aminotransferase with the elimination of water to form a Schiff base, or aldimine (Figure 13–2). The aldimine reacts with the amino group of an amino acid by transaldimination, the first step in the transamination process. The main point is that the aldimine derivative of pyridoxal phosphate and not free pyridoxal phosphate reacts with the amino group to form the intermediate Schiff base. Because α-ketoglutarate leaves the enzyme before the addition of the second substrate, pyruvate in this example, transaminases exhibit ping-pong kinetics (equation 4.12).

Transaminases or aminotransferases occur in all human cells. Aminotransferases also occur in human blood plasma in low but measurable amounts. ▶ An increase in serum transaminases occurs during hepatitis, other liver diseases, and following the tissue necrosis of a myocardial infarction. Clinical chemistry laboratories routinely measure aspartate aminotransferase (AST) and alanine aminotransferase (ALT) as noted in Chapter 4. ◀

AMMONIUM ION PRODUCTION

Oxidation-Reduction Reactions

Glutamate Dehydrogenase Reaction

The chief pathway for generating ammonium ion in humans involves the oxidative deamination of glutamate by $NAD(P)^+$; α-ketoglutarate and $NAD(P)H$ are the other products. Either NAD^+ or $NADP^+$ can serve as the oxidant for this enzyme (Figure 13–3). Although the formation of glutamate is favored under standard conditions, this is a simple oxidation-reduction reaction and is reversible. The direction that the reaction proceeds depends upon the physiological need. Glutamate plays a cardinal role in amino acid metabolism (Figure 13–4).

D- and L-Amino Acid Oxidase Reactions

Two other enzymes besides glutamate dehydrogenase oxidize amino acids to keto acids. They are

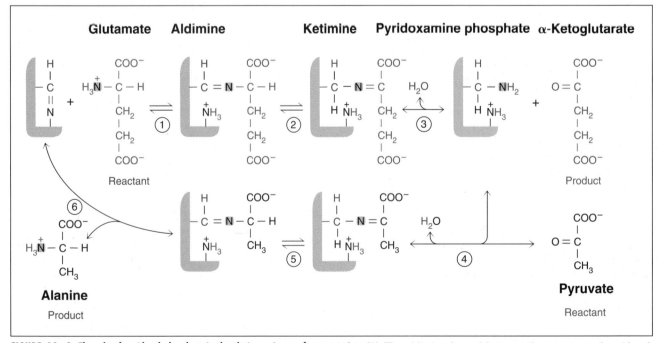

FIGURE 13–2. The role of pyridoxal phosphate in the alanine aminotransferase reaction. *(1) The aldimine formed between the enzyme and pyridoxal phosphate reacts with the amino group of the amino acid to form a new aldimine. (2) The aldimine isomerizes to form a ketimine. (3) Water adds to the ketimine, and the adduct dissociates into a keto acid and pyridoxamine phosphate. (4) The amino group of pyridoxamine phosphate forms an adduct with the acceptor keto acid that is dehydrated to form a ketimine. (5) The ketimine undergoes an isomerization, and (6) the amino acid is released and the original form of the enzyme is regenerated.*

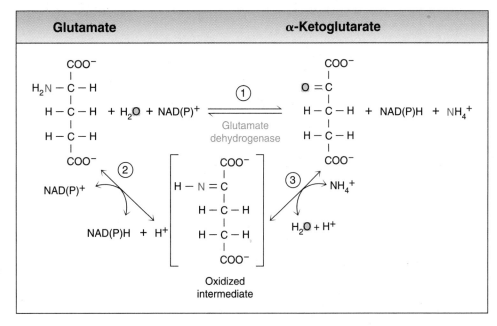

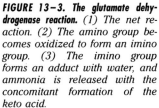

FIGURE 13–3. The glutamate dehydrogenase reaction. *(1) The net reaction. (2) The amino group becomes oxidized to form an imino group. (3) The imino group forms an adduct with water, and ammonia is released with the concomitant formation of the keto acid.*

L-amino acid oxidase (with FMN as cofactor) and D-amino acid oxidase (with FAD as cofactor). These enzymes are quantitatively less important in producing ammonium ion than is glutamate dehydrogenase. These enzymes, which are localized in peroxisomes, generate hydrogen peroxide (Figure 13–5). Hydrogen peroxide is degraded by catalase to molecular oxygen and water. The reduction of oxygen to water makes the process exergonic and irreversible (PRINCIPLE 8 OF BIOENERGETICS). Bacterial cell walls, in contrast to proteins, contain some amino acids with the D-configuration, and D-amino

FIGURE 13–4. The central role of glutamate in amino acid metabolism. *Amino acids directly or indirectly donate their amino groups to α-ketoglutarate to form glutamate. Glutamate can donate its amino group to oxaloacetate to form aspartate, and glutamate can be oxidized to form ammonium ion and α-ketoglutarate. Aspartate and ammonium ion are the nitrogen donors during urea biosynthesis.*

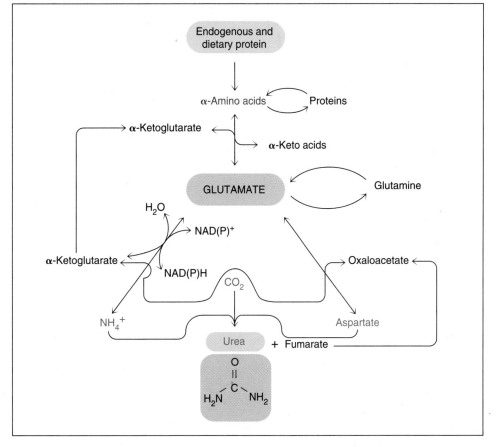

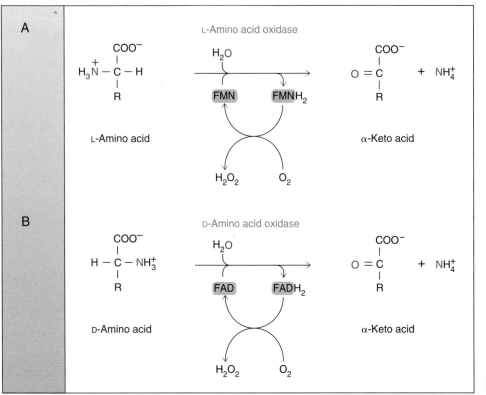

FIGURE 13–5. L- *and* D-*amino acid oxidase reactions.*

acid oxidase may function during the oxidation of D-amino acids produced by bacteria and absorbed from the gut.

Hydrolysis Reactions: Glutaminase and Asparaginase Reactions

Glutaminase catalyzes the hydrolysis of glutamine to yield glutamate and ammonium ion (Figure 13–6). The enzyme is prominent in kidney where it generates most of the ammonium ions that are ex-

creted in the urine. Asparaginase catalyzes the hydrolysis of asparagine to produce aspartate and ammonium ion. Both of these reactions are exergonic (PRINCIPLE 5 OF BIOENERGETICS). The carbon chains of glutamate and aspartate can be converted into Krebs cycle intermediates in one step by transamination.

▶ Some cells lack the ability to form adequate asparagine. This inability is the rationale for treating individuals with some malignancies with *Escherichia coli* or *Erwinia carotovora* asparaginase (Table 21–7). Given parenterally, asparaginase is

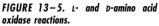

FIGURE 13–6. *Glutaminase (A) and asparaginase (B) reactions.*

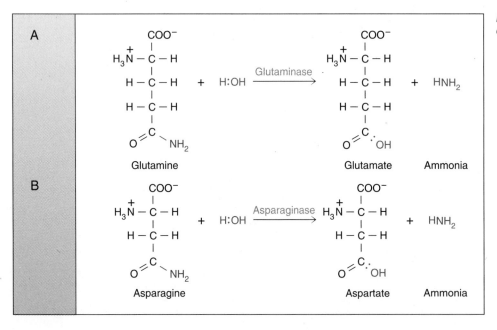

used in the treatment of some acute leukemias that fail to respond to other agents. Asparaginase catalyzes the hydrolysis of circulating asparagine and impairs the ability of sensitive cells to grow and divide owing to insufficient asparagine. The use of this enzyme is limited by its toxicity to normal cells, including those in liver, kidney, and pancreas. ◀

UREA CYCLE

A human consuming 100 g of protein daily excretes about 16.5 g of nitrogen per day. Urea, which is the chief nitrogen metabolite of humans, accounts for 80–90% of excreted nitrogen. Urate and ammonium ions are other end products. Urea biosynthesis occurs in liver cells. The amino groups of amino acids generated in other tissues are transported to the liver chiefly as alanine and glutamine. The urea cycle was elucidated in the 1930s by Hans Krebs and Wolf Henseleit. Krebs was a young physician first embarking on a medical career, and Henseleit was a medical student working on a required research project. The urea cycle was the first metabolic cycle to be described.

Overview of the Urea Cycle

The urea cycle involves the cooperation of the mitochondrion and the cytosol. **Ornithine** is the regenerating substrate in this cyclic pathway. The sequence begins with ornithine, and components are added to the parent molecule to form arginine (Figure 13–7). Arginine is hydrolyzed to produce urea and to regenerate ornithine. The overall stoichiometry of the urea cycle is shown in equation 13.1.

$$NH_3 + HCO_3^- + aspartate + 3\ ATP + H_2O$$
$$\rightarrow Urea + fumarate + 2\ ADP$$
$$+ 2\ P_i + AMP + PP_i \quad (13.1)$$

The carbon and oxygen in urea are derived from carbon dioxide. **Carbon dioxide** combines with water to produce carbonic acid as catalyzed by carbonic anhydrase. One amino group is derived from **ammonium ion,** and the second is derived from **aspartate.** The cycle is exergonic and involves the expenditure of three ATP molecules. The pyrophosphate that is generated in one step is further degraded to two moles of inorganic phosphate, thus a total of four high-energy bonds is required for the synthesis of each urea molecule.

Reactions of the Urea Cycle

The urea cycle requires carbamoyl phosphate as an activated donor. This is formed in the mitochondrion as catalyzed by **carbamoyl-phosphate synthetase I.** The reaction is complex and involves two ATP molecules. In the first step, ATP reacts with bicarbonate to form a carbonyl phosphate intermediate and ADP is released (Figure 13–8). Carbonyl phosphate is energy rich. In the second step, the carbonyl group undergoes a nucleophilic attack by the nitrogen of ammonia to produce carbamate. In the final step, a second ATP donates its γ-phosphoryl group to carbamate to form the energy-rich carbamoyl phosphate and the second molecule of ADP is released.

There are two carbamoyl-phosphate synthetases, designated I and II. Synthetase I occurs in liver mitochondria, is activated allosterically by **N-ace-**

FIGURE 13–7. Overview of the Krebs-Henseleit urea cycle.

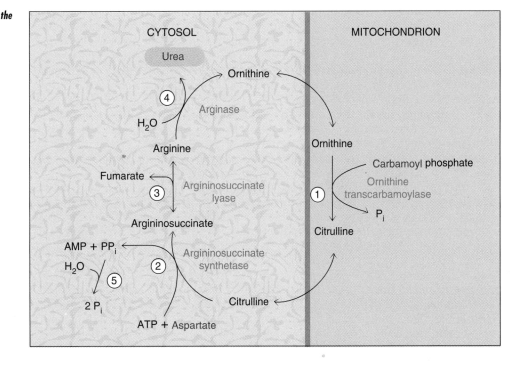

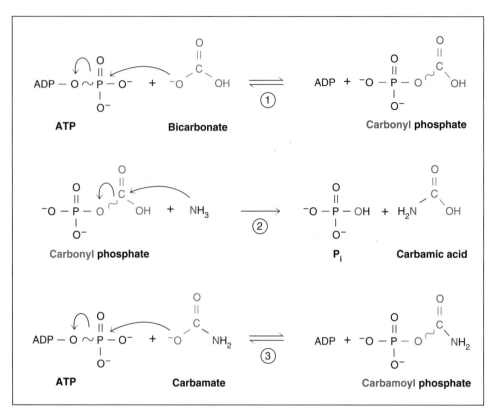

FIGURE 13–8. *Carbamoyl-phosphate synthetase I reaction. Only step 2 is exergonic.*

tylglutamate, and participates in urea biosynthesis. Carbamoyl-phosphate synthetase II occurs in the cytosol of all nucleated cells, is not activated by *N*-acetylglutamate, and participates in pyrimidine biosynthesis. Synthetase II also uses glutamine, and not ammonia, as the nitrogen donor. Carbamoyl-phosphate synthetase II is the main regulatory enzyme in pyrimidine formation as described in Chapter 14.

Ornithine, the regenerating substrate, reacts with carbamoyl phosphate in the mitochondrion in a reaction catalyzed by **ornithine transcarbamoylase.** The products include citrulline and phosphate. The reaction proceeds with the loss of the energy-rich bond of carbamoyl phosphate and is exergonic (Figure 13–9). Citrulline then enters the cytosol; this transport process may involve the exchange of citrulline for ornithine.

The next step of the cycle involves the ATP-dependent combination of aspartate and citrulline. The provision of the second nitrogen in urea involves a complex two-step process. First, citrulline reacts with aspartate in an ATP-dependent operation and produces argininosuccinate (Figure 13–9). The reaction, catalyzed by **argininosuccinate synthetase,** is exergonic and involves the dissipation of one high-energy bond. The hydrolysis of pyrophosphate by a separate pyrophosphatase results in the loss of a second high-energy bond. Second, argininosuccinate undergoes a reaction, catalyzed by **argininosuccinate lyase,** to produce arginine and fumarate. The lyase reaction is functionally isoergonic. Note that this is not a hydrolysis but a lyase reaction (Table 4–1).

The final step of the pathway consists of the hydrolysis of arginine to form urea and ornithine. **Arginase** catalyzes the exergonic hydrolysis of arginine to produce urea, the product of the pathway, and ornithine, the regenerating substrate. Ornithine enters the mitochondrion, and the process is repeated. This metabolic cycle is catalytic in the sense that small amounts of urea cycle intermediates (catalytic amounts) will sustain the synthesis of large amounts (stoichiometric amounts) of urea. Fumarate, the four-carbon compound that is produced by the argininosuccinate lyase reaction, can serve as a source for oxaloacetate and aspartate as illustrated in Figure 13–10.

Carbamoyl-phosphate synthetase I, which is activated by N-*acetylglutamate, is the main regulatory enzyme of the urea cycle* (Table 25–3). *N*-Acetylglutamate synthase is activated by arginine. The activity of the pathway is also governed by the availability of substrates.

Human Disorders of the Urea Cycle

▶ Renal disease is often associated with an elevation of the **blood urea nitrogen** (BUN). Urea is relatively nontoxic. An elevated BUN suggests renal disease, and the morbidity of renal disease is due to acid-base and electrolyte imbalance. An elevated blood ammonia concentration occurs in severe liver disease. One postulated mechanism of ammonia toxicity is related to the depletion of mitochondrial Krebs cycle intermediates as α-ketoglutarate is converted to glutamate as catalyzed by glutamate dehydrogenase. Krebs cycle function and aer-

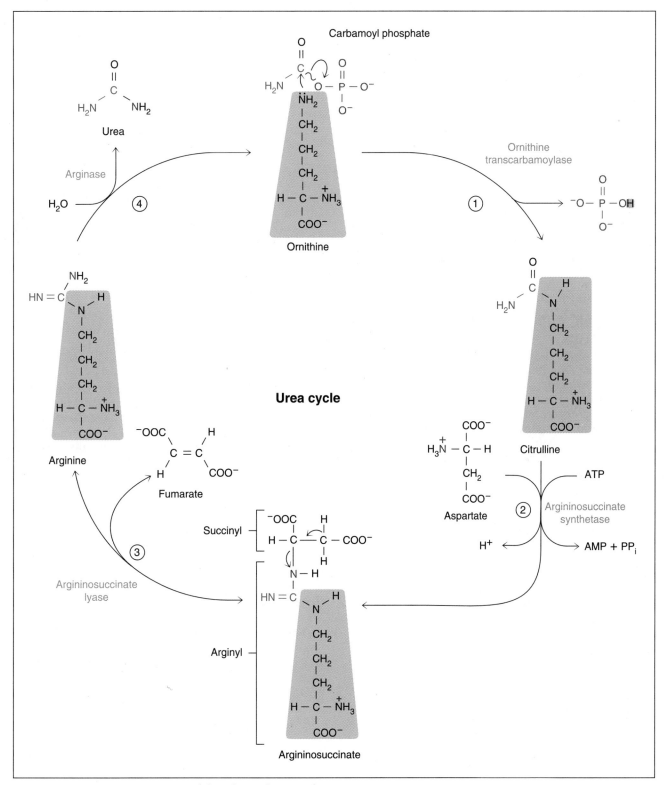

FIGURE 13–9. Reactions of the Krebs-Henseleit urea cycle. *Reactions 1, 2, and 4 are exergonic and unidirectional.*

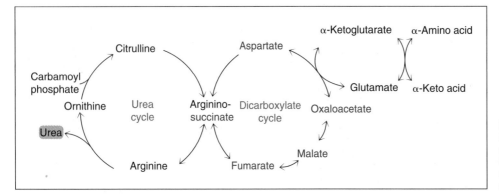

FIGURE 13–10. Interactions between the urea cycle and the dicarboxylate cycle. *The urea cycle involves both the mitochondrion and the cytosol. The dicarboxylate cycle occurs in the cytosol.*

obic metabolism are especially important in brain, and ammonia toxicity leads to hepatic encephalopathy with confusion, stupor, or even coma and death (Chapter 8).

Diseases have been described that are due to a deficiency of each enzyme of the urea cycle (Tables 13–1 and 16–5). In general, they are severe maladies associated with mental retardation, seizures, coma, and early death. ◄

GLYCOGENIC AND KETOGENIC AMINO ACIDS

There are three categories of amino acid catabolism. Amino acids are designated as **glycogenic** if they can be converted to glucose, **ketogenic** if they can be converted to ketone bodies, and **both glycogenic and ketogenic** if they can be converted to both types of compound. This classification was derived from experiments performed by administering each amino acid to dogs with experimental diabetes mellitus and determining whether there was an increase in glucose in the urine (glycogenic amino acid), an increase in ketone bodies in the urine (ketogenic amino acid), or both. Glycogenic amino acids are catabolized to pyruvate or intermediates of the Krebs cycle (Figure 10–1). Ketogenic amino acids are catabolized to acetyl-CoA, acetoacetyl-CoA, or both, while bypassing pyruvate or Krebs cycle intermediates.

The metabolic classification of amino acids is given in Table 13–2. Note that **leucine** is the sole amino acid that is ketogenic only. The aromatic amino acids plus lysine, and isoleucine (five amino acids) are both glycogenic and ketogenic, and the remainder—a majority—are glycogenic only. There are a few discrepancies in this outline of metabolism and the pathways describing amino acid metabolism that follow, and there are at least two possible explanations for any discrepancy. First, the classification of amino acid metabolism is based upon the reactions that occur under nonphysiological conditions in animals with diabetes. This experimental paradigm may bias the results. Second, the pathways described may be incomplete, and alternative routes of metabolism may exist.

ESSENTIAL AMINO ACIDS AND NITROGEN BALANCE

There are 20 genetically encoded (standard) amino acids (Table 3–1). If one is present in inad-

TABLE 13–1. Selected Disorders of Amino Acid and Urea Cycle Metabolism

Name	Enzyme Deficiency	Metabolism Affected
Amino acid metabolism		
Albinism	Tyrosinase	Tyrosine
Alkaptonuria	Homogentisate dioxygenase	Phenylalanine, tyrosine
Cystathioninuria	Cystathionine lyase	Cysteine, methionine, serine
Histidinemia	Histidine ammonia lyase	Histidine
Homocystinuria	Cystathionine synthase	Cysteine, methionine, serine
Maple syrup urine disease	Branched-chain keto acid dehydrogenase	Valine, isoleucine, leucine
Phenylketonuria (PKU)	Phenylalanine hydroxylase	Phenylalanine
Urea cycle		
Argininemia	Arginase	Urea cycle
Argininosuccinaturia	Argininosuccinate lyase	Urea cycle
Citrullinemia	Argininosuccinate synthetase	Urea cycle
Hyperammonemia I	Ornithine transcarbamoylase	Urea cycle
Hyperammonemia II	Carbamoyl-phosphate synthetase I	Urea cycle

TABLE 13–2. Metabolic Classification of Amino Acids

Glycogenic	Both Glycogenic and Ketogenic	Ketogenic
Glycine	Isoleucine	Leucine
Alanine, serine, cysteine	Phenylalanine, tyrosine	
Aspartate, asparagine	Tryptophan, lysine	
Glutamate, glutamine		
Proline, histidine, arginine		
Methionine		
Threonine		
Valine		

equate amounts, protein synthesis is correspondingly diminished. **Nonessential amino acids** can be produced from endogenous metabolites. **Essential amino acids** cannot be derived from endogenous metabolites in required amounts, if at all, and must be obtained from the diet. A relative deficiency of an essential amino acid impairs protein synthesis and leads to a **negative nitrogen balance** (nitrogen excretion exceeds nitrogen intake). In healthy adults, **nitrogen balance** exists (intake equals excretion). In growing children or pregnant women in whom nitrogen intake exceeds excretion, **positive nitrogen balance** occurs. Negative nitrogen balance occurs in a variety of nonphysiological conditions including infections, burns, and postsurgical stress. Negative nitrogen balance is related in part to increased glucocorticoid secretion from the adrenal cortex.

Experiments with normal adult volunteers (biochemistry graduate students) indicated that 8 of the 20 amino acids are essential and must be provided in the diet. A mnemonic for the essential amino acids is the acronym PVT TIM *H*A*LL* ("Private Tim Hall"). This corresponds to phenylalanine, valine, threonine, tryptophan, isoleucine, methionine, histidine, arginine, leucine, and lysine. If one remembers that tyrosine is nonessential, since it is derived from phenylalanine (essential), then the mnemonic is less ambiguous. *H*A is italicized to signify that these two additional amino acids are required by infants and children.

AMINO ACID METABOLISM BASED ON FAMILIES

The oxidative metabolism of amino acids ranges from simple to complicated. Generally, the metabolism of the nonessential amino acids is simple, and that of the essential amino acids is complicated. The metabolism of tryptophan, an amino acid that accounts for about 2% by mass of all amino acids found in proteins, involves more than 20 reactions. Tryptophan's metabolism is thus more involved than glycolysis or the Krebs citrate cycle. In contrast to glycolysis, however, tryptophan metabolism does not represent a mainstream pathway, and it is unnecessary to learn the reactions of tryptophan metabolism to the degree that the reactions of glycolysis are mastered. The metabolic fate of the 20 amino acids is illustrated in Figure 13–11, and the various families are listed in Table 13–3.

C₂ and C₃ Families of Amino Acids

Alanine, Serine, Glycine, and Cysteine

Alanine undergoes a transamination reaction with α-ketoglutarate to form pyruvate and glutamate (Figure 4–11). Transamination reactions are isoergonic and bidirectional. The oxidation of pyruvate via acetyl-CoA and the Krebs cycle is a

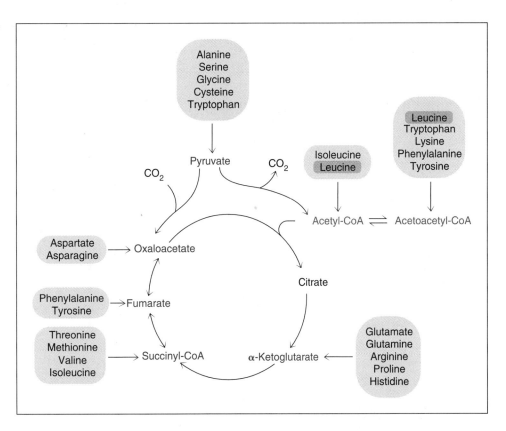

FIGURE 13–11. Overview of amino acid metabolism.

TABLE 13–3.   Amino Acid Families

Family	Amino Acids
C_2	Glycine
C_3	Alanine, serine, and cysteine
Nonessential C_4	Aspartate and asparagine
C_5	Glutamate, glutamine, arginine, proline, and histidine
Essential C_4	Threonine and methionine
Branched-chain	Valine, isoleucine, and leucine
Aromatic	Phenylalanine and tyrosine
Ketoadipate	Tryptophan and lysine

mainstream process described in Chapter 8. Pyruvate serves as a substrate for gluconeogenesis, in agreement with its metabolic classification (Table 13–2).

Serine undergoes a dehydration followed by a hydrolysis as catalyzed by serine dehydratase, a pyridoxal phosphate–requiring enzyme, to produce pyruvate (Figure 13–12). The serine dehydratase reaction is the chief enzyme responsible for the metabolism of serine. Serine can also undergo a transamination reaction to produce 3-hydroxypyruvate; this is followed by an NADH-dependent reduction to D-glycerate. These two reversible reactions are followed by an exergonic phosphorylation by ATP, catalyzed by glycerate kinase, to produce 3-phosphoglycerate. Both pathways produce a gluconeogenic intermediate that can also be metabolized by mainstream reactions.

Glycine metabolism is intimately linked to tetrahydrofolate. The structure of folate is given in Figure 2–16. We consider the biochemistry of this cofactor later in this chapter. Glycine reacts with methylenetetrahydrofolate to produce serine (Figure 13–13). Conversion of glycine to serine accounts for the glycogenic nature of glycine owing to the conversion of serine to pyruvate or phosphoglycerate (Figure 13–12).

Cysteine catabolism is intricate because of the multiple pathways that the compound can enter during the metabolism of sulfur. The amino acids cysteine and cystine are quantitatively the most important dietary sources of sulfur; although methionine contains sulfur and is essential, the methionine content of proteins is sparse. An NADH-dependent reductase interconverts cystine (the oxidized form) and two molecules of cysteine (the reduced form). Cystine is the main form found in the circulation. The sulfur of methionine is converted to that of cysteine during catabolism. The chief excretory product of sulfur is sulfate.

Cysteine reacts with oxygen to yield cysteine sulfinate (Figure 13–14). The reaction with oxygen is exergonic (PRINCIPLE 8 OF BIOENERGETICS). Cysteine sulfinate undergoes an isoergonic transamination to yield β-sulfinylpyruvate. The latter undergoes an exergonic hydrolysis to yield pyruvate and sulfite. Sulfite is oxidized to produce sulfate in a reaction catalyzed by sulfite oxidase. Oxidation of reduced cytochrome c by the electron transport chain pulls the sulfite oxidase reaction forward. Cysteine sulfinate can be converted to **taurine** in two steps (Figure 13–14). This is a quantitatively minor pathway. Taurine combines with cholyl-CoA to produce taurocholate, a bile salt (Figure 12–22). The conversion of cysteine to pyruvate accounts for the glycogenic nature of this amino acid.

Cystinuria

▶ Cystinuria is a rare autosomal recessive disease that is caused by the impairment of basic

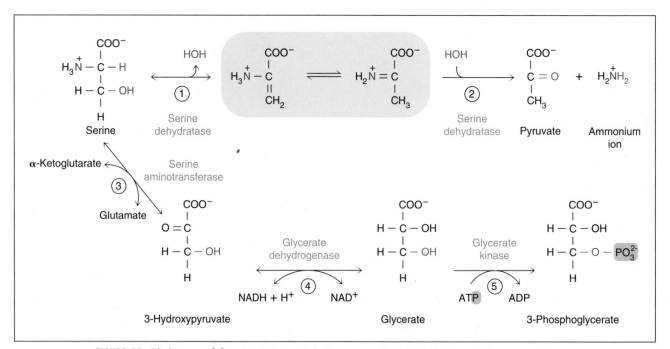

FIGURE 13–12. Serine metabolism. *(1, 2) Serine dehydratase reaction. (3, 4, 5) Phosphoglycerate pathway.*

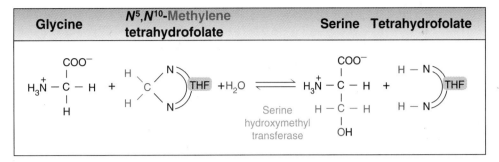

FIGURE 13–13. Interconversion of glycine and serine. *Tetrahydrofolate (THF) is required for the interconversion.*

amino acid transport in the small intestine and kidneys. Cystine, which consists of two cysteine residues linked by a disulfide bond (Figure 3–5), contains two amino groups that permit recognition and transport by this translocase. The diagnosis is made by finding elevated levels of the basic amino acids in the urine. The disorder would not be serious except for the urolithiasis (kidney stones) formed from cystine, a compound of limited solubility. Treatment is aimed at preventing urinary stone formation by maximizing fluid intake and by decreasing cystine intake. ◄

Nonessential C_4 Family of Amino Acids: Aspartate and Asparagine

Asparagine degradation involves the exergonic hydrolysis at the amide nitrogen to produce aspartate and ammonia (Figure 13–6). Aspartate undergoes an isoergonic transamination reaction to yield oxaloacetate and glutamate (Figure 4–10). As a Krebs cycle intermediate, oxaloacetate can serve as a precursor for glucose, and this explains the glycogenic nature of this amino acid (Table 13–2). The oxidative catabolism of oxaloacetate requires

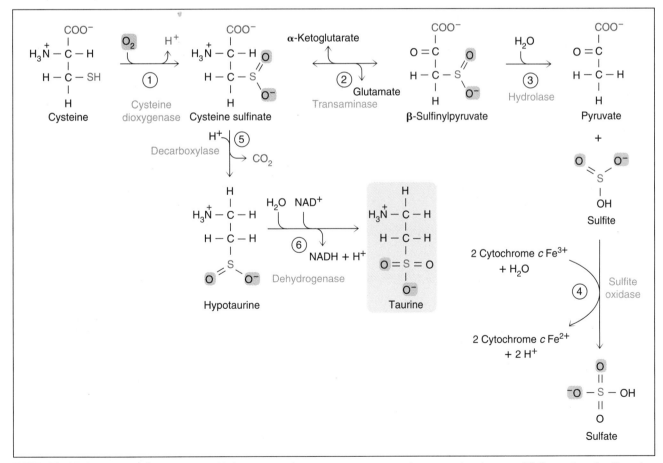

FIGURE 13–14. Cysteine metabolism. *(1, 2, and 3) Conversion of cysteine to pyruvate, a gluconeogenic substance. (4) Formation of sulfate, the chief excretory product of sulfur metabolism. (5, 6) Taurine biosynthesis. The dioxygenase (1), hydrolase (3), and decarboxylase (5) reactions are exergonic.*

the conversion of oxaloacetate to pyruvate followed by its oxidation to acetyl-CoA (Figure 11–13).

C₅ Family of Amino Acids

Glutamate and Glutamine

Glutamate can be oxidized to produce α-ketoglutarate and ammonia (Figure 13–3). α-Ketoglutarate can be converted to malate and oxaloacetate by the Krebs cycle. These compounds account for the glycogenic nature of glutamate. These compounds can also be converted to pyruvate and acetyl-CoA before complete oxidation by the Krebs cycle. Glutamate can also react with an acceptor keto acid such as oxaloacetate by transamination to form α-ketoglutarate and aspartate (Figure 4–10). This is an isoergonic and reversible reaction.

Glutamine degradation begins with the exergonic hydrolysis at the amide group to produce glutamate and ammonia (Figure 13–6). Glutamine can

also transfer its amido group to acceptor compounds, and some of these reactions are considered in Chapter 14 on nucleotide metabolism and in Figure 18–9 on amino-sugar metabolism. Glutamine functions as nitrogen donor for asparagine synthesis.

Arginine and Proline

Arginine undergoes an exergonic hydrolysis reaction as catalyzed by arginase to form ornithine and urea. Ornithine is a five-carbon amino acid that undergoes an isoergonic transamination reaction with α-ketoglutarate to form glutamate semialdehyde and glutamate (Figure 13–15). Glutamate semialdehyde is oxidized to the carboxylate state to produce glutamate. This pathway of metabolism accounts for the glycogenic nature of arginine. The conversion of an aldehyde to a carboxylate is exergonic and irreversible because the carboxylate is stabilized by resonance. To convert a carboxylate to an aldehyde requires the modification of the

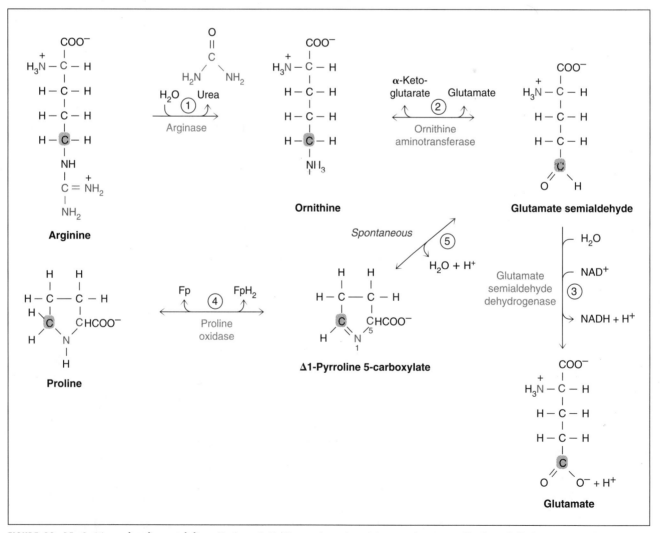

FIGURE 13–15. Arginine and proline metabolism. *(1, 2, and 3) Conversion of arginine to glutamate. (4, 5, and 3) Conversion of proline to glutamate. Fp, flavoprotein.*

carboxyl group as noted in the description of proline biosynthesis later in this chapter.

Proline catabolism begins with a flavoprotein-dependent oxidation to form Δ1-pyrroline 5-carboxylate (Figure 13–15). Water adds to the derivative, and the ring opens nonenzymatically to form glutamate semialdehyde. The semialdehyde undergoes an NAD⁺-dependent oxidation involving water to form glutamate.

Histidine

Histidine contains six carbon atoms. One atom is transferred to the one-carbon pool of tetrahydrofolate derivatives, and the other five are converted to glutamate, a glycogenic amino acid. The first step in histidine catabolism involves a lyase reaction with the elimination of ammonia and the formation of **urocanate** (originally isolated in canine urine) as illustrated in Figure 13–16. Urocanate undergoes a hydration and isomerization to form imidazolone propionate. The hydroxyl group adds to a carbon in the imidazole ring, and this process is followed by a tautomerization to yield the product. The imidazolone ring next undergoes an exergonic hydrolysis reaction to form **N-formiminoglutamate.** N-Formiminoglutamate donates the N-formimino group to tetrahydrofolate. The products of the reaction include glutamate and **N^5-formiminotetrahydrofolate.**

Essential C₄ Family of Amino Acids

Threonine and Methionine

Threonine catabolism is similar to that of serine. Serine undergoes a dehydration reaction followed by the elimination of ammonium ion to produce pyruvate (Figure 13–12). Threonine undergoes an analogous reaction catalyzed by the same enzyme: **serine/threonine dehydratase.** The product of the threonine reaction is α-ketobutyrate (Figure 13–17). **α-Ketobutyrate dehydrogenase** catalyzes a CoA-dependent oxidative decarboxylation to form propionyl-CoA. This reaction is analogous to the pyruvate dehydrogenase reaction (Chapter 8) and is exergonic and physiologically irreversible. Propionyl-CoA is converted to succinyl-CoA via methylmalonyl-CoA in a vitamin B_{12}–dependent process (Figure 11–12). Propionyl-CoA and succinyl-CoA are glycogenic, and this pathway accounts for the glycogenic nature of threonine.

Methionine plays a major role in one-carbon metabolism. Methionine also contains sulfur and serves as a source of the sulfur in cysteine. Methionine is an essential amino acid in humans, but cysteine is not. Methionine is converted to homocysteine, cystathionine, and finally α-ketobutyrate. The first step in methionine metabolism is the formation of S-adenosylmethionine (Figure 6–10). S-Adenosylhomocysteine is cleaved to form homocysteine and adenosine (Figure 13–18). Homo-

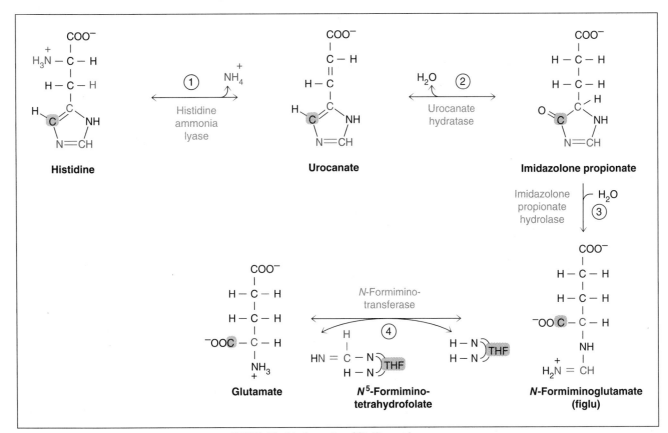

FIGURE 13–16. Conversion of histidine to glutamate.

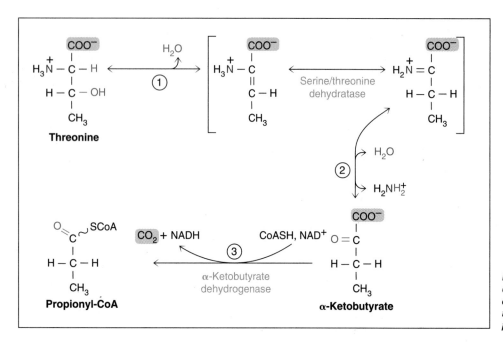

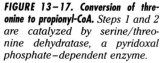

FIGURE 13–17. Conversion of threonine to propionyl-CoA. Steps 1 and 2 are catalyzed by serine/threonine dehydratase, a pyridoxal phosphate–dependent enzyme.

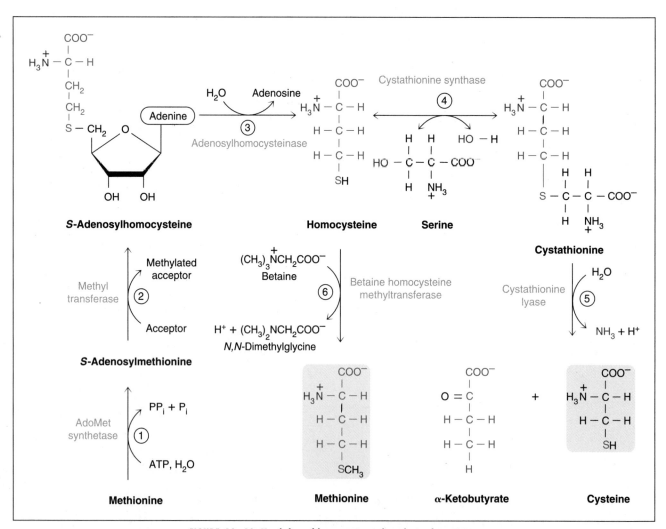

FIGURE 13–18. Metabolism of homocysteine and synthesis of cysteine.

cysteine combines with serine to form cystathionine and water as catalyzed by **cystathionine synthase,** a pyridoxal phosphate–dependent enzyme. The forward reaction is favored. **Cystathionine lyase,** also a pyridoxal phosphate enzyme, catalyzes the conversion of substrate to produce α-ketobutyrate, cysteine, and ammonia. The reaction is unidirectional. α-Ketobutyrate can be converted to propionyl-CoA (Figure 13–17). The conversion of methionine to propionyl-CoA accounts for the glycogenic nature of methionine (Table 13–2).

There are two reactions that can convert homocysteine to methionine. The first involves transfer of a methyl group to homocysteine from betaine (pronounced "beta een," *N,N,N*-trimethylglycine), a metabolite derived from choline. The second involves a reaction of homocysteine with methyltetrahydrofolate, as described later. Methionine is an essential amino acid because humans cannot synthesize homocysteine from metabolites other than methionine. The reconversion of homocysteine to methionine is a salvage pathway.

Homocystinuria and Cystathioninuria

▶ Cystathionine synthase deficiency is a rare autosomal recessive disease that produces homocystinuria (Table 13–1). Affected individuals are treated with low-methionine, cystine-supplemented diets. Some individuals with cystathionine synthase deficiency respond to pyridoxine treatment. Cystathionine lyase deficiency leads to cystathioninuria. This is an autosomal recessive disorder that is less common than homocystinuria. The clinical course is benign; pyridoxine treatment often leads to a reduction in the quantity of cystathionine in the urine. ◀

Branched-Chain Amino Acids

The metabolism of the final seven amino acids not considered thus far is intricate. An overview is given in Figure 13–19. Carbon atoms from lysine and most of tryptophan are converted to α-ketoadipate, which is metabolized to acetoacetyl-CoA, making these two amino acids ketogenic. Part of tryptophan is converted to alanine, a precursor of pyruvate, so that tryptophan is also glycogenic. Studies in whole animals indicate that lysine is also glycogenic, but the pathway used for this conversion is obscure. Tryptophan can also be converted to NAD^+, a vitamin-derivative, and this is a noteworthy property.

Valine, Leucine, and Isoleucine

Valine metabolism begins with an isoergonic transamination reaction (Figure 13–20). The product, α-ketoisovaleric acid, undergoes an oxidative decarboxylation reaction catalyzed by **branched-chain α-keto acid dehydrogenase** to form isobutyryl-CoA. This reaction is analogous to the pyruvate dehydrogenase, α-ketoglutarate dehydrogenase, and α-ketobutyrate dehydrogenase reactions. Similar to the pyruvate dehydrogenase reaction (Chapter 8), five cofactors and three protein activities participate in these exergonic and physiologically irreversible reactions. Branched-chain α-keto acid dehydrogenase is a substrate for its special kinase (branched-chain α-keto acid dehydrogenase kinase) and following phosphorylation, dehydrogenase activity is diminished (Table 25–2).

We recognize the familiar motif (β-oxidation, Krebs cycle) of oxidizing a hydrocarbon chain such as isobutyryl-CoA by an FAD-dependent process and adding water to form an alcohol. Isobutyryl

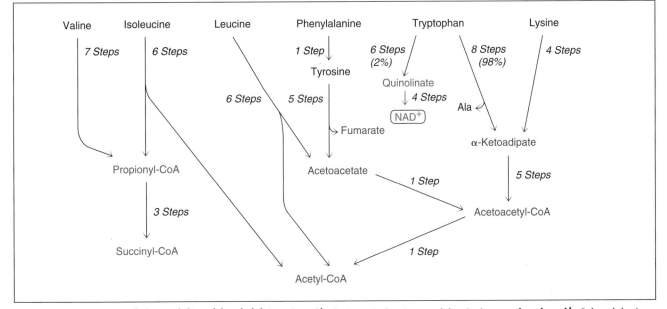

FIGURE 13–19. Overview of the metabolism of branched-chain amino acids (*valine, isoleucine, and leucine*), **aromatic amino acids** (*phenylalanine, tyrosine, and tryptophan*), **and lysine.**

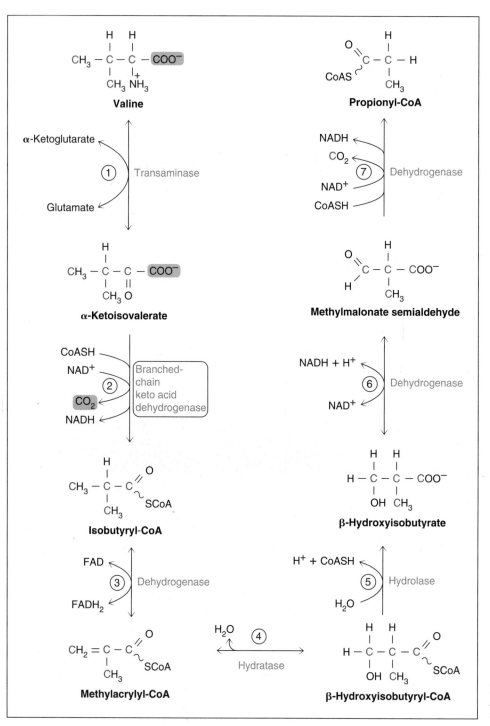

FIGURE 13–20. Valine catabolism. Reactions 2, 3, 4, and 6 resemble reactions of the Krebs cycle.

CoA undergoes an oxidation by FAD to form methylacrylyl-CoA. This is an isoergonic reaction, but it is pulled forward as $FADH_2$ is oxidized by the electron transport chain. Methylacrylyl-CoA is hydrated during an isoergonic lyase reaction. The product, β-hydroxyisobutyryl-CoA, undergoes an exergonic hydrolysis to form CoASH and β-hydroxyisobutyrate. This compound is oxidized, in a reversible, simple oxidation-reduction reaction, to produce methylmalonate semialdehyde. The semialdehyde undergoes an exergonic oxidative decarboxylation to form propionyl-CoA. Propionyl-CoA is

converted to succinyl-CoA as illustrated in Figure 11–12. Succinyl-CoA can be converted to glucose, thus accounting for the glycogenic nature of valine (Table 13–2).

Isoleucine undergoes first an isoergonic transamination. The product, α-keto-β-methylvalerate, undergoes an exergonic oxidative decarboxylation catalyzed by the branched-chain keto acid dehydrogenase (Figure 13–21). The product, α-methylbutyryl-CoA, is oxidized by an adaption of the fatty acid oxidation spiral. α-Methylbutyryl-CoA undergoes an FAD-dependent dehydrogenation of the

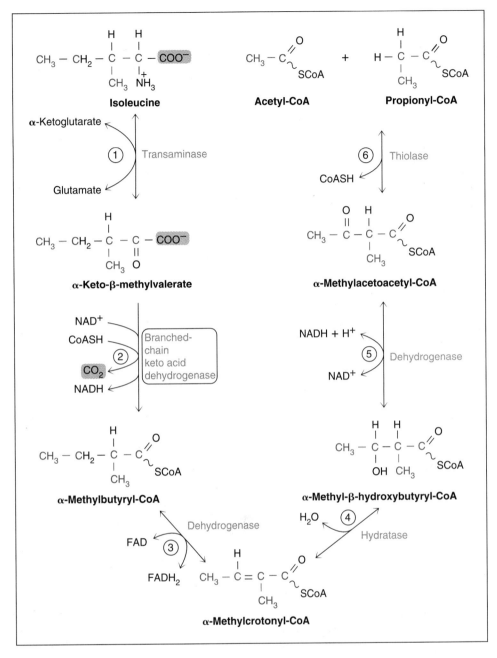

FIGURE 13–21. Isoleucine catabolism.
Reactions 3 through 6 resemble reactions of fatty acid oxidation.

alkyl side chain to form α-methylcrotonyl-CoA. This unsaturated substance is hydrated to form an alcohol, and the alcohol is oxidized by NAD$^+$ to form a ketone. α-Methylacetoacetyl-CoA undergoes an exergonic thiolytic cleavage by CoASH to form acetyl-CoA and propionyl-CoA. Acetyl-CoA is ketogenic and propionyl-CoA is glycogenic, and this accounts for isoleucine's metabolic classification (Table 13–2).

Leucine is entirely ketogenic, and this is a noteworthy property. Leucine, similar to valine and isoleucine, first undergoes an isoergonic transamination. The first three steps of leucine metabolism parallel those for isoleucine (Figure 13–22). In the fourth step, β-methylcrotonyl-CoA undergoes an ATP- and biotin-dependent carboxylation reaction

to form β-methylglutaconyl-CoA. The unsaturated compound is hydrated to form HMG-CoA. HMG-CoA undergoes a lyase reaction to form acetyl-CoA and acetoacetate. Leucine is entirely ketogenic, and the pathway outlined here accounts for its metabolic classification (Table 13–2).

Maple Syrup Urine Disease

▶ This inborn error of metabolism is due to the deficiency of the branched-chain keto acid dehydrogenase that participates in the metabolism of valine, isoleucine, and leucine. The odor of the urine resembles that of maple syrup, accounting for the name. Sweat and other body fluids also have a maple syrup odor. Symptoms begin during

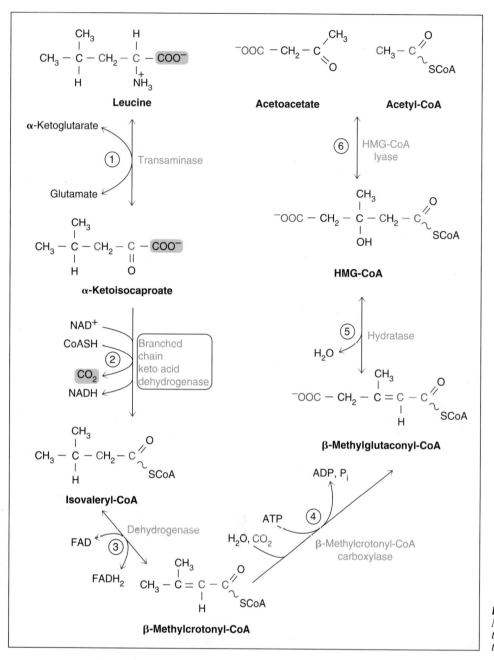

FIGURE 13–22. Leucine metabolism. Note the decarboxylation reaction in step 2 and the carboxylation reaction in step 4.

the first week of life. Common features include vomiting, acidosis, dehydration, ketosis. The odor of the urine and sweat often suggests the diagnosis. Treatment includes synthetic diets that lack the branched-chain amino acids; because these amino acids are essential, small amounts are added to the diet. Mental and neurological deficits are common. The prognosis is guarded (this is a euphemism indicating that early death usually occurs). Classical maple syrup urine disease is inherited as an autosomal recessive trait. The branched-chain keto acid dehydrogenase consists of three proteins including $E_{1\alpha}$ and $E_{1\beta}$ subunits, E_2, and E_3. Individuals with the disease can have $E_{1\alpha}$, $E_{1\beta}$, or E_2 deficiencies. The disease fortunately is rare with an incidence of 1 in 200,000 live births

and the defective gene resides on chromosome 19 (Table 16–5). Despite its rarity, it is a famous disease because of the insights into amino acid metabolism that it has provided. Mild forms (nonclassical) of maple syrup urine disease respond to high doses of thiamine. ◀

Aromatic Amino Acids

Phenylalanine and Tyrosine

Phenylalanine metabolism is initiated by its oxidation to tyrosine. Phenylalanine is an essential amino acid, but tyrosine is not. Tyrosine in the diet, however, decreases the requirement for phenylalanine, a phenomenon called **sparing. Phenylalanine hydroxylase,** located in liver, catalyzes a reaction between phenylalanine, oxygen, and tetrahydrobiopterin to form tyrosine, water, and the quinonoid form of dihydrobiopterin (Figure 13–23). The enzyme is a mixed-function oxygenase (one atom of oxygen is transferred to the substrate, and the second atom is reduced to water). The reduction of oxygen to water and the oxidation of an organic compound makes this reaction exergonic and unidirectional (PRINCIPLE 8 OF BIOENERGETICS). Tyrosine cannot be retroconverted to phenylalanine, thereby accounting for the essential nature of phenylalanine. The quinonoid form of dihydrobiopterin is converted to tetrahydrobiopterin following a reduction by NADH or NADPH as catalyzed by dihydropteridine reductase. Because the cellular [NADPH]/[NADP⁺] ratio is greater than the [NADH]/[NAD⁺] ratio, NADPH is probably the physiologically important reductant.

Tyrosine undergoes an isoergonic transamination as the first step in its catabolism (Figure 13–24). The next reaction is an irreversible dioxygenase reaction in which both atoms of oxygen are incorporated into the substrate, forming **homogentisate** (Figure 13–24). **Ascorbate** plays a role in keeping the ferrous iron of the dioxygenase in the reduced state. Paired hydroxyls on the phenyl group render it susceptible to ring opening by an oxygenation reaction. **Homogentisate dioxygenase** catalyzes the reaction of the two atoms of oxygen with adjacent ring carbon atoms to yield a ketone and the carbonyl of a carboxylate. 4-Maleylacetoacetate undergoes an isoergonic isomerization to form 4-fumarylacetoacetate. Maleate is the *cis* isomer of the four-carbon dicarboxylate, and fumarate is the

trans isomer (Figure 2–7). The fumarate derivative undergoes an exergonic hydrolysis to form fumarate (glycogenic) and acetoacetate (ketogenic), accounting for the glycogenic and ketogenic nature of these amino acids.

Disorders of Aromatic Amino Acid Metabolism

▶ **Phenylketonuria** (PKU), in its most common form, is caused by a deficiency of phenylalanine hydroxylase (Table 13–1). PKU is autosomal recessive with an incidence of 1 in 10,000 to 20,000 live births; it is the most common inborn error of amino acid metabolism. Prenatal diagnosis and carrier detection are possible. The phenylalanine hydroxylase gene is located on chromosome 12q (Table 16–5). Untreated infants with phenylketonuria exhibit neurological symptoms including hyperactive deep tendon reflexes, hyperactivity, and mental retardation. Infants are normal at birth. The Guthrie bacterial inhibition assay is widely used in the newborn period to screen for phenylketonuria; blood samples are obtained by heel prick. False positives can result from this screening test, and more accurate methods are required to establish the diagnosis. Amino acid analysis of blood reveals elevated phenylalanine (> 1.2 mM) and normal tyrosine. Phenylalanine is converted to phenylpyruvate by a transamination reaction that is inconsequential in unaffected individuals. Phenylpyruvate is excreted in the urine and accounts for the name "phenylketonuria." Phenylketonuria is treated with a synthetic diet that lacks phenylalanine.

Variant forms of phenylketonuria account for 2% of cases of hyperphenylalaninemia. These are due to deficiencies in **dihydropteridine reductase** (Fig-

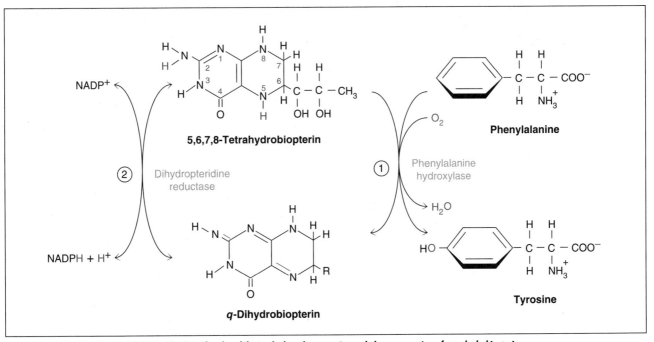

FIGURE 13–23. The phenylalanine hydroxylase reaction and the regeneration of tetrahydrobiopterin.

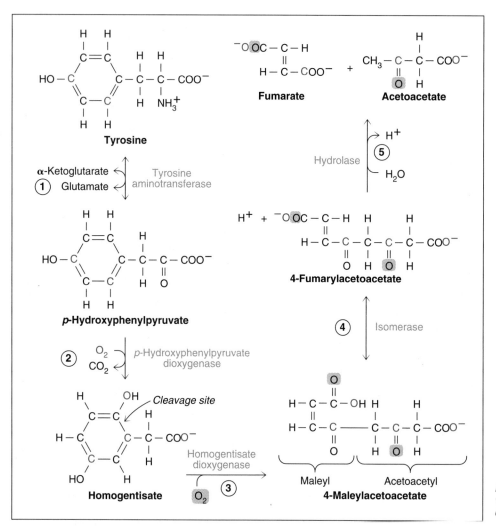

FIGURE 13–24. Pathway for the conversion of tyrosine to fumarate and acetoacetate.

ure 13–23) or one of the enzymes that catalyzes tetrahydrobiopterin synthesis from GTP. These variant disorders are treated with oral tetrahydrobiopterin.

Alkaptonuria is a rare, hereditary disease caused by a deficiency of **homogentisate dioxygenase.** Homogentisate, produced during the metabolism of phenylalanine and tyrosine, cannot be further metabolized. Homogentisate is excreted in the urine. The urine gradually turns dark as the acid is oxidized by dissolved oxygen to produce dark-colored compounds. Oxidation occurs more rapidly at alkaline pH. Washing diapers containing absorbed homogentisate in soap (an alkali) makes the stains more intense instead of removing them. Individuals with alkaptonuria develop pigmentation of the connective tissue called **ochronosis.** The name is based on the ochre color that histologic specimens exhibit. Individuals with long-standing alkaptonuria develop arthritis.

The triad of alkaptonuria includes dark urine, ochronosis, and arthritis. The clinical course of alkaptonuria is much less severe than that of phenylketonuria, and treatment is directed at minimizing the arthritic symptoms. The disease was studied by Archibald Garrod, who coined the expression "inborn error of metabolism" that is in common use today, and was important for the development of this concept. ◀

Ketoadipate Family of Amino Acids

Tryptophan

The metabolism of tryptophan is formidable. Tryptophan is converted to alanine (glycogenic) and glutaryl-CoA (ketogenic). A small fraction ($\approx 2\%$) of tryptophan is converted to nicotinate, a vitamin. That niacin deficiency symptoms occur in humans indicates that the nicotinate formed from tryptophan is not adequate to fulfill metabolic requirements. The amount of tryptophan that is metabolized daily is small, and the caloric energy derived from tryptophan metabolism is trivial, amounting to less than two calories (2 kcal) per day for 500 mg of this substance. This paragraph summarizes the essence of tryptophan metabolism, and some readers may want to skip the remainder of this section.

**CONVERSION OF TRYPTOPHAN TO AMINOCAR-
BOXYMUCONATE SEMIALDEHYDE (ACS).** Tryptophan
is converted to 3-hydroxyanthranilate, α-ketoadipate, and acetyl-CoA; alanine is also produced. The
first step in the pathway is a dioxygenase reaction
involving the addition of both atoms of molecular
oxygen to tryptophan to form N-formylkynurenine
(Figure 13–25). The reaction of oxygen with organic compounds is exergonic and physiologically
irreversible (PRINCIPLE 8 OF BIOENERGETICS). Formate
is released by an exergonic hydrolysis reaction.
Next the aromatic ring is hydroxylated during a
unidirectional monooxygenase reaction. Hydrolytic
cleavage of the side chain at the ketone group then
yields alanine (glycogenic) and 3-hydroxyanthrani-
late, which undergoes a ring-opening dioxygenase
reaction to form ACS.
   CONVERSION OF ACS TO ACETYL-COA. ACS
occurs at a crossroad of tryptophan metabolism.
Most (98%) is converted to α-ketoadipate; the remaining 2% is converted to NAD^+, a vitamin derivative. In the predominant pathway, ACS undergoes
an exergonic decarboxylation reaction that eliminates the 3-carboxylate. The resulting semialdehyde undergoes a dehydrogenase reaction involving water to form the second carboxylate in
2-aminomuconate (Figure 13–25). This compound
undergoes an NAD(P)H-dependent reduction of the
4-cis double bond and hydrolytic deamination to
form α-ketoadipate. α-Ketoadipate is the six-carbon
straight chain dicarboxylate whose metabolism is
described later with that of lysine. The formation
of alanine accounts for the glycogenic metabolism
of tryptophan, and the formation of acetoacetyl-
CoA from adipate accounts for the ketogenic nature of tryptophan (Table 13–2).
   CONVERSION OF ACS TO NAD^+. ACS undergoes
spontaneous ring closure to form quinolinate (Figure 13–25). Quinolinate undergoes a reaction with
PRPP to form quinolinate ribonucleotide (Figure
13–26). PRPP contains two high-energy bonds, and
the products contain only the energy-rich bond of
pyrophosphate. The next reaction, a decarboxylation, is also exergonic. ATP donates its adenylyl
group to nicotinate ribonucleotide to form desam-
ido-NAD^+ (a type III reaction of ATP, Figure 6–6).
The transferase reaction that produces desamido-
NAD^+ is functionally isoergonic; however, the hydrolysis of pyrophosphate pulls the reaction forward. Glutamine donates its amido group to
desamido-NAD^+, producing NAD^+ in a reaction energized by ATP.
   NAD^+ reacts with ATP in a reaction catalyzed by
NAD^+ kinase to form $NADP^+$ and ADP. A low-energy phosphate ester on the 2′ carbon atom forms
(Figure 2–13); the reaction, which occurs with the
loss of a high-energy bond, is exergonic. Nicotinate
(one form of the vitamin niacin) is converted to
nicotinate ribonucleotide following a reaction with
PRPP as illustrated in Figure 13–26. The phosphoribosyltransferase that operates on quinolinate and
nicotinate and the decarboxylase that operates on

quinolinate mononucleotide occur in the same protein. Moreover, this protein participates in pyrimidine nucleotide biosynthesis and is responsible for
the phosphoribosylation of orotate and the decarboxylation of orotidine monophosphate to uridine
monophosphate (Figure 14–4).

Hartnup Disease

▶ This rare autosomal recessive disease is
caused by the impairment of neutral amino acid
transport in the small intestine and kidneys. The
disorder is not clinically severe, which suggests
that the activity of the transport protein is defective but not absent. Diagnosis is based on finding
hyperaminoaciduria involving the large neutral
amino acids (valine, isoleucine, leucine, tyrosine,
phenylalanine, and tryptophan). There is also reduced intestinal absorption of these amino acids.
The decreased ability to absorb tryptophan in
Hartnup disease often leads to the "three D's" of
pellagra (Chapter 2): dermatitis, diarrhea, and dementia. Mild mental retardation may be present.
The dermatitis and other pellagra-like symptoms
generally respond to niacin (nicotinate), and this is
the prescribed treatment for Hartnup disease.
However, hyperaminoaciduria and intestinal transport are not corrected by this regimen. ◀

Lysine

Lysine catabolism, similar to that of tryptophan,
is intricate. These two amino acids form α-ketoadipate (Figure 13–19). Moreover, the biochemical
pathway for the catabolism of lysine does not
agree with animal studies. The pathway described
in this section indicates that lysine is ketogenic
only, and this is how lysine is classified in several
textbooks. Lysine is both glycogenic and ketogenic,
however, as assessed in experimental animals. This
discrepancy indicates that we lack complete information on the metabolism of this essential amino
acid.
   Lysine forms **saccharopine,** an adduct of lysine
and α-ketoglutarate. Saccharopine is converted to
α-ketoadipate and glutamate. α-Ketoadipate is metabolized to acetoacetyl-CoA. (The reader may
wish to skip the following paragraphs describing
lysine catabolism.)
   The ε-amino group of lysine bonds to the α-car-
bonyl group of α-ketoglutarate; water is eliminated,
and the double bond between the carbon and nitrogen is reduced to form saccharopine (Figure
13–27). **Saccharopine** is oxidized in a process that
produces glutamate and α-aminoadipate semialdehyde. After a transamination reaction, α-ketoadipate semialdehyde is oxidized by NAD^+, with water
as the oxygen donor, to form α-ketoadipate.
   Five reactions are required to yield acetoacetyl-
CoA. **α-Ketoadipate** (C_6) undergoes a unidirectional
NAD^+- and CoA-dependent oxidative decarboxylation reaction to form glutaryl-CoA (C_5); the process

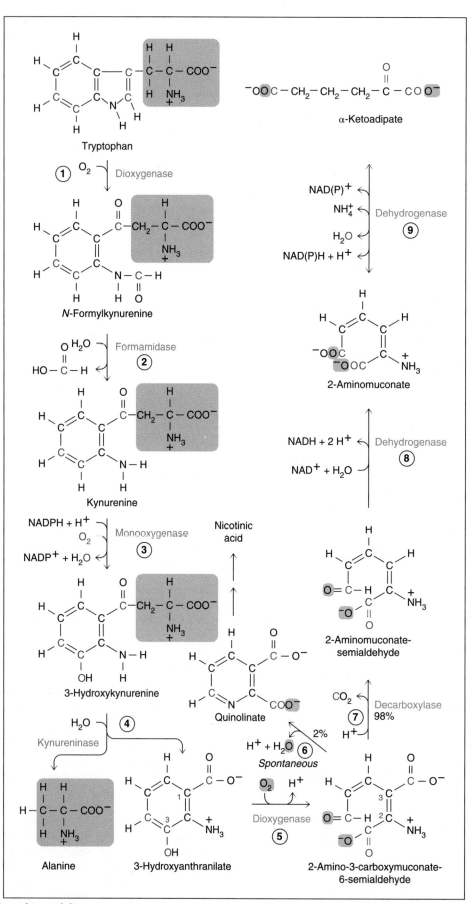

FIGURE 13–25. Tryptophan metabolism. *Most of the reactions of this pathway are unidirectional, and these are indicated by one-way arrows.*

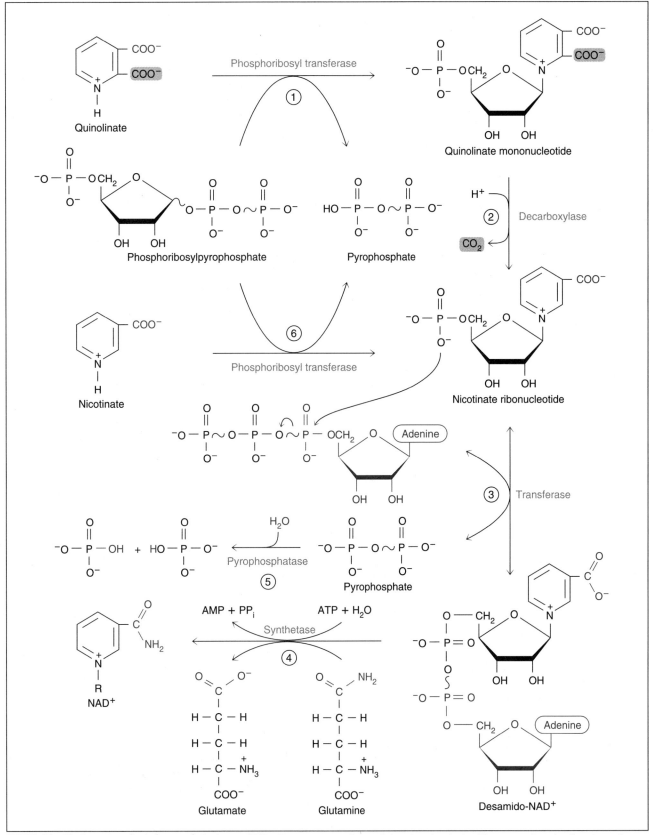

FIGURE 13–26. Conversion of quinolinate and nicotinate to NAD⁺. *Nicotinate is a form of the vitamin niacin. The same phosphoribosyltransferase catalyzes reactions 1 and 5.*

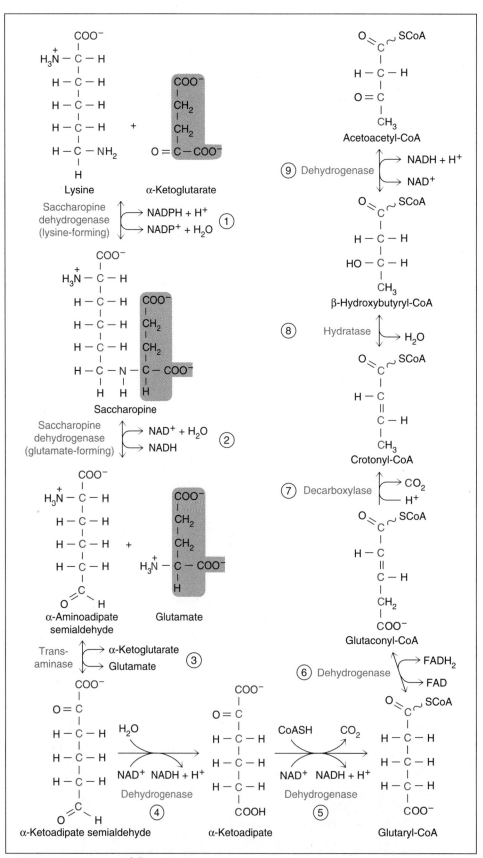

FIGURE 13–27. Lysine metabolism. *Reactions 5, 6, 8, and 9 are similar to reactions of the Krebs cycle.*

is analogous to the pyruvate dehydrogenase reaction (Chapter 8). The alkyl group is dehydrogenated in an FAD-dependent process to form a *trans* double bond in glutaconyl-CoA. Glutaconyl-CoA undergoes an exergonic decarboxylation to form crotonyl-CoA (C_4). Crotonyl-CoA is converted to acetoacetyl-CoA, a ketone body precursor, by two familiar reactions.

BIOSYNTHESIS OF THE NONESSENTIAL AMINO ACIDS

The carbon skeletons for the nonessential amino acids can be derived from glycolytic and Krebs cycle intermediates (Figure 13–28). Alanine and serine can be derived from glycolytic intermediates, and glycine can be obtained from serine. The carbon atoms of cysteine can be derived from serine via cystathionine as previously noted (Figure 13–18). The carbon atoms of aspartate and asparagine can be derived from oxaloacetate, and the carbon atoms of glutamate, glutamine, and proline can be derived from α-ketoglutarate. Tyrosine (nonessential) can be derived from phenylalanine (essential) as illustrated in Figure 13–23.

Biosynthesis of the C_2 and C_3 Families of Amino Acids

Alanine is formed by the transamination of pyruvate (Figure 4–11). **Serine** can be formed from 3-phosphoglycerate. An NAD^+-dependent dehydrogenase catalyzes the oxidation of the alcohol of 3-phosphoglycerate to the ketone of 3-phosphopyruvate (Figure 13–29). This is a simple oxidation-reduction reaction, similar to the lactate dehydrogenase reaction, and is bidirectional. 3-Phosphopyruvate undergoes an isoergonic transamination reaction with glutamate to form *O*-phosphoserine. A phosphatase catalyses the exergonic and unidirectional hydrolysis of *O*-phosphoserine to form serine and phosphate. **Glycine** is formed from serine in one step (Figure 13–13). **Cysteine** is formed during the catabolism of methionine (Figure 13–18).

Biosynthesis of the C_4 Family of Amino Acids

Aspartate can be derived from oxaloacetate from the Krebs cycle, and the amino group can be derived from glutamate as catalyzed by aspartate aminotransferase (Figure 4–10). **Asparagine** is derived from aspartate and the amide group of glutamine. The transamidation reaction requires ATP, and it is noteworthy that ATP undergoes the pyrophosphate split to form AMP and PP_i (Equation 13.2).

ATP + aspartate + glutamine + H_2O
$$\rightarrow \text{asparagine} + \text{AMP} + \text{PP}_i + \text{glutamate} \quad (13.2)$$

A suggested mechanism for the reaction is illustrated in Figure 13–30. The hydrolysis of pyrophosphate to phosphate is exergonic, and the overall process costs two high-energy bonds. The transfer of the amide group from glutamine to aspartate is nominally isoergonic owing to the sim-

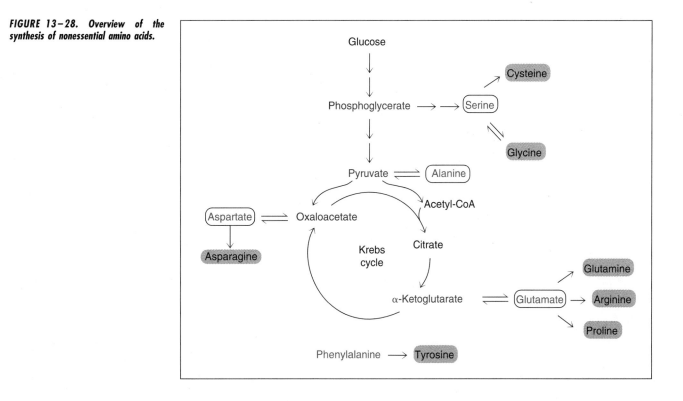

FIGURE 13–28. Overview of the synthesis of nonessential amino acids.

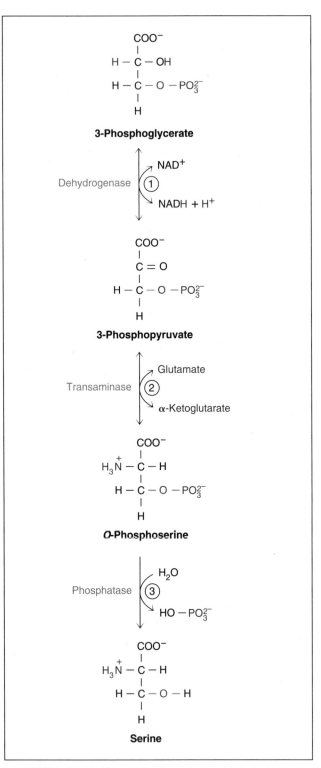

FIGURE 13–29. *Biosynthesis of serine from 3-phosphoglycerate.*

ilarity of the structures of the reactants and products. That the reaction uses two high-energy bonds makes the process exergonic and unidirectional.

Biosynthesis of the C_5 Family of Amino Acids

Glutamate can be formed by the reductive amination of α-ketoglutarate, a Krebs cycle interme-

diate, as catalyzed by glutamate dehydrogenase (Figure 13–3). This is a reversible oxidation-reduction reaction. This reaction is one of the two chief mechanisms for incorporating ammonium ion into amino acids; the second reaction involves the conversion of glutamate to glutamine. Glutamate can also be formed by the transamination of α-ketoglutarate (Figures 4–10 and 4–11).

Glutamine is derived from glutamate. The amide group is derived from ammonium ion. Glutamine synthetase catalyzes the ATP-dependent conversion of reactants to glutamine as illustrated in equation 13.3 and Figure 13–31.

$$\text{ATP} + \text{glutamate} + \text{ammonia} \rightarrow$$
$$\text{glutamine} + \text{ADP} + \text{P}_\text{i} \quad (13.3)$$

It is noteworthy that this reaction proceeds with an orthophosphate split (and not the pyrophosphate split that occurs during asparagine synthesis). The reaction proceeds through an energy-rich γ-glutamylphosphate intermediate.

Proline (C_5) can be derived from glutamate (C_5) via glutamate semialdehyde (Figure 13–32). The conversion of glutamate to the semialdehyde is intricate. Free carboxylate groups are difficult to reduce. The carboxylate must first be derivatized as the phosphate anhydride, and then reduction may proceed. Glutamate is converted first to the energy-rich γ-glutamylphosphate intermediate; the intermediate is reduced by NADPH to produce glutamate semialdehyde, phosphate, and NADP⁺. The nitrogen of the amino group adds to the carbonyl group of the semialdehyde to form a stable five-membered ring. This undergoes a dehydration to yield Δ1-pyrroline 5-carboxylate. The double bond in Δ1-pyrroline 5-carboxylate is reduced by NADPH, and proline results.

TETRAHYDROFOLATE METABOLISM

Interconversion of Tetrahydrofolate Derivatives

Tetrahydrofolate (THF) is made of tetrahydropterin, *p*-aminobenzoate, and glutamate (Figure 13–33). The glutamyl group can be covalently attached to up to five additional glutamyl residues. One-carbon groups are attached to N^5, N^{10}, or both nitrogen atoms (Figure 13–34). The group transfer potentials of the one-carbon compounds is not precisely known, but they approach the 30 kJ/mol that is characteristic of energy-rich bonds (Tables 6–1 and 6–3).

Serine is the major source of one-carbon groups, and these are derived in a reaction catalyzed by **serine hydroxymethyltransferase.** This and other aspects of one-carbon metabolism are illustrated in Figure 13–34. N^5-Formyl-THF is not physiologically important in humans. However, the compound is used as a drug called **leucovorin,** and the ATP-dependent transformation is required for leucovorin's action. N^5-Formimino-THF, formed during **histidine** catabolism (Figure 13–16), undergoes a deam-

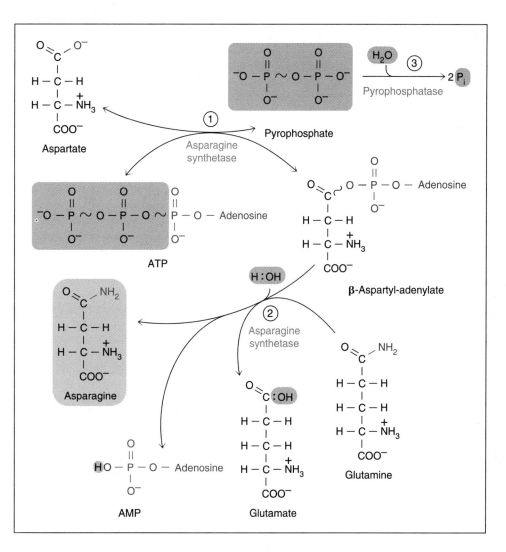

FIGURE 13–30. The asparagine synthetase reaction. AMP and pyrophosphate are formed.

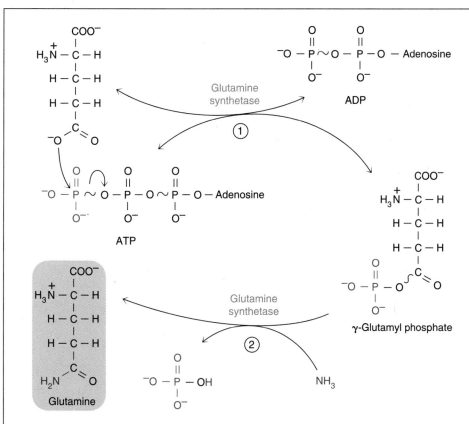

FIGURE 13–31. The glutamine synthetase reaction. ADP and P_i are formed.

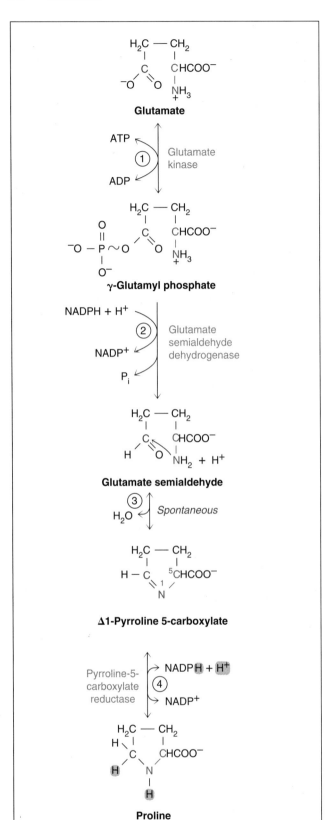

FIGURE 13–32. Synthesis of proline from glutamate.

ination reaction to produce N^5, N^{10}-methenyl-THF. ► Before the availability of methods to determine serum folate concentrations, the figlu test was used to assess folate deficiency. Following an oral dose of histidine, individuals with folate deficiency excrete increased amounts of N-formimino-glutamate (figlu) in the urine. The quantity of figlu in the urine of normal individuals after a histidine load is nil. ◄

Methylene-THF can be reduced by NADH to yield N^5-methyl-THF and NAD$^+$ (Figure 13–34). N^5-Methyl-THF can transfer its methyl group to **homocysteine** in a vitamin B$_{12}$–dependent unidirectional reaction catalyzed by **methyl-THF homocysteine methyltransferase** to form **methionine** (Figure 13–35).

Folate and B$_{12}$ Interaction: The Methyl Trap Hypothesis of Pernicious Anemia

► Because of the B$_{12}$ requirement for the homocysteine methyltransferase reaction, methyl-THF accumulates in individuals with B$_{12}$ deficiency. The methyltransferase reaction is the only significant crossroad in human metabolism involving both folate and vitamin B$_{12}$. Moreover, this is the only reaction in humans that requires methyl-THF as methyl donor. Methyl-THF cannot be retroconverted to methylene-THF because the reductase reaction is unidirectional; this represents an unusual situation for a "simple" oxidation-reduction reaction. As a result of the inability to metabolize methyl-THF, methyl-THF accumulates and tetrahydrofolate cannot be made available for other reactions.

The conversion of tetrahydrofolate to methyl-THF and the inability to metabolize methyl-THF is the "methyl trap" hypothesis that explains some of the metabolic derangements of pernicious anemia and B$_{12}$ deficiency. The anemia caused by B$_{12}$ deficiency responds to the continued administration of folate. Folate treatment, however, will not prevent or alleviate the irreversible neurological symptoms that occur in pernicious anemia. The methyl trap hypothesis, however, may represent only a partial explanation for the pathophysiology of pernicious anemia. Vitamin B$_{12}$, for example, may play a role in folate absorption, but this remains to be established. Table 13–4 lists the metabolic roles of fo-

TABLE 13–4.   Reactions of Tetrahydrofolate Derivatives

Coenzyme	Reaction
N^5-Formimino-THF	Glutamate $\rightleftharpoons$ N-formiminoglutamate
N^{10}-Formyl-THF	5-Aminoimidazole-4-carboxamide ribotide (AICAR) $\rightarrow$ 5-formamidoimidazole-4-carboxamide ribotide (FAICAR)
N^{10}-Formyl-THF	Glycinamide ribotide $\rightarrow$ formylglycinamide ribotide
N^{10}-Formyl-THF	Met-tRNA $\rightarrow$ N-formyl-Met-tRNA
N^5Methyl-THF	Homocysteine $\rightarrow$ methionine
N^5,N^{10}-Methylene-THF	Glycine $\rightleftharpoons$ serine
N^5,N^{10}-Methylene-THF	Deoxyuridylate $\rightarrow$ deoxythymidylate

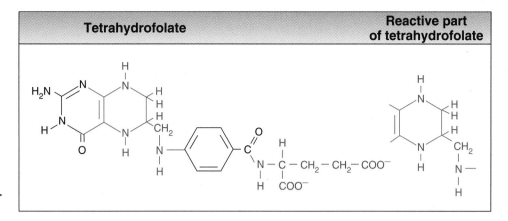

FIGURE 13–33. Structure of tetrahydrofolate and its reactive portion.

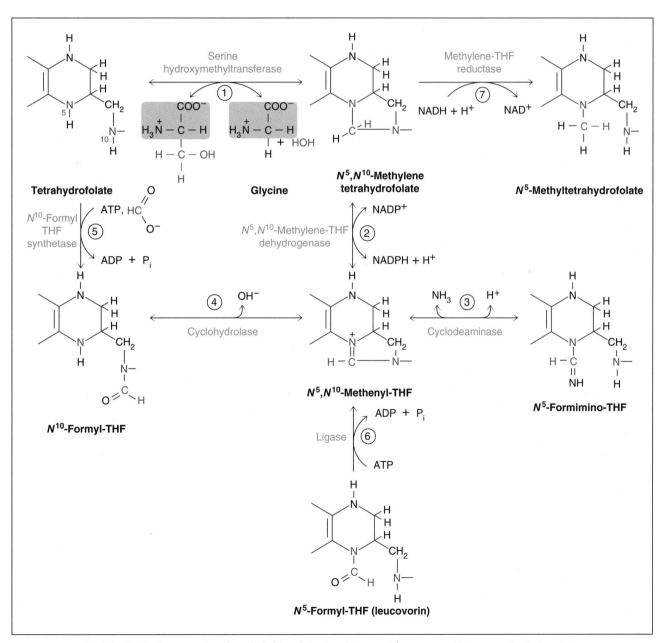

FIGURE 13–34. Interconversions of tetrahydrofolate derivatives. *The reactions are reversible except for 5, 6, and 7.*

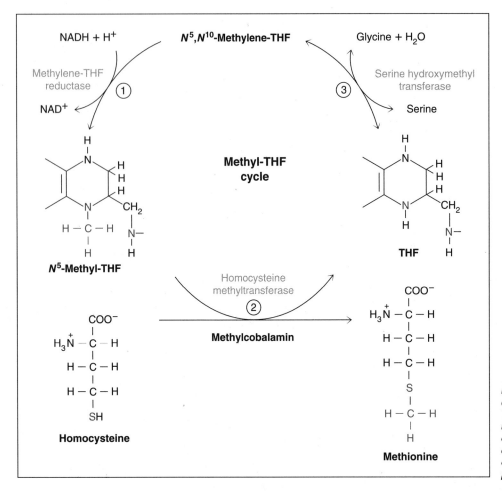

FIGURE 13–35. Conversion of homocysteine to methionine and the methyl-THF-cycle. *Reactions 1 and 2 are unidirectional. With a deficiency of vitamin B$_{12}$, N^5-methyl-THF accumulates, and this is the basis of the methyl trap hypothesis of pernicious anemia.*

late derivatives in metabolism; several of these are associated with nucleotide metabolism and are considered in the next chapter. ◄

CREATINE AND CREATININE METABOLISM

Creatine plays a pivotal role in the metabolism of high-energy phosphates (Figure 4–13). Creatine (*N*-methylguanidinoacetate) is derived from glycine, arginine, and *S*-adenosylmethionine (Figure 13–36). Creatine phosphate and creatine decompose spontaneously at low but constant rates within cells to form creatinine, a metabolite that is released into the circulation.

► Creatinine, a dead-end metabolite, has two important applications in clinical medicine. First, the amount of creatinine excreted in the urine over a 24-hour period, which correlates with muscle mass, is constant for a given individual (about 15 mg/kg of body weight). The quantity of creatinine is measured in 24-hour urine specimens to validate that the collection was complete. Second, the excretion of creatinine during a specified time in a **creatinine clearance test** serves as a test of kidney function (glomerular filtration rate). ◄

SPERMIDINE AND SPERMINE BIOSYNTHESIS

Spermidine and spermine are positively charged polyamines that complex with nuclear DNA. Spermidine and spermine are derived from ornithine and methionine. Ornithine, derived from arginine, undergoes a decarboxylation to form **putrescine** and carbon dioxide (Figure 13–37). *S*-Adenosylmethionine undergoes a decarboxylation to form **S-adenosylmethiopropylamine,** an activated propylamine donor. *S*-Adenosylmethiopropylamine donates propylamine first to putrescine and then to spermidine to form spermine. **Ornithine decarboxylase** is an enzyme with a very short half-life (on the order of 10 minutes). When cells divide, there is a large increase in the amount and activity of ornithine decarboxylase. Both **ornithine decarboxylase** and **AdoMet decarboxylase** use pyridoxal phosphate as cofactor.

CONVERSION OF TYROSINE TO MELANIN

Melanins are pigments that are derived from tyrosine. Melanin is formed in organelles called **melanosomes** that occur in pigment-producing cells

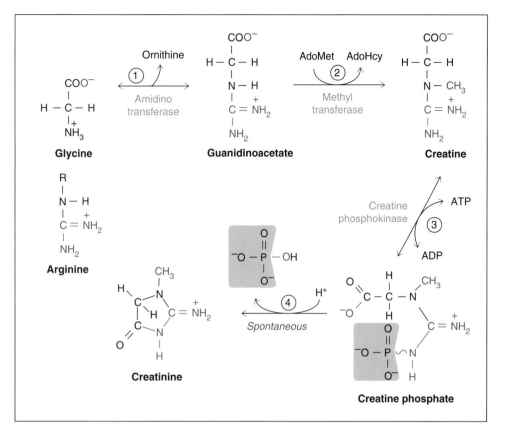

FIGURE 13–36. Creatine metabolism. (1) The transfer of the amidino group from a low-energy donor to acceptor is functionally isoergonic. (2) The loss of one high-energy bond during this transmethylation makes creatine biosynthesis exergonic. (3) The interconversion of the energy-rich creatine phosphate and ATP is functionally isoergonic and reversible. (4) The decomposition of creatine phosphate to creatinine is nonenzymatic and unidirectional.

called **melanocytes.** Melanocytes occur in skin, hair bulbs, mucous membranes, inner ear, and retina. The content of melanocytes from comparable anatomic locations does not vary by race or ethnic group. Differences in pigmentation do not depend upon the number of melanocytes but on pigment intensity. Two types of melanin occur in humans. Brown-black **eumelanins** are pigments derived from tyrosine. Yellow-red **pheomelanins** are pigments derived from tyrosine and cysteine. A series of enzymatic and nonenzymatic oxidation and coupling reactions are required to form these pigments from tyrosine. Owing to variation in the polymerization reactions and nonenzymatic interconversions, the melanins are heterogeneous compounds.

Tyrosinase, a copper-requiring enzyme, catalyzes the first two reactions of the pathway (Figure 13–38). Tyrosine reacts with oxygen to form *d*ihydroxyphenylalanine, or dopa. The same enzyme catalyzes the oxidation of dopa to form dopaquinone. Both reactions are exergonic and unidirectional because they involve a reaction of oxygen with an organic molecule (PRINCIPLE 8 OF BIOENERGETICS). Dopaquinone undergoes a series of enzymatic and nonenzymatic reactions, some of which are catalyzed by tyrosinase, to form polymeric eumelanin molecules. Dopaquinone also forms thioether (C—S—C) bonds with glutathione or cysteine; subsequent reactions not involving tyrosinase but involving other enzymes produce pheo-

melanins. The reaction that catalyzes the formation of dopa from tyrosine in nerve and adrenal medullary cells is catalyzed by an enzyme that differs from tyrosinase called tyrosine hydroxylase (Figure 19–5). Tyrosine hydroxylase requires a reducing substrate (tetrahydrobiopterin) that is not required for the tyrosinase reaction.

Exposure of skin in ultraviolet light elicits a pigmentation response called "tanning." Skin pigmentation increases during pregnancy (a reflection of altered hormonal status) and **Addison disease** (adrenocortical insufficiency). ▶ The increased skin pigmentation in Addison disease is due to increased production of adrenocorticotrophic hormone that stimulates melanocytes. Decreased skin pigmentation occurs in individuals with phenylketonuria. The elevated levels of phenylalanine inhibit tyrosinase activity and consequently melanin biosynthesis.

Albinism designates a variety of conditions that exhibit hypomelanosis based on metabolic defects in the melanocytes of the eye and skin. Melanocytes appear normal but fail to synthesize the usual amounts of melanin. Some types of albinism are due to an absence of tyrosinase. Such tyrosinase-negative individuals lack detectable pigment in the skin, hair, or eyes. For this reason, this disorder is sometimes called **complete perfect albinism.** Other forms of albinism occur in tyrosinase-positive individuals. These individuals, with **complete imperfect albinism,** have some detecta-

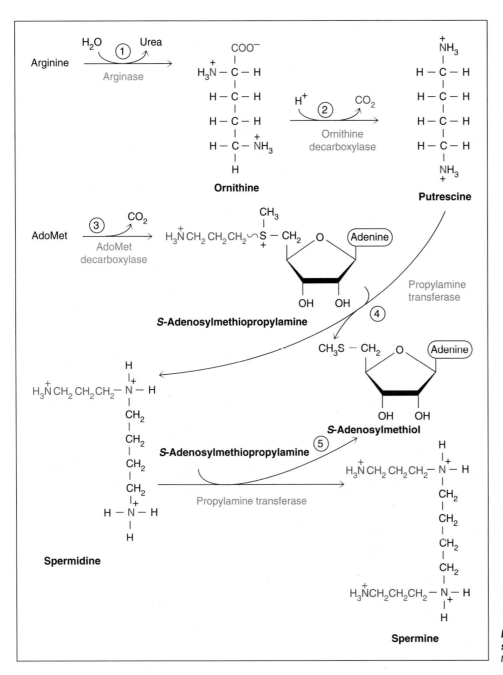

FIGURE 13–37. Polyamine biosynthesis. *All reactions are unidirectional.*

FIGURE 13–38. Overview of melanin synthesis. *The conversion of dopaquinone to eumelanins (3) and pheomelanins (4) requires several steps.*

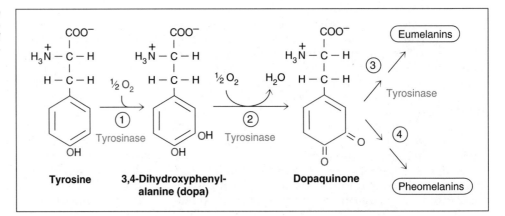

ble pigment. One defect that leads to albinism in tyrosinase-positive individuals is a deficiency in the ability to transport tyrosine from the cytosol into melanosomes. ◀

SUMMARY

Most of the proteolytic digestive enzymes are synthesized as zymogens. Pepsin is the proteolytic enzyme that is produced by the stomach. Trypsin, chymotrypsin, and elastase are the chief endopeptidases produced by the pancreas. Transamination reactions, which use pyridoxal phosphate (vitamine B_6) as cofactor, are pivotal for both the degradation and biosynthesis of the majority of the standard amino acids. The chief pathway for generating ammonium ion in humans involves the oxidative deamination of glutamate by $NAD(P)^+$.

Urea is synthesized in the liver. One nitrogen of urea is derived from ammonium ion, and the second is derived from aspartate. The carbonyl group is derived from CO_2 (as bicarbonate). The first step in the urea cycle involves the formation of carbamoyl phosphate. Its formation requires the expenditure of two high-energy bonds from two ATP molecules and is catalyzed by carbamoyl-phosphate synthetase I, a mitochondrial enzyme. This enzyme requires N-acetylglutamate as an allosteric activator. Carbamoyl-phosphate synthetase I is distinct from the cytosolic enzyme that is involved in pyrimidine formation (carbamoyl-phosphate synthetase II).

Amino acids that give rise to pyruvate and intermediates of the citric acid cycle (α-ketoglutarate, succinyl-CoA, fumarate, and oxaloacetate) are glycogenic. These compounds are able to furnish substrates for gluconeogenesis. In contrast, those amino acids that directly yield acetyl-CoA or acetoacetyl-CoA cannot support gluconeogenesis. These compounds yield ketone bodies. Four amino acids (alanine, glycine, serine, and cysteine) are converted to pyruvate. Five amino acids (proline, arginine, histidine, glutamine, and glutamate) are metabolized to α-ketoglutarate. Histidine yields N-formimino-L-glutamate (figlu) during catabolism. Valine, isoleucine, threonine, and methionine are metabolized to succinyl-CoA.

Phenylalanine and tyrosine are converted to fumarate (glycogenic) and acetoacetate (ketogenic). Asparagine and aspartate are metabolized to oxaloacetate. Leucine, lysine, and tryptophan are converted to acetoacetyl-CoA. The metabolism of tryptophan is perhaps the most complicated of all the amino acids. Both lysine and tryptophan are converted to α-ketoadipate. A small portion of tryptophan, moreover, is metabolized in humans to NAD^+, a derivative of the vitamin nicotinate.

Phenylketonuria (PKU) is due to a deficiency of phenylalanine hydroxylase. Alkaptonuria is attributable to a deficiency in homogentisate oxidase. Maple syrup urine disease is caused by a deficiency of the branched-chain keto acid dehydrogenase involved in the metabolism of valine, leucine, and isoleucine.

The biosynthesis of glutamine and asparagine requires ATP. In glutamine synthesis, ADP and P_i result. In asparagine synthesis, AMP and PP_i are formed. 3-Phosphoglycerate (an intermediate in glycolysis) is converted to serine. Proline is derived from glutamate. Cysteine is derived from methionine (essential) and serine (nonessential).

The reactions of S-adenosylmethionine, biotin, and folate derivatives are important in the transfer of one-carbon groups in metabolism. Creatine is derived from glycine, arginine, and methionine. Spermidine and spermine are derived from ornithine and methionine. Melanin is derived from tyrosine by enzymatic and nonenzymatic processes.

SELECTED READINGS

Bender, D.A. *Amino Acid Metabolism,* 2nd ed. Chichester, John Wiley & Sons, 1985.

Dennis, V.W. Investigations of renal function. *In* J. B. Wyngaarden, L.H. Smith, Jr., and J.C. Bennett (eds.). *Cecil Textbook of Medicine,* 19th ed. Philadelphia, W.B. Saunders Company, 1992, pp. 492–499.

Scriver, C.R. Hyperaminoaciduria [with a classification of the inborn and developmental errors of amino acid metabolism]. *In* J.B. Wyngaarden, L.H. Smith, Jr., and J.C. Bennett (eds.). *Cecil Textbook of Medicine,* 19th ed. Philadelphia, W.B. Saunders Company, 1992, pp. 1094–1101.

Scriver, C.R., A.L. Beaudet, W.S. Sly, and D. Valle (eds.). *The Metabolic Basis of Inherited Disease,* 6th ed. New York, McGraw-Hill Book Company, 1989.

NUCLEOTIDE

METABOLISM

Progress is made by young scientists who carry out experiments old scientists knew wouldn't work.

—FRANK WESTHEIMER

STRUCTURES OF NUCLEOSIDES AND NUCLEOTIDES

Nucleosides

Purines and **pyrimidines** are the two classes of aromatic bases found in nucleotides. Major purines include adenine and guanine, and major pyrimidines include cytosine, uracil, and thymine (Figures 6–12 and 6–13). The purines and pyrimidines are sparingly soluble in water at neutral pH. ▶ The practical consequence of this limited solubility in water is that uric acid, the main metabolite of purines, can form precipitates. As a consequence, overproduction of urate and its insolubility contribute to the pathogenesis of gout. Precipitation of urate contributes to inflammation, tophi (urate deposits in the skin, joints, and tendons), and urolithiasis (kidney stones). ◀

Nucleosides consist of a purine or pyrimidine base attached to a sugar through an energy-poor β-glycosidic bond. Naturally occurring pentose sugars include ribose and 2-deoxyribose (Figure 6–13). When the sugar is attached to a base, the numbered carbon atoms of the sugar are given a prime designation to distinguish them from positions of atoms in the base. The 2′ of 2′-deoxyribose refers to C^2 of the sugar. Ribonucleosides contain ribose, and 2′-deoxyribonucleosides contain deoxyribose.

Nucleotides

Nucleotides are nucleoside phosphate esters. There are three potential positions for esterification in ribonucleotides (2′, 3′, and 5′) and two in deoxyribonucleotides (3′ and 5′). The esters of mononucleotides are predominately 5′ in nature. Phosphodiesters of polynucleotides involve the 5′ and 3′-carbon atoms. Hydrolysis of RNA catalyzed by pancreatic RNAse or alkali yields 2′ and 3′ esters and cyclic 2′,3′ diesters. Hydrolysis by acid yields 2′-, 3′-, and 5′-derivatives. Hydrolysis of DNA catalyzed by pancreatic DNAse yields the 5′-ester derivatives. Hydrolysis by other DNAses can yield the 3′-derivative. The inability of DNA to form 2′, 3′-phosphate diesters accounts for the stability of DNA in alkali. RNA, which can form the 2′,3′-diester intermediates, is unstable in alkali.

The nomenclature used for bases and their nucleoside derivatives is given in Table 14–1. Hydrolysis at the 6-amino group of adenine yields hypoxanthine. The corresponding nucleoside (the terminology of which is a constant source of confusion for neophytes and some experts) is called inosine. Inosinate (IMP) is the key intermediate in the synthesis of AMP and GMP. Xanthine is a breakdown product of purines. The deoxyribonucleosides and deoxyribonucleotides are named by including the deoxy prefix before the corresponding ribonucleoside or ribonucleotide: for example, deoxyadenosine (dA), deoxyadenylate (dAMP). The deoxy prefix is abbreviated as "d."

Ribonucleotides are ribonucleoside monophosphates. 5′-AMP, or adenylic acid, for example, is 5′-adenosine monophosphate. Ribonucleo*side* monophosphates are often erroneously called ribonucleo*tide* monophosphates. Besides the ribonucleoside monophosphates, ribonucleoside diphosphates and ribonucleoside triphosphates are important metabolites. There are also deoxynucleoside mono-, di-, and triphosphates. The phosphates are usually esterified to the 5′-hydroxyl group. Several enzymes catalyze the phosphorylation of nucleoside monophosphates, and a single enzyme (nucleoside diphosphate kinase) catalyzes the phosphorylation of all the diphosphates (see Chapter 6).

NUCLEOTIDE BIOSYNTHESIS

Pyrimidines

Carbamoyl phosphate and aspartate are the precursors of the pyrimidine ring (Figure 14–1). Carbamoyl phosphate is derived from bicarbonate (the hydrated form of carbon dioxide) and the amido nitrogen of glutamine. An overview of pyrimidine synthesis is shown in Figure 14–2. **Orotate** is the first pyrimidine formed in the pathway, and **orotidine 5′-monophosphate** (OMP) is the first pyrimidine nucleotide. The nucleotides of uracil, cytosine, and thymine are derived from OMP, which occupies a central position in pyrimidine formation.

TABLE 14–1. Nomenclature of Bases, Nucleosides, and Nucleotides

Pyrimidine or Purine Base	Ribonucleoside	Ribonucleotide (ribonucleoside phosphate)	Deoxyribonucleotide (deoxyribonucleoside phosphate)
Adenine	Adenosine	Adenylate (AMP)	Deoxyadenylate (dAMP)
Guanine	Guanosine	Guanylate (GMP)	Deoxyguanylate (dGMP)
Uracil	Uridine	Uridylate (UMP)	Deoxyuridylate (dUMP)
Cytosine	Cytidine	Cytidylate (CMP)	Deoxycytidylate (dCMP)
Hypoxanthine	Inosine	Inosinate (IMP)	Deoxyinosinate (dIMP)
Xanthine	Xanthosine	Xanthylate (XMP)	Deoxyxanthylate (dXMP)
Thymine	Ribothymidine	Ribothymidylate (rTMP)	Thymidylate (TMP) or deoxythymidylate (dTMP)

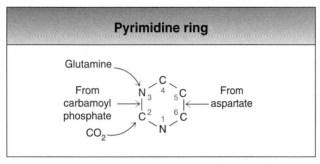

Pyrimidine ring

FIGURE 14-1. Metabolic sources of the atoms of the pyrimidine ring.

Synthesis of Carbamoyl Phosphate

Two adenosinetriphosphate (ATP) molecules are required for the synthesis of carbamoyl phosphate in an intricate reaction catalyzed by carbamoyl-phosphate synthetase II (Figure 14–3). The first ATP activates bicarbonate by forming an energy-rich carbonyl phosphate. The high-energy carbonyl phosphate reacts with glutamine, yielding carbamic acid; this reaction, which occurs with the loss of a high-energy bond, is exergonic. Reaction with a second molecule of ATP yields carbamoyl phosphate. This second reaction is functionally isoergonic because carbamoyl phosphate is an energy-rich compound with the mixed-acid anhydride linkage. The carbamoyl group is activated with a high group transfer potential (Tables 6–2 and 6–3) and is suitable for biosynthetic reactions. The overall reaction proceeds with the loss of a high-energy bond and is exergonic. *Carbamoyl-phosphate synthetase II is the rate-limiting enzyme of pyrimidine biosynthesis in humans* (Table 25–3).

Carbamoyl-phosphate synthetase II occurs in the cytosol of all nucleated cells. Carbamoyl-phosphate synthetase I that uses free ammonia (not glutamine) as the source of the nitrogen for urea synthesis (Chapter 13) occurs in liver mitochondria. Carbamoyl-phosphate synthetase II is inhibited by uridine diphosphate (UDP) and uridine triphosphate (UTP), end products of pyrimidine biosynthesis. Carbamoyl-phosphate synthetase I is not affected by UDP or UTP (Table 25–3). Carbamoyl-phosphate synthetase I, but not II, is activated by *N*-acetylglutamate.

Synthesis of the Pyrimidine Ring

The amino group of aspartate attacks carbamoyl phosphate, yielding **N-carbamoyl aspartate** and P_i in a reaction catalyzed by **aspartate transcarbamoylase** (Figure 14–4). Carbamoyl phosphate possesses an energy-rich bond; there are no high-energy bonds in the products. The reaction is exergonic and unidirectional. Next, **dihydroorotase** mediates a cyclization with the elimination of water, yielding **dihydroorotate.** This reaction is isoergonic.

The next step involves the dehydrogenation reaction converting a carbon-carbon single bond to a

double bond in **orotate.** This reaction is similar to the succinate dehydrogenase reaction of the Krebs cycle. **Dihydroorotate dehydrogenase** is an integral inner-mitochondrial-membrane flavoprotein whose active site faces the exterior (cytosol). Donation of the electrons from dihydroorotate via the flavin and coenzyme Q to the electron transport chain initiates a series of exergonic reactions that pulls the formation of orotate from dihydroorotate forward. Orotate is the first pyrimidine formed in the pathway.

Orotate next reacts with PRPP to yield OMP. This reaction occurs with the loss of a high-energy bond and is exergonic. Moreover, the formation and subsequent hydrolysis of PP_i further promote product formation. OMP, a pyrimidine nucleotide, undergoes a decarboxylation-yielding uridine 5'-monophosphate (UMP). This decarboxylation reaction is accompanied by a decrease in free energy that drives this unidirectional reaction (PRINCIPLE 6 OF BIOENERGETICS).

The overall pathway for pyrimidine biosynthesis is exergonic. Four high-energy bonds are required for the biosynthesis of UMP from carbon dioxide, glutamine, aspartate, and ribose 5-phosphate. Two are required for the synthesis of carbamoyl phosphate, and two are required for the synthesis of PRPP from ribose 5-phosphate and ATP (Figure 6–9). The oxidation of dihydroorotate provides reducing equivalents to coenzyme Q that lead to the formation of 1.5 moles of ATP per mole oxidized. This oxidative pathway from dihydroorotate to ox-

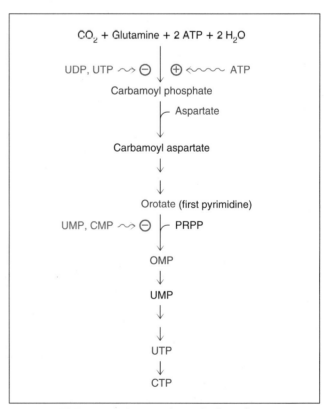

FIGURE 14-2. Overview of pyrimidine biosynthesis.

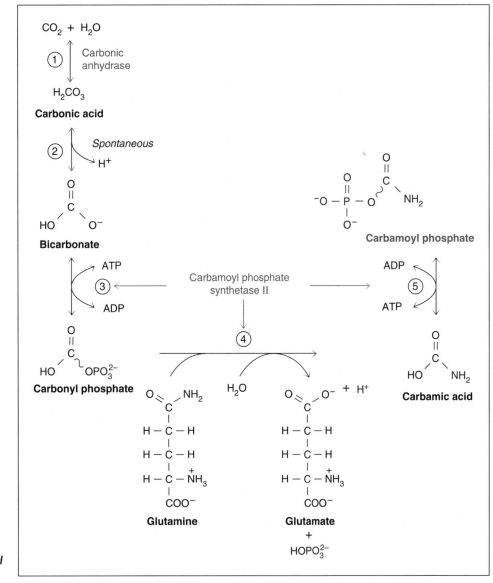

FIGURE 14–3. Synthesis of carbamoyl phosphate.

ygen, which involves the mitochondrial electron transport chain, is exergonic.

The first three enzymes of the pyrimidine pathway occur in the same cytosolic protein as a trifunctional protein or polyprotein (Table 14–2). The initial letters of each enzyme activity of this trifunctional protein are combined to form the acronym CAD, and the protein is called the **CAD complex.** The dehydrogenase, a protein with one activity, is located on the outer face of the inner mitochondrial membrane, where it can interact with cytosolic dihydroorotate. The last two enzymes of the pathway occur in the cytosol as a bifunctional protein called **UMP synthase** (Table 14–2). Besides its role in pyrimidine biosynthesis, the UMP synthase complex also catalyzes two reactions in the conversion of quinolinate, a tryptophan metabolite that resembles a pyrimidine, to NAD+ (see Figure 13–26). These sequential reactions in NAD+ formation involve phosphoribosylation and decarboxylation.

Conversion of UTP to CTP

UMP is converted to UTP in two successive phosphorylation reactions involving ATP. The first reaction is catalyzed by a nucleoside monophosphate kinase that can use cytidine monophosphate (CMP), dCMP, or UMP as substrate. The second reaction is catalyzed by a broad specificity nucleoside diphosphate kinase. These two reactions are functionally isoergonic (PRINCIPLE 1 OF BIOENER-

TABLE 14–2.   The Multifunctional Proteins of the Pyrimidine Biosynthetic Pathway

Enzymes	Designation	Disease
Carbamoyl-phosphate synthetase II Aspartate transcarbamoylase Dihydroorotase	CAD	Deficiency unknown
Orotate phosphoribosyltransferase Orotidylate (OMP) decarboxylase	UMP synthase	Orotic aciduria

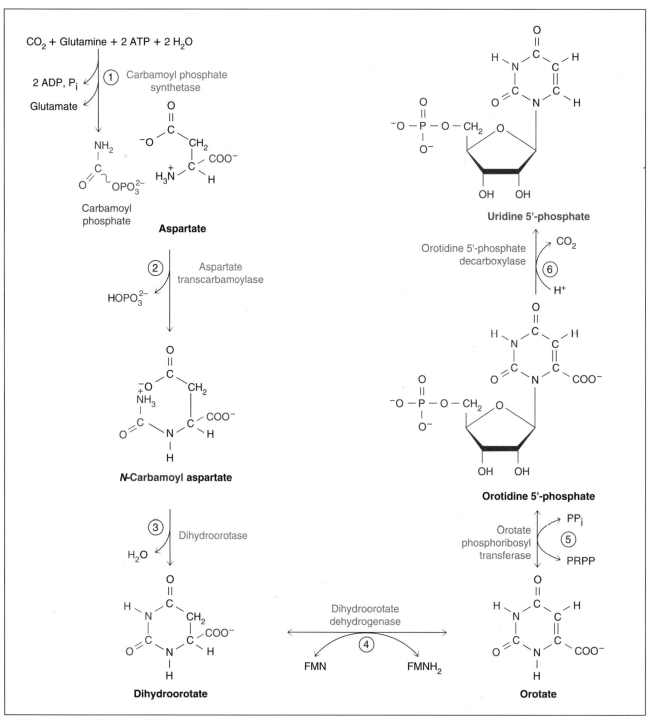

FIGURE 14–4. Pyrimidine biosynthesis. *One protein, the CAD complex, catalyzes reactions 1–3, and another protein, the UMP synthase complex, catalyzes reactions 5 and 6. Unidirectional and bidirectional reactions are indicated by the arrows.*

GETICS). UTP reacts with glutamine in an ATP-dependent reaction to form cytidine triphosphate (CTP). The oxygen on C^4 of UTP forms a hydroxyl group by enolization; the hydroxyl group is phosphorylated by ATP. Glutamine then donates its amide group, liberated by hydrolysis at the enzyme's active site, and phosphate is displaced (Figure 14–5). The reaction is not driven by the simple hydrolysis of ATP; rather ATP participates in the actual chemical transformation. The CTP synthetase reaction occurs with the loss of one high-energy bond and is exergonic and unidirectional.

Orotic Aciduria

▶ Orotic aciduria is a rare (fewer than 20 reported cases) inborn error of metabolism. Affected individuals exhibit retarded growth and development, as well as a megaloblastic anemia. The dis-

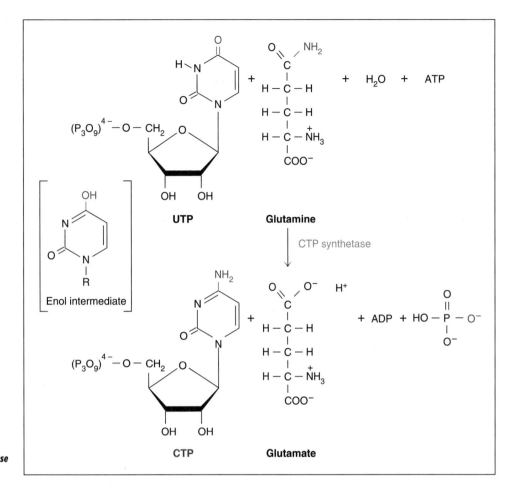

FIGURE 14–5. The CTP synthetase reaction.

ease, which is autosomal recessive, is caused by a deficiency of the UMP synthase complex (phosphoribosyltransferase and orotate decarboxylase) in the pyrimidine biosynthetic pathway (Table 14–2). The gene for UMP synthase is on the long arm of chromosome 3 (Table 16–5). Affected individuals excrete about 1.5 g of orotate daily; this is 1000 times the normal value. The anemia is due to a deficiency of nucleotides, precursors of DNA and RNA, in rapidly dividing bone marrow cells. Oral pyrimidines (synthetic or from yeast extract) provide substrates for pyrimidine nucleotide, RNA, and DNA synthesis to correct the anemia of orotic aciduria. ◀

Purines

The information in Figure 14–6, which illustrates the origin of the atoms of the purine ring, is noteworthy. The mechanism of several antimetabolites used in cancer chemotherapy and as antibiotics is based on their action on purine biosynthesis. Furthermore, a knowledge of the mechanism of action of allopurinol, a drug commonly used in the treatment of gout, requires an understanding of the pathway for purine biosynthesis and the reutilization (salvage) of existing purine metabolites. We will consider the pathway for purine biosynthesis

step by step to gain an understanding of the process. Only experts, however, know it by rote.

A flow chart shows the reactants that are required for the 10 steps in the biosynthesis of IMP, the first purine nucleotide formed *de novo* (Figure 14–7). Note that PRPP participates in the initial reaction and that the purine ring is constructed on phosphoribose. The 5-membered imidazole ring (5-aminoimidazole ribotide) is first synthesized. Successive reactions result in the formation of IMP, which is a complete purine nucleotide. IMP occurs at a crossroad in the pathway of purine biosynthe-

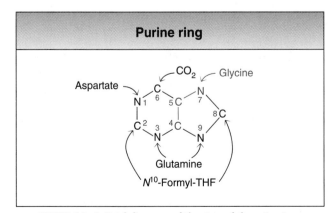

FIGURE 14–6. Metabolic sources of the atoms of the purine ring.

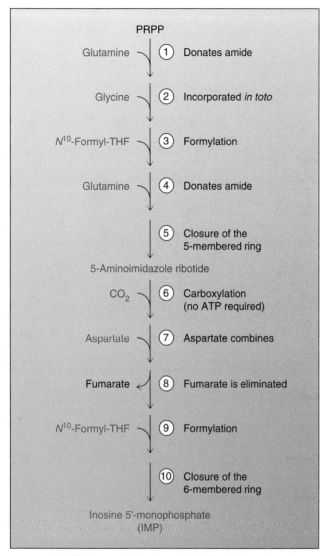

PRPP

Glutamine ─┐ (1) Donates amide

Glycine ─┐ (2) Incorporated *in toto*

N^{10}-Formyl-THF ─┐ (3) Formylation

Glutamine ─┐ (4) Donates amide

(5) Closure of the 5-membered ring

5-Aminoimidazole ribotide

CO_2 ─┐ (6) Carboxylation (no ATP required)

Aspartate ─┐ (7) Aspartate combines

Fumarate ─┐ (8) Fumarate is eliminated

N^{10}-Formyl-THF ─┐ (9) Formylation

(10) Closure of the 6-membered ring

Inosine 5'-monophosphate (IMP)

FIGURE 14–7. Overview of purine biosynthesis.

sis. Separate pathways lead to the formation of AMP and GMP.

PRPP Amidotransferase Reaction

The first and committed step in purine biosynthesis is catalyzed by glutamine PRPP amidotransferase. The reaction proceeds with inversion of configuration at C^1, yielding the characteristic β configuration that occurs in nucleotides (Figure 14–8). The amidotransferase reaction occurs with the loss of a high-energy bond and is unidirectional. The liberation of pyrophosphate followed by its hydrolysis provides additional energy for phosphoribosylamine synthesis.

Synthesis of 5-Aminoimidazole Ribotide

An ATP-dependent condensation of glycine with phosphoribosylamine occurs next. It is likely that an energy-rich acylphosphate (glycylphosphate) is an intermediate. This reaction proceeds with the

loss of a high-energy bond. Next, N^{10}-formyltetrahydrofolate donates its formyl group to glycinamide ribotide. The amido group of glutamine is then transferred to substrate in an ATP-dependent reaction. Enol keto tautomerism most likely furnishes a hydroxyl group that is phosphorylated; the resulting phosphate is a good leaving group. Hydrolysis of glutamine to glutamate occurs at the enzyme's active site. The dissipation of a high-energy bond of ATP contributes to the exergonic nature of this unidirectional reaction.

The next step involves a cyclization that produces the imidazole ring. The amino group adds to the aldehyde carbonyl group, which occurs with the formation of a hydroxyl group. The hydroxyl group is phosphorylated by ATP; elimination of phosphate results in the creation of a double bond and ring closure. This completes the first segment of the pathway.

Synthesis of IMP

5-Aminoimidazole ribotide (AIR) undergoes a carboxylation reaction. It is noteworthy that this is an **ATP-independent** process; other carboxylation reactions almost always require the input of energy. Moreover, biotin or pyridoxal phosphate is not involved in this reaction. The addition of the amino group in the next steps of purine biosynthesis is analogous to similar reactions in the urea cycle (Chapter 13). This process involves the addition of aspartate and the elimination of fumarate. Aspartate condenses with the carboxyl group of the acceptor substrate in an ATP-dependent reaction. A carboxyphosphate attached to the imidazole ring, an intermediate, reacts with the amino group of aspartate. The reaction occurs with the loss of a high-energy bond and is unidirectional. ATP undergoes an orthophosphate split during purine synthesis but a pyrophosphate split during urea synthesis. Fumarate is then discharged in an isoergonic lyase reaction.

The resulting AICAR reacts with N^{10}-formyltetrahydrofolate. For ring closure, the amino group combines with the formyl group and water is eliminated to form IMP. A substantial part of the thermodynamic driving force for the ring-closing reaction is the formation of the resonance-stabilized aromatic ring. There is no suggestion that the reaction can occur in the reverse direction.

The PRPP amidotransferase reaction is rate-limiting and the main regulatory reaction of purine biosynthesis (Table 25–3). This first enzyme in the pathway is the committed step and is irreversible. PRPP activates this enzyme allosterically and serves as a substrate. AMP and GMP, synthesized from IMP, inhibit the amidotransferase reaction. Six high-energy bonds are expended for the synthesis of IMP from ribose 5-phosphate and the other components. Purines are built on ribose phosphate; on the other hand, ribose phosphate is added to the pyrimidine after the base is synthesized.

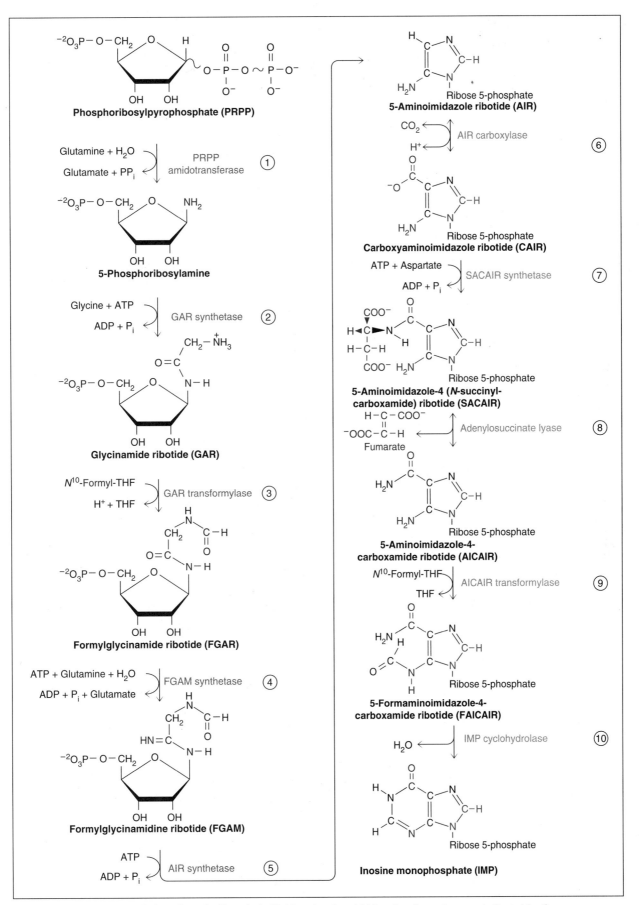

FIGURE 14–8. Pathway for purine biosynthesis. *Unidirectional and bidirectional reactions are indicated by the arrows.*

Conversion of IMP to AMP and GMP

AMP Formation. Aspartate serves as the source of the amino group attached to the adenine ring of AMP. The 6-keto group of IMP forms a 6-hydroxyl group by tautomerization. The hydroxyl group is phosphorylated by GTP; GDP is liberated. The amino group of aspartate displaces phosphate, yielding adenylosuccinate (Figure 14–9). The reaction occurs with the loss of one high-energy bond. A lyase then catalyzes the elimination of fumarate and the formation of AMP. The reaction is entropically favored as one molecule splits into two. There is no indication that the reverse reaction occurs physiologically.

GMP Formation. In the pathway for GMP synthesis, IMP is first hydrated to produce a hydroxyl group on C^2. The compound undergoes an oxidation by NAD^+, yielding xanthosine 5'-monophosphate. Glutamine next donates its amido nitrogen

to C^2 in an ATP-dependent reaction. ATP may pyrophosphorylate the oxygen on C^2, also yielding AMP. An amido group could displace pyrophosphate, resulting in the formation of GMP and PP_i. Hydrolysis of PP_i provides additional free energy in the direction of GMP formation. Conversion of IMP to GMP occurs with the loss of two high-energy bonds and is thus quite exergonic. This step completes the pathway for purine biosynthesis by *de novo* pathways.

RIBONUCLEOTIDE REDUCTASE AND DEOXYRIBONUCLEOTIDE SYNTHESIS

Ribonucleotides are converted to deoxyribonucleotides by replacement of the 2'-hydroxyl group by hydrogen. Ribonucleoside **diphosphates** serve as a substrate for **ribonucleotide reductase.** The enzyme catalyzes a reaction between reduced thio-

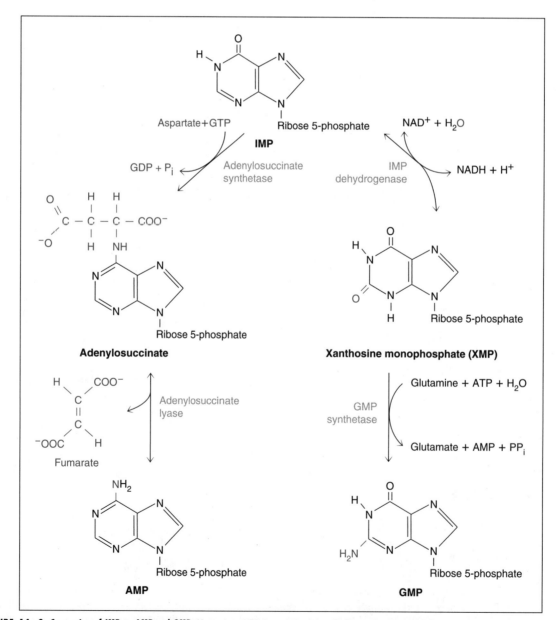

FIGURE 14–9. Conversion of IMP to AMP and GMP. *Note that ATP is required for GMP synthesis and GTP is required for AMP synthesis.*

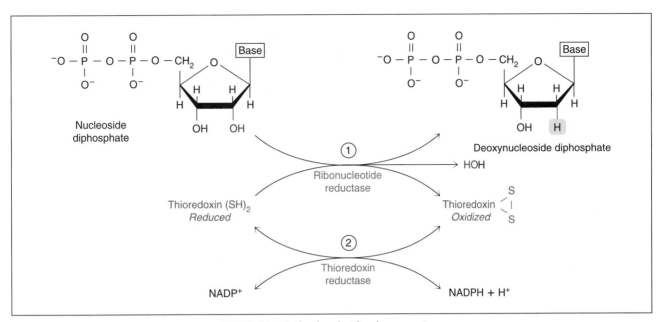

FIGURE 14–10. The ribonucleotide reductase reaction.

redoxin and ribonucleotide, yielding 2'-deoxyribo-nucleotide, oxidized thioredoxin, and water (Figure 14–10). The reduction of ribonucleoside diphosphates by thioredoxin is physiologically irreversible. The ribonucleotide reductase reaction plays an indispensable role in the biosynthesis of deoxyribonucleotides that serve as precursors of DNA.

Ribonucleotide reductase, which can reduce physiological and pharmacological diphosphate compounds, exhibits wide substrate specificity. Furthermore, the enzyme exhibits complex regulatory properties. Ribonucleotide reductase is regulated allosterically by many purine and pyrimidine nucleotides; this regulation is quite intricate and is designed to maintain appropriate concentrations of the deoxyribonucleotides for DNA synthesis. dATP serves as an allosteric inhibitor for the reduction of all nucleoside diphosphates.

Thioredoxin is a protein with two cysteines that are separated by one residue in the primary structure, and these cysteine residues serve as the source of electrons. A free radical of tyrosine is involved in ribonucleotide reductase catalysis. A disulfide bond forms in thioredoxin during nucleotide reduction. **Thioredoxin reductase** catalyzes the formation of the reduced thioredoxin using NADPH as reductant. This substrate specificity fits into the general notion that NADPH is the reductant for anabolic processes (PRINCIPLE 16 OF BIOCHEMISTRY) including cell division.

THYMIDYLATE SYNTHESIS AND THE TETRAHYDROFOLATE CYCLE

Thymidylate Synthase and Cancer Chemotherapy

Thymine, which shares base-pairing characteristics with uracil, occurs in DNA. **Thymidylate** **synthase** is the enzyme that catalyzes the methylation of dUMP to yield thymidylate (dTMP). The formation of dUMP, a reactant in the thymidylate synthase reaction, occurs by a circuitous route. UMP is converted to UDP in a reaction catalyzed by a nucleoside monophosphate kinase (Figure 14–11). UDP is converted to dUDP in the ribonucleotide reductase reaction. The next reactions were unanticipated. dUDP is next converted to dUTP by nucleoside diphosphate kinase. To prevent incorporation of this compound into DNA, cells contain a powerful **dUTPase** activity that catalyzes the formation of dUMP and PP_i. This process occurs with the loss of a high-energy bond; hydrolysis of pyrophosphate provides additional energy for the process.

Thymidylate synthase catalyzes the transfer of the one-carbon group from N^5,N^{10}-methylenetetrahydrofolate (THF), yielding thymidylate (dTMP) and DHF. This reaction has the following unusual and important characteristic. *Methylenetetrahydrofolate acts as a one-carbon donor and as a reductant;* the methylene group is reduced to a methyl group during the transfer reaction and *tetra*hydrofolate yields *di*hydrofolate (Figure 14–12). Synthesis of thymidylate occurs in a physiologically irreversible reaction. To participate in further reactions, dihydrofolate must be converted to tetrahydrofolate as catalyzed by **dihydrofolate reductase.** Tetrahydrofolate, but not dihydrofolate, can accept one-carbon groups from a variety of donors. The main source of one-carbon groups is from the amino acid serine (Figure 14–12).

Thymidylate synthase is a direct target for cancer chemotherapy and is one site of action of **fluorouracil** (FU). The basis of the inhibition is that fluorouracil is converted to fluoro-2'-deoxyuridylate, a structural analogue of dUMP (Table 14–3). Fluorodeoxyuridylate binds to the enzyme

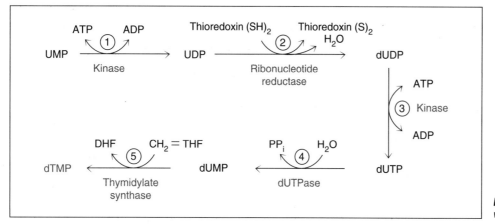

FIGURE 14–11. Pathway for the conversion of UMP to thymidylate (dTMP).

and undergoes a partial reaction. Midway through the reaction, fluorodeoxyuridylate forms a covalent adduct that bridges thymidylate synthase and N^5,N^{10}-methylene-THF (Figure 14–13). The covalent attachment of fluorodeoxyuridylate to thymidylate synthase produces irreversible inhibition. That the inhibition is based on the participation of the com-

pound in part of the enzyme-catalyzed reaction led to the concept of a **suicide-based enzyme inhibitor.** The compound *per se* is not an inhibitor; during an abortive catalytic cycle, the enzyme generates an active species that reacts with and inactivates the enzyme. In this sense, the enzyme "commits suicide."

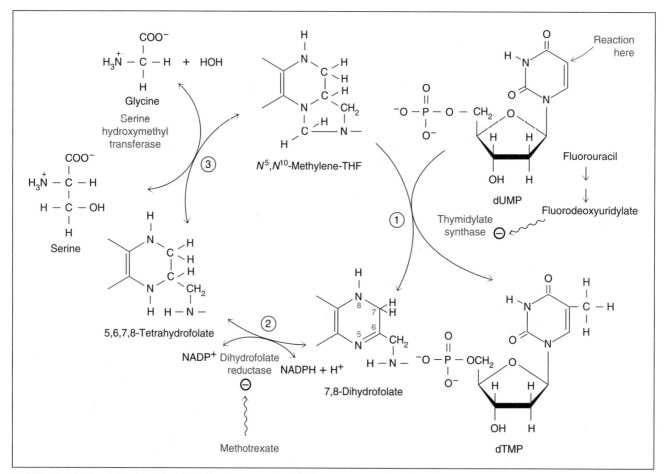

FIGURE 14–12. Thymidylate biosynthesis. *(1) Methylene tetrahydrofolate acts as a one-carbon donor and as a reductant. (2) To reenter the metabolic pool, dihydrofolate must be reduced to form tetrahydrofolate. (3) Tetrahydrofolate can accept one-carbon compounds from a variety of sources.*

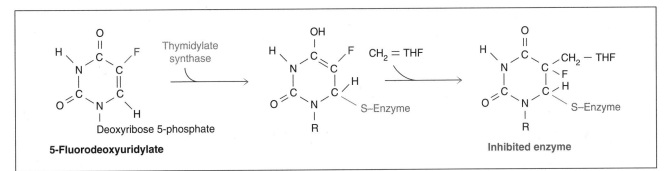

FIGURE 14–13. *Inhibition of thymidylate synthase by 5-fluorodeoxyuridylate, a suicide inhibitor.*

Dihydrofolate Reductase and Cancer Chemotherapy

Dihydrofolate reductase, which catalyzes the NADPH-dependent reduction of dihydrofolate to tetrahydrofolate, is required for nucleotide metabolism because folate functions in the tetrahydro oxidation state in one-carbon metabolism. Dihydrofolate reductase also catalyzes the NADPH-dependent reduction of dietary folate to dihydrofolate.

▶ **Methotrexate,** an inhibitor of dihydrofolate reductase, is an important drug used in cancer chemotherapy (see Figure 21–9). Acute lymphoblastic leukemia and osteosarcoma in children and choriocarcinoma in women are neoplastic diseases that are treated with methotrexate, in combination with other agents. A variety of solid tumors, including those of the breast, head and neck, ovary, and bladder, are also treated with methotrexate.

Methotrexate is a potent competitive inhibitor of dihydrofolate reductase with respect to dihydrofolate as substrate (Table 14–3). Methotrexate prevents the regeneration of tetrahydrofolate. Because of the decrease in the concentration of tetrahydrofolate resulting from methotrexate treatment, the synthesis of thymidylate and purines is inhibited. This decrease in nucleotides and deoxyribonucleotides inhibits cell replication. More rapidly dividing cells are more sensitive to its action than nondividing cells, but normal cells are also subject to the inhibitory effects of methotrexate, which results in toxicity. If it were not for the conversion of the tetrahydro form of folate to the dihydro form of folate during this methyl transfer reaction, inhibition of dihydrofolate reductase would not exert such powerful effects on dividing cells.

One strategy for the use of methotrexate in cancer chemotherapy is called **leucovorin rescue.** Individuals are given a dose of methotrexate that, if not followed by additional treatment, would be lethal. After 6–36 hours, leucovorin is administered. Leucovorin is N^5-formyl-THF (Figure 13–34); this agent is converted to N^5,N^{10}-methenyl-THF in an ATP-dependent process. The treated individual is "rescued" by the folate compound. In many cases, methotrexate rescue therapy is curative (all neoplastic cells are killed) while lower, nonlethal doses are only palliative. Resistance of tumor cells to methotrexate can occur. One mechanism for developing resistance involves the production of higher than normal levels of dihydrofolate reductase. This can occur as a result of gene amplification or the production of more than the two copies of the dihydrofolate reductase gene normally present in diploid cells. ◀

NUCLEOTIDE CATABOLISM

Pyrimidines

The pyrimidine ring, in contrast to the purine ring, can be completely degraded in humans (Figure 14–14). The hydrolytic reactions that liberate phosphate and ammonia are unidirectional. dUMP can be converted to dTMP by the thymidylate synthase reaction (see Figure 14–11). Uridine and deoxythymidine phosphorylases liberate uracil and thymine from their parent nucleosides. The phosphorylase reactions are isoergonic and reversible.

Uracil dehydrogenase catalyzes the reduction of uracil to dihydrouracil. This is an unusual reaction in catabolism because NADPH is the reductant. (NADPH is usually anabolic.) The ratio of NADPH/ NADP$^+$, which exceeds that of NADH/NAD$^+$ in cells, favors catabolism of uracil. Hydrolysis of dihydrouracil yields β-ureidopropionate during an exergonic process. β-Ureidopropionate is hydrolyzed to β-alanine, carbon dioxide, and ammonia. β-Alanine undergoes an isoergonic transamination to form malonate semialdehyde, which is converted to acetyl-CoA by an exergonic oxidative decarboxylation reaction.

Thymine is metabolized in a series of parallel reactions to form methylmalonate semialdehyde. Methylmalonate semialdehyde undergoes an exergonic oxidative decarboxylation to yield propionyl-CoA, which is metabolized by familiar reactions (Figure 11–12). The hydrolysis reactions and oxidative decarboxylation promote the breakdown of

TABLE 14–3. Selected Inhibitors of Nucleotide Metabolism

Inhibitor	Physiological Metabolite	Active Form of Inhibitor	Enzyme Target

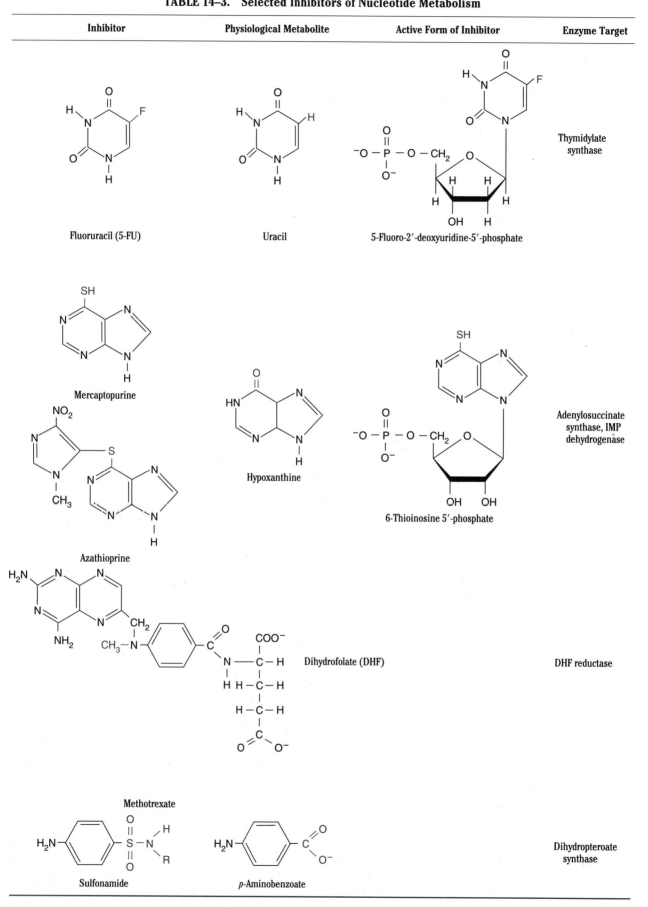

Fluoruracil (5-FU) · Uracil · 5-Fluoro-2′-deoxyuridine-5′-phosphate · Thymidylate synthase

Mercaptopurine · Hypoxanthine · 6-Thioinosine 5′-phosphate · Adenylosuccinate synthase, IMP dehydrogenase

Azathioprine

Methotrexate · Dihydrofolate (DHF) · DHF reductase

Sulfonamide · *p*-Aminobenzoate · Dihydropteroate synthase

TABLE 14–3.   Selected Inhibitors of Nucleotide Metabolism *Continued*

Inhibitor	Physiological Metabolite	Active Form of Inhibitor	Enzyme Target
			Bacterial DHF reductase
Trimethoprim	Dihydrofolate (DHF)		

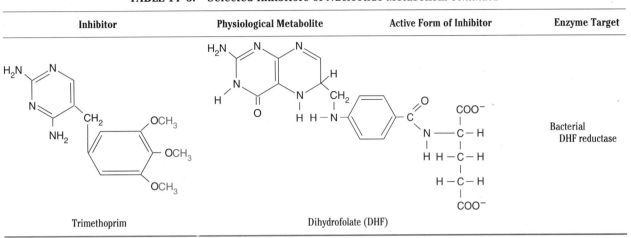

pyrimidine rings and make the pathways exergonic. Uracil can be salvaged by phosphoribosylation with PRPP as catalyzed by orotate phosphoribosyltransferase.

Purines

Reactions

Several enzymes (5′-nucleotidase, AMP deaminase, GMP deaminase, adenosine deaminase, and guanine deaminase) catalyze the hydrolysis of purine substrates. Purine nucleoside phosphorylase catalyzes the conversion of purine nucleosides to the free bases and pentose phosphates. The pathways of degradation of AMP, GMP, xanthine monophosphate (XMP), and IMP and their corresponding 2′-deoxy derivatives are shown in Figure 14–15. The hydrolytic removal of amino groups and 5′ phosphates is unidirectional. The phosphorolysis reactions, which are bidirectional, merit comment. Phosphorolysis of purine or pyrimidine nucleosides to yield (deoxy)ribose 1-phosphate is an important step in salvaging five-carbon sugars for subsequent reactions. Formation of purine and pyrimidine nucleosides from the corresponding bases in reactions catalyzed by the phosphorylases represents one mechanism for salvaging and reutilizing the bases and ribose 1-phosphate. Ribose 1-phosphate can also be converted by a mutase to ribose 5-phosphate, a substrate for PRPP synthetase.

Xanthine dehydrogenase catalyzes the conversion of hypoxanthine to xanthine and xanthine to uric acid according to the following equations.

Hypoxanthine + NAD^+ + $H_2O \rightarrow$
$$Xanthine + NADH + H^+ \quad (14.1)$$

Xanthine + NAD^+ + $H_2O \rightarrow$
$$Urate^- + NADH + 2\,H^+ \quad (14.2)$$

Xanthine dehydrogenase can be converted to **xanthine oxidase** through the oxidation of cysteine thiols. Xanthine oxidase catalyzes the following reactions.

Hypoxanthine + O_2 + $H_2O \rightarrow$
$$Xanthine + H_2O_2 \quad (14.3)$$

Xanthine + O_2 + $H_2O \rightarrow$
$$Urate^- + H^+ + H_2O_2 \quad (14.4)$$

The xanthine dehydrogenase and xanthine oxidase reactions, catalyzed by the same protein, differ, but many texts use the terms interchangeably. The oxidase reaction results in the production of hydrogen peroxide, and the dehydrogenase reaction does not. *The reaction catalyzed by xanthine dehydrogenase is the physiologically important process in purine degradation* in vivo. ▶ The conversion of xanthine dehydrogenase to xanthine oxidase occurs within hypoxic cells. This metabolic transformation produces an enzyme activity—xanthine oxidase—that generates toxic oxygen intermediates such as superoxide and peroxides (Figure 5–3). Xanthine dehydrogenase is a target for the treatment of hyperuricemia and gout, and this issue will be considered later in this chapter. ◀

Adenosine Deaminase Deficiency

▶ Adenosine deaminase deficiency is responsible for about 50% of the autosomal recessive forms of severe combined immunodeficiency disease (SCID). The gene for adenosine deaminase occurs on chromosome 20 (Table 16–5). Diagnosis of this rare disease can be made by measuring enzyme activity in erythrocytes. SCID is characterized by defective development of B and T lymphocytes, lymphopenia (low levels of circulating white blood cells), deficient antibody production (agammaglobulinemia), and deficient cell-mediated immunity. Adenosine deaminase (ADA) deficiency usually

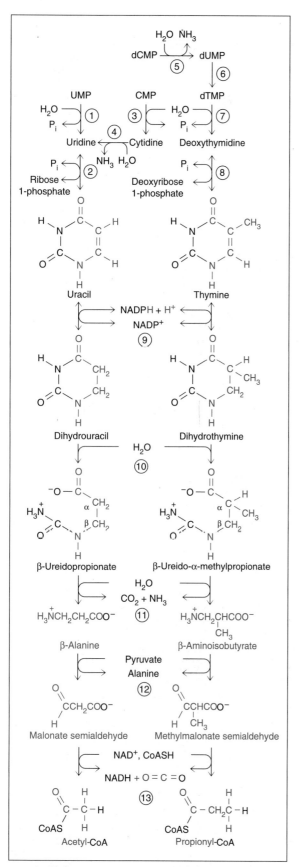

FIGURE 14–14. Degradation of the pyrimidine nucleotides.

presents during the neonatal period with diarrhea, pneumonia, otitis media, and failure to thrive.

The pathogenesis of SCID is due to altered concentrations of nucleotides. Conversion of adenosine to adenylate (catalyzed by adenosine kinase) provides a substrate for adenylate deaminase; the amino group from adenine-containing ribonucleotides can thereby be removed. Adenylate deaminase, however, will not catalyze the deamination of dAMP (Figure 14–15); high concentrations of dATP occur in adenosine deaminase deficiency. dATP inhibits ribonucleotide reductase allosterically, and the concentrations of other DNA precursors (dGTP, dCTP, and dTTP) are decreased. Although adenosine deaminase is widely distributed, lymphocytes have the highest activity. DNA synthesis is impaired, and lymphocytes are unable to divide and mount an immune response. Since both B cells and T cells are affected, the term "combined" is included in the name of the disease.

If untreated, individuals with adenosine deaminase deficiency rarely reach the age of 2 years and die of infection. Heroic measures have been employed to prevent infection in the hospital setting. Bone marrow transplantation from a suitable donor is effective. Compatible donors can be obtained, however, in only a quarter of the cases. A palliative mode of therapy is treatment with chemically modified bovine adenosine deaminase. The enzyme, modified by covalently attaching polyethylene glycol to the protein, has a longer half-life than the unmodified enzyme (days compared with minutes to hours) and is a poor immunogen. The poor immunogenicity retards the formation of antibodies against the foreign enzyme. Bovine adenosine deaminase must be given by injection. ◄

Purine Nucleoside Phosphorylase Deficiency

► A rarer form of autosomal recessive severe combined immunodeficiency is caused by a lack of purine nucleoside phosphorylase (PNP). The gene for this enzyme is located on chromosome 14 (Table 16–5). A deficiency of enzyme activity as a result of mutation leads to increased concentrations of deoxyguanosine and dGTP. The disorder is less severe than that produced by adenosine deaminase deficiency, and affected individuals present with variable susceptibility to infections. dGTP inhibits allosterically the conversion of CDP to dCDP as catalyzed by ribonucleotide reductase. dGTP stimulates allosterically the conversion of ADP to dADP. The resulting disorder and the inability to mount an appropriate immune response is postulated to result from abnormal nucleotide levels, especially in T cells. ◄

SALVAGE PATHWAYS FOR PURINE NUCLEOTIDE SYNTHESIS

A salvage pathway is a process whereby a metabolite is reutilized for the biosynthesis of a com-

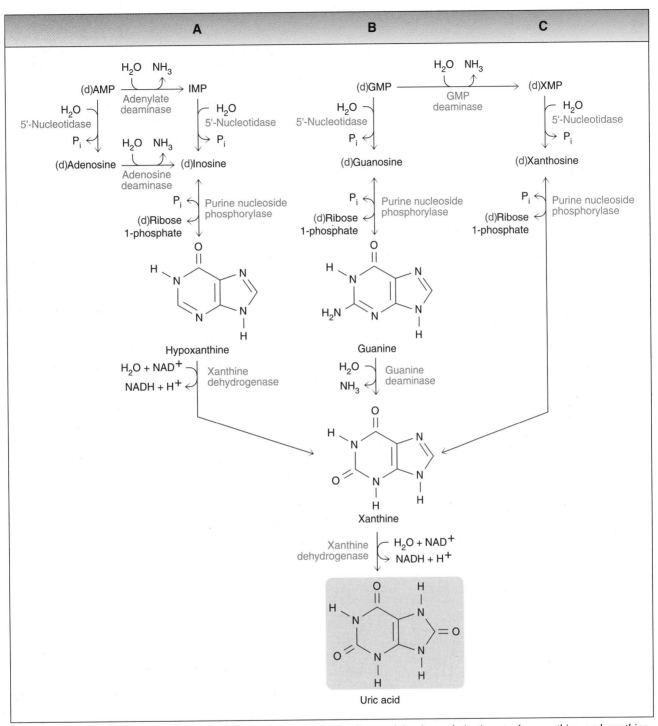

FIGURE 14–15. Purine catabolism. A. *Pathway for the conversion of adenylate and inosinate derivatives to hypoxanthine and xanthine.* B. *Pathway for the conversion of guanylate to xanthine.* C. *Conversion of xanthosine to xanthine. The hydrolysis reactions are unidirectional; the phosphorylase reactions are bidirectional. The reactions catalyzed by xanthine dehydrogenase are unidirectional.*

pound from which the metabolite was derived. For example, choline released from phospholipids can be reconverted into phospholipids by a salvage pathway (Figure 12–3). Similarly purine nucleotides are degraded to free bases, and the bases can be salvaged by conversion to purine nucleotides. Degradation of nucleotides to adenine, hypoxanthine, and guanine and their reutilization represent salvage pathways of purine biosynthesis.

Two specific phosphoribosyltransferases participate in the reutilization of adenine, hypoxanthine, and guanine. **Adenine phosphoribosyltransferase** catalyzes the reaction between adenine and PRPP to form AMP and pyrophosphate (Figure 14–16). **Hypoxanthine-guanine phosphoribosyltransferase (HGPRT)** catalyzes an analogous reaction (Figure 14–17). Both reactions occur with the loss of one high-energy bond and are exergonic. The hydroly-

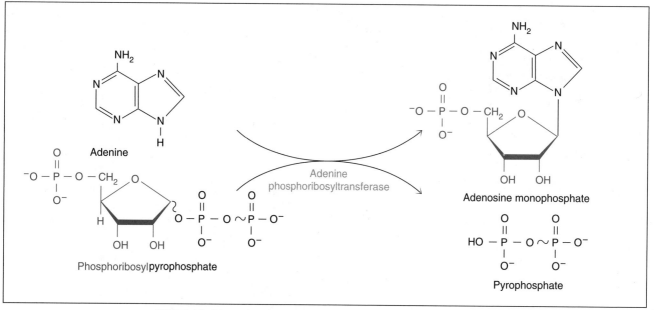

FIGURE 14–16. *The adenine phosphoribosyltransferase (APRT) reaction.*

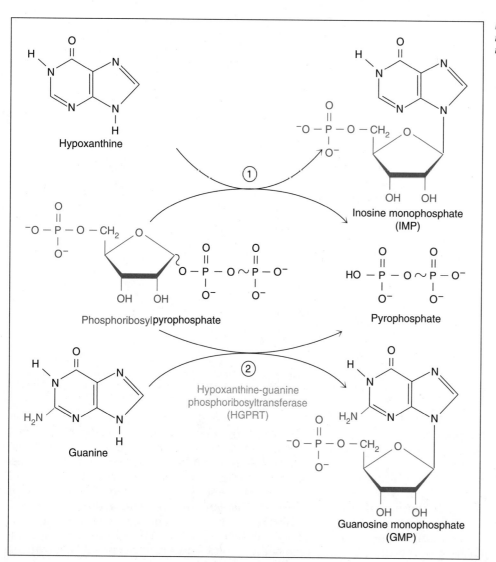

FIGURE 14–17. *The hypoxanthine-guanine phosphoribosyltransferase (HGPRT) reaction.*

sis of pyrophosphate also promotes the overall reaction.

REGULATION OF NUCLEOTIDE METABOLISM

Purines

PRPP is required for the synthesis of purine and pyrimidine nucleotides. *The committed and chief regulatory step in the pathway* de novo *for purine biosynthesis is the reaction catalyzed by glutamine PRPP amidotransferase* (Table 25–3). This enzyme is inhibited by IMP, AMP, GMP, and allopurinol ribonucleotide (Figure 14–18). Allopurinol ribonucleotide, a drug metabolite, will be considered later. PRPP synthetase plays a secondary role in the regulation of purine nucleotide biosynthesis. PRPP synthetase is inhibited by these nucleotides. PRPP, moreover, serves as a feed-forward activator of the PRPP amidotransferase reaction (Figure 14–18). High concentrations of PRPP promote purine biosynthesis.

The biosynthesis of the adenine and guanine nucleotides branches at IMP. 5'-AMP serves as a feedback inhibitor in its pathway, as does 5'-GMP in its pathway. An additional aspect of regulation past the IMP branch is that ATP is required for GMP formation. In parallel, GTP is required for the biosynthesis of AMP (Figure 14–18).

Pyrimidines

The regulatory steps of pyrimidine biosynthesis differ in animals and in bacteria. *The primary regulatory step in pyrimidine synthesis in humans is the formation of carbamoyl phosphate as catalyzed by carbamoyl-phosphate synthetase II* (Table 25–3). Carbamoyl-phosphate synthetase II is inhibited by

UDP and UTP; this enzyme is also activated by ATP. A secondary regulatory step is at the OMP-decarboxylase reaction. This enzyme is inhibited by UMP and CMP (Figure 14–2).

The primary regulatory step of pyrimidine biosynthesis in *Escherichia coli* and other (but not all) bacteria is catalyzed by aspartate transcarbamoylase (ATCase). CTP is a powerful inhibitor of aspartate transcarbamoylase in *E. coli*. The enzyme from *E. coli* is famous because its allosteric properties, which were among the first to be described, have been studied extensively. We mention the regulation of pyrimidine synthesis by this bacterial enzyme so that a knowledgeable distinction between human and bacterial *(E. coli)* pathways can be made (particularly on examination questions).

Lesch-Nyhan Syndrome

▶ The importance of salvage pathways in nucleotide metabolism was not appreciated until the discovery of a metabolic disease called the Lesch-Nyhan syndrome in the 1960s. This is a rare but famous X-linked disease. Affected boys appear normal at birth. There is a delay in motor development a few months after birth. Affected boys exhibit choreoathetosis (a sign characterized by flailing arm movements), spasticity, mental retardation, and uric acid overproduction that produces gout. They also are pathologically aggressive toward others and themselves, as shown by self-mutilating behavior. Self-mutilation is evidenced by biting and chewing lips and fingers. *The syndrome is caused by an absence of HGPRT activity.* Until the elucidation of the mechanism of the Lesch-Nyhan syndrome, scientists did not believe that purine salvage pathways were physiologically important. The severity of this disease, however, provided evidence to the contrary.

Three mechanisms account for the hyperuricemia of Lesch-Nyhan syndrome. (1) The inability to salvage hypoxanthine and guanine permits increased conversion of hypoxanthine and guanine to urate (Figure 14–19). The rate of urate production is six times normal. (2) A deficiency in the salvage pathway leads to a decrease in IMP and GMP concentrations; this removes normal feedback inhibitors of the *de novo* pathway at the level of PRPP amidotransferase and PRPP synthetase. (3) There is decreased utilization and an increase in the concentration of PRPP because less is used by the salvage pathway. The elevation of PRPP and the decline in feedback inhibitors stimulate the PRPP amidotransferase reaction and lead to a 200-fold increase in purine synthesis by the *de novo* pathway. It is unclear how altered purine nucleotide metabolism produces the signs and symptoms of the disease.

Affected individuals are treated by physical restraint and with allopurinol. Allopurinol treatment, whose action is described next, has some beneficial effect on the hyperuricemia but not on the

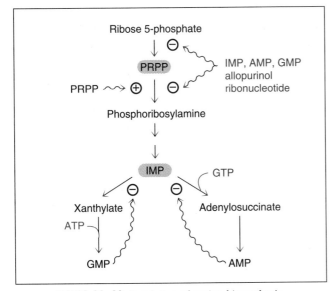

FIGURE 14–18. *Regulation of purine biosynthesis.*

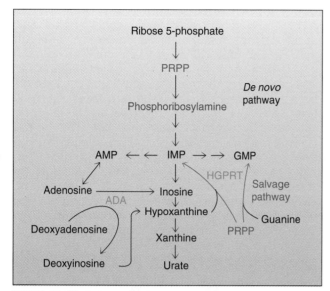

FIGURE 14–19. *Role of HGPRT in the regulation of purine biosynthesis.*

central nervous system symptoms. The prognosis is guarded, and the individuals usually succumb by 10 years of age. ◄

Gout

► Gout is the result of excess purine production. Hyperuricemia and elevated urate concentrations can lead to precipitation of sodium urate in selected tissues. Primary gout, which occurs predominantly in adult males in midlife (>90% of cases), is due to aberrations in the regulation of purine biosynthesis that are incompletely understood. In secondary gout, hyperuricemia is due to other causes. For example, hyperuricemia can result from decreased urate excretion because of renal insufficiency. Secondary gout can occur in individuals with increased cellular turnover as a result of polycythemia vera, some leukemias and lymphomas, multiple myeloma, and hemolytic anemias. Secondary gout can also result from increased urate formation because of cell death and nucleic acid degradation following treatment with antimetabolites or radiotherapy. In some cases of gout, PRPP synthetase fails to respond normally to feedback inhibition by GMP and AMP. Other cases of gout may be due to variants of PRPP synthetase with increased activity. However, the mechanisms responsible for most cases of primary gout are unknown. Hyperuricemia can lead to acute inflammation (classically in the large toe), gouty arthritis, and renal stones.

Acute inflammatory gout is treated with **colchicine.** This compound combines with microtubules. How this action leads to the dramatic and effective decrease in the pain of acute gout is unclear. Hyperuricemia is often treated with uricosuric agents (drugs that enhance renal excretion of urate). Such agents, for example, **probenecid,** inhibit renal tu-

bular absorption of urate and thereby promote excretion. Both primary and secondary gout can be treated with **allopurinol,** a purine base analogue.

The therapeutic effect of allopurinol results from three mechanisms. (1) Allopurinol is oxidized to alloxanthine by xanthine dehydrogenase (Figure 14–20), and allopurinol and alloxanthine are inhibitors of xanthine dehydrogenase. This inhibition decreases urate formation so that hypoxanthine and xanthine accumulate. These two urate precursors are more soluble than urate and have less tendency to form the precipitates that produce the symptoms of gout. Increased amounts of hypoxanthine and xanthine are excreted in the urine. Allopurinol and alloxanthine are also substrates for HGPRT (Figure 14–20). The products of the reaction are the corresponding ribonucleotides. (2) The production of allopurinol and alloxanthine ribonucleotides consumes and thereby decreases the concentration of PRPP, an activator of glutamine PRPP amidotransferase (Figure 14–18). (3) Allopurinol ribonucleotide and alloxanthine ribonucleotide are feedback inhibitors of PRPP amidotransferase.

Purines in the diet are liberated from nucleic acids following hydrolysis. The gut contains high xanthine dehydrogenase activity, and most dietary purines are catabolized to urate within the gut. Restriction of dietary purine intake can lead to small decreases in plasma urate concentration, but dietary restriction represents an ancillary treatment of gout. Caffeine, a methylxanthine, is not implicated in the pathogenesis of gout.

Only humans and a few other animal species are unable to degrade urate. Does urate have any beneficial effects? Urate is a reductant (Table 5–3) that may protect against oxygen toxicity. Urate may thus function as an antioxidant like β-carotene, vitamin C, and vitamin E. ◄

SELECTED ANTIMETABOLITES AND NUCLEOTIDE METABOLISM

► Several drugs that are used in the treatment of bacterial infections or in cancer chemotherapy act by inhibiting nucleotide biosynthesis, either directly or indirectly. Antimetabolites used in cancer chemotherapy are toxic to rapidly dividing cells including those of the bone marrow and intestinal epithelia. Consequently agents that inhibit nucleotide synthesis must be used judiciously.

Fluorouracil (5-FU) interferes with thymidylate synthesis (Figure 14–13). Inhibition of thymidylate synthase decreases cellular levels of the thymidine nucleotides. Cells lacking thymine are prone to die, a phenomenon called "thymineless death." The mechanism for this response is unclear. Fluorouracil is used in the treatment of a variety of solid tumors including carcinoma of the ovary, cervix, bladder, prostate, and gastrointestinal tract.

Mercaptopurine is a potent inhibitor of purine nucleotide biosynthesis. This agent, which is a hy-

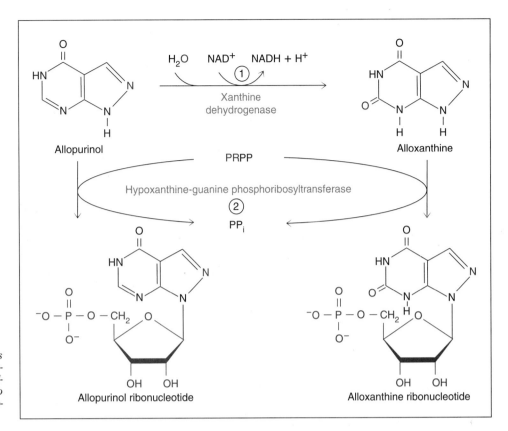

FIGURE 14-20. *Allopurinol as substrate for xanthine dehydrogenase. Both allopurinol and alloxanthine can be converted to their corresponding ribonucleotides as catalyzed by HGPRT.*

poxanthine analogue, must first be converted to 6-thioinosine 5′-monophosphate (Table 14–3). This derivative inhibits adenylosuccinate synthetase and IMP dehydrogenase. 6-Thioinosine 5′-monophosphate also inhibits allosterically the *de novo* pathway of purine synthesis at the amidotransferase reaction. Mercaptopurine is used in the treatment of some forms of leukemia. **Azathioprine** (Table 14–3) is converted to mercaptopurine following reduction *in vivo* by glutathione. Azathioprine is an immunosuppressive agent that is used to treat tissue rejection in individuals who have organ transplants. That immune cells are sensitive to alterations in nucleotide levels is evidenced by the immunodeficiency states that are produced by adenosine deaminase and purine nucleoside phosphorylase deficiency.

Sulfonamide antibiotics are used in the treatment of various infectious diseases. These agents are structural analogues of *p*-aminobenzoate, a component of folate (Table 14–3). Sulfonamides inhibit competitively the incorporation of *p*-aminobenzoate into folate. Purine biosynthesis in bacteria sensitive to sulfonamides is diminished, and 5-aminoimidazole-4-carboxamide ribotide (Figure 14–8) accumulates. Evidently, the second formyltransferase in the pathway is more sensitive to formyl-THF concentrations than the first formyltransferase. Sensitive bacteria are those that must synthesize their own folate; bacteria that can use preformed folate are not affected. Vulnerable bacteria also are incapable of transporting folate derivatives into their cells. Humans are resistant to

the action of sulfonamides because folate synthesis does not occur in human cells and preformed folate, a vitamin, is required.

Trimethoprim (Table 14–3) is an antibiotic that is prescribed together with sulfonamide antibiotics. The action of this agent is to inhibit dihydrofolate reductase in sensitive bacteria. Trimethoprim's action in bacteria resembles the action of methotrexate in humans (Figure 14–12). Human dihydrofolate reductase is resistant to the action of trimethoprim. ◀

BIOSYNTHESIS OF NUCLEOTIDE COENZYMES

Having gained an appreciation of the importance of nucleotides such as coenzyme A and FAD in metabolism, we now consider the pathway for the biosynthesis of these substances. Each of these coenzymes contains an AMP component, and this is derived from ATP. We consider the pathway for NAD^+ synthesis from tryptophan and quinolinate in Chapter 13 (Figure 13–26). The pathway, however, is not active enough to obviate the need for dietary niacin (nicotinate and nicotinamide), a vitamin. The pathway for the conversion of nicotinate to NAD^+ is also given in Figure 13–26.

Coenzyme A

Coenzyme A biosynthesis begins with **pantothenate,** a vitamin. In the first step of the pathway, ATP

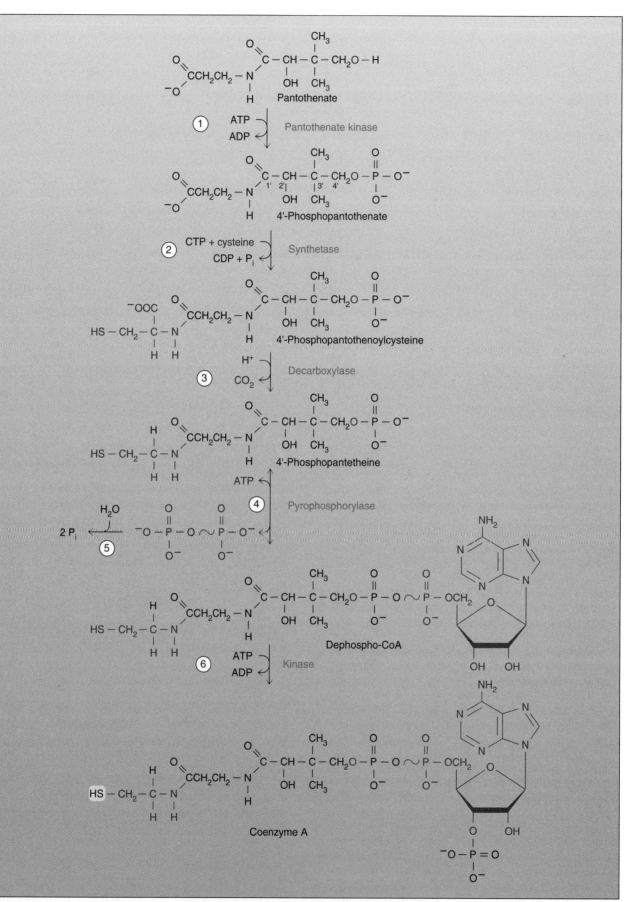

FIGURE 14–21. *Pathway for coenzyme A biosynthesis.*

phosphorylates pantothenate to yield the low-energy phosphate ester of 4'-phosphopantothenate and ADP (Figure 14–21). This reaction, which proceeds with the loss of a high-energy bond, is exergonic and unidirectional (PRINCIPLE 2 OF BIOENERGETICS). 4'-Phosphopantothenate reacts with cysteine to form the amide derivative in 4'-phosphopantothenoylcysteine. *That CTP is the energy donor in this reaction makes it unusual.* The carboxyl group is most likely activated as the energy-rich acylphosphate before amide formation. This reaction, which proceeds with the loss of a high-energy bond, is exergonic.

The subsequent decarboxylation that yields 4'-phosphopantetheine is also exergonic (PRINCIPLE 6 OF BIOENERGETICS). ATP then serves as an activated adenylyl donor to yield dephospho-CoA and PP_i. There is retention of the energy-rich simple-acid anhydride bond in dephospho-CoA, and this reaction is functionally isoergonic (PRINCIPLE 1 OF BIOENERGETICS). The hydrolysis of PP_i thus plays an important thermodynamic role (PRINCIPLE 5 OF BIOENERGETICS) in promoting the forward reaction.

The final step of the pathway involves a familiar phosphotransferase reaction involving the formation of a low-energy phosphate bond. Every step in this pathway is unidirectional except the adenylyl transfer reaction. Hydrolysis of PP_i, however, pulls the adenylyl transfer reaction forward.

FMN and FAD

We now examine the pathway for the biosynthesis of the flavin coenzymes: flavin mononucleotide (FMN) and flavine adenine dinucleotide (FAD). We begin with riboflavin, an essential nutrient or vitamin. The first step involves the phosphorylation of riboflavin by ATP to yield the energy-poor FMN (Figure 14–22). In the next reaction, ATP functions as active adenylate to yield FAD. This reaction, which occurs without a loss in the number of high-energy bonds, is functionally isoergonic. Hydrolysis of PP_i, however, serves to pull the adenylyl transfer reaction forward.

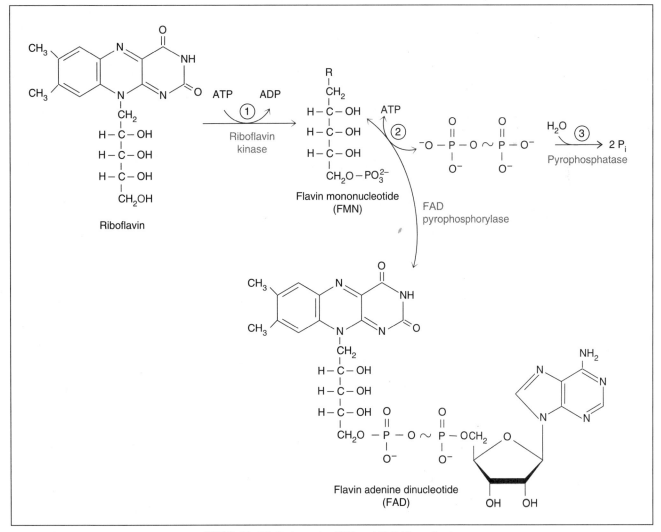

FIGURE 14–22. *Pathway for FMN and FAD biosynthesis.*

SUMMARY

Mononucleotides are derived from a nitrogenous base, a five-carbon sugar, and phosphate. The pyrimidine ring is derived from carbamoyl phosphate and aspartate. The formation of carbamoyl phosphate is catalyzed by carbamoyl-phosphate synthetase II, the rate-limiting enzyme for pyrimidine synthesis in humans. This enzyme differs in three ways from the enzyme that participates in urea biosynthesis. The pyrimidine enzyme (1) is found in the cytosol of all nucleated cells (and not just in liver mitochondria), (2) utilizes glutamine (not ammonia) as the amido donor, and (3) is not regulated by N-acetylglutamate. The first pyrimidine is orotate. Orotate reacts with PRPP to yield orotidine 5′-monophosphate. The nucleotides of uracil, thymine, and cytosine are derived from OMP. OMP is converted to UMP; UTP is converted to CTP in an ATP-dependent reaction with glutamine as the amido group donor.

The purine ring is constructed on phosphoribose. The 5-membered imidazole ring is first synthesized. Successive reactions result in the formation of IMP, which is a complete purine nucleotide. IMP occurs at a fork in the pathway of purine biosynthesis. Separate pathways lead to the formation of AMP and GMP. The first and committed step in purine biosynthesis is catalyzed by glutamine PRPP amidotransferase. This reaction is inhibited by AMP and GMP (and several purine nucleotide analogues) and is activated by PRPP.

Ribonucleoside diphosphates serve as substrate for ribonucleotide reductase. The ribonucleotide reductase reaction plays an indispensable role in the biosynthesis of deoxyribonucleotides that serve as precursors of DNA. Thymidylate synthase catalyzes the transfer of the methyl group from N^5, N^{10}-methylene-THF to dUMP, yielding thymidylate and dihydrofolate. This enzyme is the site of action of fluorouracil deoxyribonucleotide, a suicide inhibitor of this reaction. Methotrexate is an inhibitor of dihydrofolate reductase, and this prevents the conversion of dihydrofolate to tetrahydrofolate. Dihydrofolate is generated during the thymidylate synthase reaction.

Pyrimidine bases can be degraded to carbon dioxide and ammonia. Thymine is converted to propionyl-CoA, and the other pyrimidines yield acetyl-CoA. Catabolism of purines stops at urate. Gout results from altered purine metabolism. Gout is treated with allopurinol. Allopurinol and alloxanthine are inhibitors of the xanthine dehydrogenase reaction, and this action inhibits urate production. Allopurinol and alloxanthine react with PRPP to form ribonucleotides. The formation of ribonucleotides decreases PRPP concentrations to thereby decrease glutamine PRPP amidotransferase activity. Allopurinol and alloxanthine ribonucleotides also serve as allosteric inhibitors of PRPP amidotransferase.

SELECTED READINGS

Becker, M.A., and M. Kim. Regulation of purine synthesis de novo in human fibroblasts by purine nucleotides and phosphoribosylpyrophosphate. Journal of Biological Chemistry 262:14531–14537, 1987.

Blakley, R.L., and S.J. Benkovic. *Folates and Pterins,* Vols. 1 and 2. New York, John Wiley & Sons, 1985.

Elion, G.B. The purine path to chemotherapy. Science 244:41–47, 1989.

Jones, M.E. Pyrimidine nucleotide biosynthesis in animals: Genes, enzymes, and regulation of UMP biosynthesis. Annual Review of Biochemistry 49:253–279, 1980.

Reichard, P. Interactions between deoxyribonucleotide and DNA synthesis. Annual Review of Biochemistry 57:349–374, 1988.

Stout, J.T., and C.T. Caskey. Hypoxanthine phosphoribosyltransferase deficiency: The Lesch-Nyhan syndrome and gouty arthritis. *In* C.R. Scriver, A.L. Beaudet, W.S. Sly, and D. Valle (eds.). *The Metabolic Basis of Inherited Disease,* 6th ed. New York, McGraw-Hill Book Company, 1989, pp. 1007–1028.

CHAPTER FIFTEEN

DNA BIOSYNTHESIS

AND

REPLICATION

The virtuosity of the DNA polymerase first isolated from E. coli *still amazes me.*
—ARTHUR KORNBERG

The period of the 1950s was a golden age in nucleic acid biochemistry. The double helical structure of DNA was proposed by Watson and Crick, and Kornberg described the enzymatic synthesis of DNA by DNA polymerase.
—GERTRUDE B. ELION

INFORMATION TRANSFER IN MOLECULAR BIOLOGY

Crick's Law of Molecular Biology

The pivotal role of DNA in information transfer in living cells, formulated by Francis Crick, is called the central dogma of molecular biology (PRINCIPLE 25 OF BIOCHEMISTRY). The sequence of bases of cellular DNA is the source of information for the faithful copying, or **replication,** of DNA (Figure 15–1). This process produces identical molecules of DNA for each of two daughter cells. The sequence of bases in DNA is the source of information for RNA synthesis, or **transcription.** In bacteria, transcribed RNA is functional. In human cells, RNA processing, splicing, and transport from the nucleus are required to produce functional RNA (Figure 15–2). Sometimes viral RNA provides information for DNA biosynthesis by **reverse transcription.**

Conversion of the four-letter alphabet of nucleic acids to the 20-letter alphabet of proteins occurs during **translation.** Translation involves protein biosynthesis by the ribosomal system and is considered in Chapter 17. The sequence of bases in messenger RNA determines the sequence of amino acids in the corresponding protein. The genetic code is a triplet code; three nucleotides in DNA and in RNA correspond to one amino acid in a protein. The structures of the bases found in DNA and RNA are illustrated in Figure 6–12.

Genes and Molecular Medicine

Life scientists surmise that knowledge of the anatomy of the gene will be as important in medical practice as knowledge of the anatomy of the heart. DNA is the focus of attention because of its role in carrying and expressing genetic information. Inherited traits are passed from one generation to the next, and the **gene** is the unit of inheritance. A **structural gene** is a nucleotide sequence that carries the information corresponding to a specific RNA or protein. A **regulatory gene** or **element** is a nucleotide segment that alters the expression of a structural gene.

To minimize mutations (changes in base sequence), most of which are unfavorable, the cell has evolved mechanisms for avoiding errors in DNA synthesis and, when mistakes occur, mechanisms for repairing the damaged DNA. Many insults can alter DNA. These incidents include spontaneous hydrolysis, electromagnetic irradiation (ultraviolet light and x-rays), cosmic rays, and chemicals in the environment. Mutations can cause genetic diseases and cancer.

Enormous advances in the ability to manipulate and study DNA were initiated in the 1970s, and the rate of progress continues at a rapid pace. Now it is possible to determine the sequence of large segments of DNA (thousands of bases) in a few days' time. Moreover, DNA can be inserted into foreign cells, where it can be expressed as functional protein. The manipulation and expression of DNA and its protein products has facilitated major advances in medicine. Hormones and growth factors can be expressed, purified, studied, and used for human therapeutics by procedures unimaginable in 1970. People are currently receiving human (as opposed to bovine or porcine) insulin for the treatment of diabetes. Moreover, growth hormone, erythropoietin, and tissue plasminogen activator, which are scarce proteins that cannot be isolated easily from natural sources, are produced by recombinant DNA technology for use in human therapeutics.

The use of DNA per se as a therapeutic agent (gene therapy) is an emerging technology. Gene therapy has been approved for trials in adenosine deaminase deficiency (Chapter 14). Because of the importance of recombinant DNA technology in diagnostic and therapeutic medicine, we consider the biochemistry of DNA replication in bacteria (*Escherichia coli*) as thoroughly as that for human cells. Moreover, the knowledge gained from replication in *E. coli* paved the way for the advances in understanding animal cell replication. A glossary of many terms used in this and subsequent chapters appears in Box 15–1.

STRUCTURE OF DNA

Sequence of DNA

DNA is a polymer of deoxyribonucleotides consisting of thousands or even millions of monomeric residues. Deoxyribonucleotides are made up of purine (adenine, guanine) or pyrimidine (cytosine, thymine) bases covalently attached to the 1′-carbon atom of 2′-deoxyribose. A phosphodiester bond joins the 5′-hydroxyl group of deoxyribose to a 3′-hydroxyl group of an adjacent deoxyribonucleotide to form a repeating backbone (Figure 15–3).

The sequence of bases along the sugar-phosphate backbone makes up the **primary structure** of DNA, and the specific sequence distinguishes the DNA of one gene from another. The sequence of bases represents the information content of DNA.

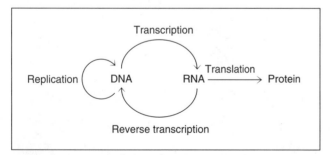

FIGURE 15–1. Direction of information transfer in cells. *Note that information does not go from protein to nucleic acid.*

BOX 15-1   GLOSSARY OF TERMS USED IN MOLECULAR MEDICINE AND GENETICS

Allele: One of the alternative forms of a gene.

Autoradiography: Localization of a radioactive substance based upon its photoactivation of an adjacent x-ray film.

Bacteriophage: A bacterial virus.

Blunt-ended DNA: A DNA duplex that ends with paired nucleotides.

cDNA (complementary DNA): A single- or double-stranded DNA that is synthesized using an RNA as template and the enzyme reverse transcriptase.

Clone: A large number of cells, molecules, or organisms that are identical with a single parental cell or molecule. To obtain a clone of a DNA molecule is to possess many identical copies. To clone a gene is to obtain the DNA corresponding to the gene in a form that can produce many copies of the gene.

Codon: A triplet of three bases in a DNA or RNA molecule that specifies a single amino acid.

Cosmid: A plasmid vector that carries the cos (cohesive) sites of bacteriophage lambda. This allows the plasmids containing DNA segments for cloning to be packaged into phage particles for efficient introduction into bacteria.

Endonuclease: An enzyme that catalyzes the hydrolysis of phosphodiester bonds that are in the interior of a nucleic acid.

Exon: The sequence of a gene that is represented in the mature RNA corresponding to the gene; the exon is expressed.

Exonuclease: An enzyme that catalyzes the hydrolysis of phosphodiester bonds that are at the end of a nucleic acid.

Genetic code: The base triplets that specify the standard 20 amino acids found in proteins.

Hybridization: The formation of a duplex molecule from two complementary single-stranded polynucleotides.

Insert: A fragment of DNA that is added covalently to bridge a discontinuity in a DNA vector; the DNA vector has the ability to replicate and form clones of itself or the covalent vector-insert molecule.

Intron: The polynucleotide sequence of a gene that is transcribed into RNA but is not expressed in the mature molecule.

Kilobase (kb): A unit of 1000 bases in DNA or RNA sequence. In double-stranded DNA, designates kilobase pairs (kbp).

Library: A group of clones of DNA that represents an entire collection of genetic sequences. A genomic library contains the entire genome of an organism. A cDNA library contains the sequences corresponding to the entire expressed mRNAs of a cell. The library is made up of many different replicating forms that together contain the whole of the starting material.

Long interspersed nuclear element (LINE): Repeated sequences found in chromosomal DNA in unit lengths of 5000 to 7000 base pairs.

Mutation: A heritable change in DNA due to an alteration in the base sequence.

Northern blot: Transferring RNA resolved by gel electrophoresis to a matrix (nitrocellulose or nylon) and identifying a specific RNA with a probe.

Oligonucleotide: A short segment of DNA or RNA (up to about 50 residues).

Palindrome: A segment of complementary duplex DNA that reads the same on both strands in the 5' to 3' direction.

Plasmid: A small, extrachromosomal, circular DNA that replicates independently from the chromosomal DNA.

Polymerase chain reaction (PCR): Cyclical denaturation of DNA, oligonucleotide priming, and elongation reactions that amplify target DNA.

Polymorphism: The occurrence of two or more alternative genotypes in a population that occur at a frequency greater than that which could be maintained by mutation alone.

Probe: A cloned or synthetic (by organic chemistry) DNA or RNA that can be labeled (with radioactivity or other indicator) and used to identify its complementary polynucleotide sequences by hybridization.

Proliferating Cell Nuclear Antigen (PCNA): An accessory protein for DNA polymerase δ.

Pseudogene: A segment of DNA that has evolved from a functional gene but has mutations that prohibit its function.

Recombinant DNA: A DNA molecule that is made by combining different segments of DNA.

Repetitive DNA: DNA sequences that are present in multiple copies in the genome.

Replication: DNA directed DNA synthesis.

Restriction enzyme: An endonuclease that recognizes and cleaves specific DNA sequences.

Restriction fragment length polymorphism (RFLP): A difference in DNA sequence between two individuals that alters the site of cleavage by restriction endonucleases.

Reverse transcriptase: An enzyme that catalyzes RNA-directed DNA synthesis.

Short interspersed nuclear element (SINE): Repeated sequences found in chromosomal DNA consisting of several to several hundred base pairs.

Single-strand conformation polymorphisms (SSCPs): Alternative forms of DNA with single nucleotide differences that can be detected by altered electrophoretic mobility of single-stranded DNA.

Single-stranded binding (SSB) protein: A protein that binds preferentially and cooperatively to single-stranded DNA.

Southern blot: Resolution of DNA molecules by electrophoresis and transfer and fixation to nitrocellulose or nylon sheets with retention of the relative position of the DNA polynucleotides. DNA is detected with a suitable probe following hybridization.

Splicing: The excision of RNA corresponding to an intron and the ligation of the ends corresponding to the exons.

Tandem: One following another, as in tandem repeats.

Telomere: The end of each chromosome arm.

Transcription: DNA-directed RNA synthesis.

Transfection: Introduction of DNA into a eukaryotic cell.

Transformation: Introduction of DNA into a bacterial cell; also, the conversion of a normal cell into a cancer cell.

Translation: RNA directed polypeptide synthesis.

Variable number of tandem repeats (VNTRs): A DNA polymorphism created by variations in the number of tandemly arranged, multiple copies of short DNA sequences.

Vector: A DNA molecule that is capable of replicating in a particular host, either alone or with an insert. Examples include plasmids, bacteriophage lambda, cosmids, and yeast artificial chromosomes (YACs).

Western blot: Electrophoresis of protein followed by transfer to a nitrocellulose matrix and identification by an antibody.

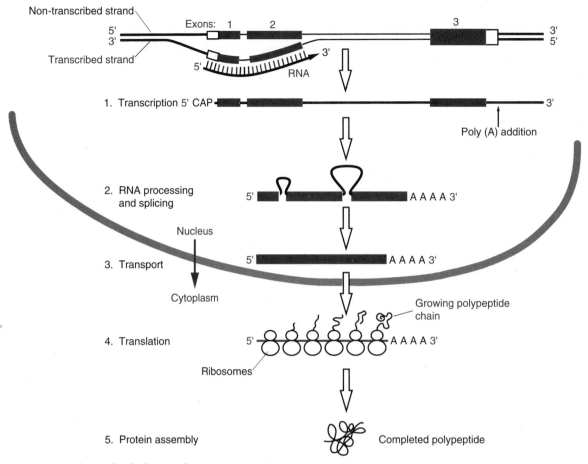

FIGURE 15–2. Steps in the transfer of information from DNA to RNA to protein. *This DNA contains a gene with three exons and two introns such as occurs for the α- or β-chains of hemoglobin. Exons are expressed in the mature RNA; introns are not expressed but are removed during RNA processing. The CAP is a modification of the 5′ end of RNA. Reproduced, with permission, from M.W. Thompson, R.R. McInnes, and H.F. Willard.* Thompson and Thompson Genetics in Medicine, *5th ed. Philadelphia, W.B. Saunders Company, 1991, p. 45.*

The polydeoxyribonucleotide chain has polarity. A 5′-hydroxyl group points toward the 5′ end, and the 3′-hydroxyl group points to the 3′ end; the 5′ → 3′ direction of a nucleic acid molecule is very important. Such polarity can be discerned even in a circular DNA lacking a free 5′- or 3′-hydroxyl terminus. To determine polarity, draw an arrow from the 5′-hydroxyl to the 3′-hydroxyl group of one deoxyribose residue, and this arrow points in the 5′ → 3′ direction (Figure 15–3).

DNA Double Helix

DNA exists as a duplex of two strands of poly-deoxyribonucleotide, except for a few bacterial viruses made up of a single-stranded DNA (or RNA) chain. The two strands exhibit **Watson-Crick complementary base pairing.** Cytosine forms three hydrogen bonds with guanine, and thymine forms two hydrogen bonds with adenine (Figure 15–4). *If the sequence of bases of one strand of DNA is known, the sequence of the complementary strand can be derived by complementary base-pairing rules* (PRINCIPLE 23 OF BIOCHEMISTRY). The complementary

chains of the double helix exhibit opposite polarity, and they are **antiparallel:** one strand progresses in the 5′ → 3′ direction, and the opposite strand progresses in the 3′ → 5′ direction.

Three forms of DNA have been identified by x-ray crystallography: A, B, and Z. The B form of DNA, which is the chief form in cells, is a right-handed double helix with 10 base pairs (bp) in each turn of the helix. The A form, which forms in low humidity in the laboratory, exists as a right-handed double helix with nearly 11 base pairs per turn. The Z form, which may occur physiologically in stretches of DNA that contain alternating purine and pyrimidines, is a left-handed double helix with 12 base pairs per turn. Its zigzag structure prompted its name. All three forms of DNA exhibit Watson-Crick complementary base pairing and are antiparallel.

In the B form, each base pair extends 0.34 nm along the axis. To determine the physiological length of DNA, multiply the number of base pairs by 0.34 nm. The haploid genome of humans consists of 2.9 billion base pairs corresponding to a length of 0.986 m (2.9×10^9 base pairs $\times$ 0.34 $\times$ 10^{-9} m/base pair = 0.986 m). The nucleus of each

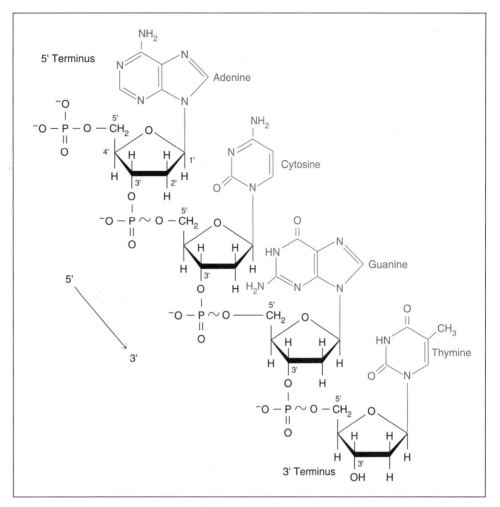

FIGURE 15–3. Covalent structure of a single DNA (deoxyribonucleic acid) strand. *The polarity of the molecule is shown in the 5' to 3' direction by the arrow.*

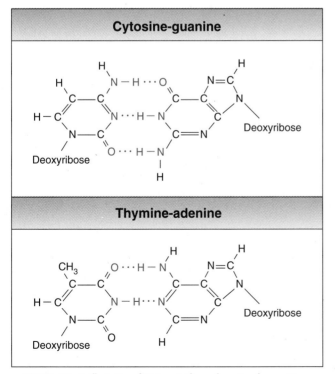

FIGURE 15–4. Illustration of Watson-Crick complementary base pairing.

cell contains about 2 m of diploid DNA. That the nucleus is 10 nm in diameter indicates that DNA is condensed.

The hydrophilic sugar-phosphate backbone of DNA occurs on the outside and the hydrophobic bases on the inside. The paired bases are stacked on one another. In the B form of DNA, the phosphodiester backbones of the two strands are separated by variable distances into **major** and **minor** grooves (Figure 15–5). The aromatic rings forming the bases interact by hydrophobic forces that stabilize the structure of the double helix. The planes of the bases are nearly perpendicular to the long axis of the helix.

The primary structure of DNA is its sequence of bases. For example, the structure in Figure 15–3 is abbreviated

5' ACGT 3'

If we know that this sequence occurs on one strand of the duplex, then we can immediately deduce the corresponding sequence of bases of its complementary strand by using the principles of Watson-Crick base pairing. Recall that the two chains exhibit opposite polarity.

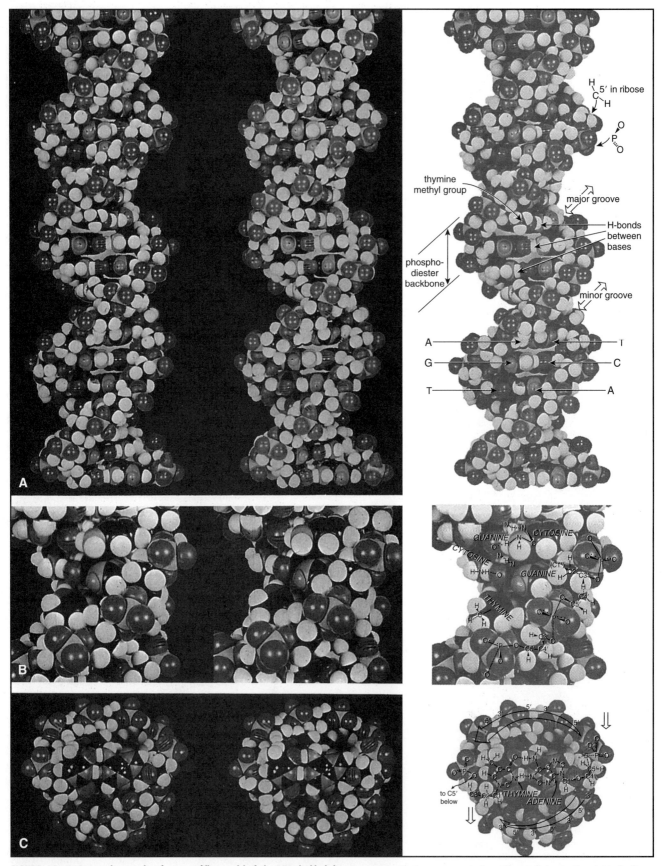

FIGURE 15–5. Stereo photographs of a space-filling model of the DNA double helix. *Significant features are noted on the models on the right.* A. *Two full turns of double helix.* B. *A close-up view of the major groove of DNA.* C. *DNA viewed from the end. To appreciate the stereo photos on the left without optical aids, bring the pictures close to the eyes, but stare into the distance through the blurred images until they fuse. Then withdraw the picture slowly, keeping the images fused, until focus is reached. Persistence and practice may be required, and some never learn the procedure. Reproduced, with permission, from R.B. McGilvery.* Biochemistry: A Functional Approach, *3rd ed. Philadelphia, W.B. Saunders and Company, 1983, pp. 54–55.*

5′ ACGT 3′   original sequence

3′ TGCA 5′   deduced complement

PRINCIPLE 28 OF BIOCHEMISTRY states that complementary base pairing is antiparallel. This includes DNA with DNA, DNA with RNA, and RNA with RNA.

Of paramount importance in explaining the predictable inheritance from one generation to another is the complementary nature of the DNA duplex and its mode of replication. Watson and Crick suggested that if the strands of a double helix separated and served as a template for the synthesis of their complement, two identical DNA duplexes would result. The daughter cells would then receive a complete set of genetic instructions. This is shown for a hypothetical case in Figure 15–6.

Bacterial Chromosomes

The DNA of a bacterial cell such as *E. coli* consists of a single duplex (double-stranded) molecule. The DNA or chromosome is a covalently closed circle. DNA from *E. coli* consists of many loops held together by proteins. The chromosome is also **supercoiled** or supertwisted. This procedure introduces negative supercoils and produces a more compact DNA form. Variations in supercoiling lead to the formation of isomers with different topologies, or **topoisomers.**

In contrast to those of human DNA, nearly all the nucleotides of *E. coli* have a genetic function. Bacteria also lack genes with intervening segments (introns) that are not expressed in the mature gene product. Bacteria additionally lack large "selfish" or "junk" DNA segments that have no apparent function. Bacterial DNA complexes with positively charged salts and polyamines such as putrescine and spermidine (Figure 13–37). Bacteria lack a prominent class of basic proteins called histones that play a structural role in forming chromatin in animal and plant cells.

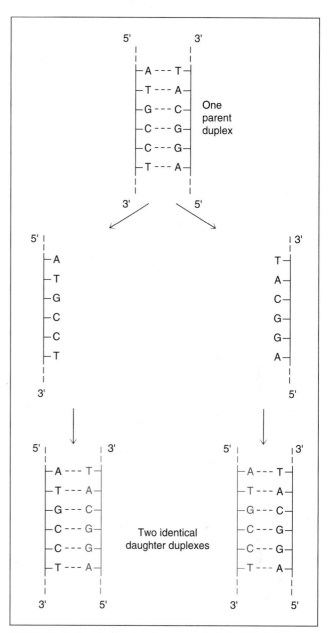

FIGURE 15–6. Template function of each strand of the DNA duplex. *DNA consists of complementary and antiparallel polynucleotides. This diagram shows that if the individual strands function as a template to form complementary strands, the result is two daughter duplexes that are exact replicas of the parent duplex.*

Human Chromosomes and Nucleosomes

Human cells contain 600 times as much DNA as *E. coli.* The entire **genome** of eukaryotic cells is divided among a number of chromosomes characteristic for each species. Human cells, for example, contain 46 chromosomes. Each chromosome contains a single DNA molecule. The sizes of the DNA associated with each human chromosome differ. Human chromosome 1 contains the largest DNA molecule (250×10^6 bp), and chromosome 23 contains the smallest DNA molecule (50×10^6 bp).

The **centimorgan** is the unit of genetic linkage and corresponds to the distance between two genetic loci where recombination occurs between them in 1% of meioses. The human linkage map contains about 3000 centimorgans of recombination units. Based upon a value of 2.9×10^9 base pairs per haploid genome, a centimorgan represents, on the average, 1 million base pairs. The centimorgan is a genetic unit, and the physical distance can vary from locus to locus.

Each chromosome contains many genes. The chromosome of *E. coli,* for example, is composed of about 3000 genes. The number of genes in humans is estimated to be between 50,000 and

100,000. In contrast to the circular DNA found in bacteria, the chromosomal DNA in humans is linear. Human DNA, similar to bacterial DNA, forms supercoils. Supercoiling of human DNA is not related to the formation of covalently closed circles but to the tethering of segments of DNA to nuclear matrix proteins. Each mitochondrion contains several copies of circular duplex DNA that is about 17,000 nucleotides in length. Human mitochondrial DNA codes for two dozen mitochondrial RNAs and about a dozen mitochondrial polypeptides.

Human DNA consists of various classes based on their copy number in a haploid genome. The main classes include nonrepetitive, or unique, DNA (75%) and repetitive DNA (25%). Unique DNA occurs once or only a few times at most. Genes for individual proteins such as trypsin occur in unique DNA. The majority of unique DNA, however, does not code for RNA or protein, and the function of this excess DNA is an enigma.

There are several types of **repetitive DNA** including interspersed and tandem sequences (Table 15–1). These repeated sequences are not exact copies of each other but vary by a few percent. **Satellite DNAs** are repeats that are arranged in tandem arrays (one behind another or head-to-tail). The name satellite refers to the resolution of this DNA from the main body of DNA by ultracentrifugation. At least six different satellite DNAs in humans can be distinguished. The distribution of satellite DNAs among the various chromosomes

differs, although each chromosome contains them at the centromere and telomeres.

There are several classes of interspersed repetitive DNA. **Minisatellite DNAs** consist of a variable number of tandem repeats, or **VNTRs** (from about 5 to 65 bp depending upon the particular repeat), and these are dispersed throughout the chromosome. VNTRs are used as genetic markers, as described later in this chapter.

Short interspersed nuclear elements (SINEs) consist of several to several hundred base pairs. The Alu family is one example of a short interspersed element (*Alu*I is a restriction enzyme that catalyzes the hydrolysis of DNA at specific sequences and is used in characterizing this family). The Alu sequence is transcribed into RNA and is postulated to have become added to the human genome by reverse transcription and reintegration. There are 500,000 copies of the Alu family in humans, and Alu constitutes 5% of the haploid genome. **Long interspersed nuclear elements (LINEs)** occur in unit lengths of 5000 to 7000 base pairs. An example of this second major family of dispersed repeats in humans is the L1 family. L1 elements constitute about 5% of the genome (Table 15–1).

Inverted repeats (fold-back DNA) are linear DNA sequences (from 100 to 1000 bases) that can form stem loops and complementary structures with just one strand of DNA (Figure 15–7). There are about 2 million inverted repeats in humans. Their function is unknown.

The function of only 10% of the DNA in the human genome is known. This includes the stretches of (1) unique DNA that encodes RNA, proteins, and genetic regulatory sequences and (2) repetitive DNA of the centromeres and telomeres. Centromeric and telomeric DNA probably plays a structural role in forming the chromosome. The function of the various repeats and noncoding unique DNA is a mystery.

Chromosomes are visible as discrete bodies during mitosis. In nondividing cells, the chromosome (chromatin) is distributed throughout the nucleus. **Euchromatin** is decondensed and light-staining during interphase. **Heterochromatin** is condensed and dark-staining during interphase. Heterochromatin, which is genetically inactive, is composed of the DNA that corresponds to centromeres, telomeres, and acrocentric short arms of chromosomes (Chapter 1). Chromatin in humans is about 35% DNA, 5% RNA, and 60% protein by mass.

The DNA of human cells is associated with basic proteins called **histones** that package DNA into nucleosomes. **Nucleosomes** occur about every 200 base pairs and resemble a string of pearls. Of these 200 base pairs, approximately 160 base pairs are wrapped around 8 molecules of histones of a specific type (two each of histones H2A, H2B, H3, and H4) as illustrated in Figure 15–8A. One molecule of histone H1 is associated with the DNA segments that link the nucleosomes together. Forma-

TABLE 15–1.	Properties of Human DNA and Human Genes
Total DNA per somatic cell	6.3 picograms*
Nuclear DNA	99.7% of total cellular DNA
Number of chromosomes	46 per diploid genome
Autosomes	44 per diploid genome
Sex chromosomes	2 per diploid genome
Nucleotides in the haploid genome	2.9×10^9 base pairs
Number of genes in the haploid genome	50,000–100,000
GC content	40%
AT content	60%
Length of DNA of haploid genome	0.986 m
Structure of DNA	Linear with histones and nucleosomes
Unique sequences	75% of total DNA
Repetitive sequences	25% of DNA
Interspersed	15% of DNA
SINEs (Alu)	5% of DNA
LINEs (L1)	5% of DNA
VNTRs	5% of DNA
Inverted repeats	
Tandem	10% of DNA
Mitochondrial DNA	0.3% of total cellular DNA
Size	≈17,000 bp (16,569 bp)
Genes	2 rRNA, 22 tRNAs, and 13 polypeptides
Structure	Circular without histones or nucleosomes

*1 picogram = 1×10^{-12} g.

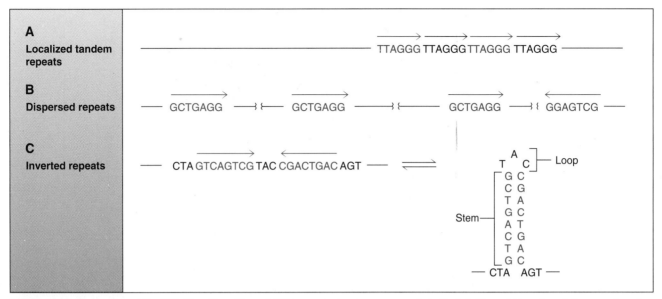

FIGURE 15–7. Classes of repetitive DNA. *The disposition of DNA repeats in chromosomes is indicated. The relative size of the repeat varies considerably. A. Tandem repeats. This example represents repeats that occur in telomeres (at the end of a chromosome). B. Dispersed repeats. These repeats occur throughout the chromosome and can have either orientation. C. Inverted repeats. The repeat sequence occurs in the complementary strand. These repeats can form a stem loop, as illustrated. Only one strand of the DNA is illustrated for simplicity, and the sizes are not to scale.*

tion of the **10-nm nucleosome fibers** achieves a packaging ratio (duplex length ÷ condensed length) of about 7. Nucleosomes form **30-nm filaments** or solenoids that contain six nucleosomes per turn (Figure 15–8B). This achieves a packing ratio of about 40. The 30-nm filaments form radial loops that contain about 100,000 bp of DNA, achieving a packaging ratio of about 1000. The coalescence of multiple loops about a center achieves a packaging ratio of 8000 or more, depending upon the particular chromosome. The packaging of DNA most likely provides constraints on its replication and transcription.

The primary structure of histones was conserved during evolution. The primary structure of pea seedling histone H4 varies from that of humans in only two of 103 amino acid positions. These alterations are conservative. A valine in the human sequence is replaced by isoleucine, and a lysine is replaced by arginine. Bacterial and mitochondrial DNA lack histones and nucleosome structure. Sperm contains **protamine,** a basic protein, in place of histones. The DNA in sperm is more highly condensed than that in somatic cells, and protamine binding to DNA produces this result.

REPLICATION OF DNA

Origin of Replication

Before considering the enzymology of DNA replication, let us examine some general aspects of DNA replication. Electron microscopy and autoradiography show that the two strands of the *E. coli*

DNA duplex do not separate completely before functioning as templates during the biosynthesis of the complementary strands as suggested in Figure 15–6. Rather, strand separation occurs while the complementary strands are synthesized. In *E. coli,* there is a single origin for DNA replication called **ori**C. Moreover, theta structures are seen by electron microscopy during replication. These structures are named for their resemblance to the Greek letter theta (Θ) shown in Figure 15–9. The Y-shaped portion of the theta structure is called the **replication fork.** Replication in bacteria occurs in both directions (clockwise and counterclockwise) and ends about 180 degrees from the origin.

In contrast to the single origin of replication in *E. coli,* there are about 40,000 initiation sites for the biosynthesis of the DNA in mammalian cells (Figure 15–10). Coalescence of the bubbles, or eyes, of replication occurs at the completion of synthesis of the daughter strands. If there were only one initiation site for the replication of each chromosome, it would take several months to synthesize the DNA of a human cell. Some blood cells and enterocytes of the gut replicate daily.

Semiconservative DNA Replication

The experiment performed by Matthew Meselson and Franklin Stahl proved that one strand of a parent duplex is associated with a newly synthesized strand in a daughter cell following replication. The Meselson-Stahl experiment is a cornerstone of DNA replication. *E. coli* cells were grown for several generations with $^{15}NH_4Cl$ as nitrogen

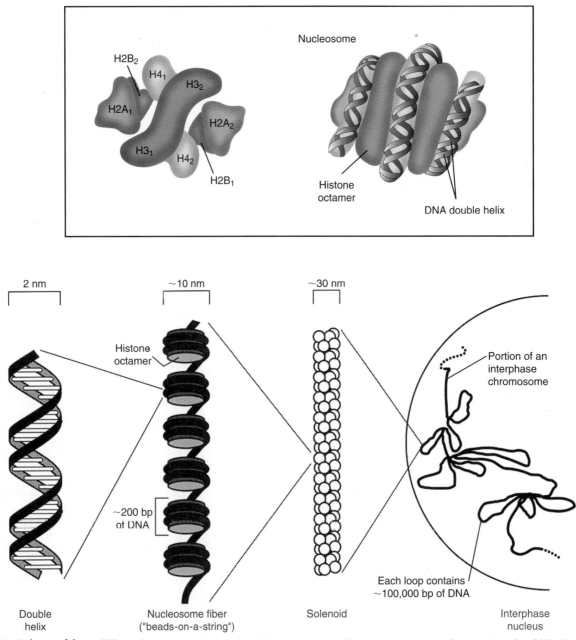

FIGURE 15-8. Packaging of human DNA. A. *Structural organization of the nucleosome. Nucleosomes consist of two turns of a DNA duplex coiled about a histone octamer. The histone octamer of the nucleosome consists of two molecules each of histone H2A, H2B, H3, and H4. Reproduced, with permission, from R. H. Garrett and C. M. Grisham.* Biochemistry. *Fort Worth, Saunders College Publishing, 1995, p. 194.* B. *Progressive levels of DNA condensation. Reproduced, with permission, from M. W. Thompson, R. R. McInnes, and H. F. Willard.* Thompson and Thompson Genetics in Medicine, *5th ed. Philadelphia, W.B. Saunders Company, 1991, p. 35.*

source. The resulting DNA had a greater buoyant density than that associated with growth in the usual isotope of nitrogen (^{14}N). After transfer of the cells from the growth medium with the heavy isotope to that of the light isotope, the DNA after one generation exhibited a density intermediate between light and heavy DNA. After two generations in the medium with the light isotope, half the DNA was of normal density and half was of the intermediate density (Figure 15–11). The results based on the observed densities are explained by **semiconservative replication;** one parent strand is distributed to each daughter duplex in combination with a newly synthesized strand. Moreover, the two strands of DNA must be synthesized with opposite polarity (Figure 15–12).

Enzymes of Replication

E. coli DNA Polymerases

PRIMER AND TEMPLATE STRANDS. The reactions that extend the polydeoxyribonucleotide

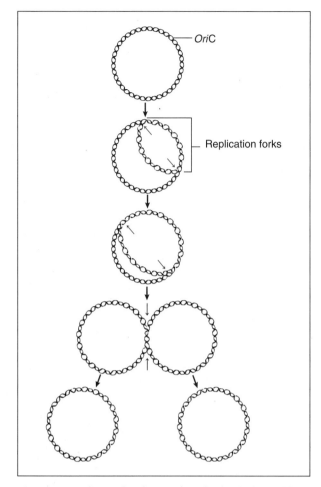

FIGURE 15-9. Bidirectional replication of circular E. coli DNA exhibiting a theta-structure intermediate. Supercoiling of the DNA is omitted in this diagram for the sake of clarity.

strands during DNA biosynthesis are catalyzed by **DNA polymerases,** a family of enzymes. *E. coli,* the organism for which the most thorough information is available, contains three DNA polymerases, which are called I, II and III, named in order of their historical discovery.

The primer and template strands participate in replication. Each DNA polymerase catalyzes the extension of an existing polynucleotide; this strand is called the **primer.** *All DNA polymerases studied thus far are unable to initiate DNA biosynthesis* de novo *and require a primer.* **Primase** catalyzes the formation of the initial primer. DNA polymerases require a template strand of DNA for activity. Physiologically, each strand of the parent DNA duplex serves as the template strand. In contrast to the primer, the **template** serves as a blueprint to direct the synthesis of the complementary strand. The template functions by directing the incorporation of nucleotides according to Watson-Crick base pairing. If cytosine is the base in the template strand, then guanine is incorporated into the primer strand at this position during the elongation reaction (Figure 15-13). Besides the primer and

template, four deoxyribonucleoside triphosphates serve as substrates. During elongation, the free 3'-hydroxyl group of the primer attacks the α-phosphorus atom (an electrophile) of the incoming deoxyribonucleoside triphosphate. Pyrophosphate is displaced, and a new phosphate ester forms.

BIOENERGETICS. The deoxyribonucleoside monophosphate group is activated by the covalent linkage with pyrophosphate. The two acid anhydride linkages in the deoxyribonucleoside triphosphates are energy rich. The elongation reaction (Figure 15-13) occurs without the loss of a high-energy bond (because the phosphodiester bonds of DNA are energy rich), and the process is isoergonic (PRINCIPLE 1 OF BIOENERGETICS). The hydrolysis of inorganic pyrophosphate is required to make the overall biosynthetic reaction exergonic. The structures in Figure 15-13 illustrate this information, and they also show that chain growth occurs in the $5' \rightarrow 3'$ direction. The 5' end of the primer strand is at the top of the figure, and the 3' end is at the bottom. *All DNA polymerases and all RNA polymerases catalyze chain growth in the $5' \rightarrow 3'$ direction* (PRINCIPLE 29 OF BIOCHEMISTRY). Because the duplex DNA is antiparallel, we will shortly consider how both strands function as templates physiologically. The polarity of the newly synthesized chain is opposite that of the template strand. Many polymerization reactions occur without the release of the enzyme from the template. Such a mechanism is termed **processive.**

PROOFREADING AND REPAIR. Besides strand elongation activity, DNA polymerases from *E. coli* possess nuclease activities. All three *E. coli* DNA polymerases possess $3' \rightarrow 5'$ exonuclease activity (Table 15-2). This activity proceeds in the direction opposite to that of biosynthesis (Figure 15-14). The 3'-terminal deoxyribonucleotide is removed by exergonic hydrolysis to yield the corresponding 5'-monophosphate and a shortened

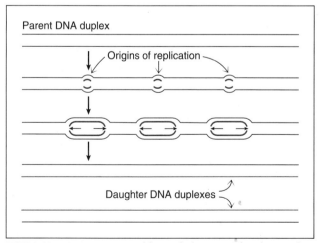

FIGURE 15-10. Human DNA exhibits multiple origins of replication along linear chromosomes. Only a very short segment of a chromosome is shown.

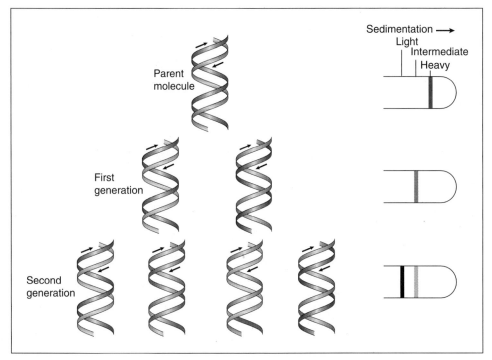

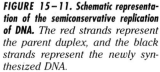

FIGURE 15–11. Schematic representation of the semiconservative replication of DNA. *The red strands represent the parent duplex, and the black strands represent the newly synthesized DNA.*

polymer (Figure 15–15). This activity serves as an **editing** or **proofreading** function to increase the fidelity with which the template strand is copied. If a base that does not form stable complementary hydrogen bonds is incorporated incorrectly, the resulting product is a poor substrate for polymerization but is a good substrate for $3' \rightarrow 5'$ exonuclease activity.

DNA polymerase I in *E. coli* possesses a $5' \rightarrow 3'$ exonuclease activity (Table 15–2). This is in the direction in which polymerization proceeds. This $5' \rightarrow 3'$ exonuclease activity may remove oligonucleotides of lengths of 10 or so from the 5' end of a nick in a duplex molecule. A **nick** refers to a discontinuity or break in the sugar-phosphate backbone. $5' \rightarrow 3'$ Exonuclease activity of DNA polymerase I plays a role in DNA repair and can remove RNA used as primer in the normal replication process. The activities of DNA polymerase I are especially suited for primer removal ($5' \rightarrow 3'$ exonuclease activity) and replacing the primer with DNA (DNA polymerase activity). The hydrolytic reactions of proofreading and repair are exergonic (PRINCIPLE 5 OF BIOENERGETICS) and are unidirectional. Selected properties of the DNA polymerases of *E. coli* are listed in Table 15–2.

Human DNA Polymerases

The enzymology of DNA polymerases from humans or other animals is not as well established as that of *E. coli* DNA polymerases. Human cells have at least five different DNA polymerases, designated α, β, γ, δ and ϵ (Table 15–2). DNA polymerase-γ is located in the mitochondrion; the four others are found in the nucleus. The five human DNA polymerases catalyze the same elongation reaction as the bacterial enzyme (Figure 15–13). Three human DNA polymerases (γ, δ, and ϵ) possess the $3' \rightarrow 5'$ exonuclease proofreading function (Table 15–2). In contrast to the bacterial polymerases, however, human DNA polymerases lack the $5' \rightarrow 3'$ exonuclease repair activity. Other proteins in the replication complex probably have the $5' \rightarrow 3'$ exonuclease activity.

DNA Ligase

To ligate means to tie together, and this is the function of DNA ligase. DNA ligase catalyzes the formation of a phosphodiester bond between a free

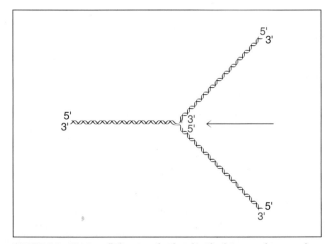

FIGURE 15–12. Overall direction of polynucleotide chain growth at a replication fork. *Because of the antiparallel nature of duplex DNA, movement of the replication fork in the indicated direction requires synthesis of strands of opposite polarity.*

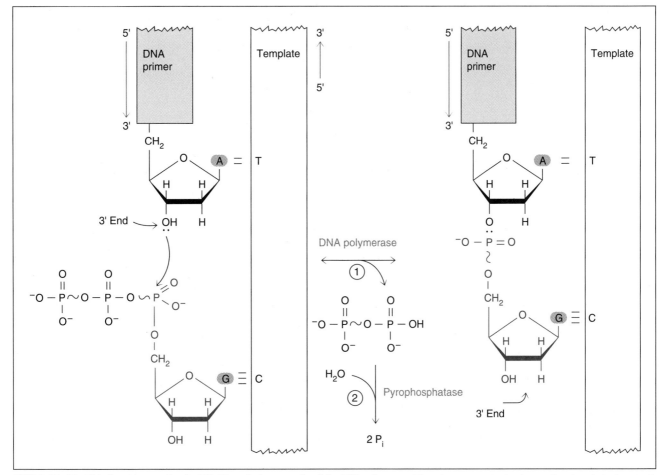

FIGURE 15–13. *The elongation reaction in DNA biosynthesis as catalyzed by DNA polymerase.* *This diagram, which shows the detailed chemical mechanism of deoxyribonucleotide addition during DNA biosynthesis, contains a deceptively large amount of information.*

TABLE 15–2.   Properties of DNA Polymerases

	DNA polymerases I, II, and III of *E. coli*		
	*pol I**	*pol II**	*pol III** (core)
Functions			
Polymerization: $5' \rightarrow 3'$	+	+	+
Proofreading exonuclease: $3' \rightarrow 5'$	+	+	+
Repair exonuclease: $5' \rightarrow 3'$	+	–	–

	Human DNA polymerases†				
	α	β	γ	δ	ε
Location	nucleus	nucleus	mitochondrion	nucleus	nucleus
Replication	yes	no	yes	yes	no
Repair	no	yes	no	no	yes
Associated functions					
$5' \rightarrow 3'$ polymerase	yes	yes	yes	yes	yes
$3' \rightarrow 5'$ exonuclease	no	no	yes	yes	yes
$5' \rightarrow 3'$ exonuclease	no	no	no	no	no
Primase	yes	no	no	no	no
Response to PCNA	no	no	no	yes	no
Strand synthesis	lagging	repair	both mitochondrial	leading	repair

*+ and – represent the presence and absence, respectively, of the property listed.
†Data from P.M.J. Burgers, R.A. Bambara, J.L. Campbell, L.M.S. Chang, K.M. Downey, U. Hübscher et al. Revised nomenclature for eukaryotic DNA polymerase. European Journal of Biochemistry 191:617, 1990.

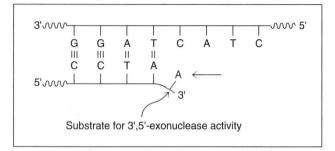

FIGURE 15–14. A mismatched base on the 3′ end of a growing DNA chain *is a substrate for the 3′-exonuclease proofreading function of* E. coli *DNA polymerases. Note that guanine (G) is the complementary base expected at this position.*

3′-hydroxyl group and 5′-phosphate group in DNA. The DNA duplex is said to possess a nick. Nicks occur during DNA replication and DNA repair. Nicks might also result from enzymatic endonuclease activity or nonenzymatic hydrolysis. The formation of a phosphodiester bond from such a reactant is endergonic and requires a source of chemical energy. ATP provides the energy for the reaction in humans; NAD⁺ provides the energy for the reaction in *E. coli.* The DNA ligase from a DNA bacterial virus of *E. coli* called T4 (type 4) uses ATP, as does the human enzyme.

Let us consider the mechanism for the human DNA ligase reaction (Figure 15–16). ATP reacts with the nicked DNA, and the adenylyl group is transferred to the 5′-phosphate to form an energy-rich acid anhydride bond. The 5′-phosphate group is thereby activated. The free 3′-hydroxyl group attacks the activated phosphate to close the nick by forming a phosphodiester bond. Although the details concerning the DNA ligase reactions are often difficult to understand on first encounter, the straightforward principles of bioenergetics aid in comprehension. Activation of the free 5′-phosphate of the nicked DNA as the pyrophosphate acid anhydride is functionally isoergonic (PRINCIPLE 1 OF BIOENERGETICS). The second step also occurs with the conservation of the number of high-energy bonds. Hydrolysis of pyrophosphate is exergonic (PRINCIPLE 5 OF BIOENERGETICS) and pulls the overall

reaction forward. Two high-energy bonds are required for the conversion of AMP to ATP, and two high-energy bonds are needed for the DNA ligase reaction. Activation of the 5′ phosphate requires one high-energy bond, and the hydrolysis of pyrophosphate consumes the second high-energy bond. The DNA ligase reaction of *E. coli* is similar except that NAD⁺ is the adenylate donor. The pyrophosphate bond in NAD⁺ is energy rich, which allows NAD⁺ to participate in this process.

DNA Topoisomerases

DNA topoisomerases are enzymes that catalyze the interconversion of topological isomers of DNA. These reactions include changes in the superhelical state of DNA. Topology refers to the degree and nature of supercoiling. *Naturally occurring DNA exists with negative supercoils.* A structure with **negative supercoils** exhibits a counterclockwise twist (Figure 15–17). All topological interconversions require the transient breakage and rejoining of the deoxyribose-phosphate backbone. DNA topoisomerases are targets for anticancer agents in humans (Chapter 21), and bacterial topoisomerases are targets for antibiotics.

For every 10 deoxyribonucleotides added during replication, the parental double helix must make one complete turn around its axis. In an *E. coli* cell where the rate of synthesis is 50,000 nucleotides per minute, each strand at each growing replication fork would have to rotate 5000 times per minute. To avoid this topological dilemma, **DNA topoisomerases** alter the superhelical structure of duplex DNA to obviate the need for rotation of the entire strand. DNA topoisomerases may play a role in the regulation of transcription (DNA-directed RNA synthesis) and in condensing or decondensing DNA.

There are two general classes of topoisomerase, designated I and II. **Topoisomerase I** makes a nick in only *one* strand and allows the intact strand to pass through the nick, which is then closed. **Topoisomerase II** makes a nick in *two* strands and allows a duplex segment of DNA to pass through

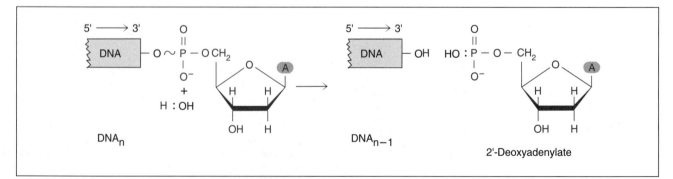

FIGURE 15–15. Hydrolytic cleavage of the deoxyribonucleoside monophosphate *by the 3′-exonuclease activity of DNA polymerase.*

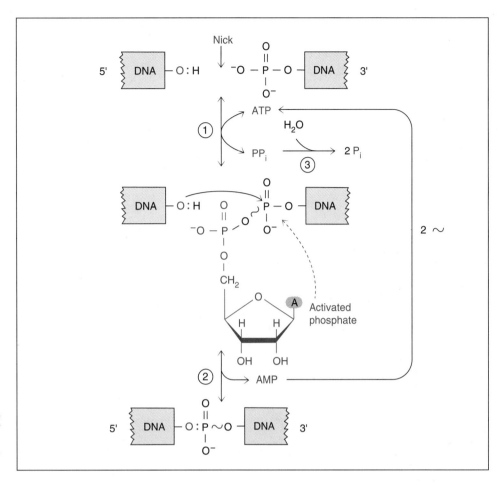

FIGURE 15–16. Steps in the human DNA ligase reaction. *Reactions 1 and 2 are catalyzed by DNA ligase. Step 3 is catalyzed by an independent pyrophosphatase.*

the open segment. The action of topoisomerase I (Topo I) is to decrease the linking number by one, and the action of topoisomerase II (Topo II) is to decrease the linking number by two (Figure 15–17). The **linking number** of DNA, which can vary in topological isomers, is the number of times that one strand of DNA winds around the other in the right-handed direction. One action of topoisomerase I and II is to relax negative supercoils during replication. Nicking and resealing of the duplex are required to change the supercoiling of DNA.

TYPE I TOPOISOMERASES. Topoisomerase I catalyzes the cleavage of one strand of DNA to form a nick through which the complementary strand passes; the enzyme then rejoins the single strand (Figure 15–18). An active site tyrosyl hydroxyl group of topoisomerase I forms a covalent phosphodiester bond with one strand of DNA. This adduct consists of a high-energy phosphodiester linkage involving an enzymic tyrosine and a hydroxyl group of a deoxyribonucleotide (Figure 15–19). The structures of the intermediates differ in humans and bacteria. (A 3′-phosphate linkage occurs in humans, and a 5′-phosphate linkage occurs in bacteria). The bioenergetics and principles of the reactions, however, are similar. Phosphotyrosine bonds are energy rich with a standard

free energy of hydrolysis of about −40 kJ per mole. Following cleavage of the phosphodiester bond of one strand, the intact strand passes through the nick (Figure 15–18). Afterward, the free hydroxyl group attacks the phosphorus atom of the enzyme-substrate covalent intermediate and displaces the enzyme's tyrosyl group and re-forms a phosphodiester bond. No additional chemical energy is required because the covalent bond between the enzymic tyrosine and 5′-phosphate forms with the retention of activation. Topoisomerase I relieves the strain in negatively supercoiled DNA.

TYPE II TOPOISOMERASES. Human topoisomerase II can relax both negative and positive supercoils in an ATP-dependent process. The precise role that ATP plays in the overall reaction is not yet understood. **DNA gyrase,** a bacterial type II topoisomerase that functions ahead of the replication fork, introduces negative supercoils into DNA molecules in an ATP-dependent fashion. The introduction of negative supercoils relieves positive supertwisting that occurs at the replication fork. Human and bacterial topoisomerase II enzymes alter the DNA linking number by two. This occurs because two strands of a duplex are broken and an intact region of DNA passes through the break. Selected properties of human and bacterial DNA topoisomerases are listed in Table 15–3.

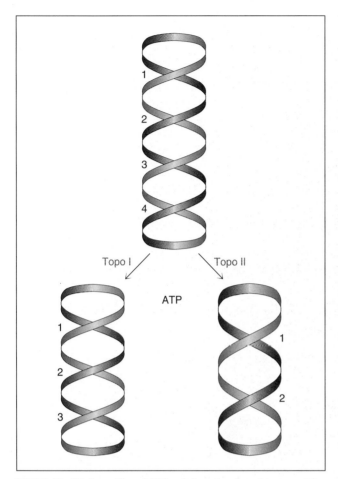

FIGURE 15–17. Supercoiling of DNA and the action of topoisomerases. *The number of supercoils is indicated.*

▶ Topoisomerase activities are targets for antibiotics. **Nalidixic acid** and **norfloxacin** are drugs used in the treatment of urinary tract infections. These compounds inhibit bacterial DNA gyrase, a type II topoisomerase, by inhibiting the strand-cutting reaction. Human type II topoisomerase is much less sensitive to the action of these two drugs. **Etoposide** and **teniposide,** which are derived from the mandrake plant, inhibit human topoisomerase II. These agents are used in the treatment of several neoplastic diseases including lymphomas, Kaposi sarcoma, and cancers of the testis, lung, and breast (Table 21–7). ◀

DNA Replication in *E. coli*

Protein Components

Many proteins and activities are required for DNA replication. Single-stranded binding **(SSB)** proteins bind preferentially and cooperatively to single strands of DNA and thereby stabilize the single-stranded state. Cooperative binding means that second and subsequent proteins bind more readily to the nucleic acid than does the first protein. Pro-

cesses that exhibit positive cooperativity exhibit sigmoid-shaped action curves and not hyperbolic curves. **Helicase** possesses ATPase activity and opens the helix in the replication fork.

DNA polymerases lack the ability to initiate DNA biosynthesis. An essential protein called **primase** initiates the synthesis of short ($\approx$5 nucleotides) strands of RNA; this RNA is complementary to DNA and serves as a primer for deoxyribonucleotide elongation reactions (Figure 15–20). Primase initiates the synthesis of both the leading and lagging strands of DNA (Figure 15–21). Many initiation events for lagging strand biosynthesis are required. The first two nucleotides of the primer are ribonucleotides. Subsequent nucleotides may be either ribo- or deoxyribonucleotides. Ribonucleoside triphosphates are substrates for the first two reactions, and ribo- or deoxyribonucleoside triphosphates are substrates for the remaining reactions. The special priming function prompted the name primase as opposed to RNA polymerase (Chapter 16). Chain growth is the $5' \rightarrow 3'$ direction, and PP_i is a product. Besides helicase, several other proteins play a preparatory role in setting the stage for primase activity. The protein components collectively form a **primasome.**

DNA gyrase, a topoisomerase II, catalyzes the ATP-dependent formation of negatively supertwisted DNA ahead of the replication fork. Negative supercoiling promotes strand separation and formation of the replication fork. Helicase mediates an energy-dependent strand separation to initiate fork formation. The unwinding of the double helix by helicase consumes about two ATP molecules per base pair (excluding the ATP required by DNA gy-

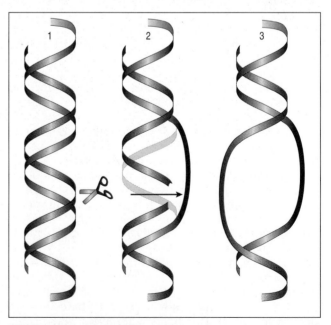

FIGURE 15–18. Action of DNA topoisomerase I. *This enzyme cleaves one strand of DNA, passes the complementary strand through the discontinuity, and reseals the strand. This process decreases the linking number by one.*

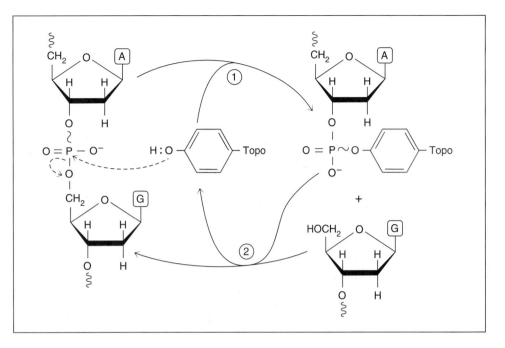

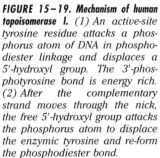

FIGURE 15–19. Mechanism of human topoisomerase I. *(1) An active-site tyrosine residue attacks a phosphorus atom of DNA in phosphodiester linkage and displaces a 5'-hydroxyl group. The 3'-phosphotyrosine bond is energy rich. (2) After the complementary strand moves through the nick, the free 5'-hydroxyl group attacks the phosphorus atom to displace the enzymic tyrosine and re-form the phosphodiester bond.*

rase). This represents a substantial energy requirement. Other major activities in replication include DNA polymerase III, DNA polymerase I, and DNA ligase.

Replication of the Leading and Lagging Strands

Let us examine the polarity of DNA strands at the replication fork. Replication proceeds into the base of the fork. Recall, however, that the two strands of DNA have opposite polarity. This means that one chain is growing in the $5' \rightarrow 3'$ direction and the opposite is apparently growing in the $3' \rightarrow 5'$ direction. DNA polymerase enzymes, however, catalyze chain growth exclusively in the $5' \rightarrow 3'$ direction. The finding of short DNA segments during replication suggests that chain

growth in the overall $3' \rightarrow 5'$ direction occurs discontinuously. These short (100 to 1000 nucleotides) DNA fragments are called **Okazaki fragments** in honor of their discoverers, R. Okazaki and T. Okazaki. Although overall chain growth occurs into the base of the fork, synthesis of the lagging strand occurs discontinuously in the opposite direction but with exclusive $5' \rightarrow 3'$ polarity (Figure 15–21).

The mechanism for the biosynthesis of the lagging strand is more difficult to understand when compared to that of the leading strand because of discontinuous synthesis (Figure 15–22). Primase initiates the biosynthesis of the lagging strand. The direction of synthesis on the lagging strand is away from the fork. DNA polymerase III catalyzes the extension of the primer. Meanwhile, synthesis along the leading strand proceeds another few hundred residues. Primase reinitiates on the newly

TABLE 15–3.   Comparison of Human and Bacterial Topoisomerases

Function	Human		Bacterial	
	Topo I	*Topo II*	*Topo I*	*Topo II*
Alter linking number by 1	+	−	+	−
Alter linking number by 2	−	+	−	+
Generate negative supercoils in an ATP-dependent process	−	−	−	+
Support replication fork movement	+	+	−	+
Aid RNA elongation by RNA polymerase	+	+	+	+
Active in dividing cells	−	+	+	+
Sensitive to nalidixic acid and norfloxacin	−	−	−	+
Sensitive to etoposide and teniposide	−	+	−	−

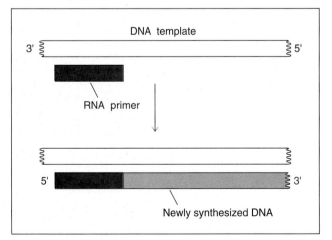

FIGURE 15–20. RNA primer function during replication.

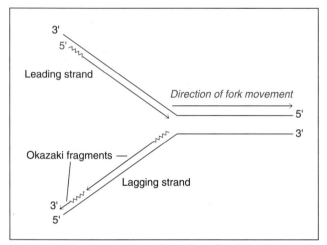

FIGURE 15–21. Primase mediates the synthesis of multiple primers on the lagging strand at the replication fork. Note that polymerization reactions on both leading and lagging strands occur in the 5' to 3' direction, and this is antiparallel to the template strand.

opened lagging strand, and DNA polymerase III extends the polymer. The DNA strand synthesized by polymerase III extends up to the primer of the previously synthesized segment on the lagging strand. The primer is excised by the 5' → 3' exonuclease activity provided by DNA polymerase I (DNA polymerase III lacks this activity). DNA polymerase I fills in the gap, and DNA ligase seals the nick. The process is repeated many times to complete the synthesis of the lagging strand. A summary of the replication process in *E. coli* is shown in Figure 15–23.

DNA Replication in Humans

The replication of human chromosomes has not been examined as extensively as that described here for *E. coli* because of the greater complexity of the cell. Overall, the process is similar. DNA polymerases (Table 15–2), DNA topoisomerases I and II, DNA helicase, SSB protein, and DNA ligase activities have been described in human cells. Human chromosomes possess multiple origins of replication about every 150 kb (Figure 15–10), in contrast to bacteria.

The DNA polymerase α complex initiates both leading and lagging strand biosynthesis with its associated primase activity. DNA polymerase α is responsible for lagging strand biosynthesis, and DNA polymerase δ and proliferating cell nuclear antigen (PCNA) are responsible for leading strand biosynthesis (Figure 15–24). PCNA, an accessory protein, is necessary for DNA polymerase δ activity. Polymerases β and ϵ function in nuclear repair synthesis, and polymerase γ carries out replication within the mitochondrion. Histones that were present in the parental cell are distributed to the leading strand. Newly synthesized histones combine with the lagging strand to form nucleosomes.

The ends of linear chromosomes (telomeres) are replicated by a novel mechanism. Telomeric DNA in humans ends with tandem repeats of TTAGGG, and the 3' end of each strand of the duplex has a short segment that lacks a complement. **Telomerase,** which contains RNA with a segment that is complementary to the tandem repeat, catalyzes the RNA template-dependent addition of multiple tandem repeats to the 3' end of telomeric DNA from deoxyribonucleoside triphosphates. The newly formed 3' end serves as template for the synthesis of DNA that will extend to the 5' end of the opposite strand by the lagging strand synthesis mechanism. ▶ Increased telomere length and telomerase activity can occur in neoplastic cells. Decreased telomere length is associated with aging. ◀

Energy Requirements for DNA Replication

We now consider the energetic costs of DNA replication from deoxyribonucleoside triphosphates. Two high-energy bonds are required to separate each base pair by the helicase in *E. coli;* this represents one high-energy bond per deoxyribonucleotide incorporated. A similar requirement for human cells seems likely. Two high-energy bonds are used for each deoxyribonucleoside triphosphate substrate incorporated because of the pyrophosphate split as illustrated in the following equations:

$$\text{n dNTP} \rightleftharpoons (\text{dNMP})_n + \text{nPP}_i \qquad (15.1)$$

$$\text{n PP}_i + \text{n H}_2\text{O} \rightarrow 2\text{n P}_i \qquad (15.2)$$

Based only on the helicase and the DNA polymerase reactions, three high-energy bonds are the minimum requirement for the incorporation of each deoxyribonucleotide. This excludes primer biosynthesis (two energy-rich bonds per nucleotide), DNA ligase activity (two high-energy bonds per reaction), and topoisomerase activity, making the energy requirements greater. Additional chemical energy is expended in proofreading to increase the fidelity of replication and to avoid production of mutations. The phosphodiester linkages in DNA are of the high-energy variety. The expenditure of more than three high-energy bonds for the synthesis of each phosphodiester bond ensures that replication is exergonic.

DNA Repair

Lesions of DNA

Each human cell loses more than 10,000 bases per day, and mechanisms exist for repairing damages in DNA resulting from spontaneous or environmental chemical or physical agents. Let us consider the types of changes that occur in the genome. Ultraviolet light (a physical agent) pro-

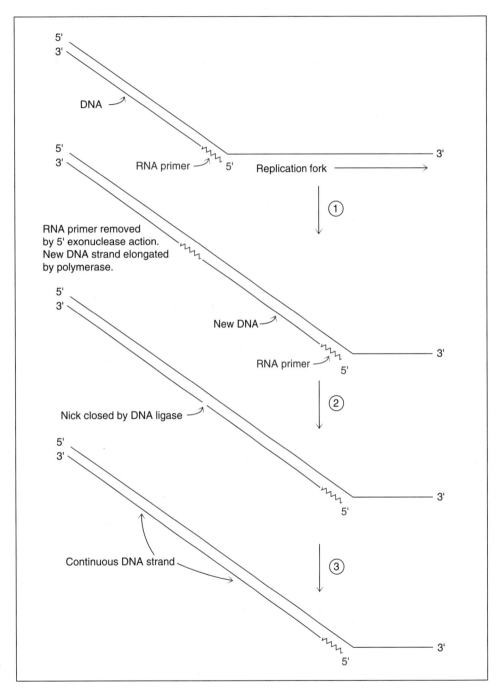

FIGURE 15–22. Discontinuous synthesis of the lagging strand.

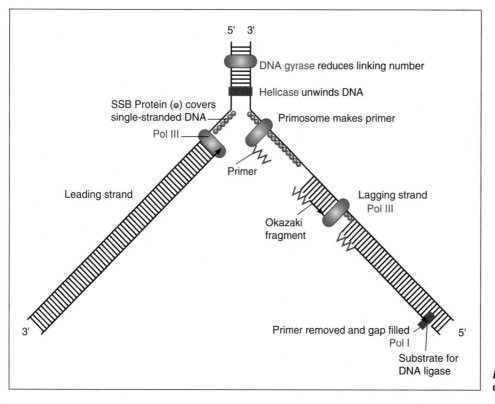

5' 3'

DNA gyrase reduces linking number

Helicase unwinds DNA

SSB Protein (○) covers
single-stranded DNA

Primosome makes primer

Pol III

Primer

Leading strand

Lagging strand
Pol III

Okazaki
fragment

3'

Primer removed and gap filled
Pol I

5'

Substitute for
DNA ligase

FIGURE 15–23. Activities at the E. coli replication fork.

motes the formation of covalent bonds between adjacent thymine bases to yield thymine dimers (Figure 15–25). Moreover, spontaneous (nonenzymatic) hydrolysis leads to the removal of adenine and guanine bases to form apurinic DNA. Spontaneous hydrolysis of the amino group of cytosine yields uracil residues. If this alteration were to persist, a C = G base pair would be converted to a T = A base pair in one of the granddaughter cells. The deamination of 5-methylcytosine results in thymine formation. Deamination occurs normally in DNA, but base-pairing is abnormal and can be repaired. X rays, γ-rays, and chemical mutagens alter DNA. The accumulation of many such changes would be deleterious to progeny cells.

Repair Mechanisms

Let us consider the **nucleotide excision repair** mechanism that removes lesions from DNA including those resulting from thymine dimer formation. The four steps in this process include (1) hydrolysis of the affected strand of the 5' side of the lesion by **excinuclease** (excision endonuclease), (2) hydrolysis on the 3' side by excinuclease to give an oligonucleotide (≈ 30 residues) containing the lesion, (3) DNA synthesis, using the 3'-hydroxyl group produced by excinuclease as primer, by repair polymerase, and (4) DNA ligation to seal the nick (Figure 15–26). In **base excision repair**, DNA glycosylases catalyze the hydrolytic removal of inappropriate bases. The abasic sugar is then removed by hydrolyses catalyzed by endonucleases,

and the gap is repaired by DNA polymerase and ligase activities.

A second mechanism for the elimination of thymine dimers is **photolyase repair.** Bacteria and many animals (but apparently not humans) possess photoreactivating enzymes called DNA photolyases that catalyze the light-dependent cleavage of the cyclobutane bonds linking thymine dimers.

The bioenergetics of DNA repair is straightforward. The hydrolytic excision of the defective base and the hydrolysis and excision of the small segments of DNA are exergonic (PRINCIPLE 5 OF BIOENERGETICS). Extension of the polynucleotide chain is accompanied by the displacement of inorganic pyrophosphate; its hydrolysis is necessary to promote the polymerization process. Closing the nick requires the expenditure of two high-energy bonds.

▶ The cell makes an appreciable investment in

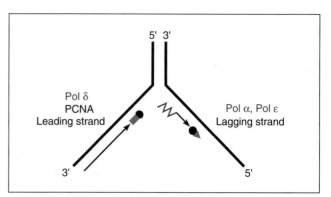

5' 3'

Pol δ
PCNA
Leading strand

Pol α, Pol ε
Lagging strand

3'

5'

FIGURE 15–24. Polymerase activities at the human replication fork.

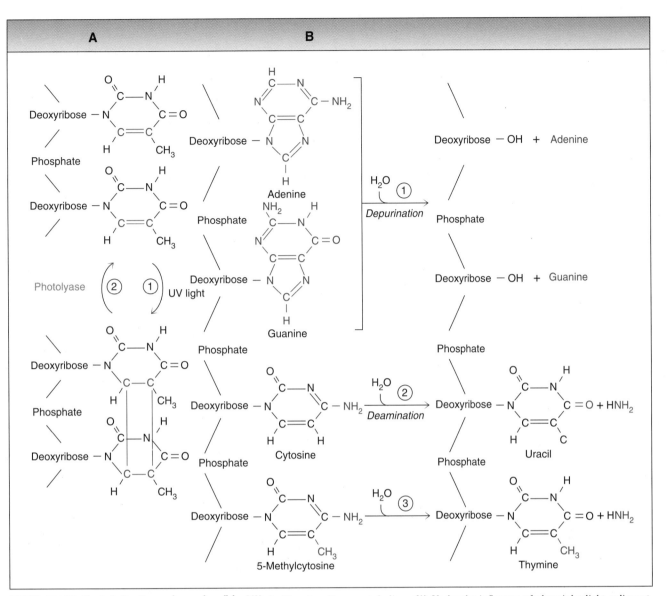

FIGURE 15–25. Chemical alterations undergone by cellular DNA. A. *Thymine dimer metabolism. (1) Under the influence of ultraviolet light, adjacent thymine bases undergo photoactivated dimerization, resulting in the formation of a covalent cyclobutane ring that fuses two thymine residues together. (2) Photolyase catalyzes the conversion of thymine dimers to thymine. B. Nonenzymatic hydrolysis of DNA. (1) The N-glycosidic linkage between purine bases and deoxyribose undergoes hydrolysis to form the free base and an apurinic site on the DNA. (2) Cytosine residues undergo nonenzymatic hydrolyses to yield uracil residues and ammonia. (3) Hydrolysis of 5-methylcytosine yields thymine.*

the production of DNA repair enzymes. Analysis of humans with a disorder called **xeroderma pigmentosum** suggests that 10 proteins may be required for the excision of damaged bases in DNA by a single repair system. Xeroderma pigmentosum is a rare autosomal recessive disease characterized by defective repair of thymine dimers. Affected individuals are prone to develop multiple skin cancers. The reduced ability to repair DNA leads to somatic mutations, some of which result in malignant transformation. ◄

Molecular Basis of Mutations

A mutation is a permanent heritable change in the sequence of genomic DNA. Mutations underlie

the normal variation in a population but can also result in disease. The rate of mutation in humans and in bacteria is about 1 nucleotide change per 10^9 nucleotides incorporated. The frequency of polymorphisms or differences in the sequence of human DNAs is about 1 in every 500 nucleotides (about 5.8 million differences per haploid genome). We consider here the nature of different mutations and their underlying mechanisms. When we consider examples of specific genetic diseases such as cystic fibrosis later in this chapter, we will see that identical phenotypes (observable traits) can be caused by different mutations. This new way of thinking about heritable diseases is the result of recent technical developments that permit elucidation of the nature of these mutants.

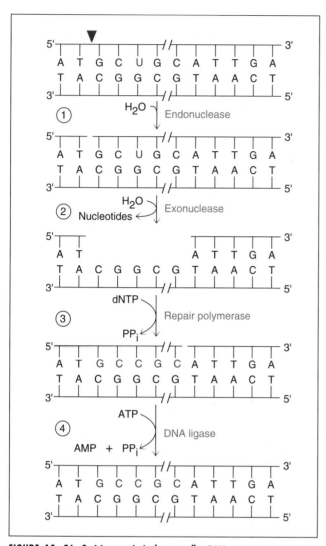

FIGURE 15–26. Excision repair in human cells. *DNA excinuclease catalyzes the hydrolysis on the 5' side and 3' side of a damaged DNA strand to liberate an oligonucleotide containing about 30 bases. DNA polymerase-β adds deoxyribonucleotides to the free 3'-hydroxyl group. DNA ligase then seals the nick. Each reaction in excision repair is exergonic.*

Nucleotide Substitutions

The simplest type of mutation involves a single base change. Substitution of one purine for another or one pyrimidine for another is called a **transition.** This involves an A ↔ G change or a C ↔ T change. The conversion of a purine to a pyrimidine or a pyrimidine to a purine (A or G ↔ C or T) is called a **transversion.** There are twice as many possible transversions as transitions. If all mutations were random, we would expect to see more transversions than transitions. The number of transitions exceeds the number of transversions, indicating that mutations are nonrandom.

A major form of modification of human DNA involves the conversion of cytosine to 5-methylcytosine in the sequence 5'-CG-3'. Spontaneous hydrolysis of the amino group of 5-methylcytosine yields thymine (Figure 15–25B). This is a transition (the

substitution of one pyrimidine for another). More than 30% of all single nucleotide substitutions that have been detected in genetic diseases are of this type. CG represents a "hot spot" for genetic mutation.

Nucleotide substitutions can have various effects on the phenotype. Perhaps the most common effect, called a **missense mutation,** involves the substitution of one amino acid in the encoded protein for another amino acid. This is the basis for sickle cell anemia, where the mutation involves an A → T transversion. A **nonsense mutation** involves formation of one of the three stop codons from a codon that corresponds to an amino acid, and this nucleotide substitution results in the formation of a truncated polypeptide chain. A **sense mutation** involves the conversion of a stop codon to one encoding an amino acid and leads to an elongated polypeptide chain. Each of the three types of nucleotide substitution are observed in the production of mutant hemoglobins.

We note in Figure 15–2 that messenger RNA undergoes splicing reactions in which a segment of RNA is removed and the two ends are covalently linked to form the mature polynucleotide. Point mutations can influence the splicing reaction in two ways. Mutations at normal donor (5') or acceptor (3') sites can interfere with physiological splicing. ▶ The failure to remove a segment of RNA occurs in phenylketonuria, Tay-Sachs disease, hemophilia B, and β-thalassemia (a hemoglobinopathy). A second class of splicing mutation involves the creation of a nonphysiological donor or acceptor site that competes with the physiological donor or acceptor site during the splicing reaction. These mutations occur in β-thalassemia. ◀

Deletions and Insertions

Deletions and insertions can involve one, a few, or many nucleotides. The insertion or deletion of one or two nucleotides results in a **frameshift mutation.** The genetic code is a triplet, and three nucleotides encode each amino acid. The change in the number of nucleotides in multiples of three does not change the reading frame of messenger RNA, and the amino acid sequence of the mutant is the same as the wild type except for the addition of one or more amino acids (insertion) or the omission of one or more amino acids (deletion). The change in the number of nucleotides that differs from multiples of three results in a completely unrelated amino acid sequence distal to the locus of the mutation. ▶ A three-base-pair deletion occurs in the most common form of cystic fibrosis. This results in a protein that is missing a single amino acid, the phenylalanine at position 508. ◀

Deletions and duplications are caused by recombination of highly similar or identical DNA sequences. These can involve repetitive DNA sequences, or they can occur in families such as the

α-globin gene family and lead to the production of α-thalassemia (Figure 24–10). When these related sequences are located in a head-to-tail fashion in the same chromosomal region, they can misalign and pair out of register in meiosis. Recombination occurring between mispaired chromosomes or sister chromatids can lead to DNA deletion, duplication, or translocation.

METHODS OF MOLECULAR BIOLOGY

Great strides in genetic chemistry have been achieved in recent years and continue at a rapid pace. These developments have led to new methods of diagnosis, better understanding of diseases, and the production of scarce human proteins as pharmaceuticals. The purpose of this section is to provide the background necessary to understand these techniques. The glossary (Box 15–1) contains many terms of molecular biology that are used in this and subsequent chapters. Several enzymes noted previously in this chapter have found practical use in molecular biology, and these are listed for general reference in Table 15–4.

It is now possible to prepare a considerable amount of DNA (hundreds of micrograms) that corresponds to a human gene. This process is called **gene cloning.** The base sequence of DNA can be determined, and the primary sequence of the protein corresponding to a gene can be deduced by the genetic code (Table 17–1). The nature of the regulation of the gene by specific DNA sequences can be determined by deleting portions of the DNA or by creating mutations (**site-directed mutagenesis**) by genetic engineering. Mutations can be produced with oligonucleotides containing the mutant sequence; these oligonucleotides are synthesized chemically in computer-controlled machines (oligonucleotide synthesizers). Mutations can be introduced by using these nucleotides as primers for DNA polymerase.

Recombinant DNA can be prepared to produce functional molecules with new properties. A gene can be inserted downstream from regulatory elements that will drive the synthesis of RNA (and protein) so that a cell (bacteria, yeast, or animal) can be made to express proteins that are not normally produced. Sometimes **reporter genes** are attached to regulatory genetic elements to monitor alterations of gene expression. Reporter genes code for proteins that can be measured conveniently and are not normally present in the recipient cell.

Mutant genes can be isolated and studied. The gene for cystic fibrosis, for example, was cloned before the nature of the protein product was known, an example of positional cloning. The cystic fibrosis gene corresponds to an integral membrane protein that functions in anion transport (Figure 22–12). After a gene is cloned, the chromosomal location can be determined. After the molecular basis of mutation is discovered, diagnostic procedures can often be developed that permit prenatal diagnosis. A description of some of the methods that made these advances possible is given in the remainder of this chapter.

Bacterial Restriction-Modification Systems

Enzymes

The general categories of restriction-modification systems in bacteria are of the type I and type II classes. Type II restriction endonucleases are a family of bacterial enzymes that catalyze the hydrolysis of DNA at specific sequences. These enzymes are important in the analysis and manipulation of DNA. They are one arm of a physiological bacterial restriction-modification system that was adapted for use in the laboratory.

The restriction-modification system allows bacteria to recognize and destroy exogenous, or "foreign," DNAs. Exogenous DNA can be introduced into bacterial cells by conjugation with other bacteria, by viral transduction, and by transformation with free DNA. The modification process involves the methylation of the amino group of particular

---

TABLE 15–4.   Enzymes Used in Molecular Biology

Enzyme	Reaction Catalyzed	Use
E. coli DNA polymerase I	Synthesizes duplex DNA using a template and primer	Elongates DNA for sequencing, fills gaps
Klenow fragment of DNA polymerase I	Synthesizes duplex DNA using a template and primer	Elongates DNA for sequencing, lacks $5' \rightarrow 3'$ exonuclease activity
Pfu polymerase	Catalyzes DNA elongation	Amplifies DNA by PCR
Taq polymerase	Catalyzes DNA elongation	Amplifies DNA by PCR
T4 DNA ligase	Eliminates nicks from duplex DNA; combines synthetic oligonucleotides to the ends of DNA fragments by blunt-end ligation	Combines complementary ends of DNA molecules
E. coli alkaline phosphatase	Hydrolyzes 5' or 3'-phosphates from DNA or RNA	Creates substrate for radiolabeling molecule; prevents self-ligation of vectors
Polynucleotide kinase	ATP phosphorylates DNA or RNA	Radiolabels DNA or RNA
Reverse transcriptase	Synthesizes DNA from an RNA template	Synthesizes cDNA from RNA
S1 nuclease	Degrades single-stranded DNA or RNA	Removes hairpin loop during synthesis of cDNA
Terminal transferase	Adds nucleotides to the 3' end of DNA	Creates polynucleotide tails on DNA

adenine or cytosine residues of endogenous DNA. The modification involves a reaction of the energy-rich methyl donor, *S*-adenosylmethionine, with DNA to form the energy-poor *N*-methyl derivative. Endogenous DNA is methylated by the modification enzymes, and this serves to mark the DNA as native. Methylated DNA is not a substrate for the restriction endonucleases. DNA that does not contain the *N*-methylated residue, however, is recognized as foreign and is hydrolyzed in reactions catalyzed by restriction endonucleases. Following the initial exergonic hydrolysis of the phosphodiester bonds, the resulting fragments of DNA are degraded by other bacterial nucleases.

There are hundreds of bacterial restriction endonucleases and modification methylases. In the type I systems, a single multisubunit protein has both methylation and hydrolysis activity. The type I enzymes do not hydrolyze at the recognition site, and they cleave at distant sites that are not sequence specific.

The type II systems are made up of independent methylation enzymes and endonuclease enzymes. The type II restriction endonucleases cleave at the recognition site, and this property is more useful for genetic engineering than cleavage at nonspecific distant sites. Some type II restriction endonucleases, for example, *Hae*III (Table 15–5), yield two blunt-end DNA chain products; the hydrolysis reactions occur at the same position in the DNA duplex. Other type II restriction endonucleases produce staggered single-strand nicks; the hydrolysis reactions occur at sites that are separated by several nucleotides (Table 15–5), and the resulting ends are complementary, cohesive, or "sticky." The names of the restriction enzymes are taken from the organism from which they were isolated. The strain, if applicable, is included along with a

number denoting the order of discovery of the enzyme. The first enzyme isolated from a strain of *E. coli* is called *Eco*RI, *Eco* for *E. coli,* R for the RY strain, and I for the first enzyme. Literally hundreds of restriction enzymes are used in genetic research.

Palindrome Recognition Sites

The great utility of the type II restriction endonucleases is that cleavage is sequence specific. The sequence recognized by restriction endonucleases is a palindrome. A **palindrome** is a word, sentence, or number that reads the same forward and backward. Examples are Otto, Able was I ere I saw elba, and 1991. A DNA palindrome occurs when the sequence on one strand of nucleic acid (from 5′ to 3′) is identical to that of its complementary strand (from 5′ to 3′). The following examples are illustrative:

5′ GGCC 3′

3′ CCGG 5′

5′ CTGCAG 3′

3′ GACGTC 5′

In each case, the sequence of the bottom strand is identical to that of the top strand. Owing to the specificity of the type II restriction endonucleases, these enzymes are valuable tools because they cleave DNA only at defined locations and produce unique DNA fragments. The type II restriction endonucleases have proved useful for research, genetic engineering, and biotechnology, and their use has revolutionized molecular biology.

The probability of having a tetranucleotide sequence of GGCC in a DNA molecule is $\frac{1}{4} \times \frac{1}{4} \times \frac{1}{4} \times \frac{1}{4}$, or 1/256. This sequence would occur randomly once every 256 nucleotides. In contrast, the probability for restriction endonuclease sites for CTGCAG is $\frac{1}{4} \times \frac{1}{4} \times \frac{1}{4} \times \frac{1}{4} \times \frac{1}{4} \times \frac{1}{4}$, or 1/4096. The number and size of the DNA fragments produced by restriction endonucleases depend upon the actual DNA sequence. SV40 DNA (from an animal virus) is 5226 nucleotides long and contains a single *Eco*RI restriction enzyme cleavage site. Bacteriophage T7 DNA is 40,000 nucleotides long, but it lacks a single *Eco*RI site.

Recombinant DNA and Clones

Vectors are DNA molecules such as plasmids or viruses that replicate independently of the host chromosome and can carry (vector) DNA segments into host cells. **Plasmids** are DNA molecules that replicate independently of the chromosome. Plasmids exist for bacteria and yeast but not human cells. Vectors such as pBR322 are used to produce clones or identical copies of DNA segments. The DNA segments that are combined with vectors are

---

TABLE 15–5. Selected Type II Restriction Endonuclease Cleavage Sites*

Source	Enzyme Designation	Sequence 5′ → 3′ 3′ ← 5′
Arthrobacter luteus	*Alu*I	AG ↓ CT TC ↑ GA
Bacillus amyloliquefaciens H	*Bam*HI	G ↓ GATC-C C-CTAG ↑ G
Brevibacterium albidum	*Bal*I	TGG ↓ CCA ACC ↑ GGT
Escherichia coli RY13	*Eco*RI	G ↓ AATT-C C-TTAA ↑ G
Haemophilus aegyptius	*Hae*III	GG ↓ CC CC ↑ GG
Haemophilus influenzae	*Hind*III	A ↓ AGCT-T T-TCGA ↑ A
Nocardia otitidis-caviarum	*Not*I	GC ↓ GGCC-GC CG-CCGG ↑ CG
Providencia stuartii 164	*Pst*I	C-TGCA ↓ G G ↑ ACGT-C

*The site of hydrolysis of each strand is indicated by the arrow.

called **inserts.** pBR322 can be used to clone DNA molecules up to 10 kb in length. Other vectors differ in the size of the allowed DNA insert, and the choice of vector is decided by the goal of the procedure. Lambda vectors can be used to clone DNA molecules up to 20 kb in length; many (but not all) genes are smaller than 20 kb. Lambda is a bacterial virus (bacteriophage). Cosmids (35–50 kb) and yeast artificial chromosomes (200–1000 kb) are used when larger DNA fragments are required for study. Cosmids contain cohesive ends, or cos sites. The *mid* of cosmid denotes that these vectors contain an origin of replication like that found in plas*mids*. Yeast artificial chromosomes contain a yeast centromere, two yeast telomere sequences, a cloning site, and genes for selectable traits (such as growth on medium lacking uracil or tryptophan). Large DNA molecules are ligated into the cloning site, and the artificial chromosomes are introduced into yeast.

Restriction enzymes can be used to produce chimeric or recombinant DNA molecules. The ends produced by *Bam*HI are self-complementary or cohesive. The product of the *Bam*HI cleavage has an extended 5'-end termed a 5'-overhang. That from the *Pst*I has a 3'-overhang. If two different DNAs (for example, human DNA and that from a bacterial plasmid) are treated with the same restriction endonuclease that produces cohesive ends, the ends of the human DNA can combine with the complementary ends of the plasmid DNA. This is one important strategy used in producing recombinant DNA molecules (Figure 15–27). The restriction endonucleases yield nicked complementary DNA strands, each with a 5'-phosphate and a free 3'-hydroxyl group. Annealed cohesive ends are bona fide substrates for DNA ligase, and recombinant strands can be covalently attached to one another.

One technical difficulty with this strategy is that many vector molecules will recombine with themselves without an insert. To minimize this possibility, the vector is treated with alkaline phosphatase

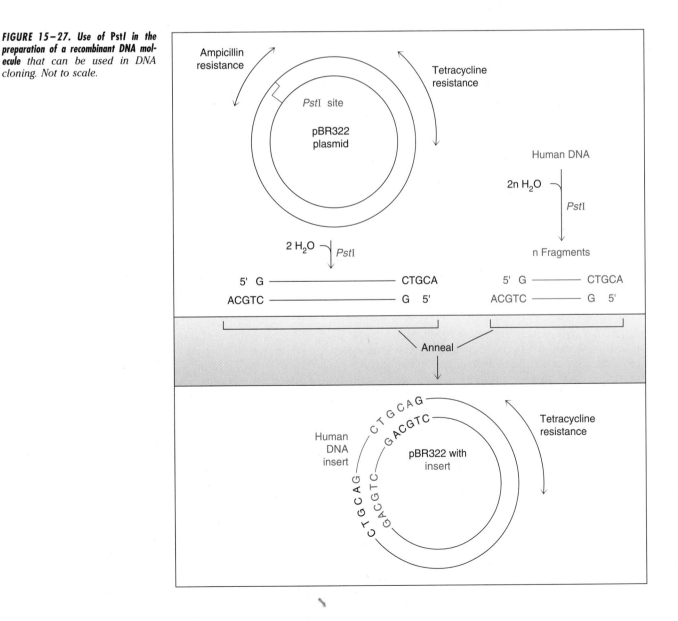

FIGURE 15–27. *Use of PstI in the preparation of a recombinant DNA molecule that can be used in DNA cloning. Not to scale.*

to catalyze the removal of the 5'-phosphate groups. The resulting vector molecules are not substrates for DNA ligase. Only vectors that have annealed with inserts with 5'-phosphates are substrates for ligation.

Natural bacterial plasmids contain genes that code for proteins that confer resistance to antibiotics. pBR322 was modified by scientists (genetically engineered) for **DNA cloning,** or the production of a large number of identical molecules (clones) for study. The ampicillin resistance gene of pBR322 contains a restriction enzyme site for *Pst*I and other restriction enzymes, and these sites do not occur elsewhere on the plasmid. Unique restriction sites for *Bam*HI and other restriction enzymes occur in the tetracycline resistance gene. Introduction of DNA into the ampicillin resistance gene of pBR322 produces bacteria that are sensitive to ampicillin but resistant to tetracycline. The bacteria are grown in tetracycline, and only those bacteria that contain a plasmid form colonies.

Immobilized Nucleic Acids

Hybridization and Dot Blots

DNA is a hybrid molecule that consists of two different but complementary polynucleotide strands. If duplex DNA molecules are heated or treated with alkali, the complementary strands separate. Strand separation is called **denaturation.** If the solution containing the denatured DNA is slowly cooled, the complementary strands reanneal to form the native double strand. Single-stranded DNA can form duplexes or anneal with any complementary DNA or RNA, whatever the source, in a process called **hybridization.** Labeled DNA or RNA, which can hybridize with complementary nucleic acids, is often used as a marker or **probe** to identify nucleic acids. *Hybridization is one of the most useful properties of nucleic acids, and this property is frequently exploited in studies of both DNA and RNA.*

Hybridization and annealing of polynucleotides following strand separation are influenced by temperature, ionic strength, and organic solvents such as dimethylformamide. When the temperature is adjusted so that complementary base pairing occurs only between perfectly matched polynucleotides, the conditions are called **stringent.** When the temperature is lowered, duplex formation can occur between polynucleotides that contain mismatches (the conditions are less stringent). Less stringent conditions might be used to promote hybridization of DNA corresponding to the same gene from related species.

Dot blots consist of samples of DNA or RNA bonded to a nitrocellulose paper matrix. RNA or alkaline-denatured DNA is fixed to the paper by heating or treatment with ultraviolet light. Binding of polynucleotides to the anchored DNA or RNA can be studied. The stringency can be adjusted so that a perfectly matched dodecamer (12 bases) will bind, but an oligonucleotide containing one mismatch will not bind to the DNA. This technique permits the identification of mutations that are the result of a single base change. The stringency of the binding of small oligonucleotides is more easily managed than that of large polynucleotides. Labeled polynucleotide probes are prepared as described later, and radioactivity bound to the immobilized DNA by hybridization is measured by exposing the blots to x-ray film in a process called **autoradiography.** An example of this procedure is illustrated in Figure 15–28.

Electrophoresis and Southern Blots

Negatively charged (anionic) DNA and RNA migrate in an electrical field toward the anode. The distance of migration is inversely related to the molecular mass or number of monomeric residues in the polynucleotide. Small molecules migrate more rapidly than large molecules. The matrix, or medium, in which the macromolecule is electrophoresed is synthetic polyacrylamide or agarose, a carbohydrate polymer. The composition of the matrix is varied depending upon the size of the nucleic acid of interest.

DNA samples can be characterized on a **Southern blot.** This procedure is useful for detecting gene rearrangements, deletions, and—in particularly favorable cases—single base changes. A sample of DNA, for example, human DNA, is treated with a restriction endonuclease and then subjected to agarose gel electrophoresis. The resulting fragments are resolved by size; smaller fragments migrate more rapidly. The DNA on the gel is transferred to a thin support such as nitrocellulose paper sheets by capillary action. Buffer moves through the slab gel and nitrocellulose; in the process, DNA is transferred from the gel and is retained by nitrocellulose. Alkali-denatured DNA is bonded to the nitrocellulose by treatment with heat or ultraviolet light. The relative positions of DNA are maintained during the transfer from the gel to the nitrocellulose paper (Figure 15–29).

The resolution of DNA by electrophoresis and transfer to nitrocellulose is called a Southern blot (named for Edwin Southern, the originator). A similar analysis of RNA was dubbed a **Northern blot.** Electrophoresis and transfer of proteins are called a **Western blot.** The principles involve electrophoretic resolution of macromolecules and transfer to a bonding agent by a method that ensures that the resolution is maintained.

Labeled Probes

Southern blotting of an *Eco*RI restriction endonuclease digest of a sample of human DNA might yield 700,000 different fragments. To identify the fragment of interest requires the use of a probe. This is generally accomplished by preparing a ra-

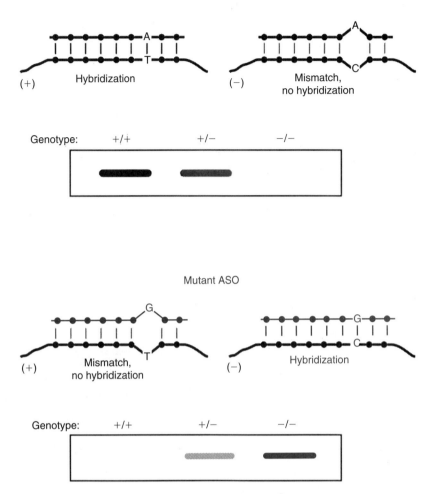

FIGURE 15–28. Hybridization on dot blots. *Single base pair mutations can be detected using oligonucleotide probes that correspond to the normal and mutant sequences. ASO, allele specific oligonucleotide. Reproduced, with permission, from M.W. Thompson, R.R. McInnes, and H.F. Willard. Thompson and Thompson Genetics in Medicine, 5th ed. Philadelphia, W.B. Saunders Company, 1991, p. 109.*

dioactive (^{32}P) DNA sample. There are several strategies for achieving this. If the primary structure of the DNA is known, complementary DNA of 15 to 25 nucleotides in length can be synthesized by oligonucleotide synthesizers. This oligonucleotide can be labeled at the free 5'-hydroxyl group in a reaction between radioactive ATP and the synthetic oligonucleotide catalyzed by **polynucleotide kinase.**

$$[\gamma^{32}P]\text{–ATP} + \text{HO–DNA} \rightarrow$$
$$\text{ADP} + {}^{32}\text{PO}_3^{2-}\text{–O–DNA} \quad (15.3)$$

If the primary structure of a segment of protein of interest is known, all of the oligonucleotides corresponding to the primary structure can be synthesized according to the genetic code (Table 17–1). Larger fragments of DNA can be labeled by using **random sequence oligonucleotides** (typically six bases in length) as primers for synthesizing labeled probe with heat-denatured DNA as template. Random sequence oligonucleotides are mixtures of oligonucleotides that contain each of the four bases at each of the six positions, and the components of the mixture can base-pair with complementary sequences on the larger DNA fragments.

Next, the blot is incubated with the radioactive probe at a specific temperature and salt concentration, which determine the stringency. During this procedure, the probe hybridizes to any immobilized complementary single-stranded DNA (a Southern blot) or RNA (a Northern blot) present on the filter. After hybridization, the blot is washed with buffer to remove nonannealed probe. The samples are then subjected to autoradiography to locate the position of the probe and the polynucleotides to which it bound. Standard nucleic acids are run in parallel so that the length or size of the DNA or RNA bands can be determined.

Polymerase Chain Reaction (PCR)

The polymerase chain reaction represents a technique that is revolutionizing genetic biochemistry. Polymerase chain reaction technology is used to amplify DNA for study. For example, the minute quantities of DNA from a few hair follicle cells can be characterized. This technique is used in molecular medicine, medical diagnostics, forensics, and genetic engineering. ▶ PCR technology is used in the diagnosis and study of several disorders including muscular dystrophy, hemophilia A, human

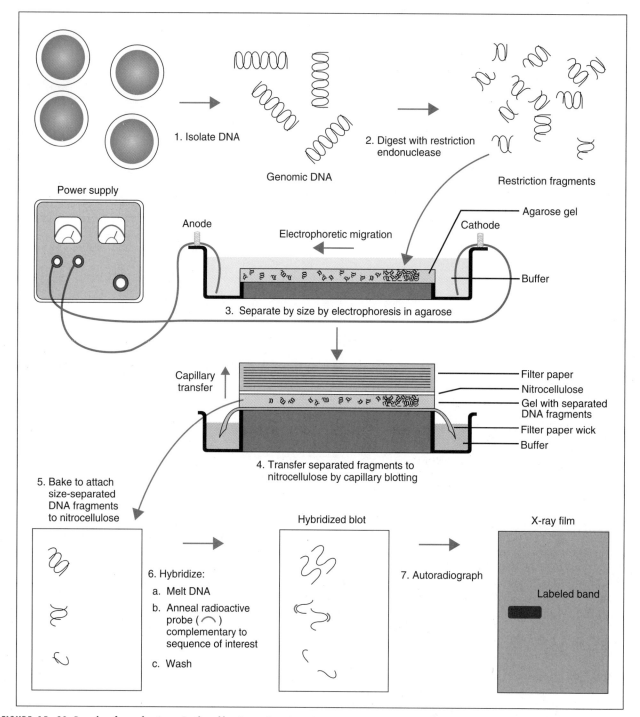

1. Isolate DNA

Genomic DNA

2. Digest with restriction endonuclease

Restriction fragments

Power supply

Anode

Electrophoretic migration

Cathode

Agarose gel

Buffer

3. Separate by size by electrophoresis in agarose

Capillary transfer

Filter paper
Nitrocellulose
Gel with separated DNA fragments
Filter paper wick
Buffer

4. Transfer separated fragments to nitrocellulose by capillary blotting

5. Bake to attach size-separated DNA fragments to nitrocellulose

Hybridized blot

X-ray film

6. Hybridize:

a. Melt DNA

b. Anneal radioactive probe (⌒) complementary to sequence of interest

c. Wash

7. Autoradiograph

Labeled band

FIGURE 15–29. Procedure for performing a Southern blot. *Reproduced, with permission, from A.K. Abbas, A.H. Lichtman, and J.S. Pober.* Cellular and Molecular Immunology, *2nd ed. Philadelphia, W.B. Saunders Company, 1994, p. 71.*

immunodeficiency virus infection, viral hepatitis, and retinoblastoma. ◄ Polymerase chain reaction technology can also be used for preparing mutant DNAs with site-specific changes.

The chain reaction refers to the use of multiple cycles (25–35) of template- and primer-dependent DNA elongation reactions. The requirements include a target DNA (the template) for amplification, two DNA oligonucleotide primers complementary to the ends of each strand of the target DNA and

extending toward the sequence that will bind the other primer, deoxynucleoside triphosphates, and heat-stable DNA polymerase. Heat-stable DNA polymerases are obtained from *Thermus aquaticus* (*Taq* polymerase) and *Pyococcus furiosis* (*Pfu* polymerase), which grow in hot springs at 100°C. These enzymes are not denatured at temperatures around 90°C; DNA polymerases from *E. coli,* on the other hand, are thermally inactivated at this temperature.

The components of a polymerase chain reaction are incubated in a thermal cycler, a heating block whose temperature can be regulated by computer. First, the temperature is elevated to about 92°C for one minute; this causes the two strands of a DNA duplex to "melt." The reaction components are cooled to 50–65°C for 1 minute so that the oligonucleotide primers can anneal with DNA. The reaction components are heated to 72°C for 1 minute so that the primers can be elongated over the length of the target DNA (Figure 15–30). A few minutes are required to produce each of these temperature changes. Each cycle is repeated 25–35 times. (The conditions given here are only approximations and have to be customized for each application.) After two cycles, fragments corresponding to target-length DNA result. The amount of target-length DNA is doubled in each subsequent cycle. This procedure can amplify the amount of DNA several million-fold. PCR technology has revolutionized genetic biochemistry in the same fundamental way as have restriction enzymes.

Oligonucleotide primers can be used to create mutant molecules. Substitutions, deletions, and insertions can be made on the 5′ end of the primer, and they will not adversely alter the amplification process. If changes that produce a noncomplementary primer occur on the 3′ end, the primer will not function properly. This property can be used to advantage to detect polymorphisms and mutations. Primers can be designed to function on target DNA molecules that correspond to a specific allele and not the polymorphic or mutant DNA.

This procedure may require, in a separate reaction vessel, a primer that will recognize and amplify the other alleles or mutant forms to serve as a control. PCR technology can be used to detect genetic variation in combination with other methods as described later.

DNA Sequence Analysis

One of the great advances in molecular biology has been the development of techniques for determining the primary structure or sequence of bases of DNA. One DNA sequencing technique, developed by Fred Sanger in England, is the **dideoxynucleotide** or **chain termination** method. Segments of the DNA of interest (up to 400 bases) are introduced into a specific site, complementary to a synthetic primer, in a single-stranded DNA bacteriophage (called M13). The primer is a short sequence of DNA (about 17 bases long) that can be produced by an oligonucleotide synthesizer.

The primer is designed to anneal to the phage DNA next to the DNA insert, and the oligonucleotide serves as primer for DNA polymerase elongation reactions. A solution containing many copies of the annealed complex is divided into four identical reaction mixtures. To each mixture is added a solution containing DNA polymerase I, pyrophosphatase, and the four deoxyribonucleoside triphosphates (one or more of which contains ^{32}P in the α-position or ^{35}S in place of oxygen on the α-phosphate). A different chain terminator is included in

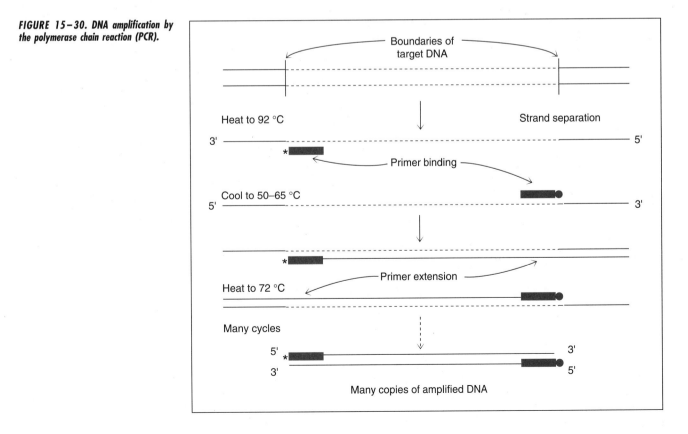

FIGURE 15–30. DNA amplification by the polymerase chain reaction (PCR).

Boundaries of target DNA

Heat to 92 °C   Strand separation

3′ ——————————————————— 5′

* ▇

Primer binding

Cool to 50–65 °C

5′ ——————————————————— 3′

Primer extension

Heat to 72 °C

* ▇

Many cycles

5′ * ▇——————————————— 3′

3′ ——————————————— 5′

Many copies of amplified DNA

each of the four mixtures. These terminators are ddATP, ddGTP, ddCTP, and ddTTP, where dd indicates dideoxy.

Dideoxynucleotides lack hydroxyl groups at both the 2′- and 3′-carbons of ribose. When these dideoxynucleotides are incorporated into the growing chain at positions complementary to the cloned insert, elongation is impossible (there is no free 3′-hydroxyl group) and chain termination results. In the case in which ddTTP is included, chain termination occurs randomly at every position complementary to an adenine residue, and a family of polydeoxynucleotides results. The incorporation of the other dideoxynucleotides indicates the positions corresponding to their complementary base.

The four mixtures are subjected to gel electrophoresis and autoradiography. The gels resolve every polydeoxynucleotide by size. It is possible, for example, to resolve a polynucleotide of 149 bases from one of 150 bases. One can read from the shortest to longest and identify the residues terminating in A, G, C, or T by the order of their appearance on the autoradiograph. The information can be entered into a computer data bank for full analysis. The steps in preparing the four samples corresponding to a given DNA sequence are shown in Figure 15–31. The figure illustrates many fundamental aspects of DNA biosynthesis per se and is therefore worth all the time it takes to understand the principles outlined. By using four nucleotides that have different attached chromophores, the sequence can be derived spectrally from a single electrophoresis lane. This technique has been automated to increase DNA sequencing capability.

▶ Analysis of a **cystic fibrosis** gene provides an example of the type of information that can be obtained from its sequence. Cystic fibrosis is a common autosomal recessive disease in Caucasian children, with an incidence in 1 of 2000 live births. Cystic fibrosis affects 30,000 people in the United States. Affected individuals, who generally succumb before the age of 40, have recurrent pulmonary infections, pancreatic insufficiency, and elevated sweat chloride. The gene is located on chromosome 7q21 (Table 16–5). The gene product is called the cystic fibrosis transmembrane regulator (CFTR) and plays a role in anion transport in cells. Cystic fibrosis can result from different mutations of this gene. The most common, accounting for about 70% of the cases, is due to a deletion of three bases (TTC). As a result, an abnormal protein that lacks a single phenylalanine residue is produced. A DNA sequencing gel illustrating the deletion of TTC is shown in Figure 15–32.

Because of defective anion transport, thick mucus secretions result in the lungs that promote the development of pneumonia (an inflammation of the lungs). These thick secretions are aggravated by viscous DNA that is released from leukocytes.

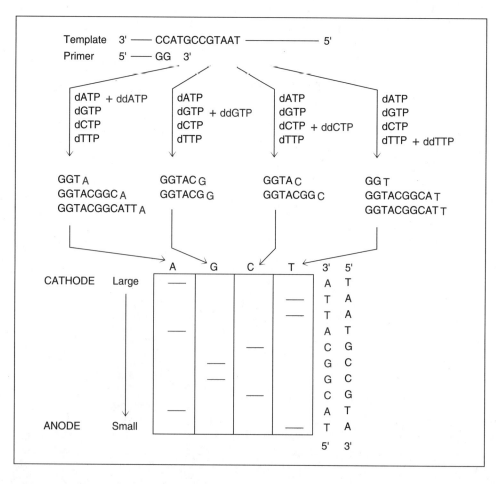

FIGURE 15–31. Procedure for DNA sequence analysis by the dideoxyribonucleotide chain termination technique. The DNA to be sequenced is inserted into a specific site in a single-stranded DNA bacteriophage called M13. The DNA insert is adjacent to an oligonucleotide primer binding site. Four independent reactions are performed in the presence of a different chain terminator. At the completion of these four reactions, the products are resolved by electrophoresis on a sequencing gel that separates products by size. Following autoradiography, the sequence can be read directly from the gel pattern. Four reactions are required to generate the polynucleotides that end with each of the four bases.

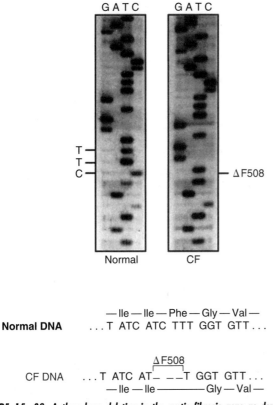

Normal DNA   — Ile — Ile — Phe — Gly — Val —
...T ATC ATC TTT GGT GTT...

ΔF508

CF DNA   ...T ATC AT_ _ _T GGT GTT...
— Ile — Ile ——————— Gly — Val —

FIGURE 15-32. A three-base deletion in the cystic fibrosis gene as demonstrated by DNA sequence analysis. *The CCT sequence present in normal individuals is absent in an individual with cystic fibrosis. As a result, the cystic fibrosis protein suffers from a deletion of phenylalanine residue 508 (Δ508). From a photograph provided by L.-C. Tsui in M.W. Thompson, R.R. McInnes, and H.F. Willard.* Thompson and Thompson Genetics in Medicine, *5th ed. Philadelphia, W.B. Saunders Company, 1991, p. 135.*

Cystic fibrosis is treated symptomatically with genetically engineered human DNAse administered by aerosol therapy, bronchodilators, and antibiotics. ◀

DNA sequencing is faster and easier than protein sequencing. To sequence a protein might require a few years' work. The cDNA corresponding to the protein can be sequenced in a few weeks. For this reason, the sequencing of whole proteins has been nearly abandoned. Considerable work may be required, however, to obtain the desired cDNA for analysis. The sequences of short segments of proteins can be used to design probes that can be used to identify the corresponding cDNA or genomic DNA for gene cloning. The protein sequence of the entire protein can be deduced from the DNA sequence analysis of the clone. The sequences of genes encoding RNA and regulatory elements of DNA can also be determined by DNA sequencing methodologies. The dideoxynucleotide chain termination strategy has been adapted for use with polymerase chain reaction methodology.

Localization of Genes on Chromosomes

Life scientists have prepared cells that are hybrids of those of humans and the mouse; these hybrid cells contain both mouse and human chromosomes. These cells are propagated in culture. Groups of such cells exist that contain between 2 and 13 human chromosomes that permit the localization of a gene to a specific human chromosome. Southern blots are performed with each type of cell found in the series, and those cell lines that contain a particular human gene can be determined. Southern blots for the α-subunit of hexosaminidase A from a panel of hybrid cells are illustrated in Figure 15-33. The results of such experiments show that the gene for the α-subunit of hexosaminidase A occurs on chromosome 15. Other studies show that the gene for the β-subunit occurs on chromosome 5. ▶ Mutations of the α-subunit result in Tay-Sachs disease (Table 12-1), and mutations of the β-subunit produce Sandhoff disease. Both diseases are sphingolipidoses. ◀

A second method for localizing genes on chromosomes involves hybridization *in situ*. DNA or RNA probes are hybridized directly to metaphase chromosomes that are spread on a slide. The DNA is denatured on the slide, and hybridization studies are performed. The probe can be radiolabeled, and the location can be determined in a photographic emulsion. Alternatively, a fluorescent label is attached to the probe, and its location is determined by fluorescence microscopy. This procedure permitted the identification of the gene for muscle glycogen phosphorylase to chromosome 11q13 (Figure 15-34). ▶ A deficiency of this protein results in McArdle disease, a glycogen storage disease (Table 10-3). ◀

Genetic Variation, Polymorphism, and Disease

Restriction Fragment Length Polymorphisms (RFLPs)

When a restriction enzyme digest of DNA from several humans is performed, the resulting Southern blots can exhibit different patterns. The differences or polymorphisms (Greek *poly*, "many"; *morphos*, "form") result from mutations that alter the restriction enzyme site. The dissimilar patterns can be due to restriction fragment length polymorphisms (RFLPs, pronounced "rif lips") that reflect different forms of a gene (alleles). ▶ One polymorphic pattern may be associated with or linked to a genetic disease. It is not necessary that the restriction enzyme cleave the defective gene. Often the altered site is near the defective gene and serves as a marker. These tests of **genetic linkage analysis** are feasible in diagnosing hereditary diseases in cells isolated from amniotic fluid following amniocentesis or from chorionic villus sampling. Extensive experimentation and painstaking effort are required to establish and validate such diagnostic tests.

The first abnormal hemoglobin to be detected was that of **sickle cell anemia,** the most widely known of all hemoglobinopathies. Sickle cell ane-

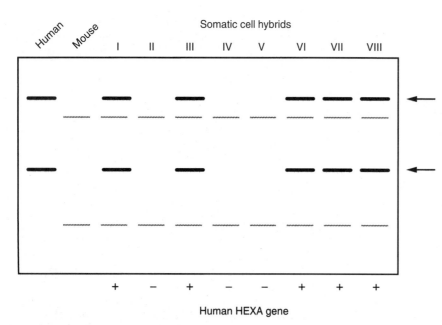

Somatic cell hybrids

Human Mouse I II III IV V VI VII VIII

+ − + − − + + +

Human HEXA gene

FIGURE 15–33. Localization of a gene on a chromosome. *Southern blots of the hexosaminidase A gene in mouse/human cell lines can distinguish between the human and mouse genes. Only those cells with human chromosome 15 give positive signals for the human hexosaminidase gene. The probe for the hexosaminidase gene hybridizes with two DNA fragments showing that there is an internal restriction enzyme site that is cleaved by the type II restriction enzyme. Reproduced, with permission, from M.W. Thompson, R.R. McInnes, and H.F. Willard.* Thompson and Thompson Genetics in Medicine, *5th ed. Philadelphia, W.B. Saunders Company, 1991, p. 172.*

mia is the cause of considerable mortality and morbidity in Africa and in every population in which there has been migration of individuals of African descent. Affected individuals are homozygous for hemoglobin S expression. Hemoglobin S differs from hemoglobin A by the conversion of an amino acid on the β-chain at the 6 position from Glu→Val. This alteration is due to the mutation that produces an A → T transversion in the triplet codon for the sixth residue of the β-globin chain on chromosome 11 (Table 16–5). Deoxygenated

sickle cell hemoglobin polymerizes and produces the characteristic sickle cell deformity. The formula for sickle cell hemoglobin can be expressed as $\alpha_2{}^A\beta_2{}^S$, where A represents normal adult hemoglobin and S represents sickle cell hemoglobin. A heterozygote with sickle cell trait who expresses both hemoglobin A and S is asymptomatic; this accounts for the designation of the disease as autosomal recessive. In heterozygotes, hemoglobin A $(\alpha_2{}^A\beta_2{}^A)$ and hemoglobin S $(\alpha_2{}^A\beta_2{}^S)$ occur together in the same cell in a ratio of 60/40.

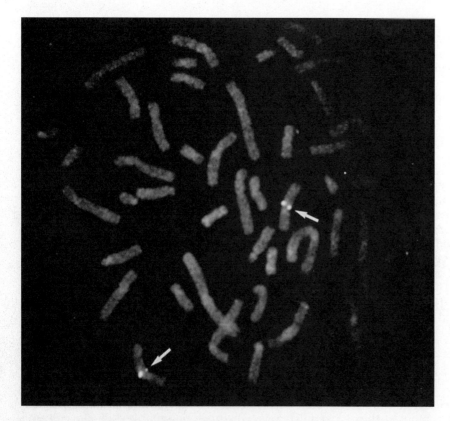

FIGURE 15–34. Localization of a gene within a chromosome by hybridization in situ. *A biotin-labeled probe for the muscle glycogen phosphorylase gene is seen over each chromatid in band q13 of chromosome 11. A fluorescent-avidin complex combines tightly with biotin to emit a fluorescent signal. From a photograph provided by Peter Lichter in M.W. Thompson, R.R. McInnes, and H.F. Willard.* Thompson and Thompson Genetics in Medicine, *5th ed. Philadelphia, W.B. Saunders Company, 1991, p. 175.*

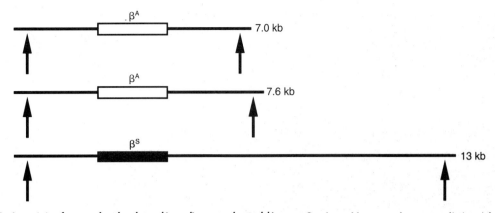

FIGURE 15–35. The HpaI restriction fragment length polymorphism adjacent to the β-globin gene. *Southern blot procedures can distinguish among the three polymorphic fragments. Reproduced, with permission, from M.W. Thompson, R.R. McInnes, and H.F. Willard.* Thompson and Thompson Genetics in Medicine, *5th ed. Philadelphia, W.B. Saunders Company, 1991, p. 256.*

Restriction fragment length polymorphisms are observed on Southern blots when the target DNA contains variable restriction sites that can be identified by different electrophoretic mobilities of the digested fragments. A polymorphism in the DNA sequence of the β-globin gene occurs in some West African populations. The normal allele contains a 7-kb *Hpa*I restriction enzyme fragment. In South African populations, a polymorphism is associated with a 7.6-kb fragment in normal individuals. A 13-kb *Hpa*I restriction enzyme fragment is associated with the sickle hemoglobin gene (Figure 15–35). This is a fortuitous but valuable association of a DNA polymorphism with the disease, and the restriction enzyme site is not in the gene nor does it directly reflect the mutant site. This RFLP provides a method for making the diagnosis of sickle cell anemia.

The mutation of the normal β^A-globin gene to form the β^S-globin gene results in the elimination of an *Mst*II restriction enzyme site (Figure 15–36). The wild type gene yields a 1.15-kb fragment, and the mutant yields a 1.35-kb fragment. Since the restriction enzyme site involves the site of mutation and is not a chance association, this procedure permits the direct identification of a normal gene or a mutated gene. Not every genetic disease is the result of a mutation that destroys a restriction enzyme site or palindrome. Single nucleotide substitutions, however, can be detected with oligonucleotide probes, as noted later. ◄

Variable Number of Tandem Repeats (VNTRs) Polymorphisms

Some DNA polymorphisms are based on the insertion or deletion of DNA rather than nucleotide

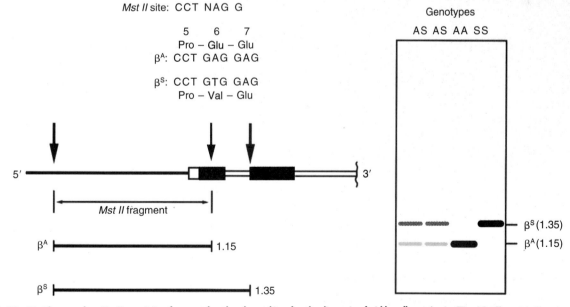

FIGURE 15–36. The use of an MstII restriction fragment length polymorphism for the diagnosis of sickle cell anemia. A. *The* Mst*II restriction enzyme site and the sequences of normal and mutant hemoglobins are shown.* B. *Cleavage sites of normal and sickle cell hemoglobin.* C. *A representation of a Southern blot showing the pattern for heterozygotes (AS), normal (AA), and individuals with sickle cell anemia (SS). Reproduced, with permission, from M.W. Thompson, R.R. McInnes, and H.F. Willard.* Thompson and Thompson Genetics in Medicine, *5th ed. Philadelphia, W.B. Saunders Company, 1991, p. 253.*

substitutions. A special class consists of a series of altered fragment lengths that are related to each other by a variable number of tandem repeated DNA segments (VNTRs) in an interval between two restriction sites. These repeats involve minisatellite DNA. These loci have many alleles or alternative gene forms. Many alleles in the normal population exist in several dozen forms. No two unrelated individuals are likely to share the same alleles. The basis of VNTR testing is illustrated in Figure 15–37. The lengths of the restriction fragments differ because of the variable number of repeats. Following a Southern blot, the fragments are identified with a probe that recognizes DNA outside the repeated segments. An example of VNTRs from monozygotic (identical) and dizygotic (fraternal) twins is illustrated in Figure 15–38. These tests can be used to establish the identity of parents and can be used in forensics.

Allele-Specific Oligonucleotide (ASO) Probe Analysis

The use of oligonucleotide probes of about 12 nucleotides permits the identification of single base changes. The efficacy of this procedure depends upon the knowledge of the normal and mutant sequences. It has the advantage of detecting single nucleotide differences and does not depend upon the chance alteration of a site on the DNA that is recognized by a restriction endonuclease. The conditions are adjusted such that the probe binds to the normal allelic DNA but does not bind to the mutant. The specificity of annealing of the probe to DNA can be manipulated easily with short oligonucleotide probes, whereas a large nick-translated DNA would bind to both wild type and mutant DNAs that differ in only a single base change. This procedure is illustrated in Figure 15–28.

Single-Strand Conformation Polymorphisms (SSCPs)

Single nucleotide differences in a DNA sequence can alter the electrophoretic mobility of single-stranded DNA. Single-strand conformation polymorphisms can be used as genetic markers in the same way that restriction fragment length polymorphisms are used. SSCPs can identify more polymorphisms or mutations than RFLPs because SSCPs detect differences that are not confined to restriction enzyme sites. This procedure can be coupled with polymerase chain reaction procedures to amplify DNA. ▶ SSCPs have been used to detect nucleotide substitutions in individuals with mild or variant forms of cystic fibrosis. ◀

Multiplex PCR

▶ Duchenne and Becker muscular dystrophy are diseases that result from disruptions within the dystrophin gene. Duchenne muscular dystrophy is characterized by progressive muscle weakness that affects the respiratory and cardiac systems. Serum creatine phosphokinase levels are elevated. Death usually occurs between 20 and 30 years. Becker muscular dystrophy is a milder disease that results from mutations of the dystrophin gene. These diseases are X-linked recessive disorders (Table 16–5).

The most common mutation that produces these diseases involves a genomic rearrangement that produces a deletion of part of the gene. The dystrophin gene is about 2.3 million bases long, contains more than 70 exons, and is one of the largest known genes, accounting for about 1.5% of the X chromosome (Table 16–6). Because of the heterogeneous nature of the rearrangement and the gene's large size, it is feasible neither to detect

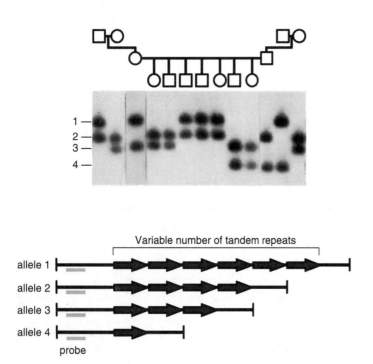

FIGURE 15–37. Genetic polymorphism based on a variable number of tandem repeats (VNTRs). Alleles 1 through 4 are related by the identical short DNA sequences (arrows). Reproduced, with permission, from M.W. Thompson, R.R. McInnes, and H.F. Willard. Thompson and Thompson Genetics in Medicine, 5th ed. Philadelphia, W.B. Saunders Company, 1991, p. 130.

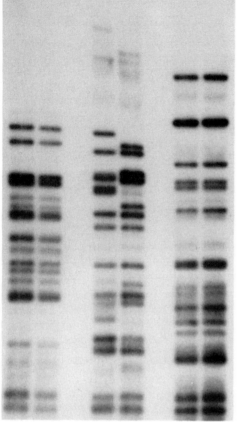

FIGURE 15–38. DNA fingerprinting of twins by means of a probe that detects VNTR polymorphisms. *Each pair of lanes contains DNA from a set of twins. The first and third sets are identical, and the second sets are fraternal. Each set is unrelated to the others and demonstrates the variation between nonidentical siblings and between unrelated people. From a photograph provided by Alec Jeffreys in M.W. Thompson, R.R. McInnes, and H.F. Willard. Thompson and Thompson Genetics in Medicine, 5th ed. Philadelphia, W.B. Saunders Company, 1991, p. 131.*

disease alleles with a single probe nor to amplify the entire gene by PCR. About 90% of the dystrophin gene deletions can be detected with multiplex PCR. This procedure involves the simultaneous use of several pairs (a multiplex) of oligonucleotide primers that anneal to different regions of the gene. With muscular dystrophies, 17 pairs of primers are used. Following PCR amplification, the products are electrophoresed in agarose. Missing products indicate deletion.

Because of the different clinical courses, Duchenne and Becker muscular dystrophy were thought to represent different clinical entities. Knowledge gained from the genetic analysis indicates that both are due to similar mutations in the same gene. Differences in clinical course are due to the production of different amounts of the gene product (dystrophin) or to dystrophins with variable biochemical activities. This is one example of

genetic analysis leading to the better understanding of the pathogenesis of disease. ◀

SUMMARY

E. coli has about 3000 and humans have 50,000 to 100,000 genes. These genes are composed of DNA. DNA forms an antiparallel double helix with complementary Watson-Crick base pairing (A with T and G with C). The information content of DNA is represented by the specific sequence of nucleotides in DNA. DNA (the genetic component of a cell) must be reproduced before cell division. DNA synthesis starts at an origin of replication. Bacteria have one origin. In *E. coli,* the origin is called *oriC.* Humans have hundreds of replication origins on each chromosome. DNA biosynthesis is semiconservative: One strand of the DNA duplex is distributed to one daughter strand, and the complementary strand is distributed to the other daughter strand. This finding was demonstrated with the use of heavy isotopes by Meselson and Stahl.

Many proteins participate in replication. A pivotal family of replication enzymes are the DNA polymerases. DNA polymerases use a DNA template to direct the sequence of incoming deoxyribonucleotides that form the new DNA chain. Chain growth is in the 5′ to 3′ direction. DNA polymerases cannot initiate synthesis of DNA; they require a preexisting primer. An enzyme, primase, catalyzes the synthesis of the primer. The primer may be an oligonucleotide containing ribonucleotides and deoxyribonucleotides. Because it contains ribonucleotides, the primer must be removed. Of the three *E. coli* DNA polymerases, pol III is the chief enzyme of replication. Pol I is the chief repair enzyme. Polymerases possess 3′ to 5′ exonuclease activity; this activity removes deoxyribonucleotides inadvertently incorporated and not complementary to the template. This action is called proofreading. DNA polymerases (in bacteria) or independent proteins (in humans) possess 5′ to 3′ exonuclease activity. This activity is important in removing primers and in participating in DNA repair.

Human cells have at least five distinctive polymerases, designated α, β, γ, δ, and ϵ to clearly distinguish them from the bacterial enzymes. Polymerase α mediates the synthesis of the lagging strand, and polymerase δ (with PCNA) catalyzes the synthesis of the leading strand. Polymerases β and ϵ function in nuclear repair synthesis, and polymerase γ carries out replication within the mitochondrion. Primase activity associated with DNA polymerase α is responsible for both leading and lagging strand chain initiation. DNA ligases catalyze the closing of nicks in DNA. DNA topoisomerases catalyze the conversion of one form of topoisomer to another. Topoisomerase I cleaves and re-ligates one strand of the DNA duplex during its action; topoisomerase II cleaves and re-ligates two strands of the DNA duplex.

Human cells, but not bacteria, contain histones, which are basic proteins that, with DNA, form nucleosomes. Nucleosomes encompass stretches of DNA about 200 base pairs in length. Histone dimers of H2A, H2B, H3, and H4 bind to regions about 160 base pairs in length. Histone H1 is found in the remaining linker region. Nucleosomes, when viewed with the electron microscope, resemble a string of pearls.

The antiparallel nature of the DNA duplex introduces complexity in the mechanism of replication. DNA polymerases catalyze the elongation reaction in the 5′ to 3′ direction. One strand, the leading strand, is synthesized continuously. The opposite strand, the lagging strand, is synthesized discontinuously as Okazaki fragments. DNA ligase links successive Okazaki fragments. Many other proteins such as topoisomerases and helicases participate in replication.

More than three high-energy bonds are required per deoxyribonucleotide linkage formed. The phosphodiester bond of DNA is energy rich. Two ATP molecules are required to separate each base pair of the parent strands through the action of DNA helicase. Two ATP molecules per base pair are equivalent to one ATP (to ADP and P_i) per deoxyribonucleotide. Deoxyribonucleoside triphosphates are the substrates for the DNA polymerase elongation reaction, and a deoxyribonucleotide and pyrophosphate are the products. The hydrolysis of pyrophosphate pulls the DNA polymerase reaction forward. An additional two high-energy bonds are thus required for the formation of each energy-rich phosphodiester deoxyribonucleotide linkage of DNA, for a minimum of three high-energy bonds. Energy must be expended to remove primers, close nicks, and interconvert topological isomers. These processes increase the energy requirements for replication.

A variety of repair mechanisms exist. Repair is based upon removal of damaged DNA segments by exergonic hydrolysis reactions, filling the gap with repair polymerase, and closing the nick with DNA ligase.

Type II restriction endonucleases catalyze the hydrolysis of DNA at palindromic recognition sites. Palindromes are complementary sequences that are the same on one strand as they are in the complement. GGCC is an example of a DNA palindrome.

DNA can be sequenced by the dideoxynucleotide chain termination technique. Dideoxynucleotides lack hydroxyl groups at both the 2′- and 3′-carbons of ribose. When these dideoxynucleotides are incorporated into the nascent chain at positions complementary to the template, elongation is impossible (there is no free 3′-hydroxyl group) and chain termination results. Analogues corresponding to each of the four deoxyribonucleoside triphosphates are used in four different reaction mixtures. Polydeoxyribonucleotides corresponding to chains terminated at each residue are identified following resolution by electrophoresis.

The polymerase chain reaction (PCR) is used to amplify and study target DNA. Primers complementary to each of two ends of target DNA sequences to be amplified are used to initiate DNA synthesis. Each synthesized strand in turn serves as a template to synthesize another DNA. The strands are separated by heating, and the temperature is lowered so that a primer will anneal. Then the temperature is elevated so that elongation can proceed. The number of strands increases exponentially, and the process is called amplification. DNA sequencing, the polymerase chain reaction, and restriction endonucleases have revolutionized research in molecular biology.

Mutations are permanent, heritable changes in the sequence of genomic DNA. They can involve single base changes, insertions, and deletions. Mutations can be detected by alterations in restriction endonuclease sites in the mutant DNAs that produce restriction fragment length polymorphisms (RFLPs). The use of allele-specific oligonucleotide probes permits detection of a change in only a single base and does not rely on the chance altering of a restriction enzyme site in the mutant DNA. Single-strand conformation polymorphisms (SSCPs) can be used as genetic markers, and this procedure will also detect a mutation that is due to a single base change. Human populations contain genes that have a variable number of tandem repeats (VNTRs). The analysis of such repeats can be used in genetic linkage studies. Multiplex PCR uses multiple primers to analyze large genes such as that for dystrophin.

SELECTED READINGS

Kornberg, A., and T.A. Baker. *DNA Replication,* 2nd ed. New York, W.H. Freeman and Company, 1992.

Lindahl, T., and D.E. Barnes. Mammalian DNA ligases. Annual Review of Biochemistry 61:251–281, 1992.

Meselson, M., and F.W. Stahl. The replication of DNA in *Escherichia coli.* Proceedings of the National Academy of Science USA 44:671–682, 1958.

Mullis, K.B. The unusual origin of the polymerase chain reaction. Scientific American 262(4):56–65, 1990.

Tompkins, L.S. Nucleic acid probes in infectious diseases. Current Clinical Topics in Infectious Diseases 10:174–193, 1989.

Wang, T.S.-F. Eukaryotic DNA polymerases. Annual Review of Biochemistry 60:513–552, 1991.

Watson, J.D., and F.H.C. Crick. Molecular structure of nucleic acids. Nature 171:737–738, 1953.

Watson, J.D., M. Gilman, J. Witkowski, and M. Zoller. *Recombinant DNA,* 2nd ed. New York, W.H. Freeman and Company, 1992.

CHAPTER SIXTEEN

RNA BIOSYNTHESIS

AND PROCESSING

Joy is not present in science as an everyday thing. What is customary is satisfaction.

—HOWARD TEMIN

RNA functions as an intermediary in the transfer of genetic information from DNA to protein as stated in Crick's law of molecular biology (PRINCIPLE 25 OF BIOCHEMISTRY). Three major classes of RNA are required for protein biosynthesis including ribosomal RNA (rRNA), transfer RNA (tRNA), and messenger RNA (mRNA). Humans and other eukaryotes possess heterogeneous nuclear RNA (hnRNA), the biosynthetic precursor of messenger RNA, and small nuclear RNA (snRNA).

Bacteria contain one class of DNA-dependent RNA polymerase, and eukaryotic cells employ three classes of nuclear RNA polymerase. RNA polymerase I mediates the synthesis of rRNA, RNA polymerase II mediates the synthesis of hnRNA-mRNA, and RNA polymerase III catalyzes the formation of tRNA and other small RNA molecules. Mitochondrial RNA polymerase is a fourth class of eukaryotic RNA polymerase.

The three steps in RNA biosynthesis include **initiation, elongation,** and **termination.** *All known RNA polymerases can initiate RNA biosynthesis* de novo. This is in contrast to the DNA polymerases, which require an existing primer. Initiation of biosynthesis in both bacteria and eukaryotic cells by RNA polymerase involves the recognition of special DNA sequences by accessory proteins and by RNA polymerase. A **promoter** is a nucleotide sequence that identifies the start site for RNA synthesis. The nature of this site depends upon the particular auxiliary proteins and the RNA polymerase.

The initial RNA product is a **primary transcript** (Figure 16–1). In a few cases, such as human 5S RNA and bacterial messenger RNA, the primary transcript is functional. For rRNA, tRNA, and eukaryotic messenger RNA, the primary transcript requires posttranscriptional processing to produce the functional form. Conversion of hnRNA to mRNA in humans requires addition of a guanine nucleotide at the 5′ end (capping), methylation, polyadenylylation at the 3′ end, and splicing.

STRUCTURE OF RNA

RNA is a polymer of ribonucleotides. The structure of an RNA tetranucleotide is shown in Figure 16–2. RNA is made up of a ribose-phosphate backbone to which the various bases are attached. RNA, like DNA, exhibits polarity. The 5′-hydroxyl group points toward the 5′ end and the 3′-hydroxyl group points to the 3′ end of the molecule. The sequence of bases along the sugar-phosphate backbone determines the primary structure (information content) of RNA, and this is the factor that distinguishes one RNA from another. Like DNA, RNA contains adenine, guanine, and cytosine. Unlike DNA, however, thymine is replaced by uracil (Table 16–1). Selected properties and the approximate sizes of the various classes of RNA are given for general reference in Table 16–2.

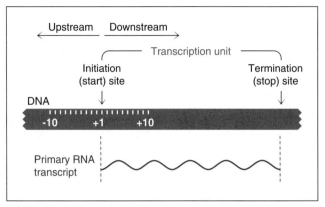

FIGURE 16–1. A transcription unit. +1 corresponds to the first nucleotide that occurs in the corresponding RNA strand.

SYNTHESIS OF RNA

RNA Polymerases

DNA-Dependent RNA Polymerases

RNA polymerase catalyzes the formation of phosphodiester bonds from a free 3′-hydroxyl group of an RNA strand and the activated α-phosphorus atom of ribonucleoside triphosphate. Chain growth occurs in the 5′ → 3′ direction (PRINCIPLE 29 OF BIOCHEMISTRY) and is antiparallel to that of the DNA template (Figure 16–3). *The sequence of the synthesized polymer is directed by the DNA template according to the Watson-Crick complementary base-pairing rules.* Adenine in DNA specifies uracil in the RNA transcript; guanine specifies cytosine; cytosine specifies guanine, and thymine specifies adenine. The structure of uracil and complementary base pairing with adenine are shown in Figure 16–4. Thymine-adenine and guanine-cytosine base pairing are illustrated in Figure 15–4. The reaction catalyzed by RNA polymerase is reversible, the number of energy-rich bonds is conserved, and the reaction is isoergonic. Hydrolysis of PP$_i$ catalyzed by pyrophosphatase, however, pulls the RNA polymerase reaction in the direction of RNA synthesis.

Although DNA consists of two strands, only one strand of DNA serves as a template for RNA biosynthesis at a given genetic locus. At some loci on a chromosome, however, one strand serves as template, and at other loci, the other strand serves

TABLE 16–1. Major Bases Found in DNA and RNA	
DNA	**RNA**
Adenine	Adenine
Cytosine	Cytosine
Guanine	Guanine
Thymine	Uracil

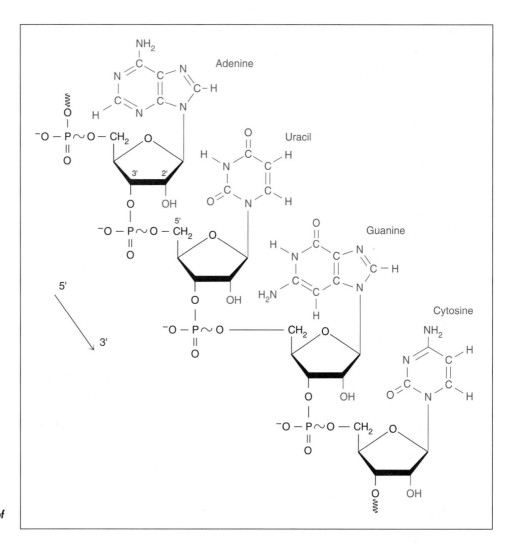

FIGURE 16–2. Covalent structure of RNA (ribonucleic acid).

TABLE 16–2.   General Classes of Human and Bacterial RNA

Class	Size	Comments
Bacterial ribosomal RNA	16S, 1500 bases	Small subunit
	23S, 2900 bases	Large subunit
	5S, 120 bases	Large subunit
Human ribosomal RNA	18S, 1900 bases	RNA polymerase I transcript, small subunit
	28S, 4700 bases	RNA polymerase I transcript, large subunit
	5.8S, 160 bases	RNA polymerase I transcript, large subunit
	5S, 120 bases	RNA polymerase III transcript, large subunit
Bacterial and human transfer RNA	75 to 95 bases	About 50 different tRNAs in the cytosol of bacterial and human cells
Bacterial messenger RNA	600 bases and greater	5% of total cellular RNA; short half-life (minutes); often polycistronic (translated into more than one protein)
Human mRNA	600 bases and greater	5% of total RNA; half-life from minutes to days; contains 5' 7-methyl G cap and polyA 3' tail Monocistronic
Human heterogeneous nuclear RNA	May contain 100 kb or more	95% degraded in nucleus. Precursor of mRNA; undergoes splicing reactions
Human small nuclear RNAs (snRNAs or snurps)	100 to 300 bases	U1, U2, U3, U4, U5, U6, U7, U8, U9, U10

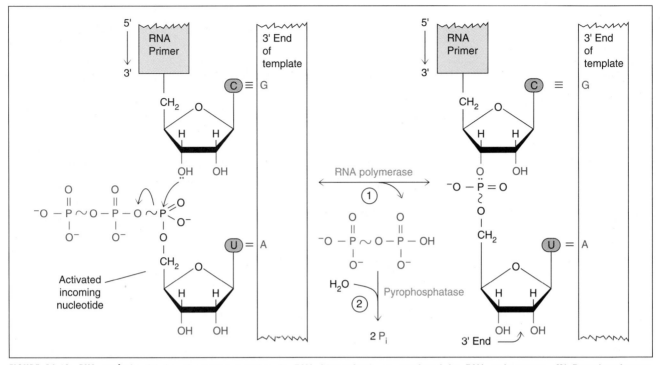

FIGURE 16-3. RNA synthesis. *(1) An elongation reaction in RNA biosynthesis as catalyzed by RNA polymerase. (2) Pyrophosphatase catalyzes the hydrolysis of its substrate.*

as template. *The DNA strand whose sequence corresponds to that of the functional RNA is called the* **sense strand.** The complementary strand is called the **antisense strand.** This nomenclature is based on the historical analysis of RNA and protein structure. The triplets, or trinucleotides, of mRNA that code for each amino acid in a protein were determined first, and these triplets correspond to information, or sense. DNA sequences are analyzed similarly, and the DNA nucleotide triplets corresponding to the RNA genetic code conform to sense. Because of the *anti*parallel nature of the DNA duplex, the DNA segment complementary to the sense strand is called *anti*sense. The antisense strand serves as the template for RNA polymerase. When regulatory DNA sequences are given, they correspond to the sense strand.

Bacterial RNA Polymerases

INITIATION AND ELONGATION REACTIONS. The protein subunit structure of the *Escherichia coli* **holoenzyme** is $\alpha_2\beta\beta'\sigma$. The β and β' subunits are unrelated despite the similarity of the designations. The length of the *E. coli* RNA polymerase molecule is 15 nm. In view of the 3.4 nm length of one turn of the DNA double helix, the polymerase can extend over the length of nearly four turns. *E. coli* RNA polymerase with a sigma (σ) subunit recognizes and binds to special sequences of DNA **(promoters)** that direct the initiation of gene transcription. Promoters include about 50 nucleotides on the 5′ side of the transcription unit and extend about 20 nucleotides into the transcription unit.

The nucleotide corresponding to the first base in the primary transcript is designated +1. Subsequent nucleotides of the sense strand corresponding to the primary transcript are designated +2, +3, and so forth. This direction is called **downstream.** The nucleotide immediately 5′ of the +1 position of the sense strand is called −1. Nucleotides in the 5′ direction are numbered −2, −3, and so forth. This direction is called **upstream** (Figure 16–1).

The exact length and sequence of bacterial promoters varies. There are two segments in the *E. coli* promoter that contain **consensus sequences.** These are centered at −10 and −30. The −10 sequence, read from the sense strand, is TATAAT; it is often called the TATA box (pronounced "tata"). The −30 region has a consensus sequence TTGACA (this is not pronounced but is read letter

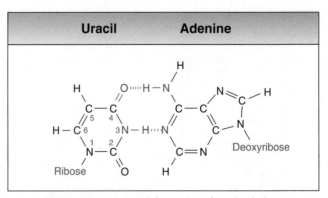

FIGURE 16-4. Watson-Crick base pairing of uracil and adenine.

by letter). The TATA box occurs in human genes; this sequence will become familiar through repetition. The -30 sequence is given for general reference, and only specialists know it by rote. Not all promoters have this precise sequence. Any given promoter, however, will vary at only a few positions—a property that led to the designation of such sequences as consensus sequences.

Bacterial RNA polymerases are classified as either **holoenzymes** or **core enzymes.** Core *E. coli* RNA polymerase consists of $\alpha_2\beta\beta'$ subunits. A σ-subunit is necessary for physiological chain initiation. Bacteria contain a several σ-subunits that differ in their DNA-recognition properties and that initiate synthesis at their cognate promoters and not at others. Five σ factors have been identified in *E. coli.* Various σ subunits are responsible for differential gene expression. A σ-subunit forms a complex with the core enzyme to form the $\alpha_2\beta\beta'\sigma$ holoenzyme. The holoenzyme scans the bacterial DNA, forming a loose complex until it binds to a cognate promoter and forms a tight complex. The initial and specific combination of the RNA polymerase holoenzyme with its promoter results in a closed complex. The **closed complex** is converted into an **open complex** as some DNA unwinds; ATP is not required for the formation of the open complex.

To initiate RNA synthesis, one nucleoside triphosphate reacts with an incoming nucleoside triphosphate; both nucleotides form complementary base pairs with the template. The 3′-hydroxyl group of the initiating nucleotide, generally ATP, attacks the α-phosphorus atom of the second nucleotide to form a phosphodiester bond. The product of the first elongation reaction is 5′-pppApN-3′ (where N is any ribonucleoside) and PP_i. The 5′ end of the molecule initially retains the triphosphate linkage. The sequence of the bases of all of the nucleotides of the RNA is determined by complementary base pairing.

After a few elongation reactions, the σ-subunit dissociates from the holoenzyme and can bind to another core RNA polymerase to reinitiate RNA synthesis at the same or different gene. The core enzyme continues the elongation process until the primary transcript is completed. Different σ subunits recognize different promoters and are responsible for differential gene expression.

The *lac* **operon** of *E. coli* consists of regulatory and structural genes that play a role in lactose metabolism. A continuous DNA segment includes an **operator** gene and the *z, y,* and *a* genes, which encode for β-galactosidase, galactoside permease, and acetylase, respectively. An *i* gene, which is separated from these genes, is also involved in regulation of gene expression. The operator gene is a regulatory gene and does not code for a protein. The other genes are structural genes and code for proteins. A group of contiguous genes controlled by a single operator is called an **operon.**

The *i* gene codes for a **repressor.** The Lac repressor is a protein that binds to the *lac* operator (a specific 17-nucleotide DNA sequence) and inhibits transcription of the *z, y,* and *a* genes. When lactose serves as the carbon source, allolactose (an intermediate produced during the hydrolysis catalyzed by β-galactosidase) binds to the repressor. The sugar-repressor complex is inactive and can no longer bind to the operator. Transcription and translation of the proteins of the *z, y,* and *a* genes then transpires. The corresponding proteins are synthesized, and their levels increase by several orders of magnitude. The three proteins participate in the utilization of lactose as a fuel to support cellular metabolism. The operator lies between the promoter and start site of the *z* gene. The binding of the repressor inhibits gene expression and is a **negative transcription element.**

A **cistron** is a unit of gene expression. In prokaryotes, the product of several contiguous genes may be transcribed to produce a **polycistronic message.** A single mRNA, for example, in *E. coli* codes for β-galactosidase, permease, and acetylase. Initiation and termination of protein synthesis from a polycistronic message occurs independently for each of the components. *Cis*-acting elements are DNA segments, and *trans*-acting elements are proteins that are encoded by a distant gene. Auxiliary factors such as cyclic *A*MP binding *p*rotein (CAP) function as positive regulators of bacterial gene transcription. The Lac repressor and CAP are examples of *trans*-acting elements.

TERMINATION REACTIONS. There are two major types of termination reaction in bacteria such as *E. coli.* One is dependent upon a ρ (rho) factor and is called **rho factor–dependent termination.** The second is independent of any factor and is called **rho factor–independent termination.** The signals for rho factor–dependent termination occur about 80 nucleotides upstream from the stop site, and they include C residues spaced 12 nucleotides apart. Rho factor has RNA-DNA helicase activity that promotes transcript release; this helicase activity consumes ATP.

Rho factor–independent signals are recognized by the core RNA polymerase and cause termination. Rho factor–independent termination occurs at specific sequences of RNA. Regions rich in GC precede a stretch of uracil residues in the primary transcript. Adenine-uracil hydrogen bonding is weaker than guanine-cytosine hydrogen bonding, and less stable DNA-RNA bonding involving stretches of A≡U promotes dissociation of the uracil-containing transcript.

Human RNA Polymerases

Human cells contain three major classes of nuclear RNA polymerase (Table 16–3). The subunit composition of human RNA polymerases is much more complicated than that of the bacterial enzymes. The molecular masses of each of the three RNA polymerases is large (500–600 kDa), and each

TABLE 16–3. Human RNA Polymerases

Polymerase	Location	Product	Polymerase Activity of Cell
RNA polymerase I	Nucleolus	35–47S pre-rRNA	≈60%
RNA polymerase II	Nucleoplasm	hnRNA/mRNA, U1, U2, U4, and U5 snRNAs*	≈30%
RNA polymerase III	Nucleoplasm	tRNAs, 5S RNA, U6 snRNA,* 7SL RNA, 7SK RNA	≈10%
Mitochondrial RNA polymerase	Mitochondrion	Products of all mitochondrial genes	≈2%

*snRNA, small nuclear RNA.

of the enzymes, like that of bacteria, contains zinc. Each enzyme contains two large subunits (molecular masses of about 200 and 140 kDa) and about 10 smaller subunits ranging in mass from 10 to 90 kDa. The reactions catalyzed by the eukaryotic enzymes are analogous to those of the bacterial enzymes. Chain growth occurs in the $5' \rightarrow 3'$ direction, and a DNA template is required (Figure 16–3). Eukaryotic and prokaryotic RNA polymerases, unlike all DNA polymerases, can initiate polynucleotide biosynthesis.

RNA POLYMERASE I. Three of the four ribosomal RNA molecules in human cells are derived from a single RNA polymerase I transcript that includes the 18S, 5.8S, and 28S RNA precursor. The fourth ribosomal RNA (5S) is an RNA polymerase III transcript. The ribosomal RNA genes occur in clusters composed of about 280 repeats (about 40 kb per repeat) of DNA clustered on five chromosomes (13, 14, 15, 21, and 22). The primary transcript is about 14 kb. About half the transcribed segments are eliminated by hydrolysis. The nontranscribed, or intergenic, segment is about 25 kb long. The substantial transcriptional activity that human cells devote toward ribosomal RNA synthesis reflects the great need of the cell for ribosomes.

Let us consider the RNA polymerase I promoter and transcription factors. The promoter of ribosomal genes surrounds the transcription start site. The region between −45 and +20 influences initiation by RNA polymerase I, and this is called the **core promoter.** The segment between −45 and −15 is important for the binding of a transcription factor called TFID (this is an abbreviation for transcription factor ID where I (one) refers to the class of eukaryotic polymerase). TFID is important for the accurate selection of the RNA polymerase I binding site. The region between −180 and −105, which is called the **upstream promoter** element, is also important in the binding of RNA polymerase I transcription factors (UBFI [upstream binding factor-I] and SL1). The SL1 transcription factor can bind to both the core and upstream promoter elements. The interaction of the promoter elements of the ribosomal RNA genes, the RNA polymerase I transcription factors, and RNA polymerase I are required for the physiological initiation of the RNA polymerase I primary transcripts. These transcrip-

tion factors can interact sequentially with several RNA polymerase I molecules and initiate the synthesis of several rRNA primary transcripts. A list of transcription factors for RNA polymerase I and their properties is given for general reference in Table 16–4.

Following initiation, multiple elongation reactions are followed by a termination event. Knowledge of the chain termination events in RNA biosynthesis is sketchy. Termination of rRNA transcripts involving RNA polymerase I appears to involve a cluster of about four T residues at the 3′ end of the gene. Other sequences, not yet identified, are also required.

RNA POLYMERASE II. RNA polymerase II, which accounts for about 30% of RNA synthesis, transcribes all the genes whose products will become translated into proteins. RNA polymerase II also transcribes some genes that encode small RNA molecules required for RNA processing (for example, U1, U2, U4, and U5 snRNA). hnRNA is the precursor of mRNA that directs protein biosynthesis.

Most commonly, only one copy of a gene per haploid genome corresponds to a particular protein. Each gene occurs at a specific location on a chromosome (Table 16–5). Note that genes for dissimilar subunits of a protein usually occur on different chromosomes. Hemoglobin, for example, contains α- and β-chains, and the corresponding genes occur on two different chromosomes. Similarly, the genes for the two different subunits of hexosaminidase A occur on different chromosomes. Synthesis of these gene products, however, is coordinately regulated. The genes for mitochondrial and cytosolic aspartate aminotransferase and the genes for different tissue forms of glycogen phosphorylase occur on different chromosomes.

TABLE 16–4. RNA Polymerase I Transcription Factors (TFI)

Factor	Characteristic
SL1	Binds to −180 to −120 region of rRNA genes; also binds to −45 to +20 region
TFIA	May be a nuclease inhibitor
TFIC	Binds to TFID-rRNA gene complex
TFID	Binds to −45 to −15 region of rRNA genes
UBFI	Binds to −120 to −105 region of rRNA genes

TABLE 16-5. Chromosomal Location of Selected Genes

Gene	Chromosome	Gene	Chromosome
Adenosine deaminase*	20	HMG-CoA synthetase	5
Argininosuccinate lyase	7	HMG-CoA reductase	5
Argininosuccinate synthetase*	9	Hypoxanthine-guanine phosphoribosyltransferase	X
Aspartate aminotransferase, cytosolic	10	α-Iduronidase*	22
Aspartate aminotransferase, mitochondrial	16	Initiator methionine tRNA	6
CAD multienzyme complex of pyrimidine biosynthesis	2	Insulin	11
Carbamoyl-phosphate synthetase I	2	Insulin receptor	19
Creatine kinase, muscle	19	Interferon α	9
Cystathionine lyase	16	*jun* protooncogene	1
Cystic fibrosis*	7	LDL receptor*	19
DNA polymerase α	X	Lecithin-cholesterol acyltransferase	16
DNA polymerase β	8	Maple syrup urine disease	19
DNA topoisomerase II	17	Muscular dystrophy, Duchenne and Becker	X
Erythropoietin	7	Myoglobin	22
Factor II (prothrombin)	11	Phenylalanine hydroxylase	12
Factor VII	13	Phosphoribosylpyrophosphate synthetase	X
Factor VIII (hemophilia A)*	X	Progesterone 21-hydroxylase	6
Factor IX (hemophilia B)*	X	Purine nucleoside phosphorylase*	14
fos protooncogene	14	Red hair color	4
α-L-Fucosidase*	1	Ribosomal RNA (18S, 28S, and 5.8S)	13, 14, 15, 21, 22
Galactocerebrosidase	17	5S ribosomal RNA	1
Galactokinase	17	RNA polymerase II, large subunit	17
Galactose-1-phosphate uridyltransferase	9	Salivary proline-rich protein complex	12
α-Globin cluster	16	Sarcomeric myosin heavy chains	17
β-Globin cluster* (sickle cell anemia, β-thalassemia)	11	Sphingomyelinase*	17
Glucagon	2	Thymidine kinase	17
Glucocerebrosidase*	1	Thyroglobulin	8
Glycogen phosphorylase, brain	20	Transfer RNAs for leucine, glutamate, and lysine	17
Glycogen phosphorylase, liver	14	Triose phosphate isomerase	12
Glycogen phosphorylase, muscle	11	Trypsin	7
Glucose-6-phosphate dehydrogenase	X	Tryptophan hydroxylase	11
α-Glucosidase	17	Tyrosinase	11
Hexokinase	10	Tyrosine hydroxylase	11
Hexosaminidase A, α-subunit	15	U1 snRNA	19
Hexosaminidase A, β-subunit	5	UMP synthase	3
Histidine ammonia lyase	12	Uroporphyrinogen synthase	11
Histone H1, H3, and H4, family 2	1	Zellweger syndrome	7
Histone H1, H2A, H2B, cluster A	7		

*Potential gene therapy candidates.

Furthermore, genes corresponding to a hormone (insulin) and its receptor occur independently. Phenylalanine hydroxylase, tryptophan hydroxylase, and tyrosine hydroxylase are evolutionarily related. Phenylalanine hydroxylase occurs on a different chromosome from the other two. Note that two of the genes for the components of a single process such as blood clotting are found on the same chromosome, and the genes corresponding to other factors occur on different chromosomes. In contrast to bacterial operons, genetic dispersion of functionally related proteins appears to be the general rule in humans.

Genes corresponding to hnRNA consist of segments that are expressed in the mature mRNA, called **exons,** and segments that are not expressed in mRNA, **introns.** The introns are removed post-transcriptionally by splicing reactions (Figure 15–2). Most genes contain considerably more intron sequence than exon sequence (Table 16–6), but the ratio varies considerably. The factor VIII gene, mutations of which cause hemophilia A, is about 187 kb in length of which 9 kb or about 5%

represents exons. The factor VIII gene contains 25 introns. The interferon α gene and histone genes, on the other hand, lack introns, but this situation is rare. The comparative sizes and numbers of exons and introns in selected human genes are illustrated in Figure 16–5.

TABLE 16-6. Exon-Intron Composition of Selected Human Genes

Gene Product	Exons *Total bp*	Introns *Number*	Introns *Total bp*
Adenosine deaminase	1,500	11	30,000
Apolipoprotein B	14,000	28	29,000
Dystrophin	14,000	79	2,300,000
Erythropoietin	600	4	1,500
Factor VIII	9,000	25	177,000
Interferon α	600	0	0
Histone	400	0	0
LDL receptor	5,100	17	40,000
Thyroglobulin	8,500	>40	100,000

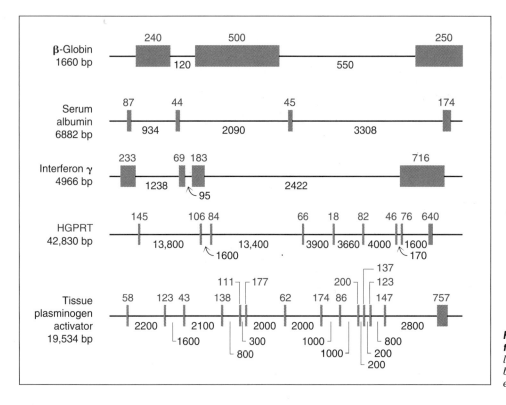

FIGURE 16-5. Exon-intron composition of selected genes. *Horizontal lines denote introns, and the boxes or vertical lines denote exons. The scale is approximate.*

Because each human cell contains many identical proteins (for so-called housekeeping functions), the promoter regions for these RNA polymerase II transcripts are expected to be similar. Other proteins, however, are cell and tissue specific. The transcription elements (TE) that regulate the expression of cell-specific and housekeeping proteins are expected to differ. As cells differentiate and development occurs, different genes are expressed. Regulation of the transcription of the various hnRNAs and their derivative mRNAs is thus an important problem in differentiation and development.

Let us consider RNA polymerase II promoters and transcription elements. **Promoters** select or determine the start site of RNA synthesis, and **transcription elements** determine the frequency of transcription. Promoter and transcription elements are modular. Different genes transcribed by RNA polymerase II may have different promoter and transcription elements. Most promoters for RNA polymerase II transcripts exhibit a TATA box about 30 nucleotides upstream from the start site. Upstream promoter elements can include one or more GC boxes around −70 to −90 and a CAAT box (pronounced "cat") at −100 (Table 16-7). The **TATA box** is called a selector, and its function is to pinpoint the start site. Mutations in the TATA box can disturb correct initiation. The TATA box precedes most (but not all) genes that are transcribed by RNA polymerase II.

Transcription elements can occur farther upstream and may be thousands of bases away from the start site. Transcription elements can also occur within the transcription unit itself (that is, downstream from the start site) or on the 3′ side of the transcription unit. Transcription elements include enhancers, silencers, and response elements. **Enhancers** are DNA sequences that increase the frequency of gene transcription. These can be located either upstream or downstream from the start site and may be in either orientation and still be active (either 5′ → 3′ or 3′ → 5′). **Silencers** ex-

TABLE 16-7.   Human RNA Polymerase II Transcription Factors (TFII)

Factor	Characteristic	Sequence Element
CREB	Binds to cyclic AMP response element	TGACGTCA
CTF	Binds to TFIID and the CAAT box	GGCCAATCT
GATA1	Functions in erythroid cells	GATA
Jun-Fos	Binds to AP1 site	TGACTCA
NF-E2	Functions in erythroid cells	TGAGTCA
NF-κB (H2-TF1)	Functions in lymphoid cells (functions in many cells)	GGGACTTTCC
OTF1	Functions in many cells	ATGCAAAT
OTF2	Functions in lymphoid cells	ATGCAAAT
SP1	Specificity factor 1 binds to GC boxes	GGGCGG
TFIIA	Stabilizes TFIID bound to the promoter	
TFIIB	Interacts with RNA polymerase II.	
TFIID (TBP and TAFs)	Binds to TATA box	TATAAAA
TFIIE	Interacts with RNA polymerase II and TFIIB	
TFIIF	Has DNA helicase activity; binds RNA polymerase II	
TFIIH	Binds after TFIIE	
TFIIJ	Binds after TFIIE	

hibit many of the same properties as enhancers except that they decrease the frequency of gene transcription. Often there are repeats of the same sequence, and the multiplicity yields more powerful regulatory effects. **Response elements** are target sequences for signaling molecules such as cyclic AMP. This target sequence (Table 16–7) is called CRE (for cyclic AMP response element). Promoter elements (TATA, GC, and CAAT boxes) identify the start site for transcription, and transcription elements alter the frequency of gene transcription. Promoters and transcription elements, however, can contain the same sequence elements and overlap (Figure 16–6).

Transcription factor IID, which plays a pivotal role in chain initiation, binds to the TATA box without the involvement of other factors or RNA polymerase II. TFIID consists of two types of component. A TATA-binding protein (TBP) recognizes the TATA box, and TAFs (TBP-associated factors) are auxiliary proteins that participate in this process. TFIID recruits the basal transcription apparatus including RNA polymerase II and factors TFIIA, TFIIB, TFIIE, TFIIF, TFIIH, and TFIIJ. TBP binds to the minor groove of DNA, and other factors bind to the major groove. SP1, a transcription factor, interacts with GC boxes in the upstream promoter region; this interaction can increase transcription fivefold. The effects of SP1 are mediated via interaction with factor TFIID. Similarly, CTF (*CAAT* box *f*actor, a family of proteins) enhances the rate of transcription via interaction with TFIID. Probably all regulatory DNA sequences that influence transcription are targets for proteins. RNA polymerase II *per se* is unable to recognize promoters without the aid of protein transcription factors (Table 16–7). The organization of several RNA polymerase II–transcribed genes is illustrated in Figure 16–6.

Regulation of the expression of the β-globin gene cluster illustrates several pertinent points. This cluster of genes is expressed sequentially in embryonic, fetal, and adult life. Expression is tissue specific: the ε-chain is produced in the yolk sac of the embryo, the δ-chain is produced by the liver of the fetus, and the β-chain and small amounts of the γ-chain are produced in the bone marrow of the newborn, child, and adult. The β-globin gene clusters have transcription elements that are upstream and downstream of their coding sequences. Some of this information is derived from a study of individuals with β-thalassemia, a disorder characterized by a deficiency of the β-chains of hemoglobin (Chapter 24).

A **locus control region** of β-globin (β-LCR) has been identified by showing that it is hypersensitive to digestion with DNAse I *in vitro*. DNAse I sensitivity is a marker for uncondensed DNA regions. The locus control region is sensitive to DNAse I in erythroid cells (yolk sac, liver, bone marrow) but not in other cells. Moreover, this region is sensitive to DNAse throughout an individual's lifetime and is not developmentally regulated. This region occurs in the segment 20 kb upstream (5′) to the ε-globin gene and involves four different hypersensitive sites (Figure 16–7). A second DNAse hypersensitive region occurs downstream (3′) from the β-globin gene. The 3′ hypersensitive region (like the β-LCR) exists in erythroid cells throughout a person's lifetime and is not developmentally regulated.

Three sequence elements have been described in the β-LCR. One element, TGAGTCA, is a binding site for the AP1 family of transcription factors that include the products of the protooncogenes named *jun* and *fos*. (Protooncogenes are genes that play a role in normal physiology but can produce cancer because of mutation or excessive expression.) The AP1 family includes an erythroid-specific factor called NF-E2. Two copies of this AP1 element occur in the β-LCR. A second sequence element, GATA, is

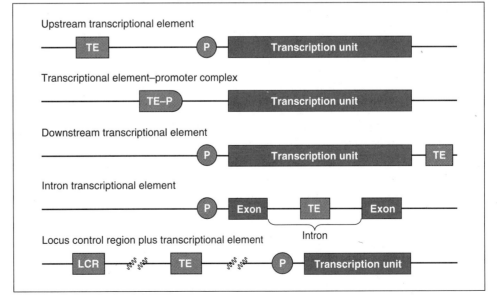

FIGURE 16–6. Design of various transcription and promoter elements for RNA polymerase II. LCR, locus control region; P, promoter; TE, transcription element.

Upstream transcriptional element

Transcriptional element–promoter complex

Downstream transcriptional element

Intron transcriptional element

Locus control region plus transcriptional element

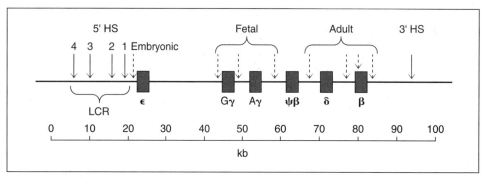

FIGURE 16–7. The β-globin gene family. *The solid arrows represent sites in DNA isolated from erythroid cells throughout life that are sensitive to DNAse digestion in vitro. The dashed arrows represent hypersensitive sites that exist only during active gene transcription in erythroid cells. HS, hypersensitive site; LCR, locus control region; G*γ *and A*γ*, two genes that encode the same fetal form of a β-like chain found in fetal hemoglobin; ψβ, a pseudogene of β-globin.*

recognized by a protein called GATA1. GATA elements replace the TATA box in a few erythroid-specific genes. A third sequence element, CACCC, is also found in erythroid-specific promoters, enhancers, and locus control regions. It is postulated that the β-LCR ensures that the globin domain of chromatin is open and available for transcription in erythroid cells but not other cells. The β-LCR presumably functions as a powerful enhancer that governs the correct temporal regulation in embryonic, fetal, and adult cells.

Other DNAse I sensitive elements are developmentally regulated and occur in the cells that actively transcribe the target DNA. A DNA hypersensitive site occurs in yolk sac cells upstream from the ε-globin gene (Figure 16–7). Hypersensitive sites occur in liver cells during fetal development and in bone marrow cells postnatally. DNAse hypersensitivity sites also occur upstream, downstream, and in the interior of the β-globin gene postnatally and in adults (Figure 16–7). Cell-specific proteins that are produced by the yolk sac, fetal liver, and bone marrow are postulated to play a role in expressing the appropriate β-like globin chain during development.

Some transcription elements respond to various physiological cues. The AP1 family of transcription factors is involved in the regulation of gene expression by various growth factors, hormones, and tumor promoters. AP1 is a heterodimer of Fos and Jun (protein products of the *fos* and *jun* protooncogenes) that interact with each other via their leucine zipper domains (Figure 3–24). The heterodimer binds to TGACTCA and enhances the transcription of target genes.

Cyclic AMP, a second messenger molecule that is produced intracellularly in response to a variety of extracellular signaling molecules, or first messengers, can activate the expression of a variety of genes including hepatic tyrosine aminotransferase and phosphoenolpyruvate carboxykinase. Cyclic AMP activates protein kinase A (where A refers to cyclic *A*MP). Protein kinase A phosphorylates and activates transcription factors that bind to a cyclic

AMP response element (CRE). One protein with CRE-binding activity is called CREB, and this protein can be phosphorylated in a reaction catalyzed by protein kinase A. The DNA sequences that respond to cyclic AMP in humans and bacteria are unrelated, and bacteria lack protein kinase A.

Initiation of RNA polymerase II transcripts follows the interaction of DNA, various transcription factors (depending on the gene), and enzyme. After multiple elongation reactions, chain termination occurs many residues (hundreds or thousands) past the 3' end of the mature RNA. The precise rules for chain termination are unknown.

RNA POLYMERASE III. tRNA, 5S RNA, and other small RNAs, whose synthesis is catalyzed by RNA polymerase III, account for about 10% of RNA synthesis. These RNAs do not encode proteins. Their products are involved in protein synthesis (tRNA and 5S RNA), intracellular protein transport (7SL RNA), and posttranscriptional processing (U6 RNA). RNA polymerase III also mediates the synthesis of RNA of unknown function including 7SK and Alu RNA. The primary transcript of 5S, 7SL, and U6 RNA requires no posttranscriptional processing reactions to generate the final product. tRNA, on the other hand, requires removal of the 5' and 3' ends to produce functional transcripts.

Three transcription factors (TFIIIA, TFIIIB, and TFIIIC) are associated with RNA polymerase III (Table 16–8). Surprisingly, the promoter region for genes transcribed by RNA polymerase III lies downstream from the transcription start site. tRNA

TABLE 16–8. Human RNA Polymerase III Transcription Factors (TFIII)

Factor	Characteristic
TFIIIA	Binds internal control region of 5S rRNA gene; a zinc-finger protein.
TFIIIB	Interacts with RNA polymerase–DNA complex via protein-protein interactions.
TFIIIC	Binds internal control region of all class III genes except the 5S rRNA gene.

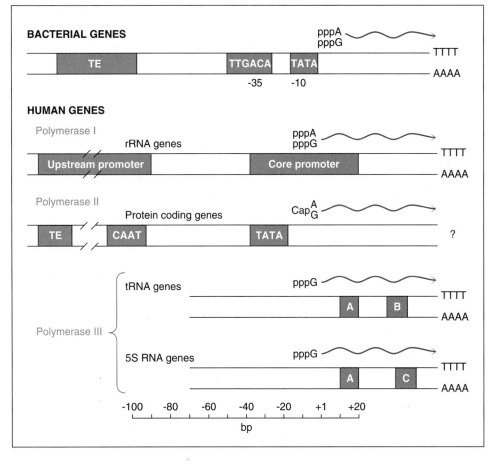

FIGURE 16–8. *Diagram of promoter and transcription elements (TEs) of bacterial and human RNA polymerases. The promoters for RNA polymerase III transcripts include A, B, and C boxes that occur in the transcribed region. The sizes of the promoter and regulatory elements are not necessarily to scale.*

genes have a promoter element just downstream from the transcription start site called the A box. The B box is a second promoter element that is farther downstream. 5S RNA genes have an A box and a C box (Figure 16–8).

Initiation of RNA polymerase III transcripts follows the interaction of DNA, transcription factors, and enzyme. Termination by RNA polymerase III of 5S RNA transcripts involves a sequence of four or more A residues in the sense strand surrounded by GC-rich sequences. Similar terminator sequences also occur after the coding regions of tRNA molecules. Terminating RNA polymerase transcripts in eukaryotic cells does not involve special protein termination factors such as those required for some bacterial transcripts. A summary of promoter elements, transcription elements, and termination signals for bacterial RNA polymerase and RNA polymerase I, II, and III transcripts is given in Figure 16–8.

Transcriptionally active chromatin differs in several respects from inactive chromatin. Active chromatin is more sensitive to digestion by DNAse I *in vitro* than is inactive chromatin. Increased sensitivity can extend over tens of kilobases and may contain arrays of related genes such as those of the α- or β-globin family. This domain of increased sensitivity may contain hypersensitive sites. The β-glo-

in locus control region of DNAse hypersensitivity occurs in all erythroid cells (whether or not they are actively expressing β-globin), but DNAse hypersensitivity is absent in nonerythroid cells. The β-globin locus of DNAse hypersensitivity, which is an example of a **constitutive** site of hypersensitivity, is present before the genes are transcribed and is independent of gene expression. **Inducible** hypersensitive sites also exist. Those sites in the β-globin that are developmentally regulated are examples. The activation of transcription by steroid hormones also induces DNAse hypersensitivity in target genes. Both constitutive and inducible hypersensitivity sites lack nucleosomes and are typically found in DNA elements such as promoters and enhancers. These sites are special targets for topoisomerase I and II activity.

Active chromatin is undermethylated. 5-Methylcytosine occurs almost exclusively in 5′-CG-3′ sequences. This sequence occurs about one-fifth as frequently as expected randomly, but 60–90% of the C residues of this sequence are methylated where they do occur. *There is a correlation between undermethylation of promoter CG sequences and gene expression.* These sequences in sperm and in inactive X chromosomes are almost fully methylated. Genes that are repressed are methylated. The mechanism for gene activation by conversion of 5-methylcytosine of DNA to cytosine is unknown.

Comparison of RNA and DNA Biosynthesis

Replication is more complicated than transcription because of the necessity for copying and completely separating both DNA strands. More proteins with diverse activities are required to initiate DNA replication than transcription. Specific DNA regulatory sequences, however, play an important role in initiating replication and transcription. All cells contain several DNA polymerases. Bacteria possess one type of RNA polymerase, and human cells possess three nuclear RNA polymerases. Sigma factors play an integral role in the initiation of RNA biosynthesis in bacteria, and a variety of transcription factors play a similar role in human cells.

Mitochondria in eukaryotic cells have an RNA polymerase and a DNA polymerase (γ) that differ from the nuclear and bacterial enzymes. Mitochondrial RNA polymerase, a monomer of molecular mass of 140 kDa, is the product of a nuclear gene. Mitochondrial RNA polymerase bears no relationship to the nuclear or bacterial RNA polymerases, and its evolutionary origin is obscure. Initiation of RNA synthesis in mitochondria appears to involve at least one transcription factor.

RNA polymerase can initiate transcription, but DNA polymerase is not able to initiate replication; this is an important difference between the two processes. RNA synthesis begins at a start site and involves a reaction between ATP and a second nucleoside triphosphate. The RNA primer for replication is synthesized by primase. The elongation reactions of RNA and DNA biosynthesis are similar and occur in the $5' \rightarrow 3'$ direction (Table 16–9).

Two high-energy phosphate bonds are used for the incorporation of each nucleotide into RNA. One energy-rich $3',5'$-phosphodiester bond is produced. The process of RNA synthesis requires the hydrolysis of pyrophosphate to pull the reaction in the forward direction. Local melting, or unwinding, of the DNA duplex does not appear to require the expenditure of two ATP molecules for base-pair separation for RNA synthesis as occurs during replication. RNA biosynthesis requires the expenditure of two high-energy bonds per nucleotide incorporated; DNA biosynthesis involves the expenditure of at least three high-energy bonds per deoxyribonucleotide incorporated.

The error frequency of RNA synthesis is about 1 in 10^4 to 10^5. The error frequency of DNA biosynthesis is estimated at 1 in 10^9. RNA polymerases, in contrast to DNA polymerases, lack the $3' \rightarrow 5'$ exonuclease proofreading activity that contributes to the fidelity of replication. RNA polymerases lack $5' \rightarrow 3'$ exonuclease activity. The rate of RNA polymerization per active site of enzyme is about 6% that of DNA polymerization (3000/min for RNA versus 50,000/min for DNA in *E. coli*). Perhaps this slower rate allows RNA polymerase to maximize the fidelity of RNA biosynthesis by not misincorporating an inappropriate nucleotide owing to the greater time the enzyme has to scrutinize the incoming nucleotide before the condensation reaction. Comparable data for human RNA polymerases are not available.

POSTTRANSCRIPTIONAL RNA PROCESSING

rRNA Processing in Human Cells

Mammalian ribosomes contain four species of RNA (Table 16–2). Transcription and processing of rRNA occurs in the nucleolus. RNA polymerase I produces a single pre-rRNA molecule that contains the 18S, 5.8S, and 28S rRNA joined by transcribed spacers. Processing involves the hydrolytic cleavage of the primary transcript of rRNA as indicated in Figure 16–9. Each of the hydrolytic reactions is exergonic and unidirectional. The 45S primary transcript of human rRNA is about 14 kb long. About 50% of the precursor occurs in the functional molecules, and the remainder is degraded.

hnRNA Processing and the Formation of mRNA

Before considering the biochemistry of hnRNA processing, we compare messenger RNAs of bacterial and eukaryotic cells. In bacteria, mRNA is synthesized in functional form and requires no additional processing. Because bacteria lack a perinuclear membrane, the transcriptional machinery is not separated from the protein synthetic machinery. Nascent mRNA can interact with ribosomes and direct protein synthesis before the completion of RNA synthesis. In human cells, the transcriptional machinery is separated from the translational machinery. The RNA is synthesized and transported from the nucleus to the cytoplasm before protein synthesis can occur. The primary transcript of eukaryotic mRNA, unlike that from bacteria, is not functional and must be processed to produce functional mRNA. Posttranscriptional modification occurs before the RNA is transported

---

TABLE 16–9. Comparison of RNA Polymerase and DNA Polymerase

	RNA Polymerase	DNA Polymerase
Similarities		
DNA template–directed	Yes	Yes
Requires 4 triphosphates	Yes	Yes
Synthesis: $5' \rightarrow 3'$, antiparallel	Yes	Yes
Differences		
Functions	Transcription	Replication, repair
Starts chains	Yes	No
Product	Single strand	Part of duplex
Proofreading	No	Yes

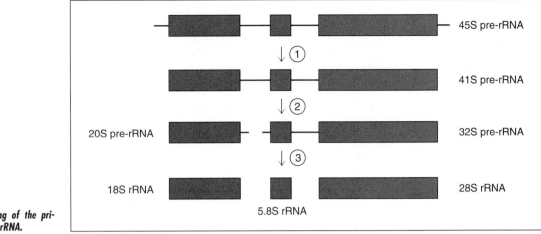

FIGURE 16–9. *Processing of the primary transcript of human rRNA.*

from the nucleus to the cytosol where protein synthesis occurs. Mature mRNA contains a special nucleotide cap, noncoding sequences, a coding sequence that corresponds to its protein, and a polyA tail (Figure 16–10). Following the formation of hnRNA, processing of the ends of the molecule occurs (Figure 16–11). The 5′ end reacts with GTP and forms a cap. The **cap** reacts with *S*-adenosylmethionine and undergoes methylation reactions. The 3′ end of hnRNA undergoes a hydrolytic cleavage reaction removing a segment of RNA. The resulting 3′ end reacts with about 200 ATP molecules to add a polyA tail. The pre-mRNA then undergoes a series of splicing reactions. Humans and other eukaryotes possess interrupted genes, and intervening RNA segments (introns) are removed during splicing and the exons are joined together (PRINCIPLE 30 OF BIOCHEMISTRY).

Capping Reactions

Mature mRNAs of eukaryotic cells have their 5′ termini blocked by a methylated guanosine cap linked to the primary transcript in 5′ → 5′ linkage, which is a rarity in nature (Figure 16–12). Human cells contain predominantly mRNAs with the cap 1 and cap 2 structures. An overview of the capping pathway, which occurs at the 5′ ends of nascent or growing transcripts, is shown in Figure 16–13. No residues are removed from the 5′ end of the primary transcript before capping. The reactants include GTP and a nascent hnRNA with a 5′-diphosphate terminus (Figure 16–14). The oxygen atom

of the diphosphate group at the 5′ end of hnRNA (a nucleophile) attacks the α-phosphorus atom of GTP. The guanylate becomes attached to the RNA by a 5′ → 5′ triphosphate bridge, and PPi is displaced.

The cap undergoes methylation by energy-rich *S*-adenosylmethionine. The methylated acceptor is low energy in nature, and the enzyme catalyzed reaction is exergonic. A consideration of the bioenergetics of the reactions involved in capping (Figure 16–13) aids in understanding these chemical transformations. The hydrolysis of phosphate from the primary transcript, the hydrolysis of pyrophosphate, and the three methyl transfer reactions are exergonic.

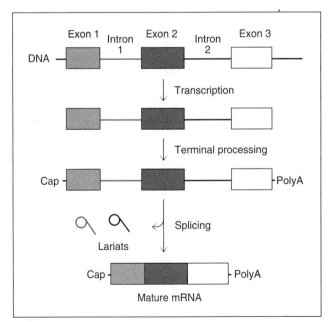

FIGURE 16–11. *An overview of the processing of eukaryotic hnRNA to form mRNA. First, RNA polymerase II catalyzes the synthesis of the primary transcript. Second, capping and the polyA tail are added during terminal processing. Third, intervening sequences are removed as lariats during splicing.*

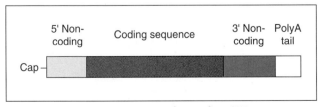

FIGURE 16–10. *Processed mammalian mRNA.*

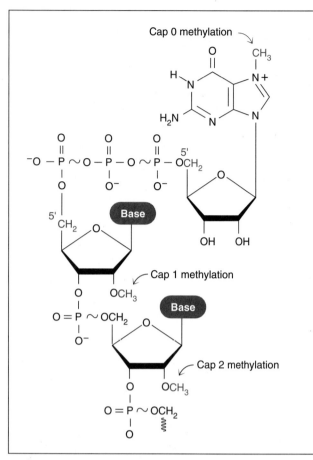

Cap 0 methylation

Cap 1 methylation

Cap 2 methylation

FIGURE 16–12. The 5′ cap of eukaryotic mRNA.

Formation of the PolyA Tail

A second event in the terminal processing of hnRNA is the addition of a polyA tail, which is not encoded by DNA. Two operations are involved. First, a segment of the 3′ end of the primary transcript is hydrolytically cleaved (Figure 16–15). This enzymatic reaction, which occurs about 20 residues downstream from a consensus sequence (AAUAAA), leaves a free 3′-hydroxyl group. In reactions catalyzed by **polyA polymerase,** about 200 adenylate residues are added to the 3′ end of RNA in 3′ → 5′ phosphodiester linkages. The free 3′-hydroxyl group of the RNA participates in a series of transferase reactions resulting in the formation of the polyA tail. *This reaction is independent of a template,* and the exact length of the polyA tail varies. ATP is the activated adenylate donor. The reaction catalyzed by the polyA polymerase is isoergonic (Figure 16–16). The reaction is pulled to completion by the action of pyrophosphatase, which catalyzes the exergonic hydrolysis of the other product of the reaction.

Nuclear mRNA Splicing Reactions

The final processing reactions of hnRNA are the splicing reactions (Figure 16–11). The location of the splice sites is determined genetically by the nucleotide sequence. The base sequence of an intron begins with GU and ends with AG. The consensus sequences surrounding the junctions of the donor and acceptor exons are shown in Figure 16–17. Introns also contain a branching site located 20 to 50 nucleotides upstream from the 3′ splice site. Introns vary in size from about 65 to greater than 10,000 nucleotides.

The stages of splicing include (1) transesterification with a branch-site adenosine, (2) displacement of exon 1, (3) transesterification of the donor and acceptor exon, and (4) displacement of lariat RNA. The final products include spliced RNA and the intron with the lariat structure (Figure 16–18).

Splicing reactions, which are intricate, occur in a complex called a **spliceosome** composed of about 45 proteins, small nuclear RNA, and the hnRNA substrate. In the first part of hnRNA splicing, a 2′-hydroxyl group of the branch-site adenosine attacks the phosphorus atom on the 5′ side of the invariant guanosine at the beginning of the intron. An isoergonic transesterification reaction results in the formation of a branch and the displacement of the 3′ end of the donor or upstream exon (Figure 16–19). In the second part of hnRNA splicing, the 3′-hydroxyl group of the donor exon (Figure 16–20) attacks the phosphorus atom on the 3′ side of

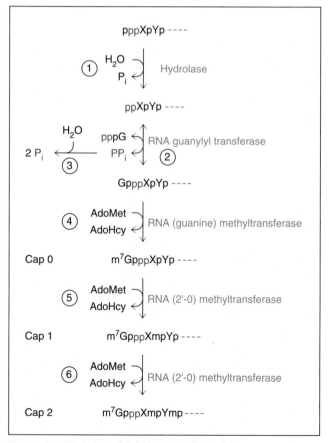

FIGURE 16–13. Pathway for the formation of capped mRNA. *The cap 0, 1, and 2 structures are formed by three successive exergonic methylation reactions. X represents the first nucleoside, and Y represents the second nucleoside of nascent RNA. m, methyl.*

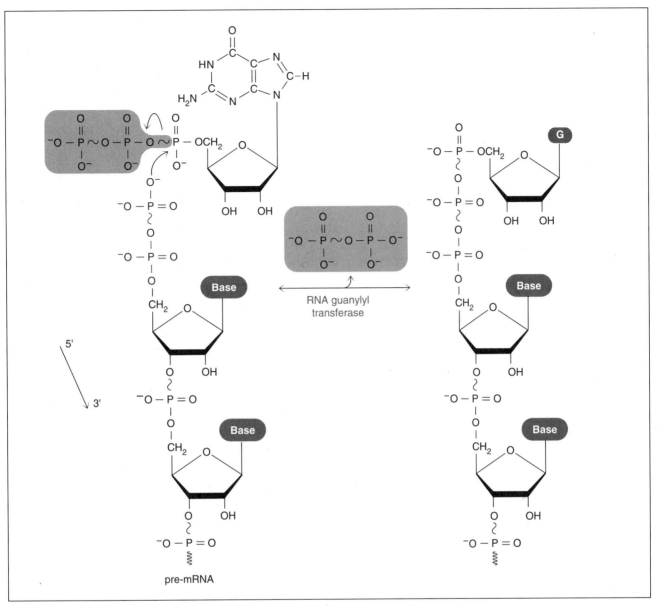

FIGURE 16–14. Guanylylation of hnRNA to form the 5' cap.

the invariant G residue at the 3' end of the intron. The intron is displaced, and a traditional 3',5'-phosphodiester bond forms. Splicing connects the donor and acceptor exons. The displaced intron contains a branch, and its structure resembles a lariat.

Small nuclear RNAs (snRNAs) complex with proteins and form small nuclear ribonucleoproteins (snRNPs). U1, U2, and U5 can form complementary base pairs with hnRNA in the region of the splice site. Moreover, pairing occurs in such a fashion that the donor and acceptor exons are in close proximity before the splicing reactions begin. Although the intervening sequence, or intron, may extend for 65 to 10,000 nucleotides, it is physically looped at the beginning of the splicing process. The role of U1 RNA in bridging the intron and exons together noncovalently by complementary base pairing is illustrated in Figure 16–21.

Formation and functioning of the spliceosome requires ATP (which is converted to ADP and P_i), but ATP does not participate in the splicing reactions *per se*. The spliceosome prevents the 5' end of the donor exon from diffusing away after its initial cleavage from hnRNA. After splicing, the intron is degraded by unspecified RNAses. All of this machinery is required to attach together exons that are separated by hundreds or thousands of nucleotides with great accuracy.

The relative size of the introns and exons of hnRNA varies considerably (Table 16–6). Occasional human mRNAs are made without any introns. The most commonly cited example is that of histone. It is noteworthy that *histone mRNAs are not polyadenylated, and they lack introns.* Sometimes introns account for a third of the total primary transcript, and in other cases introns ac-

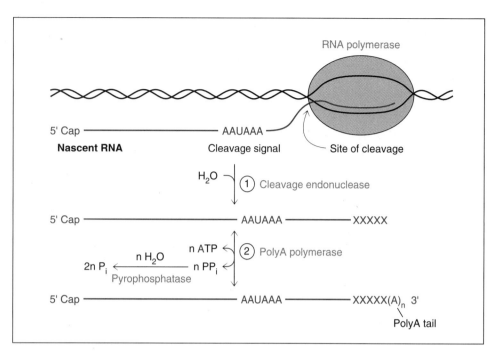

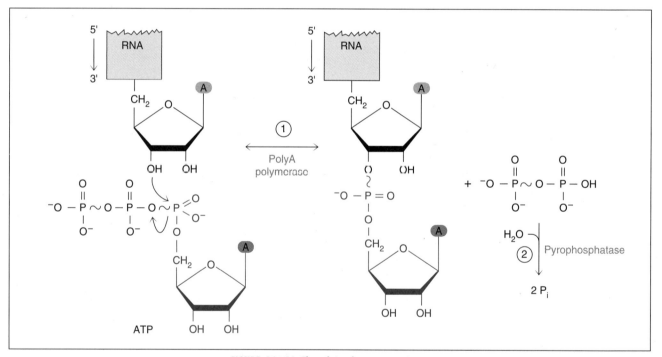

FIGURE 16–15. Cleavage and poly-adenylylation of the primary transcript of eukaryotic hnRNA. *AAUAAA on a nascent RNA serves as a cleavage signal. The hydrolysis occurs about 20 nucleotides 3' to this signal.*

FIGURE 16–16. The polyA polymerase reaction.

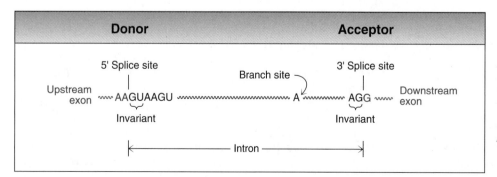

FIGURE 16–17. Consensus sequences found at eukaryotic hnRNA splice sites. *The upstream exon is also called the donor exon, and the downstream exon is called the acceptor exon. The GU at the 5' boundary of the exon and the AG residues at the 3' boundary are invariant. The branch site contains the adenosine residue that participates in lariat formation.*

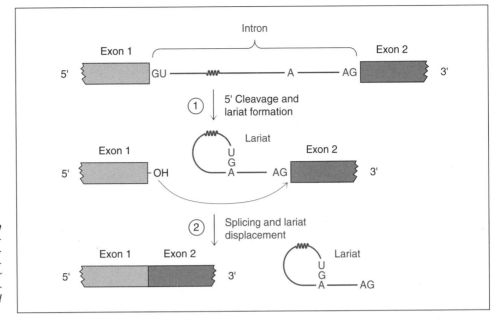

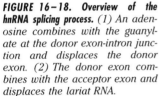

FIGURE 16–18. Overview of the hnRNA splicing process. *(1) An adenosine combines with the guanylate at the donor exon-intron junction and displaces the donor exon. (2) The donor exon combines with the acceptor exon and displaces the lariat RNA.*

count for greater than 90% of the primary transcript. Introns are not necessarily removed in the order in which they occur in the primary transcript.

The purpose or function of introns is an enigma. It has been proposed that exons encode protein domains, and that exon duplication and shuffling from gene to gene may be important in evolution by appending DNA to genes and functions to proteins. Since 90% of the primary transcript is excised and degraded in many hnRNAs, the process is energetically expensive. Eubacteria such as *E. coli* lack introns.

SYSTEMIC LUPUS ERYTHEMATOSUS. ▶ Systemic lupus erythematosus is a chronic, multisystem autoimmune disease that occurs most frequently in women between the ages of 20 and 60. The principal clinical features of this medically famous disease are skin rashes, arthritis, and glomerulonephritis. Affected individuals have antibodies that are directed toward the nucleus of the cell. Such antibodies are directed toward DNA, histone, nucleoli, and ribonucleoprotein. Antibodies from about 30% of affected individuals inhibit splicing *in vitro,* and these antibodies have provided valuable reagents for deciphering the mechanism of splicing. Whether inhibition of splicing by these antibodies plays a role in the pathogenesis of the disorder is uncertain. Antibodies directed against double-stranded DNA are specific for systemic lupus and confirm the diagnosis. Treatment is symptomatic and often includes corticosteroids to limit the immune response. ◀

Alternative Splicing Reactions

A single hnRNA can give rise to more than one mRNA by the process of alternative splicing. Alternative splicing occurs when a donor exon can be joined to different acceptor exons as illustrated by human tyrosine hydroxylase hnRNA. Tyrosine hydroxylase is the enzyme that catalyzes the conversion of tyrosine to dihydroxyphenylalanine (L-dopa) and is the first step in the pathway for catecholamine biosynthesis (Figure 19–5). Catecholamines, which include dopamine, norepinephrine, and epinephrine, function as neurotransmitters in the central and peripheral nervous systems and as adrenal medullary hormones.

The tyrosine hydroxylase gene, which is about 2 kb from the insulin gene, is about 8 kb in length. The human tyrosine hydroxylase gene contains 14 exons. There are four forms of tyrosine hydroxylase in humans, and these result from alternative splicing (Figure 16–22). The messenger RNAs for isoform 2 (12), isoform 3 (81), and isoform 4 (12 + 81 = 93) contain the designated number of additional nucleotides.

All four isoforms of tyrosine hydroxylase occur in the adrenal medulla and brain. Isoforms 1 and 2 make up about 85% of total cellular enzyme, and 3 and 4 make up the remainder. The activities of the four forms differ, and they may be regulated differently. Only humans have four isoforms. Higher primates possess two isoforms, and lower primates and other mammals have one isoform. Several other primary transcripts undergo alternative splicing including those of antibodies as described later in this chapter. Because of these reactions, one gene can give rise to more than one protein containing common and different amino acid sequences. These findings extend the one gene–one polypeptide hypothesis (PRINCIPLE 21 OF BIOCHEMISTRY).

Abnormal Splicing and β-Thalassemia

▶ β-Thalassemia is characterized by a relative or absolute deficiency of β-globin chains of hemo-

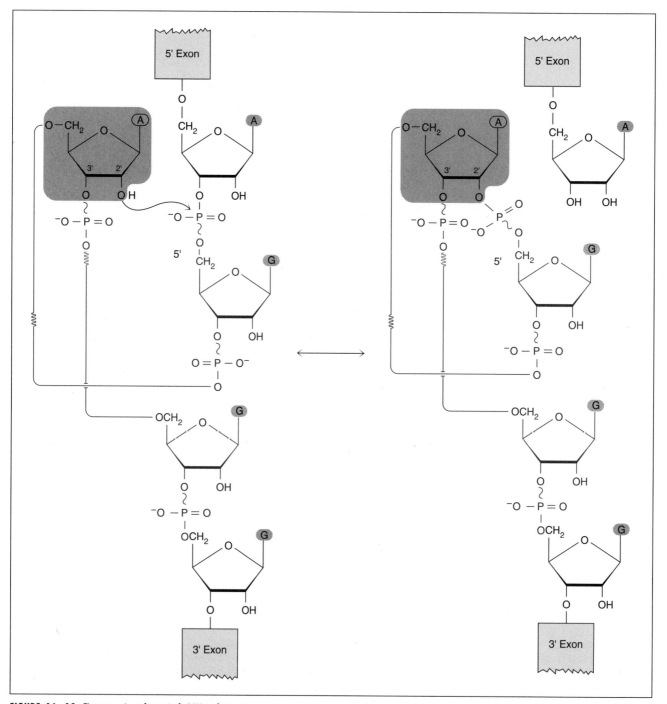

FIGURE 16–19. First step in eukaryotic hnRNA splicing. *Note that the ribose of the adenosine at the branch point forms three phosphodiesters through its 2'-, 3'-, and 5'-hydroxyl groups.*

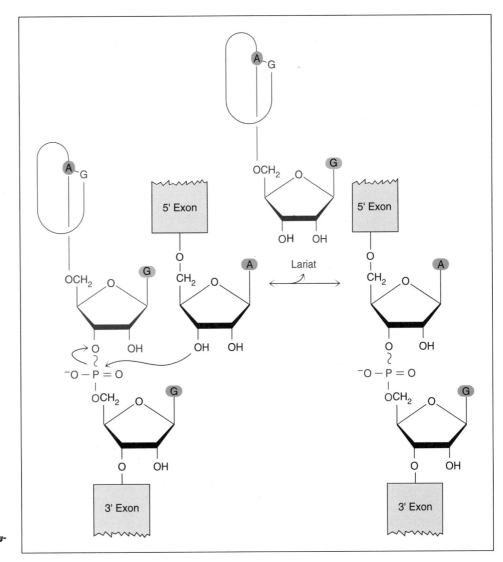

FIGURE 16–20. *Second step in eukaryotic hnRNA splicing.*

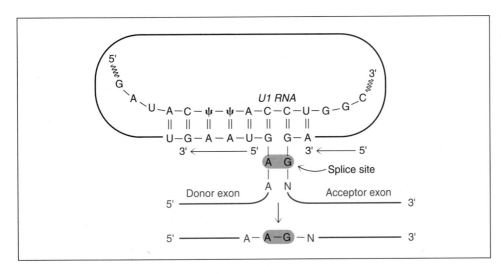

FIGURE 16–21. *A scheme for base pairing between hnRNA and human U1 snRNA.* The U1 RNA is complementary to the two boundaries of the RNA of the intron. U1 RNA brings the A residue of the donor (5′) exon adjacent to the G residue of the acceptor (3′) exon.

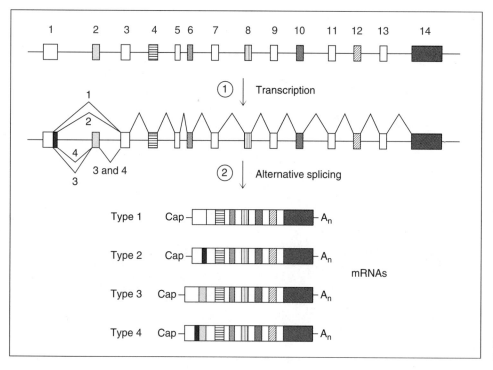

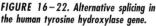

FIGURE 16–22. *Alternative splicing in the human tyrosine hydroxylase gene.*

globin. The importance of the consensus sequence surrounding the splice junctions is illustrated in variants of this disease. Mutations of the consensus sequence surrounding the donor or acceptor sites can reduce the efficiency of splicing and decrease normal β-globin mRNA levels. The critical nature of the GU in the hnRNA at the 5'-donor site and the AG dinucleotide at the 3' acceptor site was noted earlier. Individuals with mutations in any of these four nucleotides are unable to excise the affected introns normally. The conversion of the AG at the 3'-end of intron 2 of β-globin to a GG produces aberrant hnRNA. The inactivation of a normal acceptor site in this, but not all, cases elicits the use of other acceptor-like sequences elsewhere in the RNA molecule. The alternative sites are called **cryptic** (hidden) splice sites because they are not used when the correct site is available. The A → G transition mutation of the acceptor splice site results in the use of a cryptic acceptor site upstream from the normal site. Owing to aberrant splicing, the resulting RNA is unable to direct the synthesis of a normal β-globin.

Still another form of β-thalassemia is due to a mutation in an intron that converts a nonsplicing sequence into one that can participate in splicing. This can result from the generation of an AG dinucleotide from a GG dinucleotide when the surrounding sequence resembles the consensus splicing sequence. Such mutations provide an alternative acceptor site that competes with the normal acceptor site. One β-globin mRNA formed as a result of such a mutation is elongated by 19 extra nucleotides on the 5' side of exon 2, and a premature protein synthesis stop codon is introduced. This alternative form of mRNA will not direct the synthesis of normal β-globin. Some normal splicing reactions occur, however, and reduced amounts of normal mRNA are produced, leading to the expression of some normal β-chain. Current treatment of affected individuals is symptomatic. β-Thalassemia, however, is a candidate disease for future gene therapy (Table 16–5). ◄

RNA Editing and Apo-B-48

The conversion of one base to another base in hnRNA-mRNA can alter the coding properties of mRNA. The only example known in humans involves the editing of apolipoprotein B mRNA. Apo-B-48 is synthesized by the intestine, and B-100 is synthesized by the liver. Apo-B-48 is the main protein of the chylomicrons. Apo-B-100 is the predominant protein of VLDL, IDL, and LDL (Table 12–3). Intestinal cells convert a site-specific cytosine of mRNA to uracil. Because of this modification, a stop codon is created that terminates the synthesis of the growing polypeptide at 48% that of apo-B-100. The mechanism of this editing reaction is unknown, but it probably involves the deamination of cytosine. In the unedited mRNA in liver, the full-length polypeptide is produced.

tRNA

Four types of processing reactions occur during the maturation of eukaryotic tRNA. These include endonucleolytic cleavage, splicing, addition of the CCA 3' end, and base modification. Only the first three of these will be considered in this section. tRNA, 5S RNA, and a few of the small nuclear RNAs are RNA polymerase III transcripts. Only tRNAs corresponding to a few of the standard amino acids contain introns. RNAses catalyze the exergonic hydrolytic cleavage of the primary transcript to produce a shortened pre-tRNA.

The splicing reaction for tRNA of human cells is not well characterized. A linear intron is first removed in an enzyme-catalyzed reaction leaving a 3'-phosphate group on the donor exon and a free 5'-hydroxyl group on the acceptor exon. An RNA ligase catalyzes the ATP-dependent formation of the phosphodiester bond linking the donor and acceptor exon. The phosphate is derived from the 3'-phosphate group in the initial reactants.

All mature tRNAs contain CCA at the 3' terminus. This is genetically encoded in bacteria but not in eukaryotic cells. A **tRNA nucleotidyl transferase** catalyzes the addition of CCA to substrate to produce the 3' terminus. Both eukaryotic cells and bacteria possess this enzyme activity. A single enzyme catalyzes the addition of the three nucleotides. The equation for this reaction is as follows:

$$\text{pre-tRNA} + 2\ CTP + ATP \rightleftharpoons \qquad (16.1)$$
$$\text{tRNA-CCA} + 3\ PP_i$$

The reaction is template independent. It resembles the usual RNA chain elongation reactions (Figure 16–3). The formation of the new phosphodiester bonds is isoergonic. The hydrolysis of the inorganic pyrophosphate by pyrophosphatase provides the chemical energy to pull the reaction forward. Nucleases in bacteria and eukaryotic cells may catalyze the removal of one or more of these nucleotides from the 3' end during the lifetime of the molecule, and the tRNA nucleotidyl transferase can catalyze the regeneration of the functional molecule.

IMMUNOGLOBULINS

Properties of Immunoglobulins

The immune system consists of various components that protect the individual against infectious disease. Humoral immunity (*humor* is an archaic term for fluid), which is most effective against bacterial infections and some phases of viral infections, is mediated by antibodies. **Antibodies** are proteins that specifically recognize and bind to foreign, or nonself, molecules called **antigens.** Antibodies are produced by B cells, which are lymphocytes that mature in the *bone* marrow. Cellular immunity, which guards against virally infected cells, parasites, foreign cells, and neoplastic cells, is mediated by T cells, which are lymphocytes that mature in the *thymus*. Genes for immunoglobulins produced by B cells and genes that encode T-cell receptors undergo **somatic cell DNA rearrangement.** The nuclear DNA sequence of these differentiated immune cells thus differs from that of other somatic cells. Moreover, the DNA sequences of the immune cells that produce antibodies with different primary structures differ from each other. We consider only immunoglobulin gene rearrangement, but the same reorganization occurs in T-cell receptor genes.

Antibodies are made up of two light chains and two heavy chains (Figure 16–23). Light chains consist of a **variable region** (V_L) on the amino-terminal half and a **constant region** (C_L) on the carboxyterminal half. Each of these segments is about 110 amino acid residues in length. Heavy chains consist of a variable amino terminal portion (V_H) and three constant regions (C_H1, C_H2, C_H3). These segments are also about 110 amino acids long. Each antigen-binding site consists of residues derived from the variable region from one light and one heavy chain. Two heavy chains are covalently attached by two disulfide bonds. Each of the variable and constant domains of the heavy and light chains contain intrachain disulfide bonds. The constant portions of the heavy chain are responsible for complement binding and for interacting with various membrane-bound Fc receptors (Fc refers to the fragment of the heavy chain portion of antibody molecules resulting from proteolytic hydrolysis of the hinge region *in vitro*; this fragment readily forms protein crystals, hence the name).

There are five major antibody isotypes, which are determined by the heavy chain (Table 16–10). Each antibody can have a kappa (κ) or lambda (λ) light chain, but not both. The four-chain subunits of IgA and IgM are connected by a joining (J) chain of molecular mass of 15 kDa. This is an independent protein and is not to be confused with the joining region within an immunoglobulin chain as described below.

The first antibodies produced by maturing B cells are IgM followed by IgD. IgD expression ceases during terminal B-cell differentiation, and its function is unknown. **Isotype switching** describes the conversion of IgM to another isotype, and switching involves the production of a different class of heavy chain but not light chain. The structure of the variable region of the heavy chain and the antigenic specificity of the antibody are unchanged during isotype switching. Switching from IgM to IgA, IgG, or IgE involves genetic DNA rearrangement. IgD is derived by alternative splicing of hnRNA. Production of IgG follows IgM production, and IgG accounts for 80% of circulating antibodies.

Life scientists have estimated that humans can generate about 1×10^9 different antibodies, yet the haploid human genome is composed of 2.9×10^9 base pairs, and this size is not large enough to encode for this many different antibodies. The solution to this paradox is that antibodies are encoded by several genes that undergo rearrangement and recombination during B cell development that allows for the generation of this enormous diversity. Alternative splicing is responsible for the creation of soluble and membrane-bound immunoglobulins. The genes encoding the heavy and light

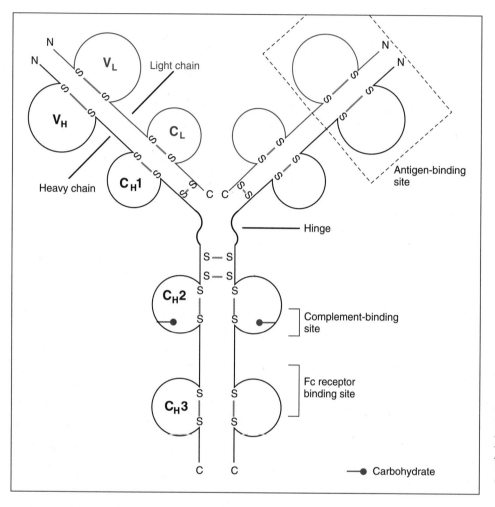

FIGURE 16–23. Schematic diagram of an immunoglobulin G molecule. *S—S refers to disulfide bonds, and N and C refer to the amino-terminal and carboxyterminal ends. Reproduced, with permission, from A.K. Abbas, A.H. Lichtman, and J.S. Pober.* Celluar and Molecular Immunology, *2nd ed. Philadelphia, W.B. Saunders Company, 1994, p. 39.*

TABLE 16–10.   Properties of Immunoglobulin Isotypes

Isotype	Heavy Chains	Light Chains	Antibody Structure	Subtype	Secretory Form	Function
IgA	$\alpha 1, \alpha 2$	κ or λ	$\kappa_2\alpha_2$ or $\lambda_2\alpha_2$	IgA1, IgA2	Monomer, dimer* Trimer*	Important in milk, saliva, tears, and intestinal secretions
IgD	δ	κ or λ	$\kappa_2\delta_2$ or $\lambda_2\delta_2$	None	None	Not clear
IgE	ϵ	κ or λ	$\kappa_2\epsilon_2$ or $\lambda_2\epsilon_2$	None	Monomer	Involved in allergic response and histamine release; may combat intestinal parasites
IgG	$\gamma 1, \gamma 2, \gamma 3, \gamma 4$	κ or λ	$\kappa_2\gamma_2$ or $\lambda_2\gamma_2$	IgG1, IgG2 IgG3, IgG4	Monomer	Combats infection, can cross placenta, chief circulating antibody
IgM	μ	κ or λ	$\kappa_2\mu_2$ or $\lambda_2\mu_2$	None	Pentamer*	First antibody expressed by each B cell

*J chain joins monomeric subunits; not to be confused with the J, or junctional, region of the heavy or light chains.

TABLE 16–11. Chromosomal Location of Human Immunoglobulin Genes

Chain	Symbol	Locus	Subdivisions per Haploid Genome
Heavy	H	14q32	$\approx 100\ V_H$, $\approx 20\ D$, $6\ J_H$, $9\ C_H$ (α_1, α_2, γ_1, γ_2, γ_3, γ_4, δ, ϵ, μ)
Kappa light	κ	2p12	$\approx 100\ V_\kappa$, $5\ J_\kappa$, $1\ C_\kappa$
Lambda light	λ	22q11	$\approx 100\ V_\lambda$, $6\ J_\lambda$, $6\ C_\lambda$
Joining	J	4q21	1

chains are located in three different chromosomes, and the gene for the joining protein that connects monomers is located on a fourth chromosome (Table 16–11). The joining protein gene does not undergo rearrangement.

Gene Rearrangements

Each heavy and light chain is encoded by multiple segments that are widely separated in the germ line DNA. Rearrangements occur during the development of somatic cells, and further rearrangements occur during B-cell differentiation. The heavy chain genes are made of four different portions including multiple variable (V), diversity (D), joining (J), and constant (C) DNA segments (Figure 16–24). The light chain genes are made of three different portions including multiple V, J, and C DNA segments.

During B-cell maturation, the DNA at the immunoglobulin loci in **stem cells** undergoes somatic rearrangement to produce transcription units. Rearrangement of the heavy chain locus occurs first, and **pre-B cells** produce heavy chains. Rearrangement of the kappa light chain occurs next. In about half the B cells in humans, the kappa chain is not expressed, and rearrangement in the lambda chain locus occurs. Expression of both the heavy chain and light chain occurs initially as IgM in the plasma membrane of **immature B cells.** Expression of both IgM and IgD then occurs in the membrane of **mature B cells.** All this activity is antigen-independent (Table 16–12). Following antigenic stimulation of cells that produce antibody which recognizes the antigen, B cells are activated and begin isotype switching. The antigen "selects" B cells that produce antibodies that recognize and bind with antigen. This is the clonal selection theory of antibody production. Membrane immunoglobulin synthesis is curtailed in **antibody-secreting cells.** All the antibody molecules that a single B cell produces contain identical antigen binding sites. The amino acid sequence of all the light chains in a single B cell is identical, and the amino acid sequence of the variable region of all the heavy chains is identical. Any variation in antibody structure is due to differences in the constant regions of the several heavy chains as IgM switches to IgA, IgD, IgG, or IgE.

V-D-J Joining and Heavy Chain Genes

Formation of the variable portion of the heavy chain region involves two DNA rearrangements. In the first process, one of the 20 D segments of chromosomal DNA is combined with one of the six J_H segments during **D-J_H joining** (Figure 16–25). The intervening DNA is eliminated and the DNA remaining is thereby different from that of other somatic cells. After this rearrangement, one of the $\approx 100\ V_H$ segments combines with the newly formed D-J_H segment during **V_H-D-J_H joining.** Because of this second rearrangement, promoter elements 5' to the V_H region are brought close to a transcriptional element that occurs in the first intron after the J_H region (Figure 16–6), and the rearranged gene is transcribed and translated.

The combination of the V_H to D and D to J_H occurs imprecisely, and inexact mergers contribute to antibody diversity. Nucleases catalyze the hydrolysis of a few nucleotides from both DNA strands, and ligases seal nicks. Exonucleases may degrade free ends, terminal transferase may add nucleotides, and DNA polymerases may catalyze the synthesis of flush ends before the DNA segments are combined. These enzymes are collectively called **recombinase,** and they recognize specific DNA sequences to initiate the process. Recombinases, which occur only in lymphocytes, function in developing B cells and are inactive in antibody-secreting cells. Two genes that stimulate immunoglobulin rearrangement, called **recombination activating genes** 1 and 2 (*RAG*-1 and *RAG*-2), are active in pre-B cells. The mechanism of their effect is not known. The enzyme called **terminal transferase,** a template-independent DNA polymerase, can add a few nucleotides to the heavy chain DNA segments. Recombination contributes to the genetic diversity of immunoglobulins.

The assembly of the V_H region coding sequences in a developing B cell occurs in a programmed order. First, D segments join to J_H segments. Second, V_H to D-J_H joining occurs. This process involves only one member of the chromosome 14 pair. After rearrangement produces a functional gene, the resulting production of complete μ chains in pre-B cells shuts down further rearrangement of V_H-region-encoding gene segments and signals the onset of V_L rearrangements. The variable region of the heavy chain corresponds to V_HNDNJ$_H$ where N refers to the addition of nucleotides that are in-

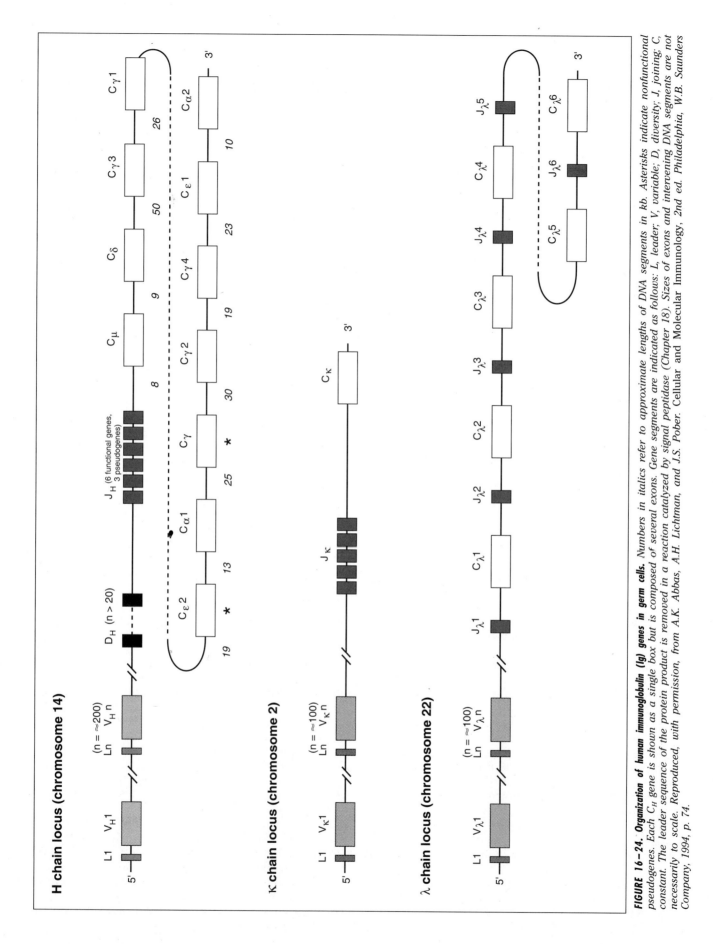

FIGURE 16–24. Organization of human immunoglobulin (Ig) genes in germ cells. *Numbers in italics refer to approximate lengths of DNA segments in kb. Asterisks indicate nonfunctional pseudogenes. Each C_H gene is shown as a single box but is composed of several exons. Gene segments are indicated as follows: L, leader; V, variable; D, diversity; J, joining; C, constant. The leader sequence of the protein product is removed in a reaction catalyzed by signal peptidase (Chapter 18). Sizes of exons and intervening DNA segments are not necessarily to scale. Reproduced, with permission, from A.K. Abbas, A.H. Lichtman, and J.S. Pober. Cellular and Molecular Immunology, 2nd ed. Philadelphia, W.B. Saunders Company, 1994, p. 74.*

TABLE 16–12. Steps in Antibody Formation

Process	Mechanism
Antigen Independent	
Heavy chain production	
D-J joining	DNA rearrangement
V-D-J joining	DNA rearrangement
Expression of heavy chain	Transcription, processing, translation
Light chain production	
V-J joining	DNA rearrangement
Expression of light chain	Transcription, processing, translation
Expression of IgM (H and L chain) in the plasma membrane	
Isotype switching to IgD	Alternative splicing
Antigen Dependent	
Secretion of IgM	Alternative splicing of the primary transcript
Isotype switching to IgA, IgG, and IgE	DNA rearrangement
Somatic rearrangement	Unknown

serted by terminal transferase; note that these nucleotides occur independently of information contained in the original DNA of the individual. The downstream heavy chain constant region that is closest to $V_H NDNJ_H$ is the μ heavy chain (Figure 16–24). Pre-B cells, which produce only a heavy chain, proliferate before the onset of light chain gene rearrangement and antibody production.

V-J Joining and Light Chain Genes

For the κ light chains, the formation of a complete variable region involves the combination of one of the more than 100 V_κ segments to any of the five J_κ segments with the loss of the intervening DNA. Once a given V_κ and J_κ are combined, the whole region is transcribed into nuclear RNA and the intervening sequences between V_κ and J_κ or between J_κ and C_κ can be removed by splicing to produce the mature mRNA for the κ protein. This process is illustrated in Figure 16–26. A similar mechanism is used for the λ light chains. Only one κ or one λ chain, however, is produced in a single B cell. There are no known functional differences between antibodies that contain κ or λ chains.

Once a cell has constructed a complete κ or λ gene, it can produce a light chain protein. The light and heavy chain proteins can be processed and targeted to the surface of the B cell where the resulting antibody molecule remains bound. A newly arisen cell with surface antibody is an immature B lymphocyte. These rearrangements and expression of antibody occur without antigenic stimulation. The lymphocyte does not divide at this stage unless it is stimulated antigenically. B cells can divide while they are undergoing genetic rearrangement. If a B cell divides after a particular D segment joins to J_H segment, the progeny will maintain this genotype. The joining of the V_H to DJ_H will usually differ in daughter cells.

Production of a membrane-bound or secreted antibody in a cell is determined by differential transcription termination and by alternative splicing. Antibodies that are secreted contain heavy chains with a hydrophilic carboxyl terminus, and antibodies that bind to the membrane contain heavy chains with a hydrophobic carboxyl terminus. The portion of the gene corresponding to the hydrophilic portion of the heavy chain occurs upstream from that of the hydrophobic domain. A short transcript produced by the first polyadenylation signal yields a primary transcript that will be processed to yield mRNA corresponding to a soluble heavy chain (Figure 16–27). A long primary transcript contains segments corresponding to both the hydrophilic and hydrophobic segments. The segment corresponding to the hydrophilic domain is excised by splicing to yield mRNA corresponding to the membrane-bound chain. The light and heavy chains of the immunoglobulin are tethered to the plasma membrane of the B cell by a hydrophobic transmembrane segment; a small hydrophilic segment occurs intracellularly.

Each B cell makes antibodies with identical antigen-binding sites. B cells, like other diploid cells, have one gene from each parent that corresponds to the heavy chain. Each B cell uses only one of the two heavy chain genes (either maternal or paternal). Expression of only the maternal or the paternal alleles of a gene in any given cell is called **allelic exclusion** and occurs in genes that encode antibodies and closely related T-cell receptors. For most other proteins that are encoded by autosomal genes, both maternal and paternal genes in a cell are expressed about equally. Only one form of light chain, λ or κ, is expressed in a given B cell. This is called **light chain isotype exclusion.**

Because of rearrangement of the heavy and light chain genes, promoter elements at the 5′ end of each immunoglobulin gene are brought close to transcriptional elements located within the intron between the variable and constant gene segments. DNA rearrangement is required to produce transcriptionally active genes. This constellation of promoter and transcription elements activates transcription of the immunoglobulin genes. Immunoglobulin genes contain a TATA box at −30 and a conserved octamer sequence 30 to 60 bases upstream from the TATA box. Lymphoid cells contain two proteins that bind to these octamers called OTF1 and OTF2 (for octamer transcription factor). A transcription factor called NF-κB (a nuclear factor first described in B cells producing kappa light chains) binds to a transcriptional element that occurs in the intron (Figure 16–28) with a 10-base consensus recognition sequence (Table 16–7). The octamer sequence and NF-κB sequence also function in nonlymphoid cells.

We can estimate the possible number of antibody molecules that can be produced from the heavy and light chain genes. For these estimates we will assume that there are 100 V_H genes per

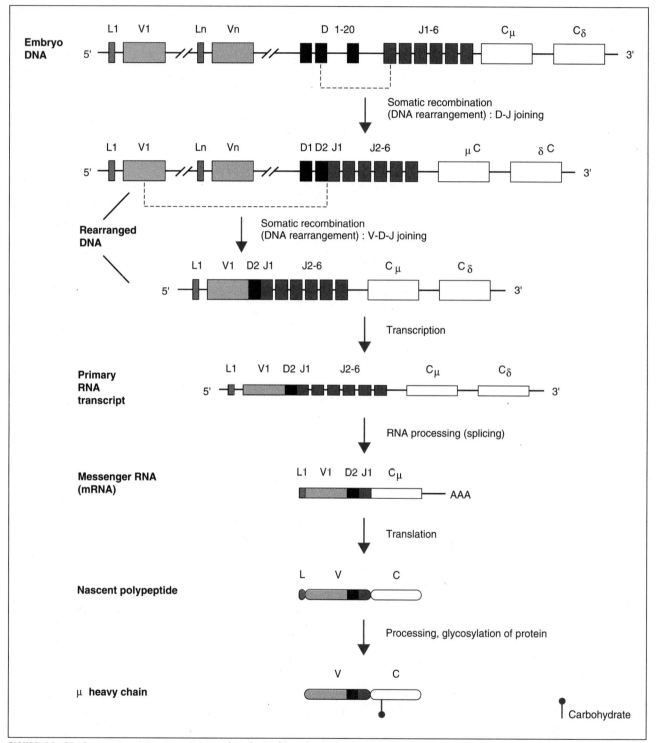

FIGURE 16–25. Gene rearrangement, transcription, and synthesis of Ig μ heavy chain. *In this example, the V region is encoded by the exons V1, D2, and J1. The location of carbohydrates is approximate, and gene segments and distances between them are not shown to scale. Modified and reproduced, with permission, from A.K. Abbas, A.H. Lichtman, and J.S. Pober.* Cellular and Molecular Immunology, *2nd ed. Philadelphia, W.B. Saunders Company, 1994, p. 76.*

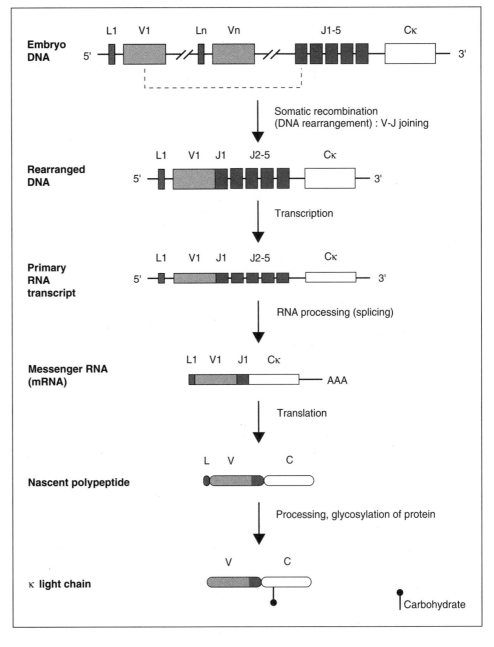

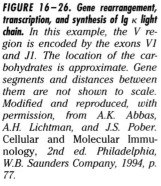

FIGURE 16–26. Gene rearrangement, transcription, and synthesis of Ig κ light chain. In this example, the V region is encoded by the exons V1 and J1. The location of the carbohydrates is approximate. Gene segments and distances between them are not shown to scale. Modified and reproduced, with permission, from A.K. Abbas, A.H. Lichtman, and J.S. Pober. Cellular and Molecular Immunology, 2nd ed. Philadelphia, W.B. Saunders Company, 1994, p. 77.

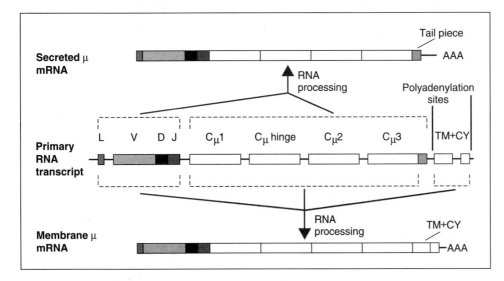

FIGURE 16–27. Expression of membrane and secreted μ chains by B lymphocytes. Dashed lines indicate the chain segments that are joined by RNA splicing. TM, transmembrane; CY, cytoplasmic. Modified and reproduced, with permission, from A.K. Abbas, A.H. Lichtman, and J.S. Pober. Cellular and Molecular Immunology, 2nd ed. Philadelphia, W.B. Saunders Company, 1994, p. 95.

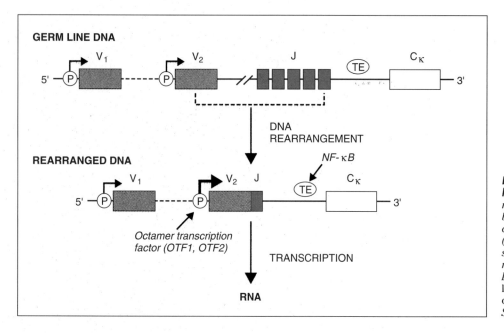

FIGURE 16–28. Transcriptional regulation of immunoglobulin genes. *Chromosomal DNA rearrangements brings promoter sequences (P) close to a transcriptional element (TE) resulting in increased transcription. Reproduced, with permission, from A.K. Abbas, A.H. Lichtman, and J.S. Pober. Cellular and Molecular Immunology, 2nd ed. Philadelphia, W.B. Saunders Company, 1994, p. 90.*

haploid chromosome, 20 D regions, and 6 J regions. This corresponds to 1.2×10^4 different combinations per haploid genome or 2.4×10^4 per diploid genome. Each DJ_H joining and V_HD joining can involve changes in the number of nucleotides. This will increase diversity by perhaps 10-fold. Thus, about $2.4 \times 10^4 \times 10 = 2.4 \times 10^5$ different heavy chains are possible. Light chains are less diverse. If there are 100 V regions, 5 J regions, and 10 ways of combining them, this represents 5×10^3 possibilities for the κ light chains. The λ light chains can encode a similar number of chains. This corresponds to about 1×10^4 combinations for both the κ and λ chains per haploid genome or 2×10^4 per diploid genome. Assuming any light chain can combine with any heavy chain, $2.4 \times 10^5 \times 2 \times 10^4 = 4.8 \times 10^9$ different antibodies could be produced. Although this calculation is an approximation, it agrees with the estimated 1×10^9 different antibodies that humans can produce.

Somatic DNA recombinations involving Ig genes occur without antigenic stimulation and lead to the appearance of B cells committed to recognizing different antigenic determinants. After antigenic stimulation of B cells, the heavy and light chain genes undergo another type of structural alteration called **somatic mutation.** The somatic mutation rate in the immunoglobulin genes is several orders of magnitude higher than that of other genes. The mechanisms responsible for these somatic mutations are unknown. As a result of somatic mutation, antibodies with higher affinity for antigen are produced.

Isotype Switching

Isotype switching involves a change in expression of the class of heavy chain by each B-cell clone. Switching does not result in loss or change in antigenic specificity; the genes encoding the variable region of the heavy and light chain are unchanged. There are two pathways for isotype switching. The first pathway is used by some members of each B-cell clone in the last step of immunoglobulin gene rearrangement. Repetitive DNA sequences in a switch (S) region upstream from the $C\mu$ gene are recombined with a downstream switch region that is 5′ of the C_H region to be expressed. This process is responsible for the generation of IgG, IgE, and IgA and occurs at the DNA level (Figure 16–29). Note that isotype switching does not alter the V-D-J gene regions and accounts for retention of identical antigen binding sites.

The second pathway describes the production of IgD, and it occurs at the RNA level. A short transcript leads to the formation of hnRNA that is processed to form a μ heavy chain. A long primary transcript consisting of VDJ-$C\mu$-$C\delta$ segments is spliced to produce VDJ-$C\delta$ mRNA that directs the biosynthesis of IgD molecules (Figure 16–30). Mature B cells use this mechanism to express surface IgM and IgD molecules with identical antigenic specificity. A summary of the steps in immunoglobulin production is given in Table 16–12.

AIDS VIRUS AND REVERSE TRANSCRIPTASE

Retroviruses such as human immunodeficiency virus (HIV) and human T-cell lymphotropic virus (Table 1–4) contain reverse transcriptase. Reverse signifies that biological information flows from RNA to DNA, opposite to the usual direction of transfer (PRINCIPLE 25 OF BIOCHEMISTRY). We consider here the properties and mechanism of replication of the AIDS retrovirus. Other retroviruses follow the same general scheme for replication but differ in detail.

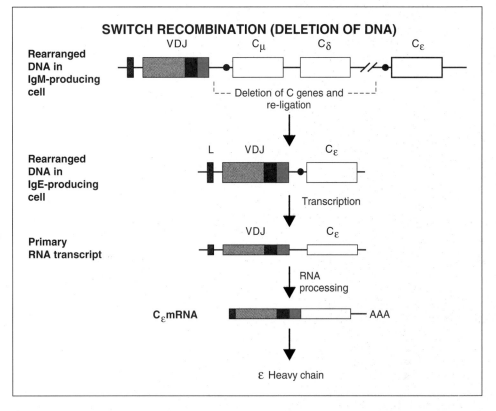

FIGURE 16–29. Isotype switching by recombination and deletion of DNA. Deletion of C_H genes, of which only $C\mu$ and $C\delta$ are shown, leads to recombination of the VDJ complex with the next (3') C_H gene, C_ϵ in this example. The $C\gamma$ genes were omitted for simplicity. Reproduced, with permission, from A.K. Abbas, A.H. Lichtman, and J.S. Pober. Cellular and Molecular Immunology, 2nd ed. Philadelphia, W.B. Saunders Company, 1994, p. 86.

Two HIV viruses produce clinical courses that are indistinguishable. HIV-1 and HIV-2, which are antigenically distinct, have about 50% sequence identity in their RNA genomes. HIV-1 is the principal causative agent of AIDS in the United States.

Each AIDS retrovirus (HIV-1 and HIV-2) contains two identical single-stranded RNA genomes of about 9700 nucleotides. The two RNAs are attached to one another at their 5' ends by hydrogen bonds. Like mRNA, each strand is capped at the 5' end and polyadenylated at the 3' end. Each HIV

particle also contains two molecules of lysine tRNA, reverse transcriptase, integrase, and a protease. The core of the virion (complete virus particle) also contains several virus-encoded proteins. The virion is enclosed in a membrane derived from the host cell, and the lipid bilayer contains glycoproteins that are specified by the virus.

The polarity of the HIV genome is identical to that of the mRNA that encodes the viral proteins, and the RNA is denoted as a + strand. In contrast, influenza viruses (Table 1–4) are a group of RNA

FIGURE 16–30. Coexpression of IgM and IgD in a B lymphocyte. Dashed lines indicate the H chain segments that are joined by RNA splicing. Reproduced, with permission, from A.K. Abbas, A.H. Lichtman, and J.S. Pober. Cellular and Molecular Immunology, 2nd ed. Philadelphia, W.B. Saunders Company, 1994, p. 84.

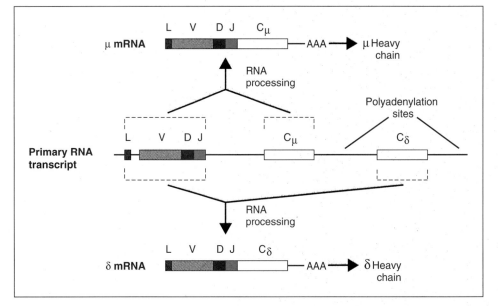

viruses whose genome is of opposite polarity to their mRNAs, and the genome is denoted as a − strand. Influenza viruses do not go through DNA intermediates in their life cycles and are not retroviruses.

The AIDS viruses infect human cells, and the RNAs and enzymes are released into the cytoplasm. HIV-1 and HIV-2 primarily infect CD4-expressing T cells. CD4 (cluster determinant 4) is a 55-kDa protein found on the surface of cells and was identified by a panel (cluster) of specific antibodies. More than 75 CD molecules are known. HIV cripples the immune system, and affected individuals are susceptible to infections from human pathogens and from bacteria which ordinarily are not pathogenic but which can cause opportunistic infections, such as *Pneumocystis carinii*. The specificity of HIV toward the immune system is due to recognition of CD4, an immune specific protein. The mechanism of viral invasion of these cells, however, is unknown.

Reverse transcriptase mediates the RNA template-dependent formation of double-stranded DNA from a single-stranded RNA by an intricate process. The double-stranded DNA product integrates into the DNA genome of the infected cell. The site of integration into the genome is random, but the sequence of the possible integration sites is specific. The integrated-viral reverse-transcribed DNA is called a **provirus.** The integrated provirus is replicated with the host cell genome. The provirus is transcribed by host cell RNA polymerase II to form mRNA for protein synthesis and virion RNA for packaging into new virus particles. The provirus can be dormant (not transcribed) for years; the mechanisms for activating transcription are obscure.

HIV-1 contains at least six genes besides the *gag, pol,* and *env* genes that are common to all retroviruses (Table 16–13). Two HIV envelope glycoproteins, gp120 and gp41, are critical for infection (the number corresponds to the molecular mass in kilodaltons). LTRs (long terminal repeats) are found at the ends of the provirus. The LTR on one end of a provirus functions as an enhancer and promoter for RNA polymerase II. The U3 region at the 5′ end of the provirus contains a TATA box, three SP1 sites, and two NF-κB sites. A silencer occurs in the −185 to −340 segment of HIV provirus. A transcription activating region (TAR) occurs in the +1 to +80 sequence (Figure 16–31), and TAR is the target of the *tat* gene product. The LTR on the other end contains a polyadenylylation signal for the transcribed RNA. The LTRs also contain sequences that serve as integration signals. The primary transcript is differentially spliced to yield several gene products. Several polyproteins (proteins that contain more than one activity) are synthesized and then cleaved to give functional molecules. The life cycle of HIV is illustrated in Figure 16–32.

TABLE 16–13.   Genes of Human Immunodeficiency Virus–1

Gene	Protein Products	Function
gag	p53 precursor	Forms structural core proteins
	p18, p24, p7, p9 mature proteins	
pol	Protease	Cleaves *gag* precursors
	Reverse transcriptase	Catalyzes proviral DNA biosynthesis from an RNA template
	RNAse H	Catalyzes hydrolysis of RNA in RNA-DNA hybrids
	Integrase	Required for proviral insertion
env	gp160 precursor	
	gp120	Binds CD4 for infection
	gp41	Required for viral fusion with cell
vpr	p15	Activates promoter
vif	p23	Involved in infection by free virus; not required for cell-to-cell infection
tat	p14	Binds to viral transcription activating region (TAR) and activates transcription of all viral genes
rev	p20	Required for posttranscriptional expression of *gag* and *env* genes
nef	p27	Inhibits HIV transcription *in vitro*; physiological function uncertain
vpu	p16	Participates in virus assembly and release

Mechanism of Reverse Transcription

Let us consider the properties and function of reverse transcriptase in greater detail. Reverse transcriptase possesses RNA-dependent DNA polymerase and DNA-dependent DNA polymerase activities at a single active site. Like other DNA synthesizing enzymes, reverse transcriptase is unable to initiate DNA synthesis *de novo*, and it requires a primer (Table 16–14). The lysine tRNAs that are packaged within the virion contain an 18-nucleotide segment that is complementary to 18 nucleotides of the viral RNA genome, and lysine tRNA functions as the primer. DNA synthesis is in the 5′ → 3′ direction. Besides the polymerizing activity, reverse transcriptase is accompanied by RNAse H activity. **RNAse H** degrades the RNA of an RNA-DNA complementary hybrid. RNAse H in the human HIV virus is separable from the polymerizing activity. In most reverse transcriptase molecules, however, the RNAse H active site is on the amino-terminal portion of the protein, and the polymerizing activity resides on the carboxyterminal portion.

The conversion of the single-stranded RNA genome into the double-stranded provirus before integration into the host genome is complicated, as described in the legend to Figure 16–33. The great diversity of the HIV genome is the consequence of hypermutability in its replication. The misincorporation rates observed experimentally are 1 in 2000 to 4000 and greatly exceed those of other DNA polymerases and also those of other reverse transcriptases.

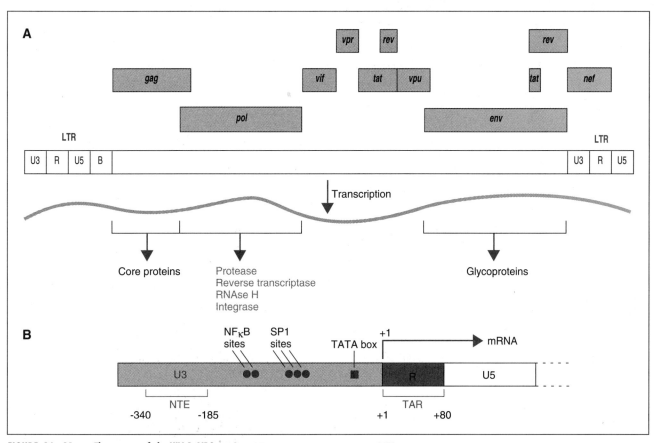

FIGURE 16–31. A. *The genome of the HIV-1 AIDS provirus.* LTR, *long terminal repeat. LTRs are extensions produced during the conversion of the single-stranded RNA genome to the double-stranded DNA prior to integration into the human genome. Several of the retroviral genes are overlapping; the information encoded in the nucleic acid sequence encodes for functions in multiple gene products.* B. *Promoter and transcription elements of HIV-1.* NTE, *negative transcription element; TAR, transcription activating region.*

As noted in Table 15–4, reverse transcriptase is widely used in the preparation of complementary DNA, and this enzyme has wide applicability in biotechnology. The enzyme used for this purpose is usually obtained from avian sources, and it is much more accurate than HIV reverse transcriptase. Eukaryotic mRNAs end with a polyA tail. To reverse transcribe such molecules, oligo dT is used as a primer. Other primers can be designed to reverse transcribe mRNA or other RNA molecules. Sometimes a strand of DNA can fold back on itself, and the end of the hairpin loop is extended by reverse transcriptase.

▶ The development of a vaccine to prevent the development of AIDS is a goal of medical scientists. The three-dimensional structure of AIDS protease has been determined by x-ray crystallography, and inhibitors of this enzyme are being developed for possible treatment. Viral polyproteins are packaged in the nascent virion. Viral protease, within the virion, catalyzes the hydrolysis of the polyprotein into functional proteins. Inhibitors of reverse transcriptase have been developed, and these are described later. Intercurrent infections are treated with antibiotics. ◀

GENE THERAPY

▶ Gene therapy is the transfer of new genetic material to the cells of an individual with resulting therapeutic benefit. Although many emphasize gene therapy in the treatment of classical genetic diseases, this technology is being applied to such diverse diseases as AIDS, cancer, and cardiovascular disease. Gene therapy protocols have been developed for adenosine deaminase deficiency using T lymphocytes and LDL-receptor deficiency (familial hypercholesterolemia) using liver cells. Only a few classic genetic diseases are currently candidates for gene therapy (Table 16–5). There are several reasons for these limitations. For example, classical genetic diseases often involve many cell types, and this presents the problem of introducing genes into a variety of cells. Moreover, methods for targeting DNA to specific cells such as brain have not been developed. This explains why Lesch-Nyhan syndrome, which is caused by a defect in HGPRT (Figure 14–17), is not a current candidate for gene therapy. Most prevailing therapy involves the removal of target cells from the individual, treating the cells in the laboratory to intro-

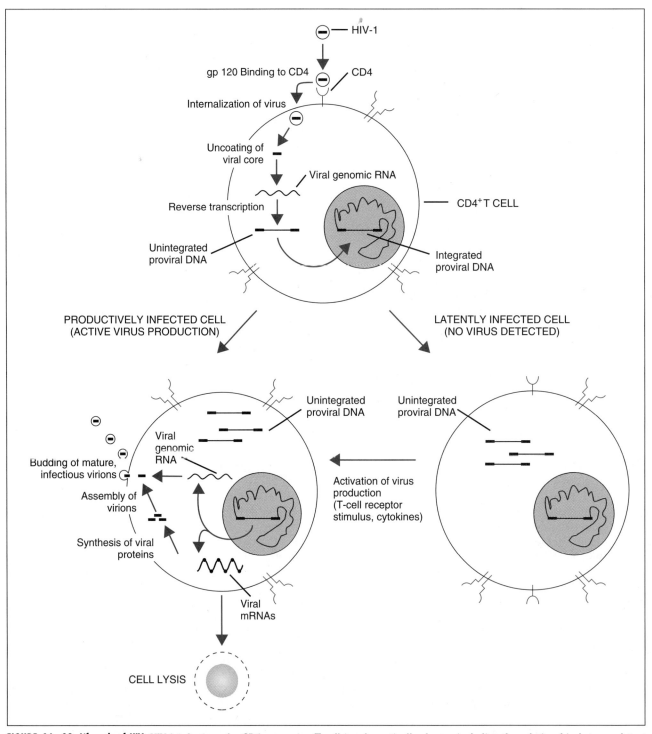

FIGURE 16–32. Life cycle of HIV. *HIV-1 infection of a CD4-expressing T cell is schematically shown, including the relationship between latent infection and productive, lytic infection. Reproduced, with permission, from A.K. Abbas, A.H. Lichtman, and J.S. Pober.* Cellular and Molecular Immunology, *2nd ed. Philadelphia, W.B. Saunders Company, 1994, p. 421.*

TABLE 16-14.   Nucleic Acid Polymerases

Enzyme	Source	Initiation Primer Required	Template	Product
DNA polymerase	Bacterial, human, virus	Yes	DNA	DNA
RNA polymerase	Bacterial, human	No	DNA	RNA
Reverse transcriptase	Virus	Yes	RNA, DNA	DNA
Primase	Human, bacterial	No	DNA	RNA
Deoxynucleotidyl terminal transferase	Human	Yes	No	DNA
PolyA polymerase	Human	Yes	No	polyA tail
tRNA Nucleotidyl transferase	Bacterial, human	Yes	No	-CCA
RNA-dependent RNA polymerase	Virus	No	Yes	RNA

duce the normal gene, and reimplanting the cells in the individual.

The ability of DNA and RNA viruses to transfer genes into cells has prompted many studies on the use of viruses for gene therapy. Almost all human gene therapy protocols currently used are based on murine (mouse) retroviral vectors. These retroviral vectors are disabled by eliminating key genes so that they cannot produce progeny virus. These systems take advantage of the virus's ability to integrate its genetic material into the chromosomes of the host cell. The gene of interest must be introduced into a packaging virion before it is taken up by the target cell.

Two steps are required to produce a retroviral gene transfer system. First, a genetically engineered **packaging-defective retrovirus** is introduced into a laboratory cell culture line. The signals for viral encapsidation are removed from the parent virus by genetic engineering to produce the packaging-defective virus. These signals occur between the LTR and the *gag* gene (Figure 16–31). The packaging-defective viral genome produces all of the proteins for virus replication and assembly, but it cannot create an infectious particle owing to the lack of the packaging signals. Second, a genetically engineered **retroviral vector** is introduced into the packaging cell line. The viral protein-coding sequences of the retroviral vector have been removed, but the packaging and replication signals are retained. In principle, any promoter-gene combination can be inserted into the retroviral vector with an upper limit of about 7000 nucleotides. The introduction of the engineered vector into the packaging cells results in the production of a retrovirus that contains the retroviral RNA vector.

The engineered retrovirus containing the desired gene is harvested from the packaging cell line and incubated with cells from the affected individual. After the virus enters the cells, RNA is reverse transcribed, and provirus integration occurs. Such cells have been shown to express adenosine deaminase or the LDL receptor, corresponding to the gene engineered into the retroviral vector. The cells containing new genetic material are reimplanted into the host. Beneficial results can be ob-

tained in some situations when only a small percentage of the host cells produce the normal protein. This strategy has been used to introduce functional LDL receptor genes into the liver cells of individuals with familial hypercholesterolemia on an experimental basis. The introduction of exogenous genes into a cell by a virus as described here is called **transduction.**

Adenovirus vectors have also been studied as potential gene transfer vectors for gene therapy. Adenoviruses are large (35 kb), double-stranded DNA viruses, and strategies for incorporating normal genes into them have been developed. After entering the cell, the DNA moves to the nucleus, where it remains extrachromosomal. This is a disadvantage because the DNA does not replicate, and cell division leads to the eventual loss of the gene from daughter cells. Adenoviruses are being studied as vector systems to deliver the cystic fibrosis transmembrane conductance regulator protein gene to respiratory epithelium. Respiratory epithelium is a usual host cell for adenoviruses.

Some cells *in vitro* take up DNA encapsulated in synthetic lipid bilayers (called liposomes), from calcium phosphate precipitates, and as a result of exposure to high voltage (electroporation). The artificial process of incorporating DNA into cells by exposing them to naked DNA by these and related processes is called **transfection.** The DNA of the cystic fibrosis gene has also been incorporated into liposomes and applied to the respiratory epithelium. Some cells take up the DNA from liposomes and express the cystic fibrosis protein. Many cell types can take DNA up from liposomes, and this may provide a method for introducing DNA into cells of several organs. ◄

INHIBITION OF NUCLEIC ACID SYNTHESIS BY DRUGS

► Bacterial RNA polymerases are inhibited by an antibiotic called **rifampin** (Figure 16–34). This antibiotic inhibits the initiation (but not elongation) of bacterial RNA synthesis. Rifampin interacts with the β-subunit of the RNA polymerase holoenzyme. Nuclear RNA polymerases are not affected by ri-

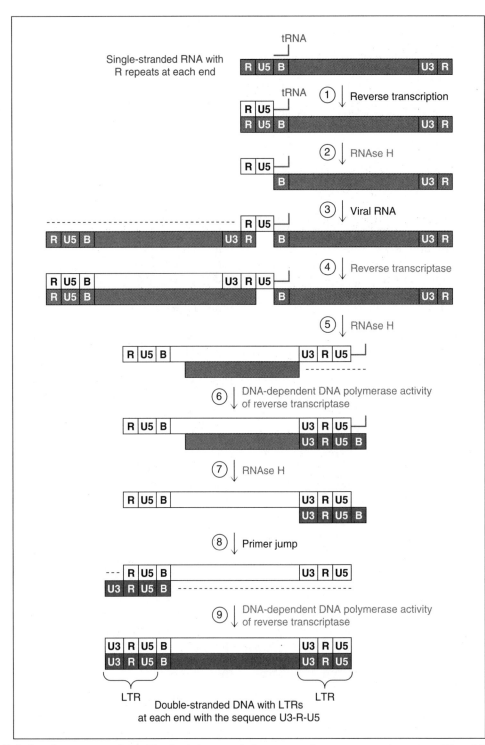

FIGURE 16–33. Mechanism of reverse transcription. *The R of the retroviral genome refers to a repeat sequence. U5 and U3 refer to unique regions on the 5' and 3' ends of the viral genome, and B is the polymerase binding site. (1) The tRNA carried into the cell by the retrovirus is complementary to the RNA genome of the virus and binds to B. tRNA serves as a primer for the elongation reactions to the 5' end of the genomic RNA template. (2) RNAse H activity catalyzes the hydrolysis of the RNA of the RNA-DNA hybrid portion of the duplex; the single- or double-stranded RNA portions are unaltered. (3) The 3'-end of the second viral RNA base-pairs with the RNAse H digest product via R. Base pairing is complementary and antiparallel. (4) The DNA portion of the tRNA-DNA hybrid molecule is extended to the end of the RNA template. (5) Considerable RNA, base pairing with DNA, is removed by the RNAse H catalyzed hydrolysis. (6) The remaining RNA base pairing with DNA functions as a primer, and DNA is synthesized to the end of the template. Note that the template is made up of newly synthesized DNA, and the end of the product has a sequence that is absent from this end of the RNA genome. (7) RNAse H removes the remainder of the genomic RNA. (8) The primer forms a new complementary structure at the opposite end of the DNA. (9) Reverse transcriptase activity completes the synthesis of each strand to yield the mature DNA. The precise order of removal of RNA by RNAse H is uncertain.*

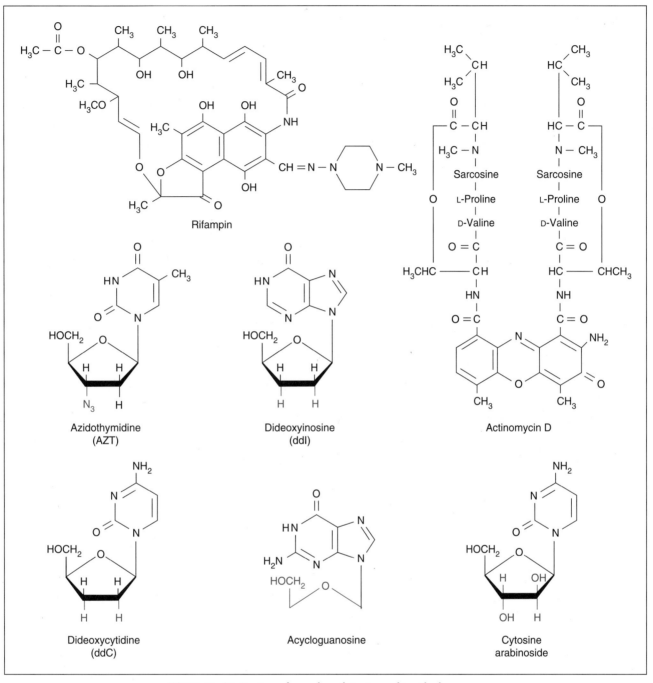

FIGURE 16–34. Structures of some drugs that act on nucleic acid polymerases.

fampin, but concentrations that are much higher than those achieved therapeutically can inhibit mitochondrial RNA biosynthesis. Rifampin inhibits the growth of most gram-positive and many gram-negative bacteria such as *E. coli*. Rifampin is the drug of choice in the chemoprophylaxis of meningococcal disease and meningitis due to *Haemophilus influenzae*.

Rifampin is one of the drugs that is currently used in the treatment of *Mycobacterium tuberculosis* infection (Table 1–2), one of the great scourges of civilization. Treatment requires the administration of a combination of drugs for 1.5–2 years. Rifam-

pin, isoniazid, and ethambutol form the cornerstone of therapy. Bacterial infections that require chronic treatment can develop resistance to a single antibiotic, and the use of a combination of drugs makes it less likely that resistance will develop. Bacteria can develop resistance to rifampin, and the resistant strains have a mutation in the β-subunit of RNA polymerase. Streptomycin can be used as an adjuvant in the treatment of tuberculosis acutely but not chronically because of ototoxicity. Streptomycin inhibits bacterial protein synthesis (Table 17–4). The mechanism of antibacterial action of isoniazid and ethambutol is unknown.

Actinomycin D is a peptide antibiotic (Figure 16–34) that inhibits DNA-dependent RNA synthesis (both human and bacterial). This antibiotic binds to the DNA template and inhibits the elongation reactions of RNA, but not DNA, synthesis. This peptide is used in the treatment of several neoplastic diseases including Wilms' tumor in children, choriocarcinoma in women, and metastatic testicular carcinoma in men (Table 21–7). Actinomycin D is not used in the treatment of bacterial infections because of its toxicity.

Azidothymidine (AZT) is a nucleoside analogue of thymidine in which the 3'-hydroxyl group is replaced by the azido group (Figure 16–34). AZT is converted to the triphosphate in reactions catalyzed by thymidine kinase, thymidylate kinase, and nucleoside diphosphate kinase (Chapter 6). AZT triphosphate is a more potent inhibitor of the reverse transcriptase of the AIDS virus than of the nuclear DNA polymerases of the host. Other potential agents for AIDS treatment include ddI (dideoxyinosine) and ddC (dideoxycytidine) illustrated in Figure 16–34. These drugs are converted to the corresponding triphosphate by cellular enzymes, and these analogues of cellular nucleotides are also inhibitors of reverse transcriptase.

Acycloguanosine is used in the treatment of herpesvirus infection (Figure 16–34). Herpesvirus is a double-stranded DNA virus (Table 1–4). Human thymidine kinase cannot use acycloguanosine as a substrate, but the herpes-coded thymidine kinase can. Cells expressing herpes proteins can phosphorylate acycloguanosine, yielding the monophosphate. Other cellular enzymes mediate the formation of the acycloguanosine triphosphate. This compound is a substrate (and not an inhibitor) of the herpes DNA polymerase. Incorporation of this nucleotide into the elongating DNA causes chain termination.

Cytosine arabinoside (Figure 16–34) is used in the therapy of acute myelogenous leukemia. It is the single most effective agent for producing remission of this disease. Cellular enzymes (deoxycytidine kinase, deoxycytidylate kinase, and nucleoside diphosphate kinase) catalyze successive phosphorylations, yielding a triphosphate substrate of DNA polymerase. High concentrations of cytosine arabinoside triphosphate inhibit human DNA polymerases, including polymerase β (repair polymerase). The compound is also incorporated into DNA, which is most likely responsible for its cytotoxic effects. The 2'-hydroxyl group interferes with the formation of the correct conformation of DNA, and this abnormality slows chain elongation. ◄

SUMMARY

RNA is a polymer consisting of ribonucleotides connected by $3' \rightarrow 5'$ phosphodiester bonds. The information content of RNA resides in the sequence of its bases. RNA polymerases are the enzymes that catalyze the DNA-template directed RNA biosynthesis. The sequence of RNA is determined by complementary base pairing (A with U, T with A, G with C, and C with G). Uracil appears in RNA and base-pairs like thymine in DNA. Unlike DNA polymerases, RNA polymerases can initiate biosynthesis and do not require a primer. Nucleoside triphosphates are the substrates, and a polynucleotide and pyrophosphate are the products. Chain elongation is in the $5' \rightarrow 3'$ direction.

Core *E. coli* RNA polymerase consists of $\alpha_2\beta\beta'$ subunits. One of five σ-subunits forms a complex with the core enzyme to form the holoenzyme: $\alpha_2\beta\beta'\sigma$. The σ-subunit is necessary for chain initiation at physiological start sites. A bacterial promoter is an RNA polymerase binding site, and these DNA binding sites are determined by the base sequence. Different σ-subunits recognize different promoters. After a few elongation reactions, the σ-subunit dissociates from the holoenzyme and can bind to another core RNA polymerase and reinitiate RNA synthesis. Rifampin inhibits the initiation of bacterial RNA biosynthesis and interacts with the β-subunit.

Eukaryotic cells contain three nuclear RNA polymerases. The subunit structure of eukaryotic RNA polymerases is more intricate than that of bacteria. RNA polymerase I, present in the nucleolus, is responsible for transcribing the genes for rRNA. RNA polymerase II is responsible for synthesizing hnRNA, the precursor of mRNA. RNA polymerase III mediates the synthesis of tRNA, 5S RNA of the ribosome, and other small RNA molecules. Mitochondria contain their own distinctive RNA polymerase.

The three polymerases each have their own promoters and transcription elements. Promoters define correct start sites, and transcription elements alter the rates of transcription from a given gene. The transcription elements are recognized by transcription factors. The promoter for RNA polymerase III occurs within the transcription unit. Promoter elements for RNA polymerase II include TATA boxes, CAAT boxes, GC boxes, octamer sequences, and NF-κB sequences.

The newly synthesized RNA polymer is called the primary transcript. A series of reactions may be required to convert the primary transcript into the functional RNA. Such processing reactions fall into a variety of classes. The primary transcript may undergo partial degradation by a combination of exonucleases and endonucleases to yield a shorter polymer and fragments (which are degraded). The bases and sugars may undergo methylation, and the polynucleotide may undergo splicing.

Following the formation of hnRNA (the primary transcript whose synthesis is catalyzed by RNA polymerase II), 5' and 3' terminal processing occurs. The 5' end reacts with GTP (to form a $5' \rightarrow 5'$ triphosphate linkage) and forms a capped structure. The cap also reacts with *S*-adenosyl-methionine and undergoes methylation reactions. The 3′ end of hnRNA undergoes a cleavage reaction removing a segment of RNA. The resulting 3′ end reacts with several ATP molecules to add a polyA tail of about 200 residues. The pre-mRNA then undergoes a series of splicing reactions. During this process, intervening sequences are removed and the exons are joined together. The splicing reactions must occur with great precision; otherwise the resulting RNA molecule would not direct the synthesis of the correct sequence of the protein. Splicing reactions occur in a macromolecular assembly called the spliceosome. Small nuclear RNAs (snRNAs) participate in this process. The location of the splice sites in human hnRNA is determined genetically by the nucleotide sequence. The base sequence of an intron begins with GU and ends with AG.

The 3′ end of bacterial tRNAs ends with the sequence 5′-CCA-3′. This sequence is encoded by the bacterial tRNA gene. The 3′ end of human tRNAs exhibits the same sequence. This sequence is not encoded by several human tRNA genes. An enzyme (tRNA nucleotidyl transferase) catalyzes the addition of CCA. Bacteria also possess this enzyme.

Antibodies are proteins that specifically recognize and bind to foreign molecules called antigens. The fundamental unit of the five isotypes of antibody consists of two heavy chains and two light chains. The heavy chain genes are made of four different portions including multiple V (variable), D (diversity), J (joining), and C (constant) DNA segments. The light chain genes are made of three different portions including multiple V, J, and C DNA segments. B cells undergo DNA rearrangements to produce genes corresponding to each antibody. Heavy chain genes rearrange first; they undergo D-J joining and then V-D-J joining. Afterward, light chain genes rearrange by V-J joining. Genetic rearrangement brings promoters close to transcriptional elements found in the first intron, and transcription occurs. Alternative splicing reactions skip exons and are responsible for the production of IgM and IgD from related transcripts. Splicing reactions also produce proteins that are secreted or membrane-bound. Isotype switching involves further DNA rearrangement as VJD regions are combined with downstream constant gene regions that correspond to IgG, IgA, and IgE.

Reverse transcriptase possesses RNA-dependent DNA polymerase and DNA-dependent DNA polymerase activity. Like other DNA synthesizing enzymes, reverse transcriptase is unable to initiate DNA synthesis *de novo,* and it requires a primer. The tRNAs that are packaged within the virion are complementary to part of the viral RNA genome, and tRNA functions as the primer. RNAse H degrades the RNA of an RNA-DNA duplex. Reverse transcriptase is a valuable tool in preparing complementary DNA (DNA complementary to RNA) and is widely used in research, biotechnology, and genetic engineering.

The bioenergetics of DNA polymerases, RNA polymerases, poly(A) polymerase, tRNA nucleotidyl transferase that adds CCA to the transcript, and primase is the same. The substrates are nucleoside or deoxyribonucleoside triphosphates, and the products are nucleotide polymers, with high-energy phosphodiester bonds, and inorganic pyrophosphate. The hydrolysis of pyrophosphate as catalyzed by pyrophosphatase is an exergonic process that pulls the nucleotidyl transferase reactions forward. The bioenergetics of other specialized nucleic acid polymerases is similar.

SELECTED READINGS

Abbas, A.K., A.H. Lichtman, and J.S. Pober. *Cellular and Molecular Immunology,* 2nd ed. Philadelphia, W.B. Saunders Company, 1994.

Coleman, J.E. Zinc proteins: Enzymes, storage proteins, transcription factors, and replication proteins. Annual Review of Biochemistry 61:897–946, 1992.

Greene, W.C. The molecular biology of human immunodeficiency virus type 1 infection. New England Journal of Medicine 324:308–317, 1991.

Guthrie, C., and B. Patterson. Spliceosomal snRNAs. Annual Review of Genetics 22:387–419, 1988.

Iseman, M.D. Treatment of multidrug-resistant tuberculosis. New England Journal of Medicine 329:784–791, 1993.

Kornberg, A., and T.A. Baker. *DNA Replication,* 2nd ed. New York, W.H. Freeman & Company, 1992.

McKusick, V.A. (ed.). *Mendelian Inheritance in Man.* Baltimore, Johns Hopkins University Press, 1991.

Morgan, R.A., and W.F. Anderson. Human gene therapy. Annual Review of Biochemistry 62:191–217, 1993.

Nagatsu, T. Genes for human catecholamine-synthesizing enzymes. Neuroscience Research 12:315–345, 1991.

Sharp, P.A. Splicing of messenger RNA precursors. *Science* 235:766–771, 1987.

Shaw, G.M. Biology of human immunodeficiency viruses. *In* J.B. Wyngaarden, L.H. Smith, Jr., and J.C. Bennett (eds.). *Cecil Textbook of Medicine,* 19th ed. Philadelphia, W.B. Saunders Company, 1992, pp. 1913–1918.

Steinberg, A.D. Systemic lupus erythematosus. *In* J.B. Wyngaarden, L.H. Smith, Jr., and J.C. Bennett (eds.). *Cecil Textbook of Medicine,* 19th ed. Philadelphia, W.B. Saunders Company, 1992, pp. 1522–1530.

Wahle, E., and W. Keller. The biochemistry of 3′-end cleavage and polyadenylation of messenger RNA precursors. Annual Review of Biochemistry 61:419–440, 1992.

CHAPTER SEVENTEEN

PROTEIN AND

PEPTIDE

BIOSYNTHESIS

The template RNA-dependent amino acid incorporation required ATP and an ATP-generating system.
—MARSHALL W. NIRENBERG AND J. HEINRICH MATTAEI

Crick's central dogma of molecular biology states that information flows from DNA → RNA → protein. The alphabet of nucleic acids consists of four letters: A, T, G, C in DNA and A, U, G, C in RNA. The alphabet of proteins contains 20 letters corresponding to the 20 standard amino acids that participate in RNA-directed protein synthesis. The translation of the nucleic acid code of four letters to the protein code of 20 letters is an intricate process that requires more than 150 components.

The three classes of RNA involved in translation include **rRNA, tRNA,** and **mRNA.** rRNA constitutes part of the ribosome, the subcellular machine where peptide bond formation occurs. tRNA molecules serve as a bridge between the nucleic acid alphabet of four bases and the protein alphabet of 20 amino acids. tRNA molecules function as **adapters** during translation of the genetic code. Amino acids, moreover, are covalently attached to their corresponding tRNA by an energy-rich bond; the amino acids are thereby activated for condensation reactions. The nucleotide sequence of mRNA determines the sequence of amino acids in proteins. A variety of proteins participate in polypeptide **initiation, elongation,** and **release** reactions. The synthesized protein may be chemically modified to yield a mature and functional protein (Chapter 18).

PROTEIN BIOSYNTHESIS

Genetic Code

The demonstration that DNA is the genetic material (PRINCIPLE 22 OF BIOCHEMISTRY) was made by Oswald T. Avery, Colin M. MacLeod, and Maclyn McCarty in the early 1940s. These three physicians showed that the molecule that converted (transformed) the R, or rough, colonies of *pneumococcus* to the S, or smooth, virulent strains was DNA. The discovery by James D. Watson and Francis H. C. Crick that DNA is made of two complementary strands (PRINCIPLE 23 OF BIOCHEMISTRY) was reported in 1953. The elucidation of the genetic code was completed in 1966. The genetic code has great predictive and correlative value, and its importance is as significant in biology as the periodic table of the elements is in chemistry.

Standard Triplet Code

Each amino acid in a protein is encoded by three bases in RNA (PRINCIPLE 26 OF BIOCHEMISTRY). A three-letter code yields 4^3 or 64 different code words, and these are more than adequate to specify the 20 different standard amino acids. Based on the methodology used to decipher the code, **codons** are expressed as a sequence of bases starting at the 5′ end of the RNA codon (mRNA is read 5′ to 3′).

AUG functions as the initiation codon and methionine is the initiating amino acid for protein synthesis

in humans, other animals, bacteria, and viruses. The genetic code is read triplet by triplet from the 5′ to 3′ direction of mRNA until a stop codon is reached. No punctuation signal is required to indicate the end of one codon and the beginning of the next (the genetic code is **commaless**). Each base of the triplet is used only once for the corresponding polypeptide, and the triplets do not overlap (the code is **nonoverlapping**). The genetic code used in *Escherichia coli* and in the cytosol of eukaryotes is identical and is called the **standard genetic code.**

Of the 64 possible codons of the standard genetic code, all but three correspond to an amino acid (Table 17–1). The three exceptions **(UAA, UAG, UGA)** produce chain termination. Two amino acids have only a single codon. These are methionine (AUG) and tryptophan (UGG), the least common amino acids in proteins. The 18 other amino acids are represented by more than one codon, and this property is called **degeneracy.** One of the consequences of degeneracy is that a mutation which produces a base change in DNA may not produce an amino acid change in the encoded protein. When reading the biomedical literature, it is helpful to remember that **AUG** corresponds to methionine and chain initiation and **UUU** corresponds to phenylalanine, the first codon identified by Nirenberg and Mattaei.

Nine of the amino acids are represented by two codons. The first two bases are the same, and the third position is a pyrimidine (Py) or a purine (Pu). The codons are XYPy or XYPu. Five amino acids are represented by four codons. The first two bases are the same, and the third base can be any one of the four (either of the two pyrimidines or two purines denoted N). The codons are XYN. Isoleucine is the only amino acid represented by three codons: AUU, AUC, and AUA. The first two

TABLE 17–1. The Standard Genetic Code

		Second letter				
		U	C	A	G	Third letter (3′)
First letter (5′)	U	UUU UUC } Phe UUA UUG } Leu	UCU UCC UCA UCG } Ser	UAU UAC } Tyr UAA UAG } Stop	UGU UGC } Cys UGA Stop UGG Trp	U C A G
	C	CUU CUC CUA CUG } Leu	CCU CCC CCA CCG } Pro	CAU CAC } His CAA CAG } Gln	CGU CGC CGA CGG } Arg	U C A G
	A	AUU AUC AUA } Ile AUG Met	ACU ACC ACA ACG } Thr	AAU AAC } Asn AAA AAG } Lys	AGU AGC } Ser AGA AGG } Arg	U C A G
	G	GUU GUC GUA GUG } Val	GCU GCC GCA GCG } Ala	GAU GAC } Asp GAA GAG } Glu	GGU GGC GGA GGG } Gly	U C A G

bases are identical, and the third base cannot be guanine because of wobble base pairing.

Wobble Base Pairing

Base pairing between the codon of mRNA and the anticodon in tRNA is antiparallel (PRINCIPLE 28 OF BIOCHEMISTRY). Nonstandard base pairing occurs between the 3′ position of the codon and 5′ position of the anticodon, and these sites are therefore designated as the wobble position. Wobble base pairing allows one tRNA to interact with more than one codon. As a consequence, cells (excluding mitochondria) contain about 50 different types of tRNA molecules and not 61 types (61 is the number of codons that represent amino acids in the standard code). Examples of wobble base pairing are illustrated in Figure 17–1. (Only individuals working in this area remember the details of this wobble base pairing scheme.) Nonstandard base pairing is possible because it does not involve the formation of a double helix and the constraints inherent in such a structure.

Inosine is less discriminating than the other nucleosides that occur in the wobble position of the anticodon; inosine base-pairs with adenosine, uridine, or cytidine (all the nucleosides except guanosine) as illustrated in Figure 17–2. Inosine contains a keto group in the 6-position, like guanosine, and is complementary to cytidine. Inosine is derived from adenosine by hydrolytic deamination. To uniquely specify AUG for methionine requires that the nucleoside which is complementary to guanosine, namely, cytidine, does not participate in wobble base pairing when it occurs in the anticodon.

To summarize the wobble base pairing for the anticodon found in tRNA, note that (1) cytidine pairs only with one base, (2) uridine and guanosine each pair with two nucleosides of the opposite type (purine or pyrimidine, respectively), and (3) inosine pairs with three nucleosides (any nucleoside except guanosine). We note that inosine does not occur physiologically in mRNA. Surprisingly, adenosine does not occur in the wobble position of tRNA from any species.

Wobble base pairing enables many tRNA molecules to recognize more than one codon and explains how the 61 codons can be read with about 50 tRNA molecules. Each of the nine amino acids with two synonym codons that differ in only the purine or pyrimidine bases in the wobble position could be recognized, in principle, by one tRNA with a U or G in the (5′) wobble position. A tRNA with inosine in the wobble position can recognize a maximum of three (but not four) codons. Those amino acids with four codons must have at least two tRNA molecules to ensure their proper recognition.

The genetic code and wobble rules for mitochondrial protein synthesis differ from the standard genetic code. In human mitochondria, all the amino acids have at least two codons, including methionine and tryptophan. AUA, which is a standard codon for isoleucine, and AUG correspond to methionine in the mitochondrion. UGA, which is a standard stop codon, corresponds to tryptophan in the mitochondrion. AGA and AGG, which are standard codons for arginine, are stop codons in the mitochondrion. There are a total of four stop codons (AGA, AGG, UAA, and UAG) in the mitochondrial code.

There are 22 human mitochondrial tRNA mole-

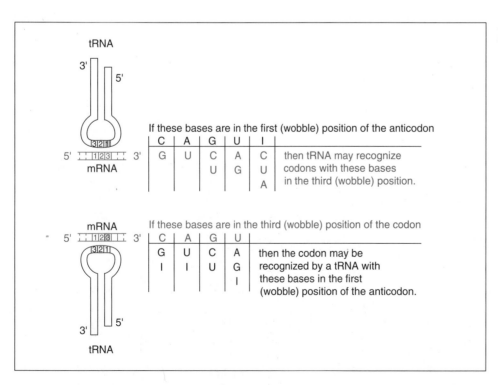

FIGURE 17–1. Codon-anticodon interaction by standard Watson-Crick and by wobble base pairing.

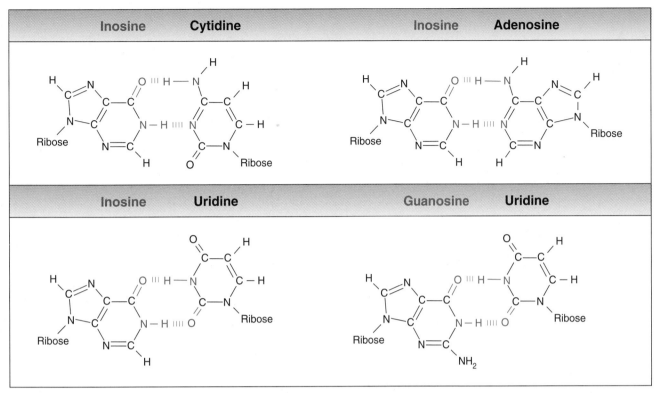

FIGURE 17–2. Wobble base pairing. *Inosine-cytidine base pairing occurs in the traditional Watson-Crick mode. The other examples represent non–Watson-Crick base pairing. Inosine occurs in the anticodon of tRNA and not in mRNA.*

cules that interact with 60 codons. This is made possible by additional wobble base pairing. When uracil occurs in the wobble position of the anticodon, it can base-pair with any of the four bases in the codon. The **standard genetic code** is (almost) universal (PRINCIPLE 27 OF BIOCHEMISTRY). The genetic codes of mitochondria, plant chloroplasts, and a few microbial species that differ from the standard code are often called dialects.

Ribosomes as the Site of Protein Synthesis

Ribosomes are the biochemical machines on which protein biosynthesis occurs. Messenger and transfer RNAs interact on ribosomes by processes that are mediated by nonribosomal protein factors, and peptide bond formation occurs on ribosomes in reactions catalyzed by ribosomes *per se*. We describe some of the properties of the ribosomes from *E. coli* because they are better understood than other ribosomes. Moreover, several antibiotics exert their effect by inhibiting bacterial protein synthesis. Protein synthesis on ribosomes in the mitochondria more closely resembles that of bacteria than that of the cytoplasm of eukaryotic cells.

Composition of *E. coli* Ribosomes

The size of ribosomes and their subunits is expressed by their sedimentation coefficient in Svedberg units, or S values. The *E. coli* ribosome is a **70S** ribosome (Figure 17–3). It is made up of one large and one small subunit that sediment at **50S** and **30S**. The RNA constitutes about two-thirds of the ribosome by mass, and the protein makes up the remainder. The small subunit contains one molecule of rRNA (16S) and 21 proteins. The proteins are named S1 through S21, the prefix "S" indicating the *small* subunit. The large subunit contains a 23S RNA and a 5S RNA. The large (L) subunit was thought to contain 34 proteins (numbered L1 to L34), but further work indicates that the large subunit contains 35 proteins. The proteins named L7/L12 differ only in that L7 is acetylated at the amino terminus and L12 is not. L8 is a complex formed from L7/L12 (which decreased the number by one, but two additional proteins called A and B were subsequently found that increased the total to 35). These values are presented to illustrate the complexity of the ribosomal machine. The ribosomal proteins are distinct, and one copy of each protein is found per functional ribosome. Note that the S values are not additive; the combined 50S and 30S subunits have a sedimentation coefficient of 70S.

The sequence of the rRNAs and bacterial ribosomal proteins has been determined. Considerable intramolecular hydrogen bonding or secondary structure of all three of the rRNAs occurs. The rRNAs are methylated (about 10 for *E. coli* and about 100 for human rRNAs). *S*-Adenosylmethionine is the activated methyl group donor that participates in the posttranscriptional methylation of rRNA.

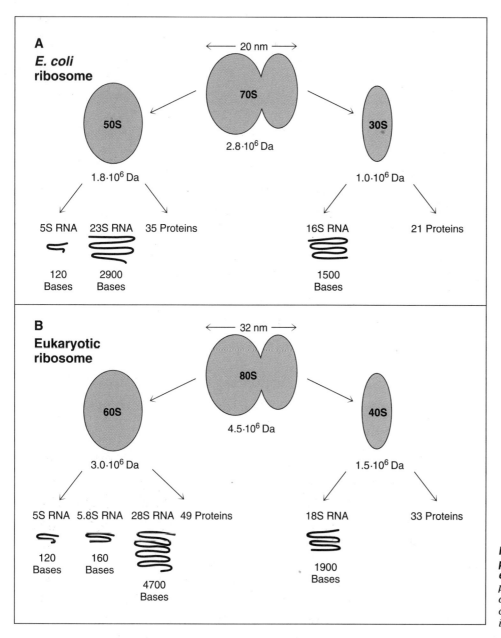

A

E. coli ribosome

← 20 nm →

70S

2.8·10⁶ Da

50S

30S

1.8·10⁶ Da

1.0·10⁶ Da

5S RNA   23S RNA   35 Proteins

16S RNA   21 Proteins

120 Bases   2900 Bases

1500 Bases

B

Eukaryotic ribosome

← 32 nm →

80S

4.5·10⁶ Da

60S

40S

3.0·10⁶ Da

1.5·10⁶ Da

5S RNA   5.8S RNA   28S RNA   49 Proteins

18S RNA   33 Proteins

120 Bases   160 Bases

4700 Bases

1900 Bases

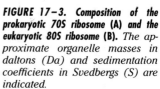

FIGURE 17–3. Composition of the prokaryotic 70S ribosome (A) and the eukaryotic 80S ribosome (B). *The approximate organelle masses in daltons (Da) and sedimentation coefficients in Svedbergs (S) are indicated.*

The 70S ribosome contains two functional sites termed the A site and the P site. *Aminoacyl-tRNA binds at the **A site**, and peptidyl-tRNA binds at the **P site.** These sites are made up of portions from both the small and large subunits (Figure 17–4). The activity that catalyzes peptide bond formation **(peptidyltransferase)** occurs in the large subunit. It is possible that rRNA, acting as a ribozyme, catalyzes the formation of peptide bonds. **Ribozymes** are catalysts that are made of RNA (PRINCIPLE 5 OF BIOCHEMISTRY).

Composition of Eukaryotic Ribosomes

Ribosomes from humans are functionally analogous to those from *E. coli.* Because of their greater complexity, however, eukaryotic ribosomes have not been characterized to the extent that those

from *E. coli* have. Human cytoplasmic ribosomes are larger, with S values of **80S** for the whole ribosome and **60S** and **40S** for the large and small subunits, respectively (Figure 17–3). The sedimentation coefficient of the mitochondrial ribosomes is about **60S**.

Amino Acid Activation for Protein Biosynthesis

Properties of Aminoacyl-tRNA

Before protein synthesis, *amino acids are activated by formation of a covalent energy-rich linkage to their corresponding tRNA.* tRNA molecules are small RNA molecules consisting of 75–95 nucleotides. The 3′ end of all tRNA molecules ends with 5′ . . . **CCA** 3′. The amino acid is attached to the

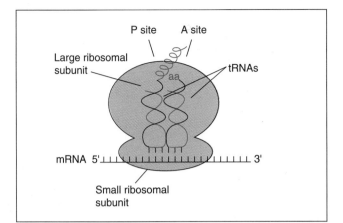

FIGURE 17–4. Schematic representation of a ribosome and its interaction with mRNA and tRNA. aa, amino acid.

ribose of the 3′ adenosine residue. The sequences of hundreds of tRNA molecules have been determined, and all of them (except mitochondrial tRNAs) can be represented as two-dimensional cloverleaf structures (Figure 17–5). The molecule contains three loops called (1) the **D-loop** (for dihydrouridine), (2) the **anticodon loop,** and (3) the **T loop** (for ribothymidine). There are four stem-

like structures in tRNA consisting of hydrogen-bonded portions of the molecule.

Note that the interaction between the anticodon of tRNA and the codon of mRNA is antiparallel (Figure 17–1). Many of the nucleosides of tRNA molecules are modified posttranscriptionally (Figure 17–6). The three-dimensional structure of tRNA molecules is L-shaped (Figure 17–7). The anticodon appears at the end of one arm of the L, and the amino acid is bound to the end of the other arm.

Formation of Aminoacyl-tRNA

The enzymes that catalyze the activation of amino acids are called **amino acyl–tRNA synthetases.** There is one enzyme for each of the 20 standard amino acids used to make proteins. Each of these enzymes catalyzes the covalent attachment of its corresponding amino acid to the specific subset of tRNA molecules that have the anticodons corresponding to that particular amino acid. These are called **isoacceptor tRNA molecules.** The two tRNA molecules illustrated in Figure 17–5 are isoacceptors for methionine, and methionine-tRNA synthetase catalyzes the addition of methionine to each of these molecules. Even though these two

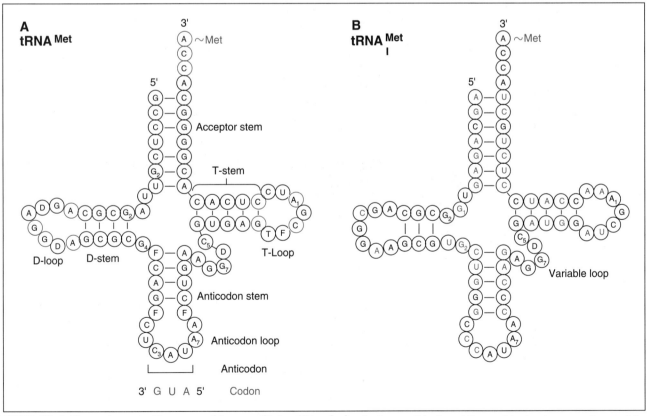

FIGURE 17–5. The complete nucleotide sequence of human methionine tRNA molecules. A. Responsible for adding methionine to a growing peptide chain. The 11 bases inside red circles are found in these positions in nearly all organisms. B. Responsible for polypeptide chain initiation. The nucleotides in red differ from those found in tRNA^Met illustrated in part A. A_1, 1-methyladenosine; A_7, ribofuranosylpurine-carbamoyl-threonine; C_2, 2-thiocytidine; C_3, 3-methylcytidine; C_5, 5-methylcytidine; D, dihydrouridine; F, pseudouridine; G_1, 1-methylguanosine; G_2, 2-methylguanosine; G_4, 2,2-dimethylguanosine, G_7, 7-methylguanosine; T, ribothymidine.

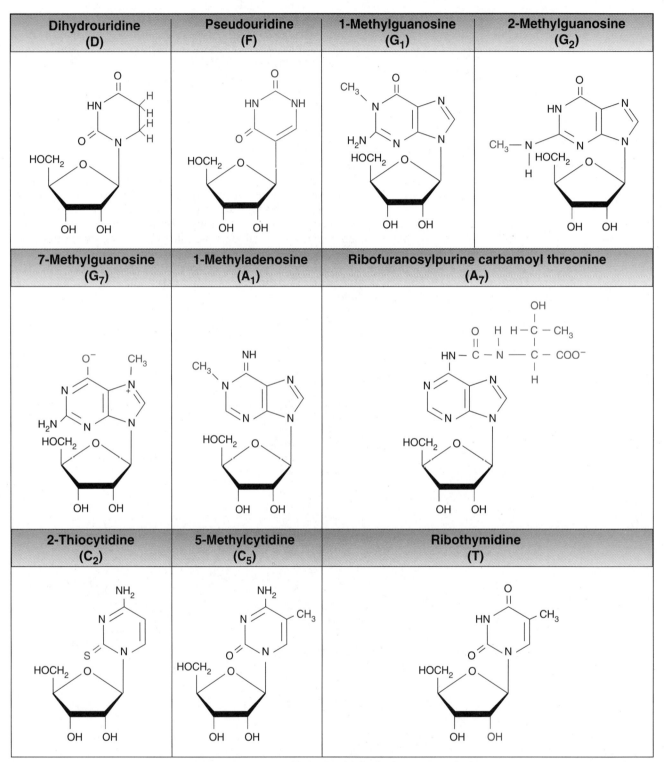

FIGURE 17–6. Common modified nucleosides found in human tRNA molecules.

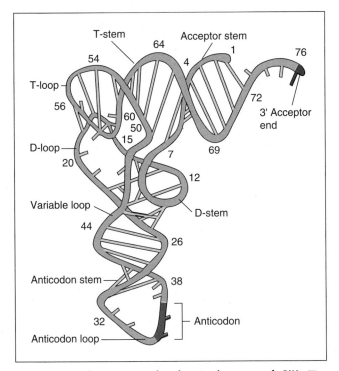

FIGURE 17–7. The tertiary, or three-dimensional, structure of tRNA. *The backbone of the tRNA is shown as a ribbon-like structure, and the hydrogen bonds as crossbars. The loops and stems correspond to those in Figure 17–5.*

isoacceptor tRNA molecules differ in 38 of the 76 positions, the enzyme recognizes these two tRNA molecules and only these two. Besides differences in 37 bases, tRNA$_I^{Met}$ contains one fewer base than tRNA^{Met}. To avoid mistakes in protein biosynthesis by misincorporating one amino acid for another, the activation reaction occurs with great accuracy.

The chemical mechanism of amino acid activation is analogous to that for fatty acid activation. Activation involves the formation of an intermediate aminoacyl adenylate and the displacement of pyrophosphate (Figure 17–8). The intermediate aminoacyl adenylate, which contains the energy-rich mixed acid anhydride bond, remains tightly bound to the active site of the enzyme. Next the activated carboxyl group of the amino acid is transferred to the 2′- or 3′-hydroxyl group of the ribose attached to the invariant adenine at the 3′ end of the tRNA molecule. This process yields an energy-rich aminoacyl∼tRNA and AMP. The acyl group may move spontaneously (nonenzymatically) between the 2′- and 3′-hydroxyl groups depending on the particular aminoacyl-tRNA, but it retains its energy-rich nature.

The number of energy-rich bonds does not change during the course of amino acid activation.

$$\text{ATP} + \text{tRNA} + \text{amino acid} \rightleftharpoons \qquad (17.1)$$
$$\text{AMP} + \text{PP}_i + \text{aminoacyl} - \text{tRNA}$$

ATP contains two high-energy bonds, and PP$_i$ and aminoacyl-tRNA each contain one (aminoacyl-tRNA + H$_2$O → amino acid + tRNA). The overall reaction is functionally isoergonic (PRINCIPLE 1 OF BIOENERGETICS). To provide the additional energy to pull the reaction in the direction of aminoacyl-tRNA formation, the familiar strategy of hydrolyzing PP$_i$ to 2 P$_i$ is employed.

Components of Protein Biosynthesis

Initiation Factors

The steps of protein synthesis include initiation, elongation, and termination or release. Protein synthesis factors transiently associate with ribosomes to perform these functions. In bacteria, the *i*nitiation *f*actors are designated **IF**, the *e*longation *f*actors are designated **EF**, and the *r*elease *f*actors are designated **RF**. The factors in eukaryotes are similarly designated with an e prefix for *e*ukaryotic (for example, eIF for *e*ukaryotic *i*nitiation *f*actor). The various factors are designated by numbers and letters, and some of their properties are given for reference in Table 17–2 (bacteria) and Table 17–3 (eukaryotes).

The two methionine tRNA molecules have different primary structures that allow initiation and elongation factors to distinguish between them. Bacterial *(E. coli)* methionine tRNA molecules differ in only three positions. Human methionine tRNA molecules differ by 38 of 76 positions (Figure 17–5). These sequence differences ensure that one tRNA will be used for initiation and the other tRNA for elongation. The two methionine tRNA molecules have the same anticodon that recognizes AUG specifically (no wobble interactions). It was the analysis of this codon-anticodon interaction which indicated that the guanine of the codon must interact with only a single base, cytosine, in the anticodon to ensure that AUG codes only for methionine.

tRNA$_I^{Met}$ refers to the initiator (I for initiator), and **tRNA^{Met}** refers to the tRNA that participates in the elongation reactions of protein synthesis. Methionine-tRNA$_I^{Met}$ initiates protein synthesis in the cytosol of humans and other eukaryotes, and methionine-tRNA^{Met} participates in the elongation reactions. In bacteria and in mitochondria, methionine-tRNA$_I^{Met}$ is converted to *N*-formyl-methionine tRNA$_I^{Met}$ prior to its use as the chain initiator (Figure 17–9). The standard free energy of hydrolysis of N^{10}-formyltetrahydrofolate, the formyl donor, to produce formate and tetrahydrofolate is − 25.9 kJ mol^{-1} and approaches the group transfer potential of a high-energy bond (Table 6–3). The amide bond of *N*-formylmethionine tRNA$_I^{Met}$ is energy poor. The formylation reaction is exergonic and irreversible.

Three initiation factors are required in bacteria, and more are required in humans. The functions of the initiation factors are similar. Both IF2 (bacterial) and eIF2 (eukaryotic) have the important role of binding aminoacylated initiator tRNA (*N*-formyl-Met-tRNA$_I^{Met}$ and Met-tRNA$_I^{Met}$, respectively) and

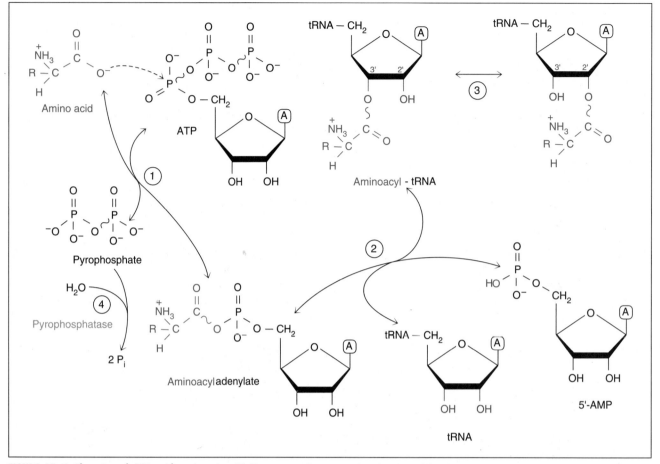

FIGURE 17–8. The aminoacyl-tRNA synthetase reaction. *(1) Formation of aminoacyl~adenylate. (2) Reaction of the aminoacyl~adenylate with its cognate tRNA. (3) Spontaneous (nonenzymatic) interconversion of the 3' and 2' aminoacyl groups. A single enzyme, aminoacyl-tRNA synthetase, catalyzes reactions 1 and 2.*

GTP. These factors place initiator methionine-tRNA into the P site of the ribosome during chain initiation. Initiation factors do not recognize or bind the methionine-tRNA^{Met} that is responsible for inserting methionine into internal positions of the growing polypeptide chain. EF-Tu in bacteria and eEF1 in humans and other eukaryotes form a complex with methionine-tRNA^{Met} and all the other aminoacyl-

tRNA molecules required for protein synthesis (one at a time) and GTP. These factors place the aminoacyl-tRNA into the A site during the elongation phase of protein synthesis.

Elongation Factors

EF-T (*elongation factor-transfer*) in bacteria consists of two components called **EF-Tu** (pronounced "ee eff tee you") and **EF-Ts** ("ee eff tee ess"). The corresponding eEF1 in eukaryotes consists of α, β, and γ subunits. EF-Tu or eEF1 each form **ternary complexes** consisting of (1) the protein factor, (2) aminoacyl-tRNA, and (3) GTP. *Transfer factors deliver (transfer) the aminoacyl-tRNA to the A site of the ribosome.* The particular aminoacyl-tRNA that is placed in the A site is the one that is determined by specific codon-anticodon base pairing. When there is a match between the aminoacyl-tRNA anticodon and the codon, binding occurs with aminoacyl-tRNA in the A site. GTP is hydrolyzed to GDP and P$_i$, and Tu · GDP or eEF1α · GDP dissociates from the ribosome. The role of GTP hydrolysis is to discharge the factor from the ribosome.

The second class of elongation factor is EF-G (bacterial) and eEF2 (eukaryotic). Both bind GTP.

TABLE 17–2. Bacterial Protein Synthesis Factors

Factor	Function
Initiation factors	
IF1	Keeps ribosome subunits dissociated
IF2	Binds GTP and formyl-Met-tRNA$_f^{Met}$
IF3	Prevents association of the small and large subunits
Elongation factors	
EF-T	*Transfer*
EF-Tu	*un*stable; binds aminoacyl tRNA · GTP
EF-Ts	stable; displaces GDP
EF-G	*G*TPase; translocates mRNA along ribosome
Release factors	
RF1	Recognizes UAA, UAG
RF2	Recognizes UAA, UGA
RF3	Binds GTP and interacts with RF1 and RF2

TABLE 17–3. Eukaryotic Protein Synthesis Factors

Factor	Function
Initiation factors	
eIF1	Assists mRNA binding
eIF2	Binds initiator Met-tRNA$_i^{Met}$ and GTP
eIF2A	AUG-dependent Met-tRNA$_i^{Met}$ binding to 40S ribosome
eIF2B	GTP/GDP exchange
eIF2C	Stabilizes ternary complex
eIF3	Binds to 40S subunit prior to mRNA binding
eIF4A	ATP-dependent helicase unwinds secondary structure of mRNA
eIF4B	Assists mRNA binding
eIF4C	Assists mRNA binding
eIF4D	Implicated in formation of the first peptide bond
eIF4E	Recognizes mRNA cap
eIF4F	Complex made of eIF4A, eIF4E, and p220
eIF5	Promotes GTP hydrolysis and release of other initiation factors
eIF6	A subunit dissociation factor
Elongation factors	
eEF1	
eEF1α	Binds aminoacyl tRNA and GTP
eEF1$\beta\gamma$	Assists in the exchange of GTP and GDP in eEF1α
eEF2	Translocates mRNA along ribosome, hydrolyzes GTP, inhibited by ADP-ribosylation catalyzed by diphtheria toxin
Release factor	
eRF	GTP binding activity and hydrolysis (GDP + P$_i$) accompanies hydrolysis of peptidyl-tRNA to form peptide and tRNA

Each participates in the movement (translocation) of peptidyl-tRNA from the A site of the ribosome to the P site. GTP is hydrolyzed to GDP and P$_i$ during the process. The role of GTP hydrolysis is to provide energy for the dissociation of these elongation factors from the ribosome.

Release or Termination Factors

Bacteria possess three release factors that participate in the termination of protein synthesis. **RF1** (UAA, UAG) and **RF2** (UAA, UGA) recognize different codons. RF3 binds GTP. **RF3** complexed with GTP facilitates the action of RF1 and RF2. Eukaryotes possess a single release factor designated **eRF**. It recognizes all three termination codons and also binds GTP. GTP hydrolysis to GDP and P$_i$ is required for chain termination in both eukaryotes and bacteria.

All the players have been introduced, and the stage is now set for a consideration of the reactions of protein synthesis.

Steps of Protein Biosynthesis

Formation of the Initiation Complex

Bacterial and eukaryotic protein synthesis are similar. Formation of the initiation complex in both cases is intricate and is the rate-limiting step. We begin with initiation of bacterial synthesis. IF1 and IF3 are bound to the small ribosomal subunit. IF2 forms a ternary complex with GTP and initiator N-formyl-Met-tRNA$_i^{Met}$. The 30S ribosomal subunit, mRNA, and the IF2 ternary complex combine. IF3 is released during the first step (Figure 17–10A). In the second step, the 50S ribosome subunit binds with the complex. GTP is hydrolyzed to GDP and P$_i$, and IF1 and IF2 are released. *At the end of this process, N-formyl-Met-tRNA$_i^{Met}$ is bound to the P site of the ribosome with its anticodon in register with the AUG initiating codon of mRNA.* Because the message is read triplet by triplet, it is essential that the interactions of the initiator tRNA and mRNA be accurate. If the binding were displaced by a single base, the amino acid sequence of the assembled polypeptide would bear no relationship to the desired product because of the altered reading frame. This requirement is part of the likely explanation for the intricacy involved in accurately forming the initiation complex.

The initiating codon (AUG) is not at the 5' end of mRNA but is often 50–100 nucleotides from the 5'

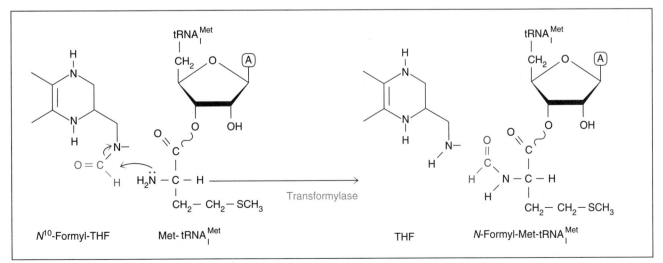

FIGURE 17–9. Conversion of methionine-tRNA$_i^{Met}$ to N-formyl-methionine tRNA$_i^{Met}$.

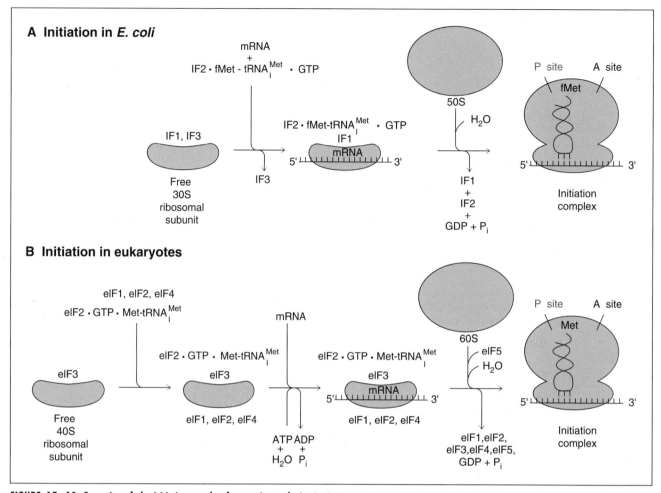

FIGURE 17–10. Formation of the initiation complex for protein synthesis. A. *Initiation events in* E. coli. *B. Initiation events in eukaryotes. At the completion of initiation, initiator methionine-tRNA resides in the P site. fMet-tRNA$_I^{Met}$ is N-formyl-Met-tRNA$_I^{Met}$.*

end. Bacterial mRNAs are polycistronic and include internal initiation sites that are far removed from the 5′ end of the molecules. Each mRNA of bacteria possesses a ribosome binding site that is upstream from the initiating codon. The message binds to a sequence of 5 bases (CCUCC) near the 3′ end of 16S RNA called the **Shine-Dalgarno** sequence. The interactions between mRNA and rRNA are antiparallel, and the interactions of mRNA with the Shine-Dalgarno site of rRNA play an important role in selecting an appropriate AUG for chain initiation. This process excludes the selection of AUG codons corresponding to methionines that occur within the protein.

Initiation of protein synthesis in eukaryotes, which involves an **AUG scanning** mechanism, is similar in outline but different in detail. Initiation differs in that Met-tRNA$_I^{Met}$ is unformylated, more initiation factors participate, and there is no comparable interaction of mRNA with a Shine-Dalgarno sequence. The functions of the numerous initiation factors are listed in Table 17–3 for the interested reader. In contrast to bacterial protein synthesis, the ternary complex formed from eIF2 · GTP · Met-tRNA$_I^{Met}$ with the small subunit occurs prior to

binding to mRNA (Figure 17–10B). eIF4E recognizes the guanosine cap of mRNA. The 40S subunit binds to the 5′ end of monocistronic mRNA and scans along the message until the first AUG is encountered. Several other initiation factors participate in binding the small subunit to mRNA. The anticodon of Met-tRNA$_I^{Met}$ plays a role in scanning. After the first AUG is encountered, the large subunit binds to form the initiation complex. eIF5 catalyzes GTP hydrolysis and the dissociation of initiation factors from the ribosomes. *At the end of the initiation process in both bacterial and animal protein synthesis, the initiator methionine-tRNA is found in the P site.* Initiator methionine tRNA is the only aminoacyl-tRNA that is delivered physiologically to the P site; the other aminoacyl-tRNAs are delivered to the A site.

Elongation and Translocation

Following the formation of the initiation complex, a series of elongation cycles occur. Let us first consider the elongation process in bacteria. A series of ternary complexes of EF-Tu · GTP · aminoacyl-tRNA interacts with the A (aminoacyl-tRNA) site of the ribosome. When a match occurs between the triplet codon immediately following the initiating AUG and an anticodon of an aminoacyl-tRNA brought to the A site as part of a ternary complex, *aminoacyl-tRNA binds to the A site* (Figure 17–11).

Hydrolysis of GTP promotes the release of EF-Tu. The role of GTP hydrolysis is to discharge the protein factor from the ribosome. GTP hydrolysis makes the overall transfer cycle exergonic. EF-Tu · GDP will not bind with another aminoacyl-tRNA until the GDP is exchanged for GTP. EF-Ts forms an EF-Tu · EF-Ts complex and displaces GDP. This complex then combines with GTP, and EF-Ts is displaced. EF-Tu · GTP can then form a ternary complex with another aminoacyl-tRNA. A similar exchange process occurs with eEF1. eEF1α binds GTP and GDP; eEF1$\beta\gamma$ mediates the exchange reaction.

Following the binding of aminoacyl-tRNA in the A site, **peptidyltransferase** (an intrinsic activity of the large ribosomal subunit) catalyzes the reaction between the amino group of the A site and the activated carboxyl group in the P site (Figure 17–12). This illustration provides a deceptively large amount of information. First, the growing portion of the polymer bears the activated group, and this activated group reacts with the amino

group of the incoming aminoacyl-tRNA. Following the condensation reaction, the energy-rich *N*-formyl-methionyl~tRNA bond is lost with the concomitant formation of an energy-poor peptide bond. The reaction is exergonic (PRINCIPLE 2 OF BIOENERGETICS), and no additional chemical energy is required for peptide bond formation. Second, dipeptidyl-tRNA is found in the A site following peptide bond formation. For further peptide bond formation to occur, it is necessary to translocate the dipeptidyl-tRNA · mRNA, in register together, to the P site. Third, the figure shows that polymerization proceeds from the amino terminus to the carboxyl terminus. The amino terminus of a protein generally has a free amino group, not in peptide linkage; here the amino group is formylated. The carboxyl terminus is that end with a free carboxyl group, not in peptide linkage; here the carboxyl terminus is attached to tRNA by a high-energy bond. This high-energy bond will be lost in the next peptidyltransferase reaction.

Following peptide bond formation, free tRNA (without an amino acid) resides in the P site and peptidyl-tRNA occurs in the A site. To prepare for the next condensation reaction, EF-G · GTP mediates the ejection of tRNA from the P site and the relative movement of peptidyl-tRNA, bonded to its codon on mRNA, from the A site to the P site

FIGURE 17–11. *Aminoacyl-tRNA binding to the A site.* (1) The transfer step in protein biosynthesis. (2, 3, 4, and 5) The exchange of GTP for GDP on EF-Tu that is mediated by EF-Ts. (6) Formation of the ternary complex.

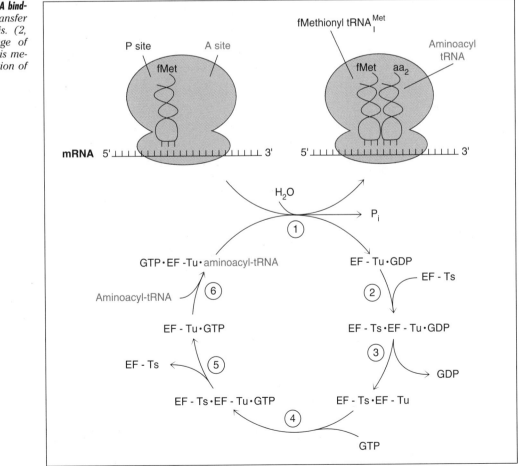

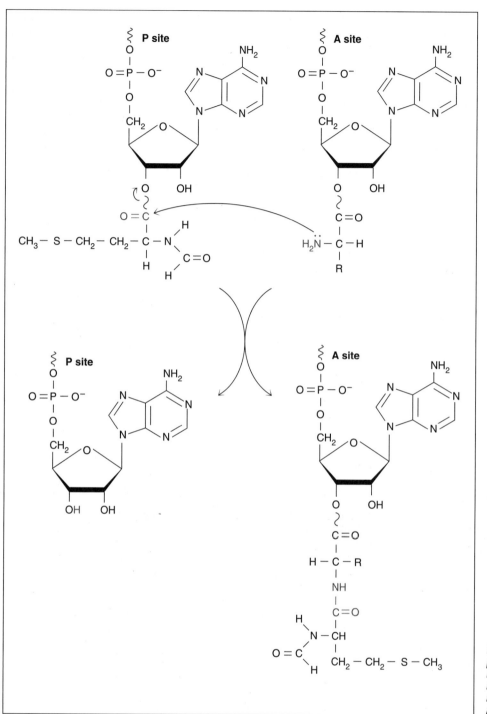

FIGURE 17–12. Chemistry of the peptidyl transfer reaction of protein biosynthesis. N-Formyl methionine tRNA or peptidyl-tRNA occupies the P site. Aminoacyl-tRNA occupies the A site.

(Figure 17–13). This process is accompanied by the hydrolysis of GTP to GDP and P_i, and hydrolysis provides energy for the dissociation of the factor from the ribosome.

Following translocation, dipeptidyl-tRNA occupies the P site. The second cycle of elongation occurs as has been described for the first cycle. The elongation reactions of protein synthesis in human and other eukaryotic cells are identical to those of bacterial cells. After about 100 nucleotides of mRNA have been translated, a second ribosome forms an initiation complex with mRNA, and biosynthesis of a second polypeptide begins. After another 100 nucleotides, a third ribosome forms an initiation complex and another polypeptide is synthesized. Structures that result from the binding of multiple ribosomes to a single mRNA are called **polyribosomes** or **polysomes.** About three or four ribosomes can bind to the short hemoglobin mRNA, and more than 30 ribosomes can bind to the long myosin mRNA. The elongation cycles continue until a stop codon occupies the A site.

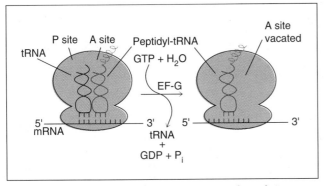

FIGURE 17–13. The translocation step in protein biosynthesis.

Release of Polypeptides

No tRNA molecules recognize the stop codon in the A site, and elongation ceases. Release factors interact with this stalled ribosome complex. In bacteria, RF1 or RF2 recognizes the termination codon. RF3 enhances the activity of RF1 and RF2. The high-energy ester bond linking the nascent polypeptide to tRNA is hydrolyzed, and the polypeptide is released from the complex (Figure 17–14). The release factor converts the peptidyltransferase activity of the ribosome to hydrolase activity that discharges the polypeptide. The tRNA, which remains attached to the mRNA-ribosome complex, is ejected by EF-G by a process that re-

quires GTP hydrolysis. IF1 participates in the dissociation of ribosomes into their 30S and 50S subunits. Although eukaryotes possess only one release factor (eRF), termination of protein synthesis is similar to that of bacteria. A summary of the steps in eukaryotic protein synthesis is shown in Figure 17–15.

UGA, which is a standard termination codon, can also encode **selenocysteine.** This amino acid, which is found in glutathione peroxidase in eukaryotes, contains selenium in place of sulfur. A rare tRNA that contains an anticodon that corresponds to UGA combines with serine. The serinyl-tRNA is converted to selenocysteinyl-tRNA. Selenocysteine is incorporated into glutathione peroxidase in response to the UGA codon. The mRNA sequence surrounding the UGA plays a role in selecting selenocysteine, and this context ensures that chain termination will not occur.

Comparison of Bacterial and Eukaryotic Protein Synthesis

BIOCHEMICAL PROCESSES. There are few mechanistic differences between protein synthesis in bacteria and eukaryotes. The major differences involve initiation. Bacteria use formylated Met-tRNA$_i^{Met}$ for initiation, and eukaryotes use unformylated Met-tRNA$_i^{Met}$. Bacteria possess a sequence in mRNA near the initiating AUG codon that binds to

FIGURE 17–14. The termination or release reaction in protein biosynthesis. *RF denotes release factor 1 or 2 plus release factor 3.*

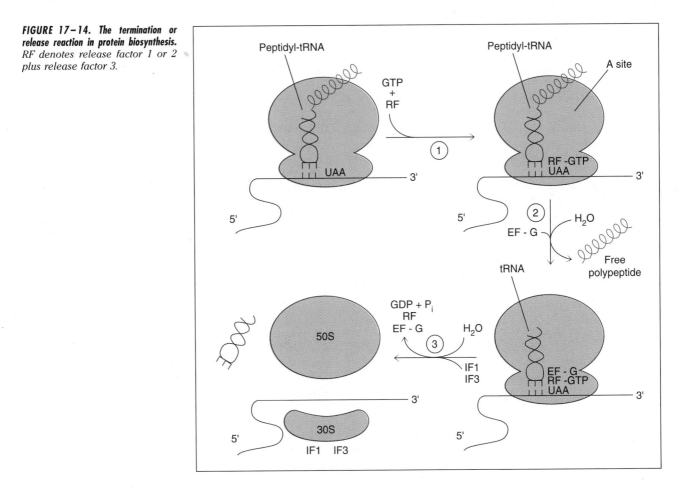

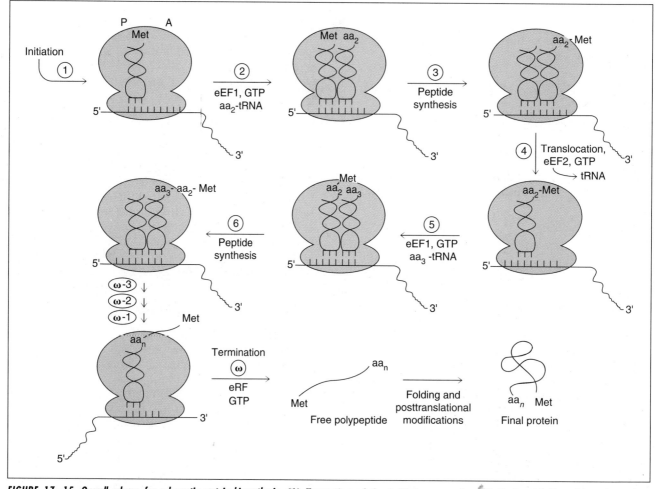

FIGURE 17–15. Overall scheme for eukaryotic protein biosynthesis. (1) Formation of the initiation complex. (2, 3, 4, etc.) Repetitive elongation cycles. Elongation continues until a termination codon occurs in the A site. (ω) eRF mediates the liberation of the polypeptide from the ribosome. aa, amino acid.

a Shine-Dalgarno sequence in 16S rRNA. Eukaryotes lack the Shine-Dalgarno sequence. The small ribosomal subunit and eIF4E of eukaryotes recognize the 7-methylguanine cap at the 5′ end of mRNA. The small ribosomal subunit with the attached initiator tRNA scans the mRNA from the 5′ end toward the 3′ end in search of the first AUG codon, which is then used in forming the initiation complex. The elongation and termination processes are similar in bacteria and eukaryotic cells. The rate of biosynthesis, however, is three-fold faster in bacteria than in eukaryotes (18 versus 6 amino acid residues per second).

Bacterial messenger RNAs can be either **monocistronic** *or* **polycistronic.** The multiple proteins encoded by the polycistronic message are synthesized independently. Initiation can occur internally on polycistronic mRNA, and this depends upon the presence of inner Shine-Dalgarno binding sequences that are near the initiating AUG (Figure 17–16).

Eukaryotic messenger RNAs are monocistronic. Eukaryotes, however, can synthesize a polyprotein from a single message. A **polyprotein** has multiple

activities. Sometimes the polyproteins function as a unit such as the CAD complex (carbamoyl-phosphate synthetase II, aspartate transcarbamoylase, and dihydroorotase) of pyrimidine metabolism (Table 14–2). In other cases, the polyproteins are cleaved by proteases posttranslationally to give multiple proteins. The *pol* gene of HIV-1, for example, encodes a polyprotein that is cleaved to form reverse transcriptase, integrase, and RNAse H (Table 16–13).

INHIBITION BY ANTIBIOTICS AND TOXINS.
▶ Several antibiotics differentially affect RNA-dependent bacterial and mammalian protein synthesis (Table 17–4). **Tetracycline** and **chloramphenicol** (Figure 17–17) are broad-spectrum antibiotics, so-called because they are effective against a number of gram-negative and gram-positive bacteria, rickettsiae, and chlamydial species. Chlamydiae are gram-negative bacteria (Table 1–3) that are obligate intracellular parasites. Chlamydiae cause atypical pneumonia. Moreover, chlamydial urethritis and cervicitis are among the most prevalent sexually transmitted diseases. Tetracycline is effective in the treatment of Lyme disease caused by the spi-

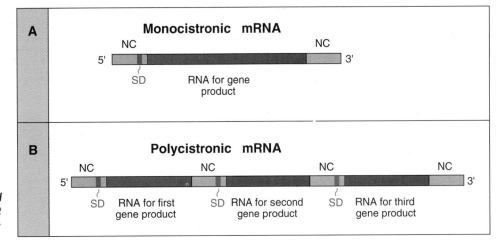

FIGURE 17–16. *Monocistronic and polycistronic mRNA.* NC, noncoding RNA; SD, Shine-Dalgarno rRNA binding sequence.

rochete *Borrelia burgdorferi.* **Erythromycin** is effective in the treatment of a variety of bacterial infections including legionnaires' disease caused by gram-negative *Legionella pneumophila.*

Corynebacterium diphtheriae, a gram-positive pleomorphic bacterium, is the causative agent of diphtheria (Table 1–2). *C. diphtheriae* produces an upper respiratory infection that can affect the tonsils, pharynx, and larynx. Only strains of *C. diphtheriae* infected by a β_1-bacteriophage that encodes the gene for diphtheria toxin produce disease. Pathogenic strains of bacteria produce a 62-kDa protein exotoxin. The toxin, which is produced and released by the bacterium, binds to host cells and undergoes proteolytic cleavage to form an A and a B chain. The A chain enters the cell by a process that requires the aid of the B chain. The A fragment catalyzes the ADP-ribosylation of eEF2. Following chemical modification, the elongation factor is inactivated. The site of ADP-ribosylation involves a posttranslationally modified histidine residue called **diphthamide** that occurs nearly exclusively in eEF2 (Figure 17–18). Entry of a single toxin molecule is sufficient to kill a cell. Bacterial EF-G lacks this sensitive residue, and bacterial protein synthesis is resistant to diphtheria toxin.

Immunization with inactivated diphtheria toxin prevents diphtheria. Immunization against diphtheria is widespread and forms part of the triad of DPT vaccine (diphtheria, pertussis, and tetanus). *C. diphtheriae* is sensitive to penicillin. After the onset of the disease, however, affected individuals are treated intravenously with antibodies directed against the toxin (diphtheria antitoxin) because too much time is required for penicillin to abolish the infection. The mortality of diphtheria in untreated children ranges from 30 to 50% and accounts for the dread of this malady. ◄

Regulation of Eukaryotic Protein Synthesis

As much as one-third of cytoplasmic mRNA is not bound to ribosomes when greater than 90% of the ribosomes are translationally active. Thus, mRNA is not limiting translation. The process for selecting mRNAs for translation, however, is unknown. All mammalian cellular mRNAs are capped with the methylated guanosine, and such a structure enhances translation. When the cap is shielded from eIF4E because of the conformation of the 5′ end of mRNA, translation of such mRNAs is decreased. The primary and secondary structures of the 5′ end of mRNA therefore represent a potential selective and regulatory mechanism of protein synthesis.

Phosphorylation and dephosphorylation of numerous protein components play a role in controlling the rate of protein synthesis in animal cells. Initiation factors, elongation factors, ribosomal proteins, and several amino acid–tRNA synthetases are phosphorylated by protein kinases. The phosphorylation of eIF2B, eIF3, eIF4B, eIF4F, and

TABLE 17–4.   Action of Antibiotics That Inhibit Bacterial Protein or Peptidoglycan Synthesis

Antibiotic	Site of Action	Mechanism	Use
Aminoglycoside (streptomycin, gentamicin)	30S subunit	Inhibits initiation; produces translation errors	Gram negative
Cephalosporin	Cell wall	Inibits transpeptidase cross-linking	Gram positive and gram negative
Chloramphenicol	50S subunit	Inhibits peptidyltransferase activity	Broad spectrum
Erythromycin	50S subunit	Inhibits translocation	Gram positive and gram negative
Penicillin	Cell wall	Inhibits transpeptidase cross-linking	Gram positive
Tetracycline	30S subunit	Inhibits aminoacyl-tRNA binding to the A site	Broad spectrum
Vancomycin	Cell wall	Blocks transfer of pentapeptide from cytoplasm to cell membrane	Gram positive

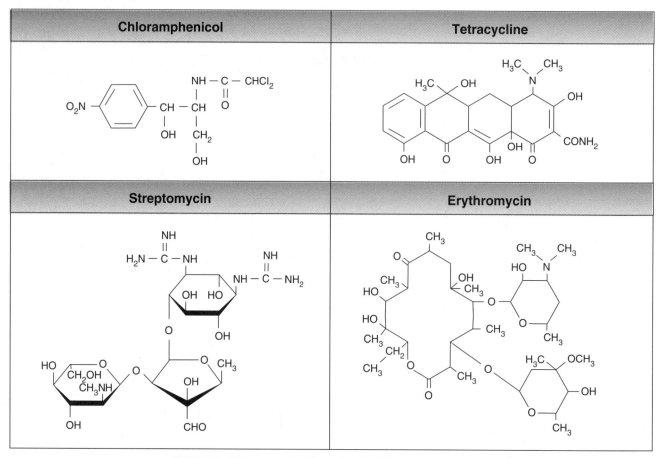

FIGURE 17–17. Structures of antibiotics that inhibit bacterial protein synthesis.

ribosomal protein S6 is associated with activation of protein synthesis.

Phosphorylation of other components of the translational apparatus diminishes the rate of protein synthesis. For example, the phosphorylation of the α-subunit of eIF2 results in repressed protein synthesis. In reticulocytes, **heme** *inhibits* a **heme-regulated eIF2 protein kinase.** In the absence of heme, phosphorylation of eIF2 by this kinase constrains the initiation of protein synthesis. This process coordinates heme and globin synthesis. Human cells contain another eIF2 protein kinase that is *activated* by **double-stranded RNA** that is formed during viral infection. This is a protective mechanism that limits protein synthesis in some virally infected cells. Phosphorylation catalyzed by both of the eIF2 protein kinases inhibits protein synthesis. Phosphorylation of eEF2 also diminishes protein synthesis. The enzyme that catalyzes this reaction is **calcium/calmodulin-dependent protein kinase III.** Protein kinase III, unlike calcium/calmodulin-dependent protein kinase II, has narrow substrate specificity and is specific for eEF2.

Bioenergetics of Protein Biosynthesis

The activation of each amino acid as aminoacyl-tRNA requires the expenditure of two high-energy bonds (ATP $\rightarrow$ AMP + 2 P_i). Placement of aminoacyl-tRNA in the A site requires hydrolysis of GTP to GDP and P_i (the expenditure of one high-energy bond). Similarly, translocation is also accompanied by the hydrolysis of GTP to GDP and P_i. *A minimum of four high-energy bonds is thus required for the synthesis of each peptide bond during protein biosynthesis.* The participation of chaperones (Chapter 3) in the formation of the active conformation of a protein results in the expenditure of additional ATP to form a functional protein. The large amount of energy needed for peptide bond formation is the price required for converting the four-letter alphabet of nucleic acids to the 20-letter alphabet of proteins.

MITOCHONDRIAL DNA, RNA, AND PROTEIN SYNTHESIS

DNA Synthesis

Each nucleated human cell contains between 100 and 1000 mitochondria. Each mitochondrion contains between 5 and 10 copies of supercoiled circular DNA. Human mitochondrial DNA contains 16,569 base pairs and 37 genes. Mitochondrial DNA codes for 13 essential genes of oxidative phosphor-

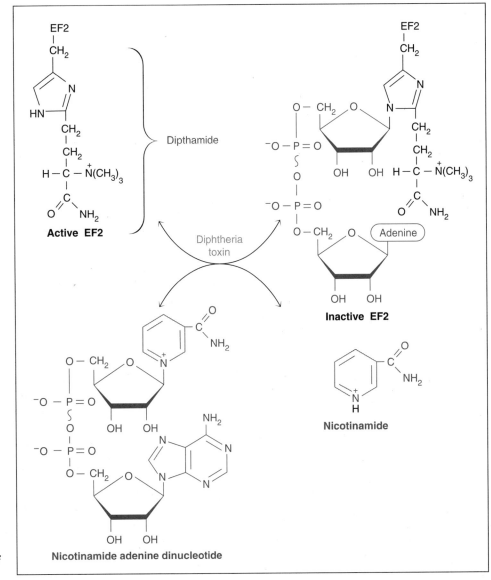

FIGURE 17–18. *ADP-ribosylation of eEF2.*

ylation, two rRNAs, and 22 tRNAs. Mitochondria contain their own replication, transcription, and translation systems. The majority of mitochondrial proteins, however, are encoded in nuclear genes. These nuclear encoded proteins are synthesized on cytoplasmic ribosomes and imported into the mitochondrion.

The two strands of mitochondrial DNA differ in their base composition. The strand that contains most of the guanine residues is called the heavy, or **H, strand,** and the complementary strand that contains most of the cytosine residues is called the light, or **L, strand.** Mitochondrial DNA uses two origins of replication, one for each strand, that are separated by two-thirds of the genome. DNA polymerase γ is the mitochondrial polymerase. Like other DNA polymerases, it is unable to initiate DNA replication alone and requires a primer.

Replication of the H strand is initiated with a short RNA primer whose synthesis is catalyzed by

mitochondrial RNA polymerase at the normal promoter for the L-strand template. The RNA is either elongated into a full-length mRNA, or it is hydrolyzed at a defined position and the 5′ fragment of the resulting RNA with its 3′-hydroxyl group is elongated to form a 7S DNA primer. DNA polymerase γ elongates the primer, and the resulting DNA displaces the parental H strand, forming a displacement loop, or **D-loop** (Figure 17–19). H strand synthesis continues past the origin of replication of the light strand to complete the first daughter duplex. After the origin of replication of the light strand is exposed, light strand synthesis is initiated by a primase containing, paradoxically, the 5.8 S rRNA of the cytosol. L-strand elongation proceeds along the free H-strand template until the second daughter duplex is completed. Replication is bidirectional but asynchronous (Figure 17–19). Each strand is synthesized continuously (no Okasaki fragments).

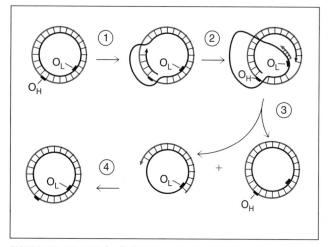

FIGURE 17–19. Mitochondrial DNA synthesis. *(1) Initiation of heavy chain synthesis. The displaced heavy chain forms a D-loop. (2) Heavy chain synthesis extends past the origin of replication for the light chain, and light chain synthesis begins. (3) Heavy chain synthesis is completed. (4) Light chain synthesis is completed. O_H, origin of heavy chain replication. O_L, origin of light chain replication.*

Mitochondrial DNA replication occurs throughout the cell cycle. The average rate of deoxyribonucleotide incorporation is 100 times less than that of bacterial DNA synthesis. Moreover, the fidelity of mitochondrial DNA synthesis is less than that of nuclear or bacterial DNA synthesis. RNA is alkali labile, but DNA is not cleaved by treatment with alkali. Mitochondrial DNA, but not nuclear DNA, is degraded into a few fragments by alkali. Thus, each strand of mitochondrial DNA contains a few ribonucleotides that are not removed by DNA repair.

Mitochondrial DNA exhibits **maternal inheritance.** Furthermore, human cells can harbor mixtures of mutant and normal mitochondrial DNAs, and the proportion of mutants can range from 0 to 100%. The rate of evolution of mitochondrial DNA is 10–20 times more rapid than that of nuclear DNA. This increased rate may be related to a less effective mitochondrial DNA repair system. Any two human mitochondrial DNAs will differ by about four nucleotides per 1000 or about 70 nucleotides per mitochondrial genome of 16,569.

RNA and Protein Synthesis

Both strands of mitochondrial DNA are transcribed from a unique heavy and a unique light strand promoter that occurs in the D region of the genome. Both transcripts encompass the entire genomic circle. The L strand is transcribed in the clockwise direction, and the H strand is transcribed in the counterclockwise direction (these directions are arbitrary). The small and large rRNAs, 14 tRNAs, and messages for 12 proteins are transcribed from the H-strand template. Eight tRNAs and the message for one protein are transcribed from the L-strand template. Each primary transcript is processed to yield the final RNA products. Processing involves the excision of dispersed tRNA molecules, and this process generates the two rRNA molecules and the mRNA that encodes proteins.

The mitochondrial genome is compact, and the mRNAs lack introns. The first trinucleotide of each mRNA is an initiating codon for protein synthesis, and this is an unusual property. mRNA molecules in mitochondria are not capped. Chain initiation for mitochondrial protein synthesis thus differs from that of bacteria (with Shine-Dalgarno rRNA-mRNA interaction) or eukaryotes (with the AUG scanning process). The initiating amino acyl-tRNA in mitochondrial protein synthesis is *N*-formyl-Met-tRNA^{Met}, thereby resembling bacterial initiation. There is but a single mitochondrial gene for tRNA^{Met}, and the same gene product subserves both initiation and elongation functions. PolyA tails are added posttranscriptionally and contribute to the production of UAA termination codons. There are no untranslated codons between the termination codon and the polyA tail.

The mitochondrion contains all of the genes for mitochondrial tRNA molecules and rRNAs. The mitochondrion contains about 20% of the genes for the proteins of the electron transport chain and ATP synthase. The nucleus, however, contains all of the genes for mitochondrial ribosomal proteins and initiation, elongation, termination factors, and the proteins required for replication and transcription. The nucleus also contains all of the genes for the proteins of the Krebs cycle, β-oxidation, and the other enzymes of intermediary metabolism (Table 1–1). The amino-terminal sequence of proteins that are imported into the mitochondrion has positively charged amino acids that are recognized by mitochondrial receptors, and only these proteins are imported.

Mitochondrial DNA and Human Disease

▶ The location of DNA within the mitochondrion may promote age-related somatic mutations based upon the generation of reactive oxides (Chapter 5). Oxygen radicals are natural by-products of oxidative phosphorylation, and they account for about 1% of total oxygen uptake. The most likely cause of age-related mitochondrial DNA damage is oxidation by superoxide anions and hydrogen peroxide. These substances react with lipids, proteins, and nucleic acids. Mitochondrial DNA is 15 times more sensitive to oxidative damage than is nuclear DNA. This increased sensitivity of mitochondrial DNA to oxidative damage is due to its location, the lack of protective histones in mitochondria, and limited DNA repair. The major sources of radical generation are between complex I and CoQ and CoQ and complex III. Reduced flavins and quinones react with oxygen to yield oxygen radicals at these sites.

In cardiac ischemia that is secondary to coronary artery disease and atherosclerosis, there is a buildup of reduced flavins and quinones that can react adventitiously with oxygen to produce oxygen radicals. Postmortem studies indicate that there is a large increase (from 8- to 2200-fold) in the amount of abnormal mitochondrial DNA in the hearts from individuals with ischemia when compared with hearts from individuals not experiencing ischemia. Such changes in mitochondrial DNA may impair cardiac function.

The optic nerve is dependent upon mitochondria for energy production. **Leber hereditary optic neuropathy** (LHON) is a maternally inherited form of adult-onset blindness due to death of the optic nerve. This rare disorder is due to missense mutations of mitochondrially encoded proteins that occur in complex I or complex III (cytochrome *b*). There is an age-dependent decrease in the expression of proteins participating in oxidative phosphorylation, accounting for the onset of blindness in adulthood. A missense mutation involving one of the proteins of ATP synthase also leads to blindness.

The antibiotic **chloramphenicol,** which inhibits the peptidyltransferase of bacterial ribosomes, also inhibits mitochondrial peptidyltransferase and protein synthesis. This inhibition is thought to explain the toxicity to humans of this agent. **Azidothymidine** (AZT), which is converted to the corresponding triphosphate, is used in the treatment of AIDS. The triphosphate metabolite inhibits reverse transcriptase (Chapter 16). This metabolite also inhibits mitochondrial DNA polymerase. A side effect of this drug is the development of a red fiber myopathy associated with a 20 to 70% decrease in mitochondrial DNA. ◄

BACTERIAL CELL WALL BIOSYNTHESIS

Properties of Bacterial Cell Walls

Cell walls surround the periplasmic space of bacteria, and peptidoglycans occur in bacterial cell walls. **Peptidoglycans** are heteropolymers made up of amino acids and sugars (glycans). This heteropolymer is cross-linked to form one gigantic molecule that encompasses each cell. In gram-positive bacteria, the peptidoglycan makes up their characteristic thick cell wall. In gram-negative bacteria, the peptidoglycan forms the innermost aspect of the multilayered cell wall (Figure 1-10). Peptidoglycans contain *N*-acetylmuramic acid (MurNAc) and diaminopimelic acid (DAP) as shown in Figure 17–20. **N-Acetylmuramate** is made from *N*-acetylglucosamine to which lactate is attached via an O^3-ether linkage. **Diaminopimelate** (ε-carboxylysine) is an

intermediate in the pathway for bacterial lysine biosynthesis.

Peptidoglycan contains *N*-acetylglucosamine and *N*-acetylmuramate as a repeating disaccharide unit (Figure 17–21). In *Staphylococcus aureus*, a pentapeptide (L-Ala-D-Glu-DAP-D-Ala-D-Ala) extends initially from the carboxyl group of *N*-acetylmuramate (the fifth amino acid is displaced in the last stage of peptidoglycan synthesis). The lactyl group furnishes the carboxyl group through which a peptide is attached to each disaccharide. Peptide bonds in peptidoglycans in various species can involve the γ-carboxyl group of glutamate, or the ε-amino group of lysine or diaminopimelate, depending upon the organism. A pentaglycine chain branches from diaminopimelate. Pentaglycine cross-links the ε-amino group of the penultimate residue (diaminopimelate) of one chain to the carboxyl group of the last residue (D-alanine) of an adjacent chain. Terminal D-Ala is displaced during the formation of this cross-link, and the peptide side chain contains four amino acids (Figure 17–22). The occurrence of the nonstandard amino acids and nonstandard peptide bonds indicates that these peptides are not synthesized by genetically encoded mRNA and the ribosomes. Each strand contains 10–65 repeating disaccharide units in β-1,4-linkage. Individual strands are connected by pentaglycine cross-links to form a single molecule that surrounds each cell.

Peptidoglycan Biosynthesis

Let us consider the biosynthesis of *N*-acetylmuramate. The 3-*O*-lactyl side chain of *N*-acetylmuramate is derived from phosphoenolpyruvate in a two-step process. First, the hydroxyl group on C^3

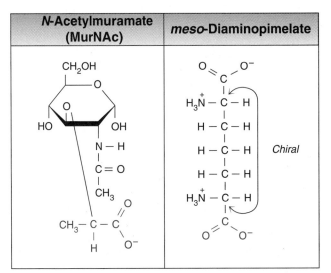

FIGURE 17–20. Structure of N-acetylmuramate and meso-diaminopimelate. *Although diaminopimelate (DAP) contains two chiral carbon atoms, the isomer that is shown is not optically active because of the symmetry of the whole molecule; thus, it is designated as a meso compound.*

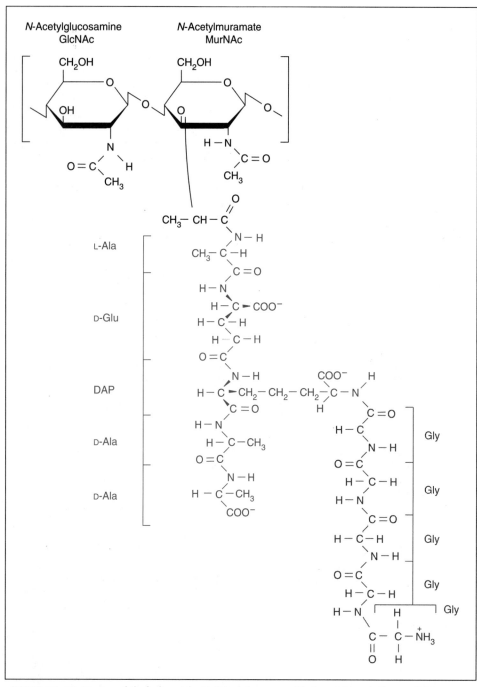

FIGURE 17–21. Structure of the fundamental unit of Staphylococcus peptidoglycan before peptide cross-linking occurs.

of UDP-*N*-acetylglucosamine attacks C^2 of phospho-enolpyruvate and displaces P_i (this is not a hydrolysis reaction). The resulting ether is a low-energy compound, and this reaction is exergonic. Second, NADPH reduces the carbon-carbon double bond to form UDP-*N*-acetylmuramate (Figure 17–23).

First Stage: Peptide Synthesis

The biosynthesis of peptidoglycan can be divided into three stages: (1) synthesis of a pentapeptide on UDP-*N*-acetylmuramate, (2) synthesis of

the disaccharide and pentaglycine side chain of the peptidoglycan repeating unit, and (3) cross-linking the disaccharide-peptide repeating units to form cell wall polysaccharide. In stage 1, which occurs in the bacterial cytosol, five amino acids are added to UDP-*N*-acetylmuramate. ATP provides the energy for this process. In stage 2, which occurs on the plasma membrane, the sugar pentapeptide is transferred to undecaprenol phosphate, a phospholipid. After adding *N*-acetylglucosamine to form the repeating disaccharide unit, a pentaglycine side chain derived from five glycine-tRNA molecules is

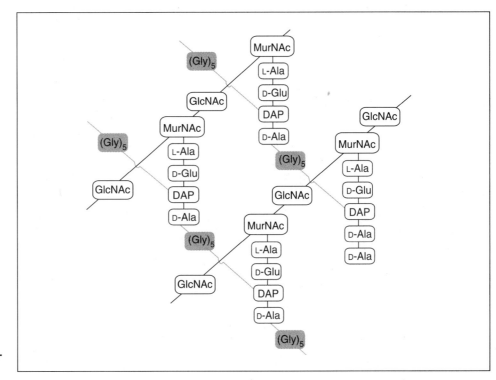

FIGURE 17–22. Structure of cross-linked Staphylococcus peptidoglycan.

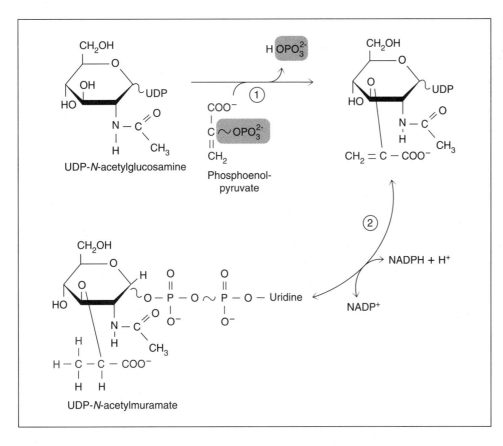

FIGURE 17–23. Synthesis of UDP-N-acetylmuramic acid from UDP-N-acetyl-glucosamine and phosphoenolpyruvate.

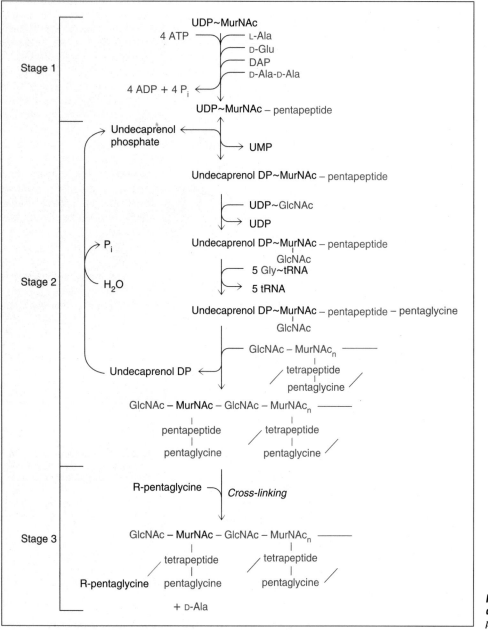

FIGURE 17–24. Overview of peptidoglycan biosynthesis. DP, diphosphate.

added to the pentapeptide formed during the first stage. The disaccharide-peptide unit is transferred to the growing peptidoglycan outside the cell. In stage 3, the pentaglycine chain of one disaccharide-peptide unit forms a peptide cross-link with another unit (Figure 17–24). Cross-linking involves a transpeptidation reaction and occurs without additional chemical energy. The cross-linking reaction is sensitive to β-lactam antibiotics, including penicillin.

The sequence of the amino acids linked to *N*-acetylmuramate varies in different bacteria. ATP serves as the source of chemical energy for the synthesis of these bonds, and the product of each reaction is ADP and P_i. The carboxylate groups are activated as the acyl~phosphate (and not as the adenylate) as illustrated in Figure 17–25. The high-energy acylphosphate undergoes a nucleophilic attack by the amino group of the incoming amino acid, and a low-energy bond forms. The overall process occurs with the loss of a high-energy bond and is exergonic.

Each of the covalent peptide bonds that forms during stage 1 of peptidoglycan biosynthesis follows this same ATP-dependent mechanism. Each step, however, is catalyzed by a different enzyme. The second amino acid in the pentapeptide precursor of *S. aureus* is D-glutamate. A pyridoxal phosphate-independent **glutamate racemase** catalyzes the isoergonic conversion of L-glutamate to D-glutamate. The third amino acid residue of the pentapeptide, which is derived from an intermediate in the pathway for lysine biosynthesis in the bacteria, is *meso*-diaminopimelate. An epimerase

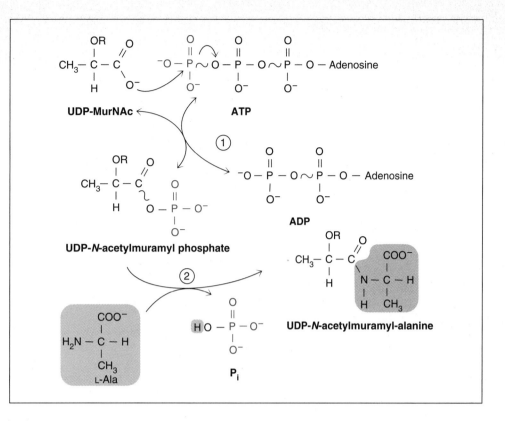

FIGURE 17–25. *Addition of the first amino acid to N-acetylmuramate during stage 1 of peptidoglycan biosynthesis.*

catalyzes the functionally isoergonic conversion of L,L-diaminopimelate (the intermediate) to *meso*-diaminopimelate.

The fourth and fifth residues of the pentapeptide are derived from D-alanyl-D-alanine. This dipeptide is synthesized in two steps. The first step involves the isoergonic racemization of each of two L-alanines catalyzed by a pyridoxal phosphate–dependent **alanine racemase.** The dipeptide is synthesized during the second step and requires ATP. One of the molecules of D-alanine is converted to the acylphosphate (Figure 17–26). The dipeptide forms after the incoming D-alanine amino group attacks the acylphosphate. To complete the synthesis of the pentapeptide chain, the free amino group of the dipeptidyl D-alanyl-D-alanine attacks the carboxyl group of the third amino acid, diaminopimelate, that has been activated as the acylphosphate. The last step in this stage is catalyzed by a **D-alanine–adding enzyme.** These reactions, which constitute the first stage of peptidoglycan biosynthesis, occur in the cytosol of the bacterial cell.

Second Stage: Repeating Unit Synthesis

The next series of reactions involves the plasma membrane. The membrane contains **undecaprenol phosphate,** an isoprenoid alcohol phosphate. *Undeca*prenol phosphate (so-named because it contains 11 isoprenoid units) reacts with UDP-*N*-acetylmuramyl-pentapeptide to form undecaprenol diphosphate *N*-acetylmuramyl-pentapeptide and UMP. The number of high-energy bonds is the same in the

reactants and products, and the reaction is functionally isoergonic (PRINCIPLE 1 OF BIOENERGETICS) (Figure 17–27). The formation of the disaccharide derivative follows a familiar pattern. The C^4 alcohol of the sugar of the undecaprenol diphosphate-*N*-acetylmuramate-derivative attacks the activated glycoside bond in UDP-*N*-acetylglucosamine to form the low-energy disaccharide bond.

Glycine residues are added sequentially from five high-energy glycine~tRNA molecules. The ε-amino group of diaminopimelate reacts with the activated carboxyl group of glycine-tRNA to form a peptide bond (Figure 17–28). This reaction occurs with a decrease in the number of high-energy bonds, and the reaction is exergonic. The free amino group of the first glycine in peptide linkage reacts with second glycine-tRNA to form the diglycine derivative. This process occurs sequentially until a pentaglycine chain is attached to diaminopimelate. Note that the growing portion of the glycine peptide chain bears a free amino group and the incoming glycine-tRNA bears the activated group. *The direction of peptide chain growth in cell wall biosynthesis is from the carboxyl to amino terminus* and is opposite to that of mRNA-directed peptide biosynthesis.

The uridine nucleotide derivatives are synthesized in the cytosol. The undecaprenol phosphate compounds are synthesized on the interior face of the plasma membrane. The growing peptidoglycan polymer is outside the cell and external to the plasma membrane, and the peptidodisaccharide chain is translocated through the plasma mem-

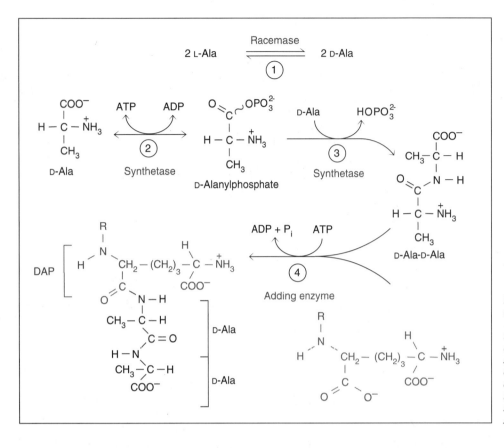

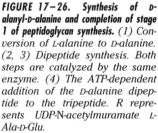

FIGURE 17–26. Synthesis of D-alanyl-D-alanine and completion of stage 1 of peptidoglycan synthesis. (1) Conversion of L-alanine to D-alanine. (2, 3) Dipeptide synthesis. Both steps are catalyzed by the same enzyme. (4) The ATP-dependent addition of the D-alanine dipeptide to the tripeptide. R represents UDP-N-acetylmuramate L-Ala-D-Glu.

brane but tethered to it via the undecaprenol phospholipid. The reaction of the activated peptidodisaccharide with the preformed polymer occurs on the external face of the plasma membrane. Although the structures of the reactants and products are intricate, the addition of the peptidoglycan unit involves the formation and cleavage of only a single bond. The chemistry and bioenergetics involve principles already considered. The free hydroxyl group on C^4 of N-acetylglucosamine on the preformed polymer attacks the glycosyl bond attached to the diphosphate of the activated precursor. The high-energy diphosphate~sugar bond is converted to a low-energy glycosidic bond, and the reaction is exergonic (Figure 17–29). The products include undecaprenol diphosphate and the elongated heteropolymer. Undecaprenol diphosphate undergoes a hydrolysis reaction to form undecaprenol phosphate and P_i. This hydrolysis reaction helps to make the overall process exergonic. Undecaprenol phosphate can participate in another cycle of peptidoglycan biosynthesis (Figure 17–24).

Third Stage: Cross-linking Reaction

The cross-linking reaction occurs in the periplasmic space surrounding the plasma membrane. The reaction that accomplishes the cross-linking process is an isoergonic transpeptidation reaction; one peptide bond replaces a second peptide bond. Transpeptidase, which catalyzes the reaction, dis-

places the terminal D-alanine from the acceptor peptide and forms a covalent bond with the carboxyl group of the peptide side chain (Figure 17–30). The amino group of the donor pentaglycine chain displaces the enzyme to form the covalent peptide bond that cross-links the two peptide chains. The effective concentration of the D-alanine product is low, and the forward reaction is favored.

Let us summarize the bioenergetics and biochemical strategy of peptidoglycan biosynthesis. Glycoside diphosphates contain two energy-rich bonds. The attachment of a diphosphate to the hemiacetal bond of the sugar results in one energy-rich bond, and the simple acid anhydride of the diphosphate is the second high-energy bond (Figure 17–27). The remainder of the diphosphate component is immaterial and can be an ester formed with uridine or undecaprenol. The sugars are activated as the nucleoside diphosphate or the corresponding undecaprenol diphosphate derivatives. The formation of the low-energy glycosidic bonds in the heteropolymer of peptidoglycan occurs with a decrease in the number of high-energy bonds and thus follows familiar bioenergetic principles.

The serial addition of the pentapeptide side chain involves new considerations. Earlier in this chapter we discussed amino acid activation as the aminoacyl adenylate. A second mechanism for activating carboxyl groups involves the formation of the acylphosphate linkage. ATP is the phosphoryl

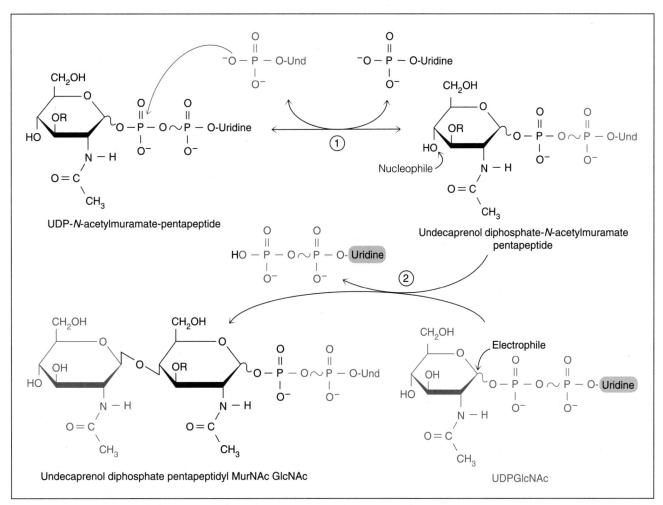

FIGURE 17−27. Synthesis of the disaccharide repeating unit of peptidoglycan. *Und, undecaprenol.*

FIGURE 17−28. Addition of glycine to the diaminopimelate side chain of undecaprenol diphosphate compound.

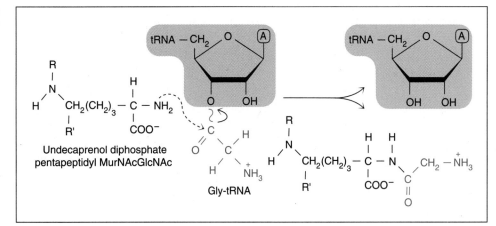

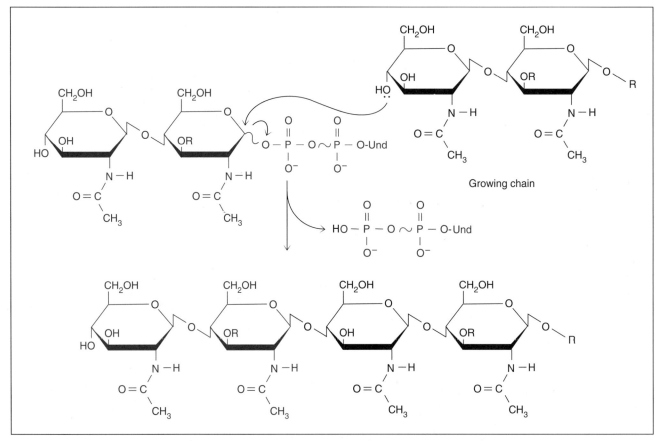

FIGURE 17-29. Addition of the disaccharide-peptide to the growing peptidoglycan chain. *Und, undecaprenol.*

donor to form the energy-rich intermediate. Free amino groups attack the activated acylphosphate to form a new peptide bond. The synthesis of D-alanyl-D-alanine occurs by a similar process.

The bioenergetics of the cross-linking reaction is unusual. The carboxyl group of D-alanine is only modestly activated because it is a low-energy peptide bond. The modestly activated carboxyl group participates in the cross-linking transpeptidation reaction. The exergonic hydrolysis of undecaprenol diphosphate helps make the overall pathway exergonic.

Penicillin and Cephalosporin Action

The transpeptidation reaction has been scrutinized because this is the site of action of the **β-lactam antibiotics** including the penicillins and cephalosporins. The β-lactam ring resembles the D-alanyl-D-alanine peptidyl group attached to other amino acids of the peptidoglycan core. Transpeptidase forms a stable covalent adduct with penicillin that results in the irreversible inactivation of transpeptidase (Figure 17-30).

▶ Gram-positive bacteria are generally more sensitive to penicillin than gram-negative bacteria. The cell wall of gram-negative bacteria prevents the entry of penicillin into the periplasmic space

and thus provides protection. The penicillins are used in the treatment of infections produced by *Streptococcus* species (gram positive), *S. aureus* (gram positive), *Neisseria* species (gram negative), and others. Some bacteria have penicillinase activity that destroys the antibiotic, and this is one mechanism of penicillin resistance.

Cephalosporins are effective against a wide spectrum of bacteria (Table 17-4) and are used for the treatment of infections caused by *Klebsiella, Enterobacter, Proteus,* and *Haemophilus* species, which are all gram-negative bacteria. The sensitivity of gram-negative bacteria to cephalosporins is related in part to the ability of the antibiotic to traverse many gram-negative bacterial cell walls. Cephalosporins can also be used as alternatives in individuals who cannot tolerate penicillins for the treatment of infections produced by *Streptococcus* and *Staphylococcus* species. Cephalosporins lack reliable activity against penicillin-resistant *Streptococcus pneumoniae* or *S. aureus*. This pattern of sensitivity agrees with a similar mechanism of action of the two classes of antibiotics. ◀

SUMMARY

The translation of the nucleic acid alphabet of four letters to the protein alphabet of 20 letters

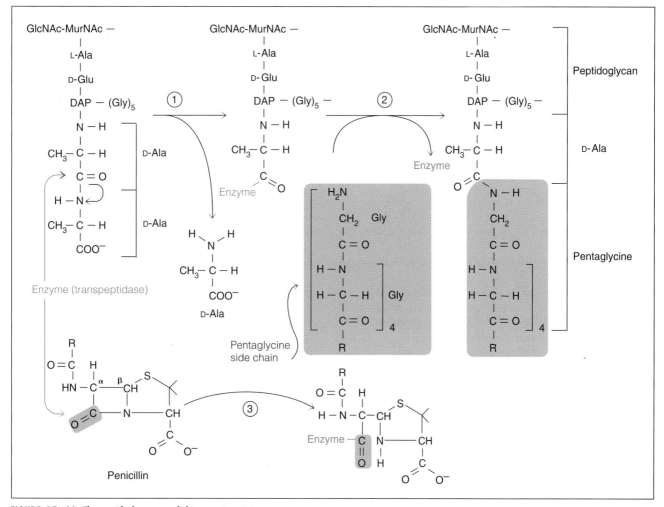

FIGURE 17–30. The peptidoglycan cross-linking reaction. (1) Peptidoglycan transpeptidase (Enzyme) reacts with the carbonyl peptide bond at the end of the pentapeptide chain to form a covalent adduct with the concomitant displacement of the terminal D-alanine. (2) The free amino-terminal group of the pentaglycine chain reacts with the peptidyl-Enzyme to form a new cross-linking peptide bond, and the initial Enzyme is regenerated. (3) The transpeptidase reacts with the lactam group of penicillin to form a stable covalent adduct that is enzymatically inactive.

requires elaborate machinery consisting of more than 150 components. The three classes of RNA involved in the translation process are rRNA, tRNA and mRNA. The rRNA constitutes part of the ribosome that is the subcellular machine where peptide bond formation occurs. The tRNA molecules function as adapters. tRNA interacts specifically with mRNA via antiparallel codon-anticodon interaction. Amino acids, moreover, are covalently attached to their corresponding tRNA and are thereby activated as the energy-rich, special oxygen ester. The nucleotide sequence of mRNA specifies the sequence of the amino acids during the polymerization reactions of protein synthesis.

The triplet genetic code is commaless, nonoverlapping, and degenerate. AUG codes for methionine, the initiating amino acid of protein synthesis. UAG, UAA, and UGA are the standard stop codons. UUU, the first codon determined experimentally, codes for phenylalanine. The third codon position, corresponding to the first position of the anticodon, is the wobble position. This position is associated with nonstandard base pairing. In consequence, some tRNA molecules can recognize two or three codons.

Amino acids are activated as the energy-rich aminoacyl~tRNA. An amino acid-tRNA synthetase catalyzes the addition of an amino acid to its corresponding tRNA. The activation requires ATP and is accompanied by pyrophosphate cleavage. Two high-energy bonds are used to form the single energy-rich bond corresponding to aminoacyl~tRNA. The activated amino acid is linked to the 2'- or 3'-hydroxyl group of adenosine at the 3' end of the tRNA molecule.

N-Formylmethionine-tRNA$_I^{Met}$ is the initiating compound in bacteria. Methionine-tRNA$_I^{Met}$ is the initiating compound in the cytosol of nucleated cells. A different methionine-tRNA^{Met} inserts internal methionines into proteins. Several protein factors assist in the formation of the initiation complex involving the ribosome, mRNA, and the initiating aminoacyl-tRNA$_I^{Met}$.

Bacterial initiation involves the interaction of the

Shine-Dalgarno sequence of rRNA and mRNA. Eukaryotic initiation involves recognition of the cap of mRNA followed by scanning of the message until the first AUG initiation codon is found. The initiator tRNA is placed in the P site of the ribosome.

Two elongation factors are required for polypeptide synthesis. Transfer factors deliver aminoacyl-tRNA to the A site of the ribosome. GTP is hydrolyzed at the end of the process and occurs when the transfer factor is released from the ribosome. Peptide bond formation is catalyzed by the ribosome. The growing polypeptide chain is activated as peptidyl-tRNA as the incoming amino group of the aminoacyl-tRNA condenses with the growing polypeptide. Another elongation factor moves the peptidyl-tRNA mRNA complex to the P site, and GTP is hydrolyzed. When a termination codon is reached, peptidyl-tRNA is hydrolyzed to yield the peptide and tRNA. Bacteria possess three release factors, and eukaryotes possess one. Four high-energy bonds are expended per peptide bond synthesized. Two are required for the activation of each amino acid, the third is expended after the transfer reaction, and the fourth is expended after translocation.

Mitochondrial replication, which is catalyzed by DNA polymerase γ, is bidirectional and asynchronous. Each strand is synthesized continuously (no Okasaki fragments). The genetic code used by the mitochondria differs from the standard genetic code used by the cytosolic ribosomes and bacterial ribosomes. There are at least two codons for all the amino acids plus four termination codons. Wobble is more extensive in mitochondria; uracil in the wobble position of the anticodon position can base-pair with all four bases found in mRNA. Toxicity of chloramphenicol is due to the inhibition of mitochondrial protein synthesis. Oxygen free radicals and peroxide, which are generated in the electron transport chain, damage mitochondrial DNA in an age-dependent process.

The peptidoglycan found in bacteria is composed of N-acetylglucosamine (GlcNAc) and N-acetylmuramate (MurNAc). A tetrapeptide is attached to the carboxyl group of each N-acetylmuramate. In staphylococci, a pentaglycine chain cross-links nearby tetrapeptide chains. The amino acids are added in ATP-requiring reactions; the products are ADP and P_i and the new peptidyl residue. Two D-alanine residues are added as a dipeptide. Pentaglycine addition involves five sequential reactions with glycine-tRNA, the activated form of glycine. The resulting 12-membered derivative condenses with an acceptor peptidoglycan chain in an exergonic process. The final stage of biosynthesis involves a cross-linking reaction in which the amino group of glycine reacts with a peptide bond on an adjacent chain by transpeptidation to produce the cross-linked product. Penicillin inhibits this transpeptidation reaction.

There are two mechanisms of amino acid activation. The most common and predominant method involves the formation first of an aminoacyl adenylate. In mRNA-dependent protein synthesis, the aminoacyl adenylate reacts with tRNA to form aminoacyl-tRNA. In the second method for amino acid activation, ATP reacts with the amino acid carboxyl group with the formation of an acylphosphate and ADP. The acylphosphate reacts with an amino group to form a peptide bond.

SELECTED READINGS

Hershey, J.W.B. Translational control in mammalian cells. Annual Review of Biochemistry 60:717–755, 1991.

Moldave, K. Eukaryotic protein synthesis. Annual Review of Biochemistry 54:1109–1149, 1985.

Nirenberg, M.W., and J.H. Matthaei. The dependence of cell-free protein synthesis in E. coli upon naturally occurring or synthetic polyribonucleotides. Proceedings of the National Academy of Science USA 47:1588–1602, 1961.

Noller, H.F. Ribosomal RNA and translation. Annual Review of Biochemistry 60:191–227, 1991.

Wallace, D.C. Diseases of the mitochondrial DNA. Annual Review of Biochemistry 61:1175–1212, 1992.

Walsh, C.T. Enzymes in the D-alanine branch of bacterial cell wall peptidoglycan assembly. Journal of Biological Chemistry 264:2393–2396, 1989.

Waxman, D.J., and J.L. Strominger. Penicillin-binding proteins and the mechanism of action of β-lactam antibiotics. Annual Review of Biochemistry 52:825–869, 1983.

CHAPTER EIGHTEEN

POSTTRANSLATIONAL

MODIFICATION OF

PROTEINS

You and your family must clearly understand that the great and ultimate healer is always nature itself and that the drug, the physician, and the patient can do no more than assist nature, by providing the very best conditions for your body to defend and heal itself.

—Hans A. Krebs

Newly synthesized proteins often undergo reactions designated as **posttranslational modification** or **processing.** The precise pathway of processing depends upon the identity of the protein and the cell type. The principles of bioenergetics will guide us along the processing pathways. Hydrolytic processing reactions and reactions of organic molecules with molecular oxygen are exergonic. With other modifications, high-energy donors react with acceptor proteins to form a new product. These reactions are also exergonic.

Besides processing reactions that alter the chemical structure of a protein, two other enzyme systems participate in conversion of the newly synthesized polypeptide into its final three-dimensional conformation. **Prolyl isomerase** catalyzes the isoergonic *cis-trans* interconversions of polypeptidic prolines. Proline occurs chiefly as the *trans* isomer in proteins, but it occurs as the *cis* isomer in selected positions. **Chaperones** are proteins that bind to hydrophobic regions of proteins and promote proper folding to the thermodynamically most stable protein conformations. Chaperones require ATP for their activity. The primary structure of a protein determines its secondary, tertiary, and quaternary structures (PRINCIPLE 6 OF BIOCHEMISTRY), but these two enzyme systems accelerate the attainment of equilibrium.

PROTEOLYTIC PROCESSING

A prominent posttranslational processing event involves hydrolytic cleavage. The amino-terminal formyl group of proteins synthesized in bacteria and mitochondria is removed by hydrolysis. The amino-terminal methionine residue that participates in the initiation process is removed from most proteins by a methionine-specific aminopeptidase (Figure 18–1).

Signal Sequences

The cellular location of a protein is determined by its structure. A key choice for the eventual location of a protein is made shortly after synthesis begins. Ribosomes occur in the cytosol, or they are bound to the endoplasmic reticulum membrane. These ribosomes are all the same, and ribosomes are free unless they are directed to the endoplasmic reticulum by a signal sequence in the protein being synthesized. The growing peptide chain is directed into the lumen of the endoplasmic reticulum. Proteins are transported to the Golgi and are sorted for delivery to lysosomes, secretory vesicles, or the plasma membrane. Different pathways, not involving the endoplasmic reticulum and Golgi, are responsible for targeting proteins to the nucleus, mitochondrion, or peroxisome.

Ribosomes bound to the endoplasmic reticulum synthesize proteins that will be secreted from the cell or will be inserted into membranes. These proteins initially contain an amino-terminal **signal sequence** of 15 to 40 amino acid residues. The signal contains at least one positively charged residue and a hydrophobic stretch of 10 to 15 residues. This signal sequence directs the protein to the endoplasmic reticulum in the following fashion. After the initiation of protein synthesis and about 70 elongation reactions, about 30 amino acid residues of the growing polypeptide extend from the ribosome. A **signal recognition particle** (SRP) binds to the signal peptide. The signal recognition particle consists of several proteins and 7SL RNA (an RNA polymerase III transcript consisting of about 300 nucleotides). The signal recognition par-

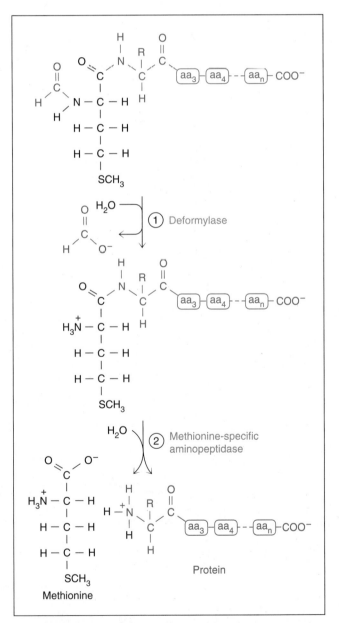

FIGURE 18–1. Hydrolytic protein processing. *aa, Amino acid.*

ticle requires GTP for activity and is a G-protein (guanine nucleotide binding protein). The signal recognition particle interferes with both entry of aminoacyl-tRNA to the A site and peptidyltransferase activity, and protein synthesis is temporarily stalled. The signal recognition particle, nascent polypeptide, and ribosome diffuse to a **signal recognition particle receptor** on the endoplasmic reticulum (Figure 18–2). The ribosome also binds to two integral membrane **ribosome receptors.** GTP, which is bound to SRP, is hydrolyzed to GDP and P_i, and the signal recognition particle is released. Protein synthesis resumes. After transit through the endoplasmic reticulum membrane, a **signal peptidase** catalyzes the exergonic hydrolysis of the signal peptide from the nascent polypeptide chain. Polypeptide chain elongation and release occur as described in Chapter 17.

Proteins that will be secreted from the cell or that will be targeted to lysosomes are translocated entirely into the lumen of the endoplasmic reticulum. Some integral membrane proteins have one membrane-spanning segment, and other proteins have several membrane-spanning segments. The amino and carboxyl termini can be on either side of the membrane, depending upon the protein. A single polypeptide can have several transmembrane segments. Those integral membrane proteins with a single transmembrane segment and a carboxyl terminus that does not cross the membrane have membrane anchor sequences that stop membrane translocation at a defined position in the protein. An example of such a protein is the LDL receptor (Figure 12–28). Other mechanisms generate more complex membrane-protein topologies. Processing of signal peptides also occurs in bacte-

ria. Bacteria, which lack an endoplasmic reticulum, direct proteins with a signal sequence to or through their plasma membrane.

Mitochondrial proteins are synthesized in the cytosol and are imported into the organelle. The **mitochondrial entry sequence,** which can vary from 10 to 70 residues at the amino terminus, consists of a stretch of hydrophobic residues interrupted by multiple serines, threonines, and positively charged residues. Proteins that occur in the outer mitochondrial membrane have the mitochondrial entry sequence, a membrane anchoring sequence, and a second positively charged sequence. These proteins are not cleaved by proteolysis. Matrix proteins, inner membrane proteins, and intermembrane proteins are transported into mitochondria at specialized **adhesion sites** where the inner and outer membranes adhere to one another. Metal-dependent proteases remove the targeting sequence from these imported proteins.

Peroxisomal ketoacyl thiolase and lipid transport protein are synthesized on cytoplasmic ribosomes and undergo amino-terminal proteolytic processing when they are imported into the peroxisome. The prepeptides, which consist of 10 to 25 amino acids, are cleaved to produce the mature protein. In contrast, catalase and several other peroxisomal proteins do not undergo proteolytic processing. The carboxyterminal 30-amino-acid sequence directs these proteins to the peroxisome.

The proteins of the cell nucleus, like mitochondrial and peroxisomal proteins, are synthesized by cytosolic ribosomes. The **nuclear localization sequence** is short, is positively charged, and contains a helix-destabilizing amino acid such as proline or glycine. The localization sequence may

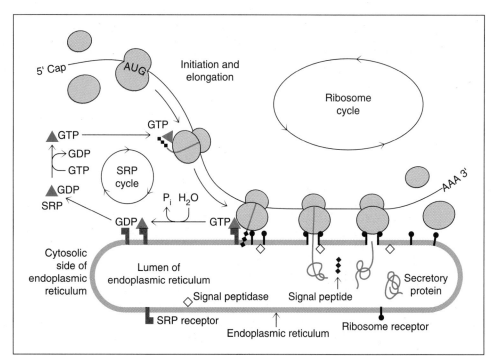

FIGURE 18–2. Role of the signal sequence of a nascent polypeptide in directing a protein to the endoplasmic reticulum. Modified, with permission, from Walter, P., Gilmore, R., and Blobel, G. Protein translocation across the endoplasmic reticulum. Cell 38:5–8, 1984.

occur anywhere in a protein. The length ranges from 6 to 16 residues. There are multiple nuclear localization sequences, and they are not cleaved from their proteins following entry into the nucleus. Thus, these proteins can reenter the nucleus at the end of each mitosis.

Insulin Biosynthesis

Insulin is a hormone synthesized in the β-cells of the pancreas. Insulin requires specific proteolytic processing during the production of functional hormone. Although insulin consists of two polypeptide chains, called A and B, that are linked by two disulfide bonds (Figure 3–17), insulin is first synthesized as a single polypeptide chain called preproinsulin. **Preproinsulin** contains a 24-residue signal peptide attached to an 86-residue **proinsulin** molecule discovered by Donald F. Steiner, a physician and biochemist. Preproinsulin is the translation product of a single mRNA. After the initiation of its synthesis, preproinsulin is directed to the endoplasmic reticulum by the signal sequence. A signal peptidase catalyzes the removal of the signal peptide. The "pre" of preproinsulin and other prepropeptides refers to the polypeptide with the signal sequence. Cysteine residues undergo **protein disulfide isomerase**–catalyzed reactions forming the disulfide bonds of proinsulin.

Proinsulin is converted to insulin by specific proteolytic reactions. Processing enzymes with trypsin-like specificity catalyze the hydrolytic removal of the connecting, or C, peptide (Figure 18–3). The enzymes that catalyze the endoproteolytic cleavage of proinsulin are analogous to bacterial subtilisin (a serine protease). Subtilisin contains the catalytic triad consisting of serine, histidine, and aspartate that is found in chymotrypsin (Figure 4–7). Enzymes that participate in proinsulin processing include **prohormone convertase 2** (PC2) and **prohormone convertase 3/1** (PC3/1). The hydrolytic reactions catalyzed by these enzymes occur on the carboxyterminal side of paired basic residues (for example, Lys-Arg, Arg-Arg). **Carboxypeptidase H,** an enzyme with the specificity of carboxypeptidase B, catalyzes the removal of basic residues from the carboxyl terminus of the prohormone to form the mature protein hormone and connecting peptide. The sites of action of prohormone convertases and the four sites of hydrolysis required for the removal of three arginines and lysine are illustrated in Figure 18–3. Some connecting peptide is release along with insulin from secretory vesicles by exocytosis, but the connecting peptide has no known biological function.

The driving force for the proteolysis processing reactions is the exergonic reaction of hydrolysis (PRINCIPLE 5 OF BIOENERGETICS). Processing of other protein and peptide hormones involves the generation of the active protein from a precursor polypeptide chain. Pathways similar to the pathway described for insulin are used in the biosynthesis of many other peptide hormones such as glucagon and parathyroid hormone. The two-chain structure and connecting peptide of insulin, however, is unusual. Prohormone convertases, which require Ca^{+2} for activity, are expressed only in neuroendocrine cells. These enzymes participate in **regulated secretory pathways.** Secretion occurs in response to a stimulus.

Furin is a processing enzyme that participates in unregulated or **constitutive secretory pathways.** Secretion is continuous and is not regulated by stimuli such as hormones, neurotransmitters, or metabolites. Furin is expressed in high levels in liver and kidney and low levels in neuroendocrine cells. Preferred substrates for furin consist of pep-

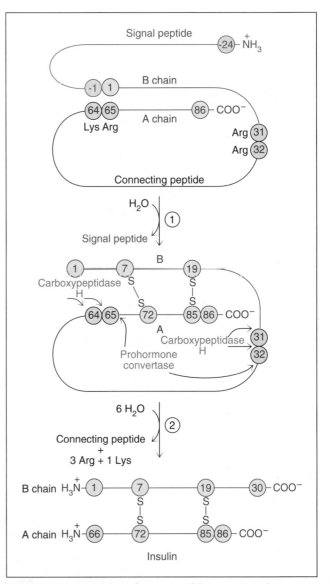

FIGURE 18–3. Posttranslational processing of human preproinsulin. *(1) Hydrolysis of the signal peptide. (2) Hydrolytic cleavage of the connecting peptide to form insulin. The sites for prohormone convertases (PC) are indicated. Additional activity of carboxypeptidase H removes residues 31 and 32 from the insulin precursor and residues 64 and 65 from the connecting peptide precursor.*

tides with tribasic and tetrabasic amino acid sequences at the cleavage sites. In liver, substrates for furin include proalbumin and blood-clotting proteins. The regulated and constitutive secretory pathways involve transport of proteins from the rough endoplasmic reticulum to the Golgi. Proteins are sorted and distributed to the appropriate secretory vesicles, organelles, or plasma membrane (Figure 18–4). A family of about a dozen related G-proteins (GTP-binding proteins) called **Rab** participates in the directionality and control of vesicular transport.

ACYLATION

The amino terminus of many human proteins is blocked by an acetyl group. Following the synthesis of human hypoxanthine-guanine phosphoribosyltransferase, for example, the amino-terminal methionine is removed by hydrolysis, and the remaining amino-terminal alanine becomes acetylated. Acetyl-CoA is the energy-rich donor in these reactions; the amino-terminal amide bond is energy poor, and so the reactions proceed with the liberation of free energy.

$$\text{Acetyl}\sim\text{CoA} + \text{H}_2\text{N-protein} \rightarrow \qquad (18.1)$$
$$\text{Acetyl-NH-protein} + \text{CoA}$$

The amino terminus of a few mammalian proteins is blocked by a 14-carbon myristoyl group. The activated donor of this 14-carbon saturated fatty acyl group is myristoyl-CoA, and the bioenergetics is identical to that described for acetylation. Proteins that bear a myristoyl group include the catalytic subunit of protein kinase A and the gag and pol proteins of HIV-1. Mutation of the amino-terminal glycine of the HIV gag precursor, which abolishes myristoylation, completely disrupts virus assembly.

METHYLATION

Specific lysines in various acceptor proteins undergo *N*-methylation. Monomethyllysine and dimethyllysine occur in cytochrome *c*, and trimethyllysine occurs in calmodulin. The activated methyl donor is energy-rich *S*-adenosylmethionine (Figure 12–4). The *N*-methyl derivatives are energy poor. The methylation reaction proceeds with the loss of one high-energy bond and is exergonic (PRINCIPLE 2 OF BIOENERGETICS).

PROTEIN KINASES AND PHOSPHORYLATION

A common posttranslational modification in animal cells is that of protein phosphorylation. The enzymes that catalyze protein phosphorylation are called **protein kinases.** Based upon the number of protein kinase complementary DNAs discovered thus far, projections suggest that perhaps 1–3% of the human genome consists of protein kinase genes. Based upon an estimate of 100,000 genes, this suggests that there are about 1000–3000 protein kinases. Protein kinases catalyze the following general reaction.

$$\text{ATP} + \text{protein} \rightleftharpoons \text{phosphoprotein} + \text{ADP} \quad (18.2)$$

Protein kinase nomenclature is intricate, in part because of the large number of protein kinases that have been described. Protein kinases are classified by (1) the amino acid phosphorylated, (2) the identity of the protein substrate that is phosphorylated, or (3) the agent that regulates protein kinase activity. Protein phosphorylation catalyzed by protein kinases and dephosphorylation catalyzed by phosphatases provide a mechanism for altering the activity of the substrate protein by a reversible process. The substrates of the protein kinases generally play a rate-limiting and regulatory role in their corresponding metabolic function.

Phosphorylated Amino Acids

Let us consider the nature of the protein side chains that may serve as acceptor substrates for protein kinases. In animal cells, serine is the most commonly phosphorylated amino acid residue of proteins, and threonine is the next most commonly phosphorylated residue. The phenolic group of tyrosine in some proteins can be phosphorylated. The ratio of protein phosphoserine/phosphothreonine/phosphotyrosine in mammalian cells is about 1000/10/1. Although protein phosphotyrosine is a quantitatively minor phosphorylated residue, its importance is profound. The insulin receptor, the epidermal growth factor receptor, and several oncogenes (cancer-causing genes) have protein-tyrosine kinase activity.

Bioenergetics

Let us consider the bioenergetics of phosphorylation of polypeptidic serine or threonine and contrast this with the bioenergetics of phosphorylation of polypeptidic tyrosine. Phosphoserine and phosphothreonine, which are phosphate esters, are energy poor. In contrast, phosphotyrosine is energy rich with a standard free energy of hydrolysis of about -40 kJ mol^{-1}. The phenolic hydroxyl group is modestly acidic with a pK_a of about 10. This phosphate tyrosine adduct may resemble in part a mixed acid anhydride to account for its energy richness.

Phosphorylation of polypeptidic serine or threonine by ATP occurs with the loss of a high-energy bond and is exergonic (Figure 18–5). The specific serine or threonine in a protein that is phosphorylated is determined by the surrounding

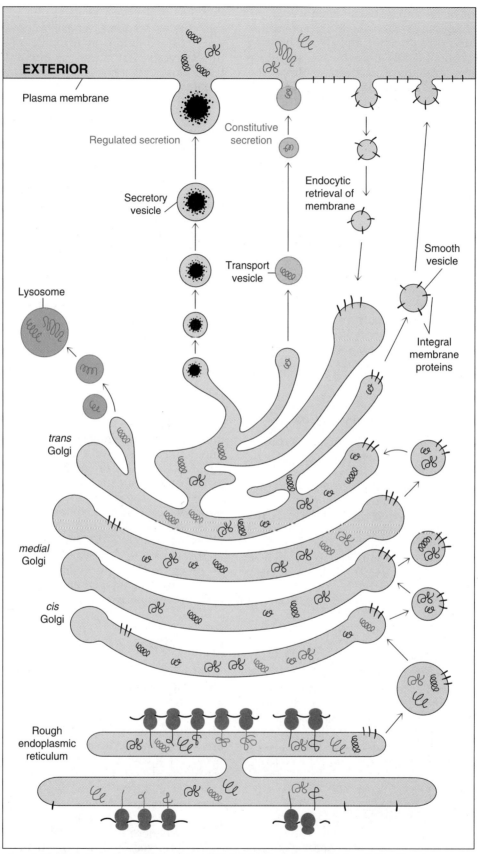

FIGURE 18–4. Overview of the distribution and sorting of proteins synthesized in the rough endoplasmic reticulum. *Proteins are transported from the endoplasmic reticulum to the* cis, medial, *and* trans *Golgi. Sorting occurs in the* trans *Golgi, and proteins are targeted to the regulated or constitutive secretory pathways, membranes, or lysosomes.*

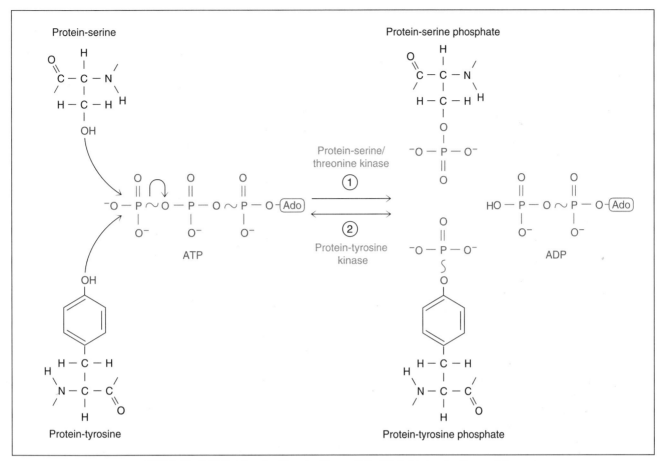

FIGURE 18-5 *(1) Protein-serine/threonine kinase activity. (2) Protein-tyrosine kinase activity.*

amino acid sequence and by aspects of the secondary and tertiary protein structure. The phosphorylation of polypeptidic tyrosine, on the other hand, proceeds without a change in the number of high-energy bonds (Figure 18–5). The reactions are functionally isoergonic (PRINCIPLE 1 OF BIOENERGETICS). The equilibrium constant for these reactions is less than one. Under physiological conditions, phosphorylation is promoted by a high ATP/ADP ratio. Because phosphorylation of protein-tyrosine is bioenergetically less favorable, this may be the reason that phosphotyrosine is the least predominant phosphorylated amino acid residue. The basis for determining substrate specificity for protein-tyrosine kinases depends upon the overall conformation of the protein and aspects of the primary structure surrounding the phosphorylated tyrosine.

Protein phosphorylation is often called a reversible process. With protein serine-threonine kinases, the reaction of phosphoprotein and ADP is endergonic. To reverse the process, phosphoprotein phosphatases (named 1, 2A, 2B, and 2C) catalyze the hydrolysis of the phosphate ester to form phosphate and the protein. Such hydrolytic reactions are exergonic. The phosphate of polypeptidic tyrosine is also removed by hydrolysis. The class of protein phosphatases that catalyze the hydroly-

sis of polypeptidic serine or threonine in animal cells differs from the many protein phosphatases that catalyze the hydrolysis of protein-tyrosine residues. Rare proteins, however, contain both phosphorylated threonine and phosphorylated tyrosine. An enzyme has been described that removes phosphate groups from both threonine and tyrosine. Unusual enzymes, called dual-specificity protein kinases, catalyze the phosphorylation of specific protein-threonine and protein-tyrosine in acceptor substrates.

Regulation

Besides the name of the amino acid of the protein that is phosphorylated, protein kinases are classified by the nature of the protein substrate that is phosphorylated (Table 18–1). Protein kinases are also classified by their regulatory properties. One family of enzymes, called protein kinase A, is activated by cyclic AMP. The phosphorylation and dephosphorylation of fructose-6-phosphate 2-kinase/phosphatase and phosphorylase kinase by protein kinase A is described in Chapter 10. Other regulatory substances include cyclic GMP, calcium/calmodulin, and diglyceride (Table 18–1).

TABLE 18–1. Classes of Protein Serine/Threonine Kinases

Kinase	Alternative Designation	Comments
Based On Second Messenger Activation		
AMP-dependent protein kinase	AMPK	AMP occurs with low energy charge
Calcium/calmodulin-dependent protein kinase	CAM kinase	Consists of types I, II, and III
Cyclic AMP–dependent protein kinase	Protein kinase A	Consists of several isozymes and gene products
Cyclic GMP–dependent protein kinase	Protein kinase G	
Cyclin-dependent protein kinase	CDPK	Consists of a family of enzymes that regulate checkpoints in the cell cycle
Diglyceride-dependent protein kinase	Protein kinase C	Requires calcium; consists of several isozymes
Based On Substrate Specificity		
Glycogen synthase kinase		Consists of a family of enzymes that are inhibitory
Myosin-light-chain kinase	MLC kinase	Activates smooth muscle contraction
Phosphorylase kinase		Contains calmodulin as an integral component (δ-subunit)
Pyruvate dehydrogenase kinase	PDH kinase	Activated by acetyl-CoA, NADH, and ATP; action of PDH kinase is inhibitory
Keto acid dehydrogenase kinase	KAD kinase	Action of kinase is inhibitory

SULFATION

Sulfate, which is covalently attached to tyrosyl hydroxyl groups, occurs in a few mammalian proteins such as fibrinogen (a blood-clotting component). Sulfate occurs in proteins that are secreted from cells. *The universal donor of sulfate (active sulfate) is **3'-phosphoadenosyl-5'-phosphosulfate, or PAPS.*** The metabolism of PAPS is illustrated in Figure 12–12. A sulfotransferase catalyzes the reaction of PAPS and the acceptor protein (Figure 18–6). Because of the very large group transfer potential of PAPS (– 75 kJ/mol), the sulfation reaction is exergonic (the standard free energy of hydrolysis of sulfate esters, however, has not been determined). Unlike protein-phosphate, protein-sulfate apparently does not undergo turnover. Sulfate is added to the protein and remains attached during the lifetime of the protein. This observation suggests that sulfate plays a structural role (sulfate is necessary for the biological activity of the hor-

mone gastrin) and not a regulatory role. Sulfation reactions occur in the Golgi.

GLYCOSYLATION

Overview

Many proteins undergo glycosylation. Most membrane proteins and proteins that are secreted from cells bear carbohydrate. Almost all plasma proteins, for example, are glycoproteins. An important exception is albumin, the predominant plasma protein that is produced by the liver. There are two varieties of glycoproteins in humans: *O*-linked and *N*-linked. **O-linked oligosaccharides** consist of carbohydrate bound via α-linkage to an oxygen derived from a polypeptidic serine or threonine. **N-linked oligosaccharides** consist of carbohydrate bound to the amide group of polypeptidic asparagine via a β-linkage (Figure 18–7). *N*-linked oligo-

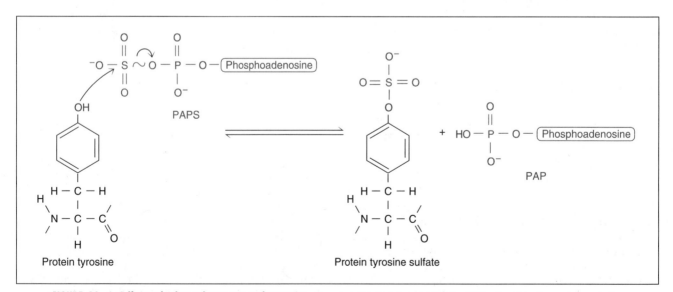

FIGURE 18–6. Sulfation of polypeptidic tyrosine residues. *PAPS, phosphoadenosylphosphosulfate; PAP, phosphoadenosylphosphate.*

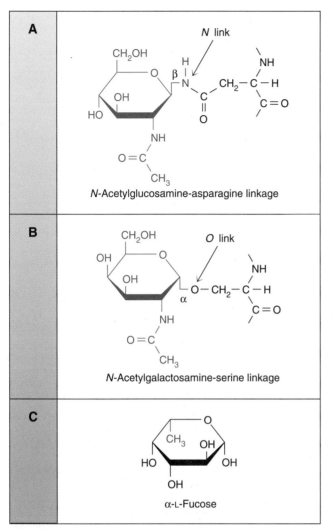

FIGURE 18–7. Selected sugars in glycoproteins. A. N-linked N-acetylglucosamine. B. O-linked N-acetylgalactosamine. C. L-Fucose.

saccharides are composed of three classes: **high mannose, complex,** and **hybrid** (Figure 18–8). A given protein, such as the LDL receptor (Chapter 12), may contain O-linked and N-linked oligosaccharides. Influenza virus protein contains high mannose, complex, and hybrid N-oligosaccharides. All human cells and body fluids contain glycoproteins.

The oligosaccharides stabilize some proteins, and they can aid in protein folding. Carbohydrates are hydrophilic and ensure that a region of a protein in which they occur is not buried in a membrane. Carbohydrates can also participate in molecular targeting and cell-cell recognition.

Some potential glycosylation sites are unoccupied. Pancreatic ribonuclease exists in two forms: RNAse A and B. The primary structure of the proteins is identical. RNAse A is nonglycosylated, and RNAse B contains a single glycosylated site. This site in different RNAse B molecules contains more than six different but related oligosaccharides, and these related glycoproteins are called **glycoforms.**

Nucleotide sugars participate in the synthesis of O-linked and N-linked compounds. Moreover, **dolichol phosphate,** which is a lipid-soluble, membrane-associated glycoside carrier, participates in the synthesis of the N-linked oligosaccharides. Protein glycosylation occurs in the endoplasmic reticulum and Golgi.

Protein glycosylation is a widespread modification. Proteins expressed in bacteria, however, are not glycosylated, because bacteria lack the required metabolic machinery. In humans, a failure to glycosylate normally may yield a nonfunctional protein or one with abnormal properties. Proteins that are not glycosylated are sometimes recognized as abnormal, taken up by the liver, and destroyed. Such observations limit the strategies that can be used in biotechnology for expressing biologically active pharmaceutical proteins. If glycosylation is required for biological activity, then therapeutic proteins must be expressed in yeast or animal cells where processing can occur. Human tissue plasminogen activator and erythropoietin are examples of pharmaceutical glycoproteins that are produced by animal cells in culture. Human insulin and growth hormone, which are not glycoproteins, are pharmaceuticals that are produced by bacteria (*Escherichia coli*).

Monosaccharide Synthesis

The intricate scheme for the synthesis of the activated nucleotide sugars used in the biosynthesis of oligosaccharides found in glycoproteins in humans is illustrated for the interested reader in Figure 18–9. Glucose and galactose are converted to their activated uridine diphosphate derivatives **(UDP-galactose** and **UDP-glucose). UDP-glucuronate** and **UDP-xylose** are formed from UDP-glucose. A single enzyme catalyzes the oxidation of UDP-glucose on C^6 from the alcohol to the carboxylate in two steps. The first reaction (alcohol to aldehyde) is reversible. The second reaction (aldehyde to carboxylate), which involves NAD^+ and water, is irreversible. The ionization of the carboxylic acid to carboxylate contributes to the overall decrease in free energy, forming UDP-glucuronate. UDP-glucuronate undergoes an exergonic decarboxylation reaction to yield carbon dioxide and UDP-xylose.

Fructose 6-phosphate is the precursor of the common amino sugars. The *amino* group is derived from the *amide* group of glutamine. **Glutamine–fructose-6-phosphate amidotransferase** catalyzes the synthesis of glucosamine 6-phosphate (Figure 18–9). The reaction is unidirectional, and part of the energy for the reaction results from the ionization of glutamic acid to glutamate. The amino group is almost always acetylated (common) or sulfated (rare). The respective donors are acetyl-CoA and PAPS. The N-acetyl or N-sulfuryl linkages that result are energy poor, and so the reactions are exergonic and physiologically irreversible.

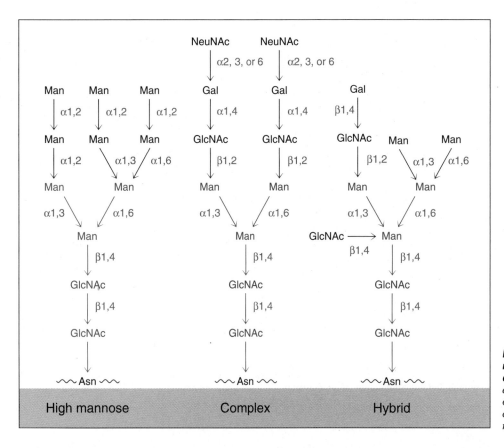

FIGURE 18-8. *Structures of high-mannose, complex, and hybrid N-linked oligosaccharides. There is considerable variability in the structures of these three classes of oligosaccharides, and the examples represent prototypes.*

UDP-*N*-acetylglucosamine and **UDP-*N*-acetylgalactosamine** are activated glycoside donors in biosynthetic reactions.

Fructose 6-phosphate also serves as a precursor of mannose and fucose (Figure 18-9). L-Fucose is L-6-deoxygalactose (Figure 18-7). These compounds are activated as **GDP-mannose** and **GDP-fucose,** the guanosine diphosphate derivatives. **CMP-*N*-acetylneuraminate** (Figure 12-15) is one of the rare examples (if not the only one) of a nucleoside monophosphate that functions as a glycoside donor. It is derived from UDP-*N*-acetylglucosamine (Figure 18-9). The *N*-acetyl derivative of neuraminic acid is called **sialic acid.**

Bioenergetics

About 80 different kinds of glycosidic linkages occur in the complex carbohydrates of humans. This variety stems from the use of many different sugars, the existence of both α- and β-glycosidic linkages, and the use of hydroxyl groups attached to different carbon atoms for chemical bonding. A consideration of the bioenergetics greatly aids in our comprehension and analysis of the biosynthetic processes associated with glycoprotein formation. There are five main sugar donors in the biosynthesis of the oligosaccharides of glycoproteins: **uridine diphosphate sugars** (Chapter 10), **guanosine diphosphate sugars, dolichol diphos-**

phate sugars, dolichol monophosphate sugars, and **CMP-*N*-acetylneuraminate.**

Dolichol phosphate is composed of five-carbon isoprenoid units (Figure 18-10). Dolichol phosphate contains a hydrophobic portion that dissolves in the endoplasmic reticulum membrane and a hydrophilic phosphate ester that participates in reactions on the membrane surface. Glycoside diphosphates contain two high-energy bonds. The nucleoside diphosphate sugars and the dolichol diphosphate sugars are such compounds. The pathway for the biosynthesis of *N*-acetylglucosamine dolichol diphosphate is illustrated in Figure 18-11A. The reactants contain two high-energy bonds, and both are found in UDP-GlcNAc (pronounced "eu dee pee glook nack"). The products also contain two high-energy bonds, and both are found in the *N*-acetylglucosamine dolichol diphosphate as indicated by the squiggles (∼). The overall process is functionally isoergonic. Product removal (conversion of UMP to UDP and UTP) pulls the reaction toward dolichol diphosphate *N*-acetylglucosamine. Dolichol diphosphate sugar derivatives are energy rich and serve as activated donors for biosynthetic reactions in glycoprotein biosynthesis.

Dolichol monophosphate sugars are a second type of dolichol derivative (Figure 18-11B). The standard free energy of hydrolysis of the monophosphate derivatives is not as great as that of the diphosphate derivatives. It is about -20 kJ mol^{-1}

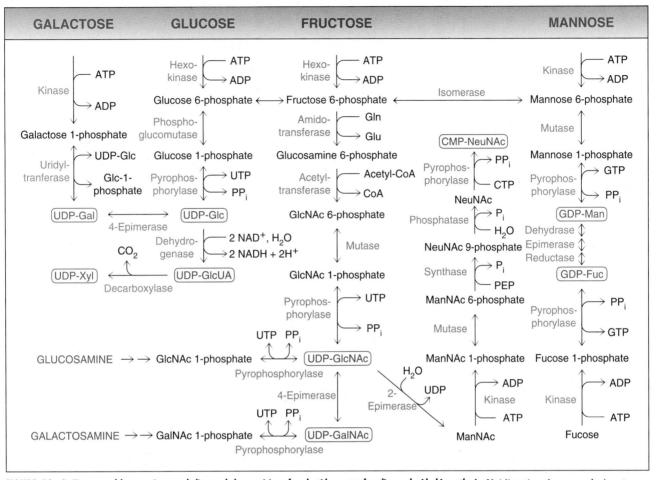

FIGURE 18–9. Hexose and hexosamine metabolism and the provision of nucleotide sugars for oligosaccharide biosynthesis. *Unidirectional arrows designate an exergonic reaction. Bidirectional arrows indicate that a reaction is functionally isoergic. Although the pyrophosphorylase reactions are functionally isoergic, pyrophosphate hydrolysis pulls the reactions in the direction of the nucleotide sugar. Fuc, fucose (L-6-deoxygalactose); Gal, galactose; Glc, glucose; GlcUA, glucuronic acid; GlcNAc, N-acetylglucosamine; NeuNAc, N-acetylneuraminic acid (sialic acid); Man, mannose; ManNAc, N-acetylmannosamine; Xyl, xylose.*

and resembles the standard free energy of hydrolysis of glucose 1-phosphate. The glycosidic bonds of the oligosaccharides exhibit a standard free energy of hydrolysis of about −10 to −20 kJ mol^{-1}. The group transfer potential of the dolichol monophosphate sugars is sufficient to energize oligosaccharide synthesis. A high ratio of dolichol monophosphate sugar to dolichol monophosphate promotes sugar transfer. CMP-*N*-acetylneuraminate is also a glycoside monophosphate. *In glycoprotein biosynthesis, the reactants are more energy rich than*

the products and the reactions are exergonic. In contrast to nucleic acids and proteins, the sequences of oligosaccharides are determined by the specificity of the various glycosyltransferase enzymes and not by a template mechanism. Each glycosidic linkage formed in the biosynthetic process is catalyzed by a different enzyme.

N-Linked Oligosaccharide Synthesis

In the **first stage** of biosynthesis of the oligosaccharide component of a glycoprotein, 14 sugars are attached sequentially to dolichol diphosphate. Nucleoside diphosphate and dolichol monophosphate glycosides are the sugar donors. The oligosaccharide is transferred *en bloc* from the energy-rich dolichol diphosphate to the asparagine amide group in an acceptor protein. In the **second stage,** the oligosaccharide is processed by exergonic hydrolysis reactions and several terminal sugars are removed. In the **third stage,** the oligosaccharide is completed by reactions with several energy-rich nucleoside diphosphate sugars. Although the pro-

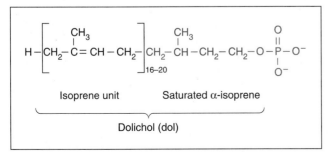

FIGURE 18–10. Dolichol phosphate.

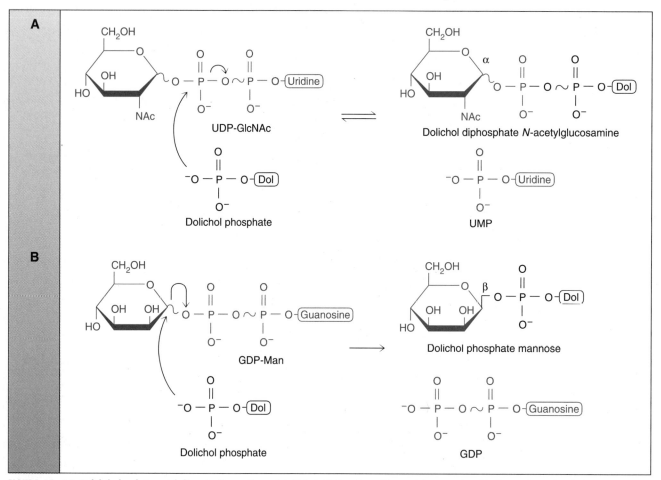

FIGURE 18–11. Dolichol phosphate metabolism. A. *Formation of dolichol diphosphate* N-*acetylglucosamine.* B. *Formation of dolichol phosphate mannose.*

cess is long and complicated, the bioenergetics is straightforward and involves familiar biochemical strategies.

First Stage

The first stage in the biosynthesis of *N*-linked glycoproteins is the formation a 14-membered core saccharide linked to dolichol phosphate. In the first reaction, UDP-GlcNAc donates its *N*-acetylglucosamine 1-phosphoryl group to dolichol phosphate. UMP and dolichol diphosphate *N*-acetylglucosamine are the products (Figure 18–11A). Next, a second molecule of UDP-GlcNAc donates its sugar to the hydroxyl group of C^4 of the previous *N*-acetylglucosamine (Figure 18–12). The glycosidic bond is converted from an energy-rich to an energy-poor linkage, and the process is exergonic (PRINCIPLE 2 OF BIOENERGETICS). This reaction pulls the previous isoergonic reaction in the direction of biosynthesis of the disaccharide derivative. A series of five exergonic reactions with GDP-mannose yields a seven-membered oligosaccharide attached to the dolichol diphosphate (Figure 18–12).

A series of seven condensation reactions occurs with dolichol monophosphate sugars to form the 14-membered oligosaccharide. The synthesis of dolichol monophosphate sugars is driven by exergonic transfers from nucleoside diphosphate sugars. The 14-membered group is then transferred *en bloc* to an acceptor protein with the appropriate primary sequence and three-dimensional conformation (Figure 18–12). The acceptor asparagine is two residues on the carboxyterminal side of serine or threonine. The reaction proceeds with the loss of one high-energy bond and is exergonic. The dolichol diphosphate oligosaccharide has two high-energy bonds; dolichol diphosphate contains one high-energy bond, and the *N*-linked glycoside bond is energy poor. A phosphatase catalyzes the hydrolytic removal of one phosphate to yield dolichol monophosphate in an exergonic process (PRINCIPLE 5 OF BIOENERGETICS). Dolichol monophosphate participates in another series of biosynthetic reactions. Note that CTP is the phosphoryl donor for the phosphorylation of dolichol.

Second Stage

The second stage involves the processing of the protein-bound oligosaccharide. The oligosaccharide, covalently attached to the protein, next un-

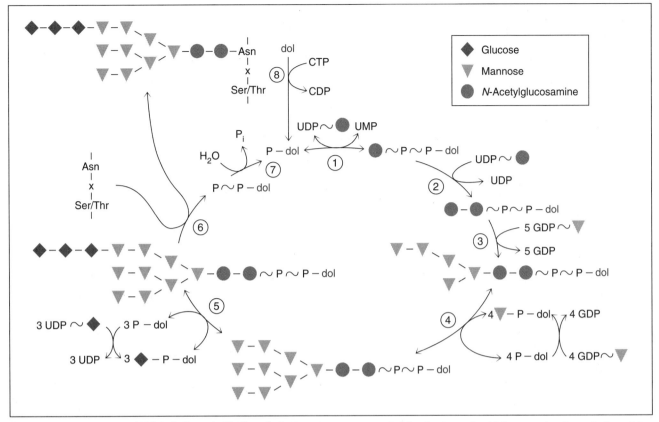

FIGURE 18–12. First stage of N-linked oligosaccharide biosynthesis. *Reactions accompanied by the loss of a high-energy bond are indicated by one-way arrows. Reactions involving low-energy compounds are indicated by two-way arrows.*

dergoes a series of exergonic hydrolysis reactions. One glucosidase catalyzes the hydrolysis of the terminal glucose; another enzyme catalyzes the removal of the second and third glucosyl groups (Figure 18–13). The product is a **high-mannose** N-linked oligosaccharide (Figure 18–8). Processing stops here with HMG-CoA reductase, an enzyme that is normally found in the endoplasmic reticulum, and other high mannose glycoproteins.

Third Stage

Additional steps are required to form N-linked **complex** and **hybrid** oligosaccharides (Figure 18–13). A mannosidase catalyzes the hydrolytic removal of mannose (reaction 3 of Figure 18–13). A second enzyme catalyzes the removal of three additional mannose residues. This creates a substrate for a reaction with energy-rich UDP-GlcNAc. Reaction 5 is followed by two hydrolysis reactions that remove mannose. The nascent glycoprotein then undergoes a series of condensation reactions yielding a complex oligosaccharide (Figure 18–13). The donors include UDP-N-acetylglucosamine, UDP-galactose, and CMP-N-acetylneuraminate. The nucleoside diphosphate sugars possess a high group transfer potential, and the reactions in which these compounds participate are exergonic. The CMP-N-acetylneuraminate possesses a moderate group

transfer potential. The process for the synthesis of the hybrid N-linked oligosaccharides is similar to that outlined for the complex class.

What is the value of synthesizing a core oligosaccharide, transferring it to protein, and then eliminating half the sugar residues? On the one hand, this seems a wasteful process. On the other hand, it provides a mechanism for making the overall pathway very exergonic, and this bioenergetic feature favors the biosynthesis of the final product. François Jacob, a French physician and molecular biologist, stated that evolution is a tinkerer. Perhaps the addition of several residues and their subsequent removal, besides making the process exergonic, amounts to tinkering with one molecule to produce a second with desired properties.

Targeting Enzymes to Lysosomes

The enzymes within the lysosomal compartment of mammalian cells contain N-linked oligosaccharides with terminal **mannose 6-phosphates.** The lysosomal enzymes include specific glycosidases, proteases (cathepsins), and other hydrolytic enzymes (Table 1–1). Mannose 6-phosphate on these enzymes targets them to the lysosomal compartment. Lysosomes contain receptors that recognize mannose 6-phosphate on oligosaccharides. The phosphorylation of mannose occurs by an unusual

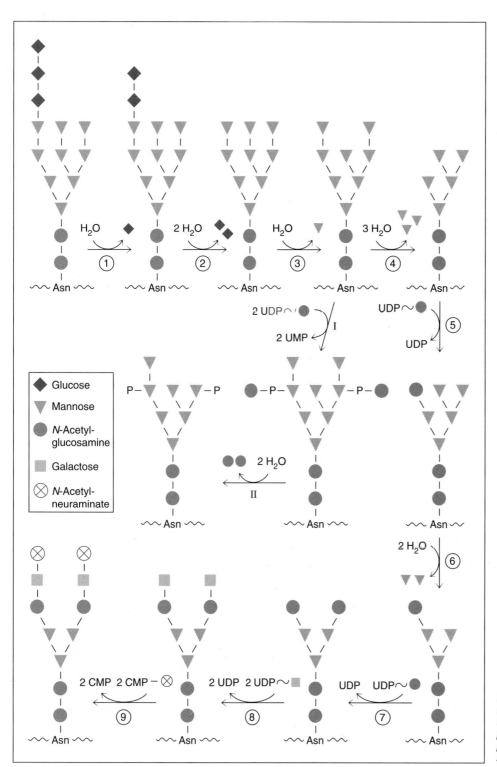

FIGURE 18–13. Second and third stages of N-linked oligosaccharide biosynthesis (1–9). *(I, II) Biosynthetic pathway for the formation of 6-phosphomannosyl residues in lysosomal glycoproteins.*

mechanism. A transferase catalyzes a reaction between UDP-GlcNAc and a terminal mannose residue of the acceptor oligosaccharide (which is, in turn, covalently linked to protein). One product of the reaction is a phosphodiester between *N*-acetylglucosamine and the 6-hydroxyl group of mannose, and the other product is UMP (Figure 18–14). Next, a phosphodiesterase catalyzes the hydrolytic removal of the terminal sugar, leaving the 6-phos-

phomannosyl group linked to the oligosaccharide (Figure 18–13, II). Both reactions are exergonic. The first proceeds with the loss of two high-energy bonds of UDP-GlcNAc, and the second is a hydrolysis reaction. The net result of the two reactions is the phosphorylation of mannose.

Instead of phosphorylating the mannose residue with ATP, an indirect pathway accomplishes this phosphorylation. This indirect process is required

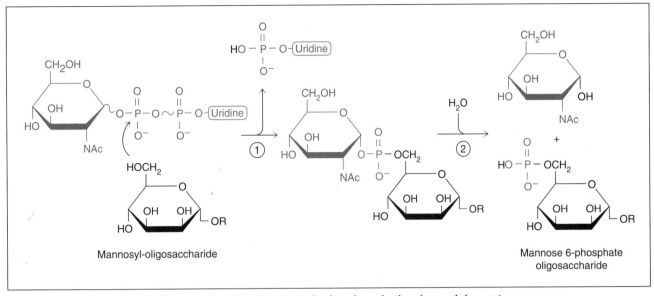

FIGURE 18–14. *Synthesis of mannose 6-phosphate oligosaccharide on lysosomal glycoproteins.*

because the reaction occurs in the Golgi, an organelle lacking ATP. The Golgi contains a translocation system that allows the nucleotide sugars to enter and the spent nucleotides to exit. Up to five phosphomannosyl residues may be found on a lysosomal enzyme, and two such reactions are illustrated in Figure 18–13, I and II. The pathway for the transport of lysosomal proteins from the rough endoplasmic reticulum to the lysosome is illustrated in Figure 18–4. A **mannose 6-phosphate receptor** recycles between the Golgi and lysosome and participates in the translocation of lysosomal enzymes.

▶ Deficiency of *N*-acetylglucosaminyl-1-phosphotransferase produces **I-cell disease.** In I-cell disease, enzymes lacking phosphorylated mannose groups are not properly packaged in the lysosomes. Cells of individuals lacking the transferase contain numerous abnormal lysosomes or *i*nclusions (hence the name I-cell). The inclusion bodies contain numerous substances that are degraded by lysosomes in normal individuals but not in affected individuals. The serum of affected individuals contains high levels of lysosomal enzyme activity. Lysosomal proteins are synthesized, but they leak from the cell because of the inability to transport them to lysosomes. The transferase can be measured for pre- and postnatal diagnosis. The inability to produce functional lysosomes has serious sequelae, and this rare disease affects many organ systems. Affected children die from pneumonia or congestive heart failure at 2–8 years of age. ◀

O-Linked Oligosaccharide Synthesis and ABO Blood Groups

The biosynthesis of *O*-linked oligosaccharides is simpler than that of the *N*-linked variety. We use

blood group antigens of the ABO system to illustrate *O*-linked glycoprotein synthesis. Human blood can be assigned to one of four types by two antigens, A and B, on the surface of erythrocytes and by two corresponding antibodies, anti-A and anti-B, in the plasma. The major phenotypes include O, A, B, and AB. The O blood group substance corresponds to an H antigen. The genotypes and phenotypes are given in Table 18–2.

▶ The primary biomedical importance of ABO blood groups is in blood transfusion and organ transplantation. There are compatible and incompatible combinations of blood from donor to recipient. A compatible combination is one in which the red blood cells of a donor lack an A or a B antigen that corresponds to the antibodies in the recipient's serum. Individuals are transfused with blood of their own ABO group, except in emergencies. In tissue and organ transplantation, ABO compatibility of donor and recipient and human leukocyte antigen (HLA) compatibility are essential to graft survival. ◀ The ABO blood groups are determined by a locus at chromosome 9q34. Three alleles are present at this locus, and they determine the ABO blood group. The antigens are composed of three different antigenic oligosaccharides: type A, type B, and type H (corresponding to the O blood type)

TABLE 18–2. ABO Blood Group Phenotypes and Genotypes

Phenotype	Genotype	Reaction with Anti-A	Reaction with Anti-B	Antibodies in serum Anti-A	Anti-B
O	O/O	–	–	+	+
A	A/A, A/O	+	–	–	+
B	B/B, B/O	–	+	+	–
AB	A/B	+	+	–	–

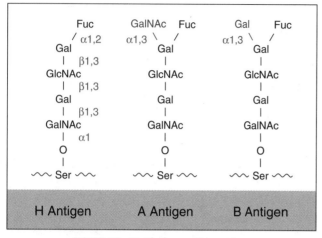

FIGURE 18–15. Blood group glycoproteins.

illustrated in Figure 18–15. These oligosaccharides are linked to glycoproteins that occur in the membranes of many cells and in several secretions (saliva, tears, milk, gastric juice); the oligosaccharide is also attached to ceramide in glycolipids that are present in cell membranes (Figure 12–17).

O-linked oligosaccharide synthesis involves the sequential addition of carbohydrate from nucleotide donors to the protein core and then to *O*-linked sugar residues. A serine or threonine hydroxyl group of the protein serves as the acceptor, and the energy-rich UDP-GalNAc (pronounced "eu dee pee gal nack") as the donor (Figure 18–16). A series of exergonic transferase reactions results in the formation of the H antigen. *O*-linked oligosaccharide synthesis does not involve dolichol or the trimming of sugars from oligosaccharides by hydrolysis.

The antigenic specificity of the blood group substances is established by the terminal sugars. The activity of the final gene product determines whether the oligosaccharide is converted to an A or a B antigen or remains unchanged as an H antigen. The A allele codes for a glycosyltransferase that catalyzes the addition of **N-acetylgalactosamine** from UDP-GalNAc to the H antigen. The B allele codes for a glycosyltransferase that catalyzes the addition of **galactose** from UDP-Gal. There are four nucleotide differences in the genes that encode these two proteins, and the resulting differences in enzyme structure account for the altered substrate specificity.

The O allele has a single base-pair deletion in the coding region. This mutation results in changes in the amino acid sequence following the mutation (a frame-shift mutation) and the introduction of a termination codon close to the site of mutation. The product of this gene is an inactive truncated protein. Because of this mutation, no additional sugars are added to the H antigen. The H antigen occurs normally in all individuals owing to the incomplete reactivity of the H antigen in reactions catalyzed by the A and B gene products.

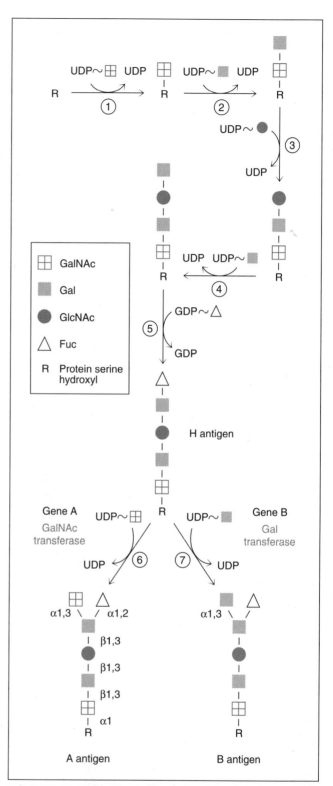

FIGURE 18–16. Pathway for the biosynthesis of the O-linked oligosaccharide of the ABO blood group substances. *Reactions 1–7 are catalyzed by different glycosyltransferases.*

Rh BLOOD GROUPS

▶ The Rh blood group ranks with the ABO blood groups because of its role in hemolytic disease of the newborn (erythroblastosis fetalis).

The name Rh comes from the rhesus monkeys used in the experiments that led to discovery of the system. The population is divided into Rh-positive individuals (homozygotes or heterozygotes) and Rh-negative individuals (homozygotes only). Rh-positive individuals possess the Rh antigen, and Rh-negative individuals lack the antigen. The Rh locus is on chromosome 1. Studies indicate that the Rh system consists of three genetic loci, each with two possible alleles. The antigens have been designated C, c, D, E, and e. No antiserum corresponding to d has been found. Individuals are classified as Rh positive or Rh negative by testing their red cells with anti-D antiserum because significant disease is associated primarily with the D antigen. In contrast to the ABO blood system, where the antigens are oligosaccharides (attached to protein or lipid), the Rh antigens are proteins of molecular mass of 7–10 kDa that are located on the erythrocyte membrane. Rh-negative individuals can form anti-Rh antibodies after exposure to Rh-positive red cells. In pregnant Rh-negative women, the risk of immunization by Rh-positive fetal red blood cells can be minimized by injection of Rh immune globulin postpartum (or during pregnancy, if necessary).

Hemolytic disease of the newborn was once the most common genetic disease. Now it is relatively rare because Rh immune globulin usually prevents its development, a practice introduced in 1968. In this hemolytic disorder, the life span of the fetal blood cells is shortened by the action of antibodies formed by the mother against antigens of the fetus. There are two main types of hemolytic disease of the newborn. One is due to Rh incompatibility, and the second to ABO incompatibility. ABO incompatibility occurs when the mother is type O and the fetus is type A or B. ABO incompatibility, which involves IgG, tends to be mild and requires no treatment. Rh incompatibility, which involves IgM and IgG, can cause severe anemia and hepatosplenomegaly in the fetus and can result in stillbirth. Perinatal survival of this now rare disorder is about 90% with intrauterine transfusion. ◀

PRENYLATION

An important posttranslational modification of proteins involves the addition of the 15-carbon farnesyl group or the 20-carbon geranylgeranyl group to acceptor proteins. The addition of either of the two isoprenoid compounds to proteins is called prenylation. The pathway for farnesyl pyrophosphate synthesis, a part of the cholesterol pathway, is illustrated in Figure 12–21. Geranylgeranyl pyrophosphate is formed in a reaction of farnesyl pyrophosphate with isopentenyl pyrophosphate. Farnesylation and geranylgeranylation reactions are catalyzed by different enzymes: farnesyl-protein transferase and geranylgeranyl-protein transferase. The reactants include farnesyl pyrophosphate or geranylgeranyl pyrophosphate and the specific acceptor protein. The stoichiometries of these two modifications are indicated by the following chemical equations.

$$\text{Farnesyl-PP}_i + \text{HS-acceptor}_f \rightarrow \tag{18.3}$$
$$\text{farnesyl-S-acceptor}_f + \text{PP}_i$$

$$\text{Geranylgeranyl-PP}_i + \text{HS-acceptor}_{gg} \rightarrow \tag{18.4}$$
$$\text{geranylgeranyl-S-acceptor}_{gg} + \text{PP}_i$$

The isoprenoid groups become linked to a polypeptidic cysteine through a thioether (C–S–C) bond. The reactants contain one high-energy bond, and the products also contain one high-energy bond (Figure 18–17). The hydrolysis of pyrophosphate makes the overall process exergonic and pulls the transferase reactions forward.

Although proteins are modified by different isoprenoids (farnesyl versus geranylgeranyl), the nature and sites of prenylation catalyzed by farnesyl-protein transferase and geranylgeranyl protein transferase are the same: the prenyl group is linked through a thioether bond to a cysteine residue initially positioned four amino acids from the carboxyl terminus of the protein. The carboxyterminal amino acid sequence of a protein that is or can be prenylated is called a CAAX box: C refers to cysteine (which forms the thioether with the isoprenoid), A refers to nearly any aliphatic residue (not necessarily alanine), and X refers to the terminal amino acid. Cells contain distinct farnesyl transferase and geranylgeranyl transferase enzymes. The specificity of the two enzymes depends upon the X residue of the CAAX box. Proteins that end with leucine are good substrates for geranylgeranyl-protein transferase, and proteins that end with methionine or serine are good substrates for farnesyl-protein transferase.

Prenylation is the first step in a sequence of posttranslational events. Following prenylation, the distal three amino acids (AAX) are eliminated by proteolysis, an exergonic process. The cysteine carboxyl group is then methylated to form an ester. The activated donor for this methylation reaction is *S*-adenosylmethionine. The resulting methyl ester is low energy in nature. The reaction thus proceeds with the loss of one high-energy bond and is exergonic. The overall pathway for the three modifications of the CAAX box by isoprenylation, proteolysis, and methylation is illustrated in Figure 18–17.

Some nearby cysteine residues may form a covalent thioester bond with palmitate. Palmitoyl-CoA is the activated and high-energy donor. The resulting thioester is high energy in nature, and the reaction is isoergonic. The high ratio of palmitoyl-CoA/CoA promotes the forward reaction. Prenylation, methylation, and palmitoylation render the protein more hydrophobic and enhance interaction with the cell membranes. These reactions occur in the cytosol.

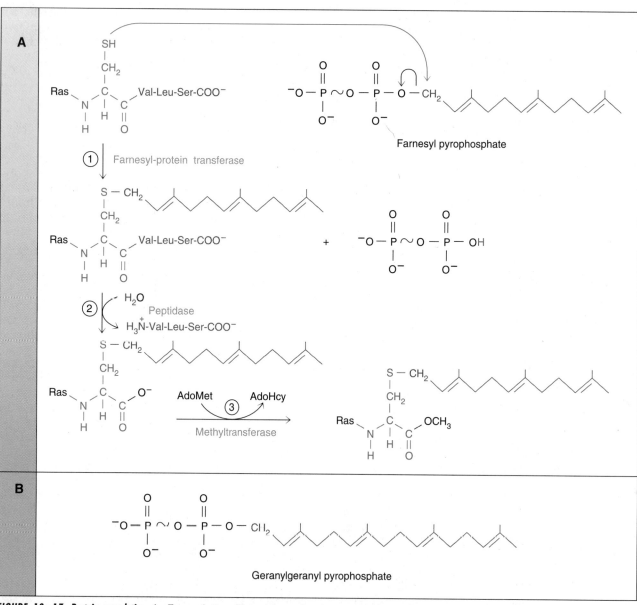

FIGURE 18–17. Protein prenylation. A. *Farnesylation. The pathway for the posttranslational modification of the CAAX box at the carboxyl terminus of polypeptides involves (1) farnesylation, (2) proteolysis, and (3) methylation. B. Geranylgeranyl pyrophosphate. Modification of acceptor proteins by this 20-carbon derivative follows the three steps outlined in part A.*

Protein prenylation is important because of the nature of the acceptors. Protein substrates for farnesylation include the cell-transforming GTP-binding protein called **Ras** and the γ-subunit of **retinal transducin,** a protein that is required for vision. Protein substrates for geranylgeranylation include the γ-subunit of **G-proteins** involved in signal transduction called G_s, G_i, and G_o (Chapter 19). These proteins must be prenylated as a prerequisite for membrane association, which, in turn, is required for activity. The G-proteins play an integral role in controlling the activity of adenylyl cyclase and phospholipase C.

▶ Ras is a protein with GTPase activity that is involved in signal transduction. The *ras* gene undergoes mutations that result in a product lacking GTPase activity that exists in a perpetually acti-

vated state. About 50% of colorectal and 90% of pancreatic carcinomas have *ras* mutations. Such mutant *ras* genes occur in 10–20% of all human cancers. Inhibitors of farnesyl-protein transferase are being sought as potential drugs for the treatment of these malignancies. ◀

VITAMIN C–DEPENDENT MODIFICATIONS

Protein Hydroxylation

The hydroxylation of prolyl and lysyl residues occurs posttranslationally in collagen. **Collagen** is a protein found in bone, muscle, tendons, teeth, skin, blood vessels, and other organs and tissues. *Collagen is the most abundant protein in mammals*

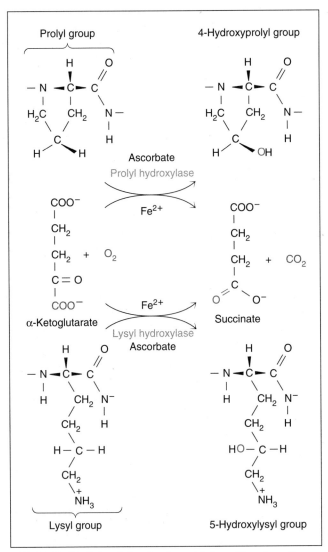

FIGURE 18–18. *Hydroxylation of proline and lysine residues of procollagen.*

and accounts for one-third (by mass) of all protein. Not all prolines or lysines of the collagen molecule are hydroxylated; the sites of hydroxylation are determined by protein conformation, which may delimit potential hydroxylation sites, and by the specificity of the hydroxylating enzymes, which occur in the Golgi. The primary structure of collagen is also important in determining hydroxylation sites catalyzed by **prolyl hydroxylase** because residues only on the amino-terminal side of glycine are hydroxylated. Reactants include oxygen, α-ketoglutarate, and collagen. Products include polypeptidic 4-hydroxyproline, carbon dioxide, and succinate (Figure 18–18). One atom of oxygen forms the 4-hydroxyl group of proline, and the second atom is incorporated into the carboxyl group of succinate. The reactant, α-ketoglutarate, undergoes a decarboxylation reaction.

Both oxidation of the substrate by molecular oxygen (PRINCIPLE 8 OF BIOENERGETICS) and the decarboxylation (PRINCIPLE 6 OF BIOENERGETICS) make this reaction highly exergonic and biochemically irre-

versible. **Ascorbate** keeps the iron of prolyl hydroxylase in the reduced (Fe^{+2}) state. The hydroxylation of lysyl residues on C^5 also occurs in collagen. The process is catalyzed by a distinct **lysyl hydroxylase** that catalyzes a reaction that parallels the one described for proline (Figure 18–18).

▶ Studies indicated that ascorbate promotes tissue repair after surgery, before this role of vitamin C in collagen hydroxylation was discovered. The importance of ascorbate in collagen synthesis provides an explanation for its beneficial effects in wound healing. ◀

Protein Amidation

Several peptide hormones possess an amidated carboxyl terminus. These hormones include oxytocin and vasopressin (hormones of the posterior pituitary gland). The amide group is derived from the amino group of a carboxyterminal glycine. Two enzyme activities, which occur in the Golgi, catalyze the amidation reaction (Figure 18–19). The substrates for the first reaction include peptidylglycine, molecular oxygen, and ascorbate. Copper is a cofactor. The products include the amidated

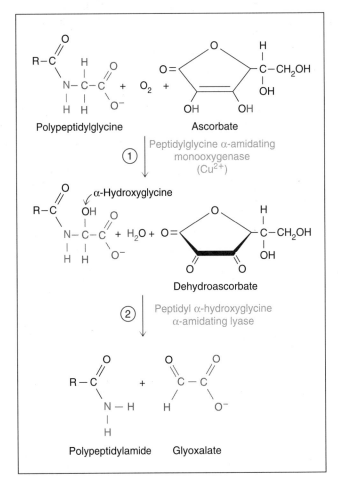

FIGURE 18–19. *The two-step process for amidating the carboxyl terminus of a protein or peptide.*

peptide, glyoxylate (derived from glycine), water, and dehydroascorbate (Figure 18–19). The reaction of organic compounds with molecular oxygen is exergonic (PRINCIPLE 8 OF BIOENERGETICS). In the second step of the process, a lyase catalyzes the cleavage of the nitrogen-carbon bond. The products include the amidated carboxyl group and glyoxylate. Lyase reactions are favored at low concentrations of products, and the concentration of glyoxylate is quite low.

An indirect method achieves this amidation. The glycine residue is genetically encoded, and the α-amidating enzymes convert the amino group of glycine to the amide group at the new carboxyl terminus of the peptide. The reaction is driven by the free energy change of an oxidation-reduction reaction.

VITAMIN K–DEPENDENT CARBOXYLATION

Another posttranslational modification of proteins involves the carboxylation of polypeptidic glutamate residues. The glutamates that are modified are located within the first 40 to 45 amino acids of the amino terminus. In the biotin-dependent carboxylation of pyruvate, acetyl-CoA, and propionyl-CoA, ATP is required to furnish chemical energy. An entirely different strategy is employed to provide the chemical energy for the carboxylation of polypeptidic glutamates. The driving force for these carboxylation reactions is a highly exergonic oxidation-reduction process.

The carboxylation of polypeptidic glutamate requires carbon dioxide, vitamin K, and molecular oxygen and is catalyzed by **vitamin K–dependent carboxylase,** which occurs in the Golgi. The products include protein γ-carboxyglutamate, water, and vitamin K 2,3-epoxide (Figure 18–20). Vitamin K acts as a reducing agent, and the two hydrogen atoms in water are derived from vitamin K. Vitamin K, moreover, reacts with one oxygen atom. The reaction of organic compounds with oxygen is exergonic and irreversible. Another reaction, which is catalyzed by **vitamin K–epoxide reductase,** is required to regenerate vitamin K. During the carboxylation of protein-glutamate, one molecule of oxygen and two molecules of NADPH are consumed, and two molecules of water are formed. This net process, which involves the reduction of oxygen to water, is highly exergonic.

▶ Vitamin K–epoxide reductase is inhibited by dicumarol and warfarin. Dicumarol inhibits the blood-clotting process by inhibiting the carboxylation of several blood-clotting components that are synthesized in liver. When individuals are treated with anticoagulants for venous thrombosis, pulmonary emboli, myocardial infarction, unstable angina, or atrial fibrillation, oral dicumarol often is prescribed. ◀

THYROID HORMONE BIOSYNTHESIS

We noted in Chapter 2 that thyroid hormones are tyrosine derivatives that contain iodine (Figure

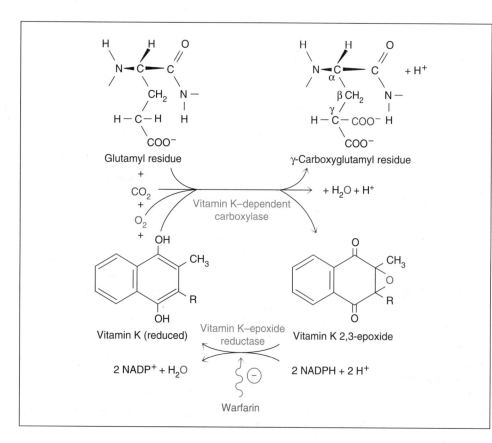

FIGURE 18–20. Formation of γ-carboxyglutamate in proteins by vitamin K–dependent oxidation.

2–2). Tetraiodothyronine (thyroxine, T_4) and triiodothyronine (T_3) are not synthesized by the iodination and coupling of free tyrosine. Rather, these compounds result from the posttranslational processing of thyroglobulin, a thyroid protein. A heme-containing **thyroperoxidase** has two functions in thyroid hormone biosynthesis (Figure 18–21). First, it catalyzes the iodination of tyrosine residues in thyroglobulin. Second, it catalyzes the condensation of two protein iodotyrosine residues to form protein-bound T_4 and T_3 (in a ratio of about 10/1). The hydrogen peroxide required by the thyroperoxidase is generated by NADPH and molecular oxygen. Thyroperoxidase is an integral membrane protein with the active site in the extracellular domain in the thyroid follicle.

Thyroglobulin is a large glycoprotein dimer made up of two polypeptide chains each containing about 2800 amino acids. Coupling of two diiodotyrosine residues yields protein-tetraiodothyronine and protein-dehydroalanine. The coupling of monoiodotyrosine with diiodotyrosine yields protein-linked triiodothyronine. Other tyrosines are iodinated that do not contribute to T_4 or T_3 biosynthesis, and these represent storage forms of iodine. Two to four hormone molecules are derived from each thyroglobulin dimer.

Modified thyroglobulin, which occurs in the thyroid follicle and is extracellular, is the storage form of T_4 and T_3. Thyroglobulin is degraded by cathepsins in lysosomes to produce free amino acids and the active thyroid hormones, T_4 and T_3, and monoiodotyrosine and diiodotyrosine. A deiodinase catalyzes the release of iodide from the

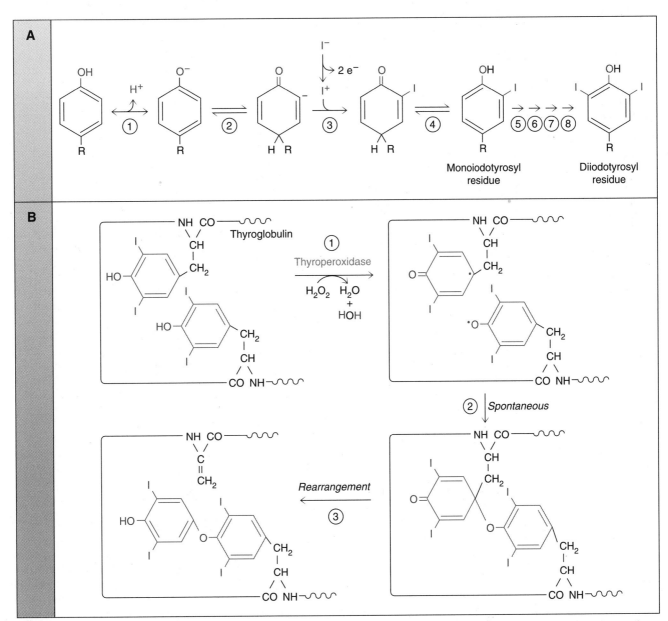

FIGURE 18–21. Thyroid hormone synthesis. A. *Iodination of the tyrosine residues of thyroglobulin.* B. *Coupling of iodinated residues to form thyronine derivatives. Both of these processes are catalyzed by thyroperoxidase.*

monoiodotyrosine and diiodotyrosine compounds. The iodide can be recycled and converted into T_3 and T_4 in subsequent cycles.

The biosynthesis of T_4 and T_3 is bioenergetically expensive. Assuming that four molecules of thyroid hormone are formed from each thyroglobulin dimer, each molecule is derived from a polypeptide with about 1400 amino acids. At four high-energy bonds per peptide bond, a total of 5600 high-energy bonds are required per T_4 molecule. The value of 5600 high-energy bonds for a small molecule may be a record.

DEGRADATION

Ubiquitin-Mediated Degradation

The two main systems for protein degradation are that of the lysosome and the ubiquitin-based system that occurs in the cytosol and nucleus of eukaryotic cells. Ubiquitin is a polypeptide that contains 76 amino acid residues. The protein is abundant and ubiquitous in its distribution (hence its name). Its sequence is highly conserved. The protein found in humans, other vertebrates, and the fruit fly *Drosophila* is identical in primary structure.

Proteins that are selected for degradation by the ubiquitin-dependent pathway are first covalently linked to this protein in an ATP-dependent process. Following ubiquitinylation, a multiprotein complex catalyzes the hydrolysis of the modified target protein. Proteins that are degraded by the ubiquitin system include Myc and Myb (nuclear proteins), p53 (a tumor suppressor protein), and cyclins (proteins involved in cell division).

The attachment of the carboxyl terminus of each ubiquitin molecule to the ϵ-amino group of a lysine residue of the target protein occurs in three stages. These steps resemble the activation of fatty acids as the coenzyme A thioesters (Figure 6–8) and involve the conversion of ATP to AMP and PP_i. First, the carboxyl terminus of ubiquitin is activated as the adenylate, and the activated group forms a thioester with the ubiquitin activating enzyme (E1) as shown in Figure 18–22. The hydrolysis of pyrophosphate, as catalyzed by an independent pyrophosphatase, pulls this reaction forward. Second, ubiquitin is transferred to E2, forming another high-energy thioester bond. E2 is a ubiquitin-carrier protein. A third protein component, E3, catalyzes the formation of a covalent isopeptide bond with the side chain of a lysine residue that occurs in the target protein. This reaction occurs with the loss of a high-energy bond. The resulting bond is called an **isopeptide bond** because it involves the ϵ-amino group of a protein lysine and an amino acid carboxylate; the α-amino group of lysine is in peptide linkage in the target protein. Several ubiquitin molecules can be attached to the target protein by multiple lysine residues by this process.

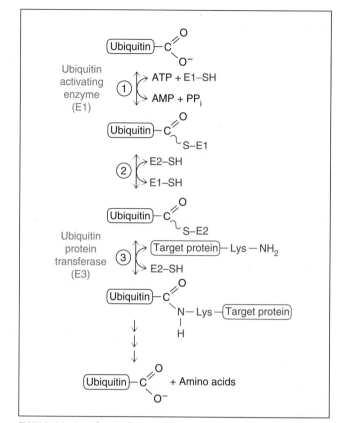

FIGURE 18–22. Ubiquitinylation and hydrolysis of target proteins. *Two-way arrows signify functionally isoergonic processes, and one-way arrows signify exergonic and unidirectional reactions.*

Furthermore, several ubiquitin molecules can be attached to each other via lysine 48 of ubiquitin.

After marking the protein target by ubiquitinylation, a **ubiquitin conjugate–degrading enzyme** catalyzes the hydrolysis of the targeted protein. This degrading enzyme is part of a large multiprotein complex with a molecular mass of greater than one million daltons. The conjugate-degrading enzyme is made up of three conjugate factors (CF1, CF2, and CF3). ATP is required for proteolytic degradation (ATP + H_2O → ADP + P_i). ATP plays a role in promoting the association of the three factors to form the degrading enzyme, and the hydrolysis reactions do not require additional energy. Cells contain **ubiquitin C-terminal hydrolase** activity that catalyzes the hydrolysis of the linkage between the carboxyterminal glycine of ubiquitin and the ϵ-amide group, linking it to target proteins. Free ubiquitin recycles to select other proteins for degradation.

A protein's half-life is partially determined by its amino-terminal residue. Some amino acids stabilize and others destabilize. The amino terminus of proteins influences their interaction with E3 of the ubiquitinylation system. E3 interacts with proteins that begin with basic residues (arginine, histidine, lysine) and with hydrophobic residues (leucine, phenylalanine, tryptophan, and tyrosine). The target proteins of ubiquitinylation are generally short-lived (an hour or less). Some proteins with stabilizing amino-terminal amino acids can have arginine from Arg-tRNA^{Arg} added to their amino terminus posttranslationally. Such proteins become targets for ubiquitinylation.

Lysosomal Degradation

The second process for degrading proteins involves the lysosomes. These organelles contain a variety of proteolytic enzymes called **cathepsins** that catalyze the hydrolysis of proteins. Lysosomes fuse with membrane-enclosed bits of cytoplasm and degrade their contents. Lysosomes also degrade substances that cells take up by endocytosis as described for LDL receptor-mediated endocytosis (Figure 12–29). Turnover of proteins facilitates the regulation of various metabolic pathways.

Lysosomes participate in the physiological involution of the uterus postpartum. The weight of the uterus decreases from 2 kg to about 50 g over the first 9 days postpartum, providing the mother with valuable nutrients. The breakdown of endogenous proteins eliminates abnormal proteins that are produced as the result of deamidation of asparagine or glutamine or other environmental insults.

Almost all short-lived proteins contain one or more sequences of proline (P), glutamate (E), serine (S), and threonine (T), called a **PEST** sequence. Neither the mechanistic basis by which the PEST signal targets proteins for degradation nor the system that recognizes the signal has been identified. Some proteins with the PEST sequence can be degraded by the ubiquitin system (at least *in vitro*), and other PEST proteins cannot. The amino-terminal sequence is not involved in the degradation of most cellular proteins, and our knowledge concerning the mechanisms for selecting proteins for degradation by the ubiquitin pathway, the lysosomal pathway, or other pathways is incomplete.

SUMMARY

A newly synthesized polypeptide often undergoes enzyme-catalyzed chemical reactions designated as posttranslational modification or processing. Such reactions include hydrolytic cleavage of the amino-terminal methionine or a signal peptide. The B chain, connecting peptide, and A chain make up proinsulin. Prohormone convertases catalyze the hydrolytic removal of the connecting peptide at paired basic residues. Carboxypeptidase H catalyzes the removal of the basic residues to yield mature insulin and connecting peptide.

Perhaps 1–3% of the human genome corresponds to genes for protein kinases, the enzymes that catalyze protein phosphorylation. Protein kinases are classified (1) by their substrate, such as pyruvate dehydrogenase kinase; (2) by their activator, such as cyclic AMP and protein kinase A;

and (3) by the protein amino acid that is phosphorylated, such as protein-tyrosine kinase.

There are two varieties of glycoproteins in mammals: O-linked and N-linked, O-linked oligosaccharides consist of carbohydrate bound to an oxygen derived from a polypeptidic serine or threonine. N-linked oligosaccharides consist of carbohydrate bound to the amide group of polypeptidic asparagine. N-linked oligosaccharides are composed of three classes: high mannose, complex, and hybrid.

There are five main sugar donors in the biosynthesis of the oligosaccharides of glycoproteins. These include the uridine diphosphate sugars, guanosine diphosphate sugars, cytidine monophosphate N-acetylneuraminate, dolichol diphosphate sugars, and dolichol monophosphate sugars. The first segment in the synthesis of N-linked oligosaccharides involves the formation of a 14-membered core saccharide linked to dolichol diphosphate. The 14-membered group is transferred *en bloc* to the acceptor protein-asparagine residue. This glycosyltransferase reaction proceeds with the loss of one high-energy bond and is exergonic. The acceptor asparagine is two residues on the carboxylterminal side of serine or threonine. Following a series of hydrolytic reactions that remove several sugar residues, the product is a high-mannose N-linked oligosaccharide. Additional steps are required for the formation of the N-linked complex or hybrid oligosaccharide. The oligosaccharide-protein complex undergoes a series of condensation reactions catalyzed by glycosyltransferases and utilizing nucleotide sugar donors. The nucleoside diphosphate sugars possess a high group transfer potential, and the reactions in which these compounds participate are exergonic. CMP-N-acetylneuraminate and dolichol monophosphate sugars possess a moderate group transfer potential.

O-linked glycosylation occurs by a simpler process. Nucleotide sugars serve as the activated donors. Polypeptidic serine and threonine are the acceptors. Blood group substances include O-linked glycoproteins. The differences in the A, B, and O blood groups are based on the specificity and activity of glycosyltransferases that are encoded by different alleles.

Certain proteins that end with the sequence cysteine–aliphatic residue–aliphatic residue–X (CAAX) often undergo a series of posttranslational modifications that involve farnesylation or geranylgeranylation. The donors for these reactions are farnesyl pyrophosphate and geranylgeranyl pyrophosphate. The donors react with the acceptor polypeptide to form a thioether involving the side chain of cysteine. Next, the terminal three amino acids are removed during an exergonic hydrolysis reaction. Finally, the terminal carboxylate of cysteine reacts with S-adenosylmethionine to form the methyl ester and S-adenosylhomocysteine.

Lysine and proline residues of collagen are hydroxylated by lysyl or prolyl hydroxylases. The reactants include oxygen, α-ketoglutarate, and collagen. The products include the hydroxylated collagen molecule, succinate, and water. Vitamin C plays a role in maintaining ferrous ion of the hydroxylase enzymes in its reduced state. Several proteins and peptides in animal systems contain a carboxyl terminus blocked with an amide group. The amide group is derived from glycine by posttranslational modification. The glycine is originally at the carboxyl terminus. In an exergonic oxidation reaction involving oxygen, the protein, and ascorbate (vitamin C), a peptidyl-α-hydroxylglycine, dehydroascorbate, and water are the products. The peptidyl-α-hydroxylglycine undergoes a lyase cleavage reaction to form the α-amidated peptide and glyoxylate.

A few calcium-binding proteins in animals undergo a vitamin K–dependent carboxylation reaction. The reactants include a protein-glutamate, oxygen, carbon dioxide, and vitamin K. The products include protein γ-carboxyglutamate, water, and vitamin K 2,3-epoxide. The vitamin K epoxide is reconverted to reduced vitamin K by reduction with two moles of NADPH. Reactions with molecular oxygen are exergonic, and this is the bioenergetic basis for three posttranslational reactions (protein hydroxylation, amidation, and carboxylation). Vitamin K–dependent carboxylation, removal of signal peptides, sulfation, glycosylation, collagen proline and lysine hydroxylation, and protein amidation occur in the endoplasmic reticulum and Golgi.

Thyroglobulin is iodinated in a reaction that depends upon the generation of activated iodine intermediates. Cross-linking of mono- and diiodotyrosyl residues in thyroglobulin occurs. Thyroperoxidase plays a role in the iodination reactions and also in the coupling of the protein-monoiodotyrosine and protein-diiodotyrosine. The derivatized thyroglobulin is degraded by hydrolysis in the lysosomes, and free amino acids and T_3 and T_4 are formed.

Some proteins are degraded by lysosomal cathepsins. Others are degraded in the cytosol following their conjugation with ubiquitin. The covalent attachment of ubiquitin is an ATP-dependent process that involves thioester intermediates. The covalent attachment of ubiquitin to target proteins involves the carboxyterminal glycine of the ubiquitin polypeptide with the ϵ-amino group of lysyl residues in the target.

Posttranslational modification of proteins represents a varied group of reactions. Although the details of the reactions are innumerable, the bioenergetics of each of the processing reactions is generally straightforward. The hydrolytic processing reactions are exergonic reactions, a property that underpins the bioenergetics of many posttranslational modifications. Acyl-CoA is the activated donor for exergonic acyltransferase reactions, S-adenosylmethionine is the activated donor for methylation reactions, ATP is the activated donor for phosphorylation reactions, PAPS is the activated donor of sulfate, and nucleoside diphosphate sugars and dolichol diphosphate sugars are the activated donors for glycosylation reactions. Dolichol monophosphate sugars and CMP-N-acetylneuraminate are moderately activated donors for glycosylation reactions.

SELECTED READINGS

Clarke, S. Protein isoprenylation and methylation at carboxy-terminal cysteine residues. Annual Review of Biochemistry 61:355–386, 1992.

Eipper, B.A., D.A. Stoffers, and R.E. Mains. The biosynthesis of neuropeptides: Peptide α-amidation. Annual Review of Neuroscience 15:57–85, 1992.

Hershko, A., and A. Ciechanover. The ubiquitin system for protein degradation. Annual Review of Biochemistry 61: 761–807, 1992.

Kornfeld, R., and S. Kornfeld. Assembly of asparagine-linked oligosaccharides. Annual Review of Biochemistry 54:631–664, 1985.

Kornfeld S. Trafficking of lysosomal enzymes. FASEB Journal 1:462–468, 1987.

Rose, J.K., and R.W. Doms. Regulation of protein export from the endoplasmic reticulum. Annual Review of Cell Biology 4:257–288, 1988.

Scott, J.R. Immunologic disorders in pregnancy. In J.R. Scott, P.J. DiSaia, C.B. Hammond, and W.N. Spellacy (eds.). Danforth's Obstetrics and Gynecology, 6th ed. Philadelphia, J.B. Lippincott, 1990, pp. 461–493.

Steiner, D.F., S.P. Smeekens, S. Ohagi, and S.J. Chan. The new enzymology of precursor processing endoproteases. Journal of Biological Chemistry 267:23435–23438, 1992.

NEUROTRANSMITTERS

Research is the hardest and finest game.
—ERNEST HENRY STARLING

FIRST AND SECOND MESSENGERS

Extracellular signaling molecules are called **first messengers** and include neurotransmitters, hormones, growth factors, and local mediators. The primary function of extracellular signaling molecules is intercellular communication. A **neurotransmitter** is a substance that is secreted by neurons and diffuses a short distance to target cells (Figure 19–1) where it produces a physiological response such as muscle contraction. The neurotransmitter may alter ion flow to produce depolarization or hyperpolarization, or it may alter the metabolism of the target cell. A **hormone** is a substance that is secreted by cells in trace amounts and is transported by the bloodstream to target cells where it regulates metabolism and thereby produces its physiological effects.

Growth factors, cytokines and interleukins (white

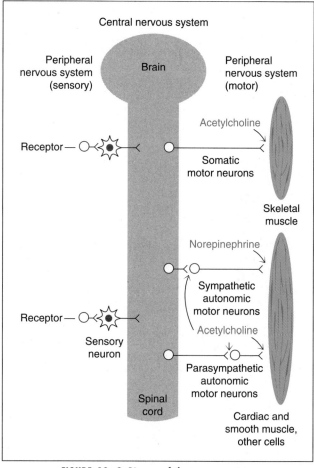

FIGURE 19–2. *Diagram of the nervous system.*

blood cell–signaling molecules), and eicosanoids (Chapter 12) are **local mediators.** These substances are released from cells and act on nearby target cells. Local mediators can be subdivided into autocrine and paracrine groups. **Autocrine** cells release an extracellular signaling molecule that acts on the cell which released the substance. **Paracrine** cells release an extracellular signaling molecule that diffuses to and acts on nearby cells. A cell also may be autocrine (acting on itself) *and* paracrine (acting on adjacent cells). The distinction between hormones, neurotransmitters, growth factors, and local mediators has blurred because these agents act by similar signal-transduction mechanisms. **Signal transduction** is the process by which an extracellular signal alters intracellular events. The effects of hormones and local mediators may last for minutes, hours, or days. Neurotransmitters can alter postsynaptic ion currents in milliseconds. The effects of neurotransmitters, however, can produce recollections that last for decades.

Sensory neurons carry signals into the central nervous system. **Interneurons** carry signals from one cell to another cell within the central nervous system, while **motor neurons** carry signals from the central nervous system (brain and spinal cord)

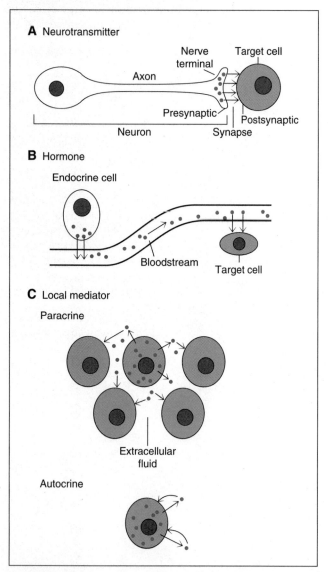

FIGURE 19–1. *Sites of action of neurotransmitters (A), hormones (B), and local mediators (C).*

to target cells outside the nervous system. The two divisions of the motor nervous system are (1) nerves to skeletal muscle and (2) autonomic nerves to smooth and cardiac muscle, endocrine and exocrine glands, and other cells (Figure 19–2).

Some specialized molecules, such as the catecholamines, act as extracellular signaling molecules (Figure 19–3). These substances function as first messenger molecules, and they lack other metabolic roles. Some common metabolites also act as extracellular signaling molecules. Glutamate, for example, is the chief excitatory neurotransmitter in the central nervous system (Table 19–1). Polypeptides also function as neurotransmitters, as hormones, and as growth factors.

The distinction among the endocrine, nervous, autocrine, and paracrine systems is not physiologically or biochemically absolute. The hypothalamus and posterior pituitary gland are neuroendocrine organs that have properties of both nerve and endocrine cells. Many chemical compounds are both hormones (produced by endocrine cells) and neurotransmitters (produced by nerve cells). Norepinephrine, for example, is one of two hormones produced by the adrenal medulla (the other is epinephrine), and norepinephrine is the neurotransmitter of the postganglionic sympathetic nervous system. Norepinephrine and epinephrine function as neurotransmitters in the central nervous system.

All of the extracellular signaling molecules interact with specific recognition proteins called **receptors.** A substance that binds to a protein while not undergoing chemical transformation is called a ligand, and the formation of a ligand-receptor complex is the first step in producing a physiological response, where the first message is the ligand. The ligand-receptor complex initiates the physiological response. Some neurotransmitter receptors form ligand-activated **ion gates.** Following activation, ions flow through these receptors. Some receptors increase the sodium current and depolarize the postsynaptic cell. Other receptors increase the chloride current and hyperpolarize the postsynaptic cell. Some receptors for first messenger molecules are **metabolotropic** and alter the activity of intracellular enzymes and metabolism.

All cells maintain a negative intracellular electromotive force under resting conditions. Moreover, excitable cells such as nerve cells and muscle cells can propagate an electric current called an action potential. When an excitable cell is depolarized, sodium flows into the cells by a voltage-gated sodium channel that is activated by a change in electrical potential across the membrane. The cell is repolarized as potassium flows out of the cell via a voltage-gated potassium channel. Voltage-gated calcium channels occur in nerve and muscle cells. *The movement of calcium into nerve cells triggers release of neurotransmitter by calcium-dependent exocytosis.*

Many extracellular signaling molecules, after interaction with their receptor, cause the generation of cyclic AMP. Epinephrine and glucagon are examples of first messengers that activate adenylyl cyclase. Cyclic AMP is an example of a **second messenger** (the extracellular signaling molecule is the first messenger). Other second messengers include cyclic GMP, calcium, inositol trisphosphate, and diglyceride (Figure 19–4). One of the main functions of second messenger molecules is to activate their cognate protein kinases. Cyclic AMP activates

FIGURE 19–3. Catecholamines.

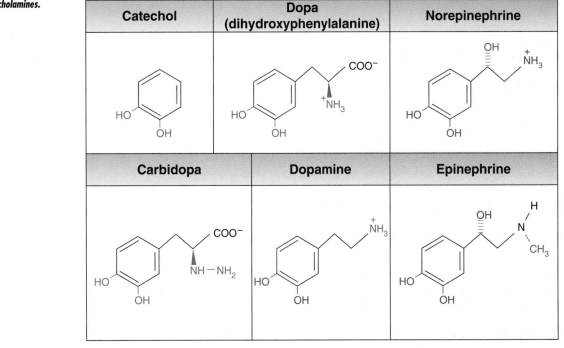

TABLE 19-1. Selected Neurotransmitters

First Message	Origin	Comments
Acetylcholine	Cholinergic neurons	Neurotransmitter at neuromuscular junction and at preganglionic and postganglionic parasympathetic and preganglionic sympathetic nervous system junctions
Dopamine	Dopaminergic neurons	Deficiency in the nigrostriatal tract results in parkinsonism. Excess action in the prefrontal (limbic) cortex produces schizophrenia
Epinephrine	Adrenergic neurons	Role in the regulation of arterial pressure
GABA	GABAergic neurons	γ-Aminobutyric acid; chief inhibitory neurotransmitter in brain
Glycine	Glycinergic neurons	Chief inhibitory neurotransmitter in spinal cord
Glutamate	Glutamatergic neurons	Chief excitatory neurotransmitter in the central nervous system
Histamine	Histaminergic neurons	Possibly functions in sleep-wake cycle
Norepinephrine	Noradrenergic neurons	Neurotransmitter of the postganglionic sympathetic nervous system. Deficiency in brain produces mental depression
Serotonin	Serotonergic neurons	Deficiency in brain produces mental depression. Involved in sleep and arousal

protein kinase A, and cyclic GMP activates protein kinase G. Diglyceride is the second message, which activates protein kinase C (Table 18–1). Calcium in combination with calmodulin activates several protein kinases called calcium/calmodulin protein kinases I, II, and III (based on the order of their discovery).

DOPAMINE, NOREPINEPHRINE, AND EPINEPHRINE

Biosynthesis

The **catecholamines** include dopamine, norepinephrine, and epinephrine (Figure 19–3). There are several neural pathways in the brain that use dopamine as neurotransmitter including the nigrostriatal pathway.

▶ A deficiency of dopamine in the nigrostriatal pathway is associated with Parkinson disease. An excessive action of dopamine in the limbic cortex is associated with schizophrenia. Deficiencies of norepinephrine or serotonin or decreased actions of these substances are associated with mental depression. ◀

The first step in catecholamine synthesis involves a reaction of tyrosine, oxygen, and tetrahydrobiopterin as catalyzed by **tyrosine hydroxylase** (Figure 19–5). L-Dopa (*d*ihydr*o*x*y*phenyl*a*lanine) is one product. The process is analogous to the phenylalanine hydroxylase reaction (Figure 13–23). These reactions, which involve reaction of molecular oxygen with organic molecules, are physiologically irreversible (PRINCIPLE 8 OF BIOENERGETICS). The second step, catalyzed by **aromatic amino acid decarboxylase,** involves the decarboxylation of dopa to produce dopamine. Decarboxylation reactions are exergonic (PRINCIPLE 6 OF BIOENERGETICS), and this reaction is physiologically irreversible. The enzyme, like many others that catalyze decarboxylation reactions, contains pyridoxal phosphate (vitamin B_6) as cofactor. In nerve cells that secrete dopamine as the neurotransmitter, the pathway ends at this step.

The third reaction in the pathway is catalyzed by **dopamine β-hydroxylase.** The reactants include dopamine, oxygen, and ascorbate. Products include norepinephrine, water, and oxidized ascorbate (as a free radical). This oxygenation reaction is physiologically irreversible (PRINCIPLE 8 OF BIOENERGETICS). This process is notable because **vitamin C** is a reactant. The end product in noradrenergic cells is norepinephrine, and the pathway ends here. The fourth reaction in the pathway is catalyzed by **phenylethanolamine *N*-methyltransferase.** Norepi-

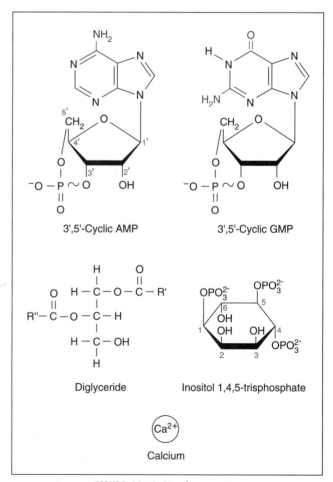

FIGURE 19–4. Second messengers.

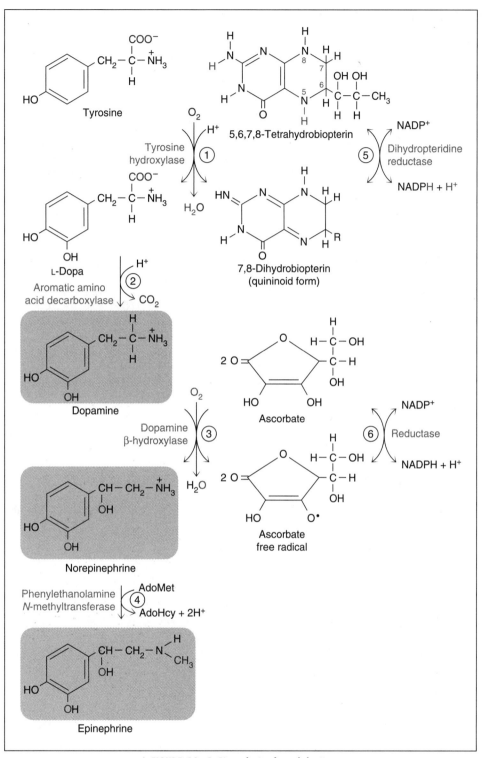

FIGURE 19–5. Biosynthesis of catecholamines.

nephrine and *S*-adenosylmethionine form epineph-rine and *S*-adenosylhomocysteine. *S*-adenosylmethi-onine contains an energy-rich bond, and the prod-ucts are energy poor. The reaction proceeds with the loss of a high-energy bond and is exergonic. Enzymes catalyze the reduction of dihydrobiop-terin and oxidized ascorbate to regenerate sub-strates for the hydroxylase reactions (Figure 19–5).

The rate-limiting step in catecholamine synthesis is catalyzed by tyrosine hydroxylase, the first and committed step in the pathway. The activity of this enzyme is increased by several protein kinases and by induction. Human tyrosine hydroxylase consists of four isoforms that are generated by alternative splicing of hnRNA (Figure 16–22).

Catecholamines are transported into secretory

vesicles by an amine transporter that contains 12 transmembrane segments. *Many transport proteins contain 12 transmembrane segments.* Dopamine β-hydroxylase, moreover, is found in vesicle membranes, and minute amounts of enzyme occur within the vesicles. Influx of calcium at the nerve terminal is prompted by the depolarizing nerve action potential. The catecholamines are released from their neurons by calcium-dependent exocytosis. ATP, chromogranin, and dopamine β-hydroxylase, which occur in the vesicles, are released with the catecholamine. **Chromogranin** is an acidic protein that complexes with positively charged catecholamines. The action of catecholamines is terminated by a sodium-dependent transport protein that removes the catecholamines from the synaptic region and transports them into the cells that released them. These molecules can be transported into vesicles and recycled. Alternatively, they can be metabolized and degraded as described in the next section.

Catabolism

The pathway for the degradation of the catecholamines is intricate because it involves a network of reactions that uses four enzymes. These enzymes include monoamine oxidase (MAO), catechol-*O*-methyltransferase (COMT), aldehyde reductase, and aldehyde oxidase. These enzymes are widely distributed and have their greatest activity in the liver and kidney.

Humans possess two **monoamine oxidases,** called MAO-A and MAO-B, that differ in their substrate specificity and sensitivity to different inhibitors. Both MAO-A and MAO-B, which are located in the outer mitochondrial membrane, catalyze a reaction of the amino group of the catecholamines with water to produce the aldehyde and ammonia (Figure 19–6). The cofactor for these enzymes is FAD. **Clorgyline** is an inhibitor of the A-type enzyme that prefers norepinephrine and serotonin. **Deprenyl** is a selective inhibitor of the B-type enzyme that operates on a broad spectrum of amines including *N*-methylhistamine and dopamine.

Cathechol-*O*-methyltransferase catalyzes the reaction between the energy-rich *S*-adenosylmethionine and catechol derivatives to produce the methylated derivative. The reaction proceeds with the loss of a high-energy bond and is exergonic (Figure 19–6). The aldehyde can be acted upon by **aldehyde dehydrogenase** to produce a carboxylate or by **aldehyde reductase** to produce an alcohol.

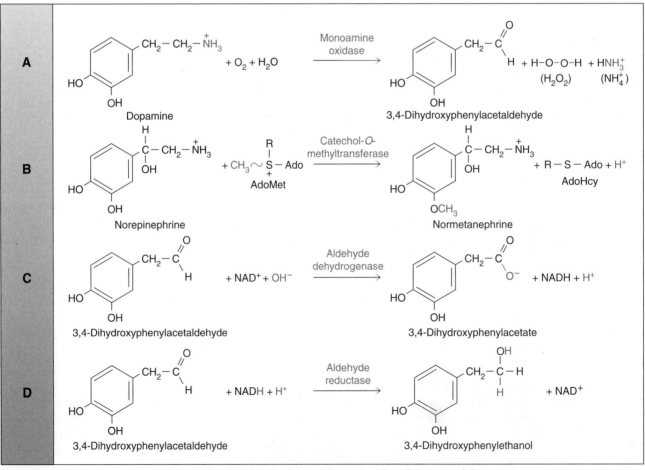

FIGURE 19–6. A through D. The four catabolic reactions of catecholamine metabolism.

End products of catecholamine metabolism are excreted in the urine. The chief metabolite of dopamine is **homovanillate** (HVA), and the chief metabolite of norepinephrine is **vanillylmandelate** (VMA). The metabolism of dopamine and norepinephrine, which is intricate, is driven by exergonic monoamine oxidase and catechol O-methyl transferase reactions. These are illustrated in Figures 19–7 and 19–8 for the interested reader. Only experts know these pathways by rote, and they are provided for reference.

▶ Urinary VMA is commonly measured by the clinical chemistry laboratory as a diagnostic test in individuals who may have a catecholamine-secreting tumor of the adrenal medulla called a pheochromocytoma. 3-Methoxy-4-hydroxyphenylethyleneglycol is a major metabolite of norepinephrine in the brain (but not the periphery). Measurement of this metabolite in cerebrospinal fluid and urine affords an index of norepinephrine metabolism in brain. ◀

Adrenergic Receptors and G-Proteins

Adrenaline was the name of an extract isolated from adrenal glands; such extracts contained both epinephrine and norepinephrine. Adrenergic receptors interact with these compounds. The prefix "nor" means without a chemical group. Norepinephrine lacks the methyl group found in epinephrine (whose structure was determined first). The responses of various tissues to catecholamines were divided into two groups called α and β based upon the potency of a few adrenergic agents. The two types of adrenergic receptors were further subdivided (Table 19–2). Each of the receptors has seven transmembrane segments, and such receptors interact with G-proteins.

Activation of Adenylyl Cyclase

Following the binding of epinephrine to the β-receptor, the receptor undergoes a conformational change that produces activated receptor. The fifth transmembrane segment of the human β_2-**adrenergic** receptor, containing serines 204 and 207, provides the site for binding norepinephrine or epinephrine (Figure 19–9). The third intracellular domain is responsible for activation of adenylyl cyclase. The third and fourth intracellular domains contain serines that are sites for phosphorylation by protein kinase A. The fourth intracellular domain contains phosphorylation sites for β-adrenergic receptor protein kinase. These phosphorylations, which convert the receptor to a less active form, participate in desensitization, making the receptor less responsive to norepinephrine and epinephrine.

The β-adrenergic receptor does not directly interact with and activate adenylyl cyclase. This and other receptors interact with G-proteins that activate or inhibit enzymes or ion channels. **G-proteins** bind and hydrolyze GTP. Several classes of G-proteins have been described. They include $\mathbf{G_s}$ (stimulatory) and $\mathbf{G_i}$ (inhibitory). These proteins regulate adenylyl cyclase. $\mathbf{G_P}$ activates phospholipase C. $\mathbf{G_K}$ and $\mathbf{G_{Ca}}$ regulate potassium and calcium channels, respectively. Other G-proteins ($\mathbf{G_0}$) have been described.

G-proteins consist of three polypeptide subunits named α, β, and γ. Under basal conditions, the α-subunit contains bound GDP and exists in an inactive state (Figure 19–10). Following the interaction of the activated receptor with the G-protein heterotrimer, GTP exchanges with GDP and the αG-GTP dissociates from the $\beta\gamma$-dimer and acts on its target protein. αG-GTP has intrinsic GTPase activity that leads to the formation of the inactive

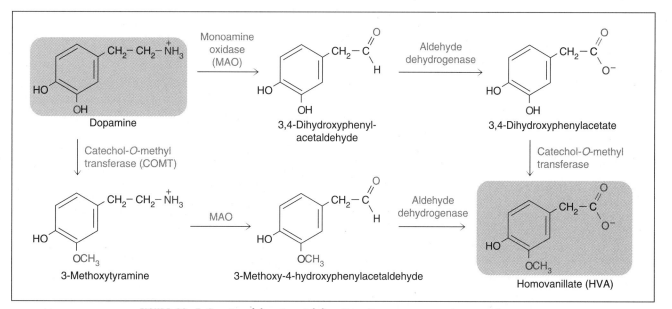

FIGURE 19–7. Overview of dopamine catabolism. *Not all reactants or products are shown.*

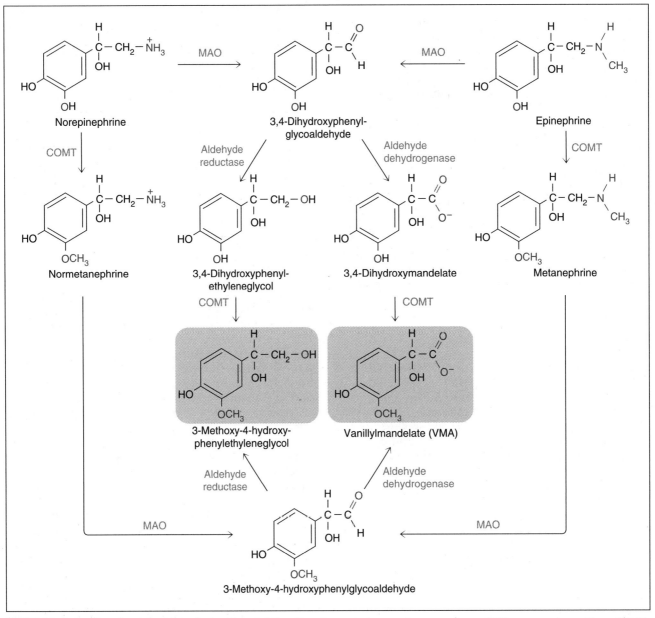

FIGURE 19–8. Overview of norepinephrine and epinephrine metabolism. *Not all reactants or products are shown. MAO, monoamine oxidase; COMT, catechol-O-methyltransferase.*

αG-GDP complex. This complex reassociates with the $\beta\gamma$-dimer to form inactive trimer that can be activated again. *Receptors that activate heterotrimeric G-proteins possess seven transmembrane segments,* including the β-adrenergic receptors.

Activated β-receptors mediate the formation of active αG$_s$-GTP. αG$_s$-GTP interacts with adenylyl cyclase and activates the enzyme (Figure 19–11). Adenylyl cyclase is an integral membrane protein with 12 transmembrane segments. The following steps reverse the activation process. The α-subunit of the G-protein complex possesses GTPase activity that catalyzes the exergonic hydrolysis of bound substrate to GDP and P$_i$. The resulting αG$_s$-GDP complex, which lacks stimulatory activity, reassociates with the $\beta\gamma$-subunit to form the heterotrimer. Adenylyl cyclase assumes its basal state

and activity. A cell may possess receptors for different first messengers that activate adenylyl cyclase, and these receptors interact with the same G$_s$ proteins.

Adenylyl cyclase catalyzes the conversion of ATP to 3',5'-cyclic AMP and pyrophosphate. The number of high-energy bonds in the reactants and products is the same (two), and the reaction is functionally isoergonic (Figure 19–12). Inorganic pyrophosphatase, an independent enzyme, catalyzes the exergonic breakdown of pyrophosphate, pulling the cyclase reaction forward. Phosphodiesterases that catalyze the conversion of cyclic AMP to inactive 5'-AMP are inhibited by high concentrations (millimolar) of caffeine and theophylline. Inactivation of phosphodiesterase leads to an increase in cyclic AMP concentration.

TABLE 19–2.   Classification of Neurotransmitter Receptors

Receptor Type	Function
Acetylcholine	
Muscarinic	
M_1 and M_4	Inhibit adenylyl cyclase; activate potassium channels
M_2 and M_3	Activate phospholipase C
M_5	Inhibits adenylyl cyclase and may couple to phospholipase C
Nicotinic	
N_1	Forms an ion channel at the neuromuscular junction
N_2	Forms an ion channel at autonomic ganglia and in the central nervous system
Adrenergic	
α_1	Activates phospholipase C
α_2	Inhibits adenylyl cyclase
β_1, β_2, and β_3	Activate adenylyl cyclase
Dopamine	
D_{1A} and D_{1B}	Activate adenylyl cyclase
D_{2S} and D_{2L}	Inhibit adenylyl cyclase; open potassium channels
D_3 and D_4	Unknown
GABA	
$GABA_A$	Increases chloride conductance
$GABA_B$	Inhibits adenylyl cyclase and affects calcium and potassium channels via G-protein action
Glutamate	
Glu_1 (NMDA)	Activated by N-methyl-D-aspartate, a synthetic drug; functions as a cation channel and may play a role in memory
Glu_2 (AMPA)	Activated by α-amino-3-hydroxy-5-methyl-4-isoxazole propionate, a synthetic drug; functions as a cation channel and is responsible for most "fast" excitatory neurotransmission in brain and spinal cord
Glu_3 (kainate)	Activated by kainate, a synthetic drug; functions as a cation channel
Glu_4 (ACPD)	Activated by 1-amino-cyclopentane-1,3-dicarboxylate; activates phospholipase C
Glu_5 (AP4)	Activated by phosphonylglutamate; activates cyclic nucleotide phosphodiesterase in retina and hyperpolarizes cells
Histamine	
H_1	Linked to G-protein and phospholipase C activation
H_2	Linked to G-protein and adenylyl cyclase activation; blocked by cimetidine
H_3	Linked to G-protein and calcium and potassium ion fluxes
Opioid	
μ (mu)	Morphine (and β-endorphin) receptor; linked to G_i
δ (delta)	Enkephalin receptor; linked to G_i
κ (kappa)	Dynorphin receptor; linked to G_i
Serotonin	
$5\text{-}HT_{1A}$	Inhibits adenylyl cyclase and opens potassium channels; activates adenylyl cyclase in some cells
$5\text{-}HT_{1B}$	Inhibits adenylyl cyclase
$5\text{-}HT_{1C}$	Activates phospholipase C
$5\text{-}HT_{1D}$	Inhibits adenylyl cyclase
$5\text{-}HT_2$	Activates phospholipase C and closes potassium channels
$5\text{-}HT_3$	Ligand-gated cation channel depolarizes cells
$5\text{-}HT_4$	Activates adenylyl cyclase and closes potassium channels

▶ Theophylline is used in conjunction with β-receptor agonists in the treatment of asthma. These agents produce bronchiolar smooth muscle relaxation by elevating cyclic AMP levels. ◀

Inhibition of Adenylyl Cyclase

The α_2-adrenergic receptor and many other receptors inhibit adenylyl cyclase activity with the assistance of a G-protein (Table 19–2). The activated receptors bind to G_i proteins (where i designates inhibitory). This class of G-proteins also consists of three polypeptide subunits named α, β, and γ. The α-subunit of G_s, but not the $\beta\gamma$-subunit complex, differs from that found in G_s. The activated α_2-adrenergic receptor promotes the exchange of GTP for GDP, and the αG_i-GTP subunit dissociates from the $\beta\gamma$-dimer. αG_i-GTP binds to and decreases adenylyl cyclase activity. The inhibitory process is terminated by GTPase activity of αG_i. αG_i-GDP binds to free $\beta\gamma$-dimers, and the trimer complex is inactive.

Activation of Phospholipase C

The α_1-adrenergic receptor activates phospholipase C via a G-protein that is called G_p. $\mathbf{G_P}$ also consists of three subunits ($\alpha\beta\gamma$). The mechanism of action of this G-protein parallels that of G_s. **Phospholipase C** catalyzes the hydrolysis of phosphatidylinositol 4,5-bisphosphate to form inositol 1,4,5-trisphosphate and diglyceride (Figures 12–6 and 12–7). **Inositol 1,4,5-trisphosphate** is a second messenger that interacts with a receptor on the endoplasmic reticulum and promotes calcium transport into the cytosol (Figure 19–13). Calcium can then effect varied cellular responses. **Diglyceride** is a second messenger that remains membrane bound and activates protein kinase C. Although protein kinase C requires phosphatidylserine and calcium for the full expression of activity, these agents are present at effective levels under basal conditions. Regulation of protein kinase C is thus under the regulatory control of diglyceride.

Cholera and Pertussis Toxins

▶ The major symptom of cholera, an intestinal disorder caused by the gram-negative *Vibrio cholerae* (Table 1–3), is massive diarrhea, which can cause death by dehydration. Although rare in the United States, cholera is responsible for about 750,000 deaths annually in the world. The bacteria colonize the intestine and produce a toxin that causes loss of more than one liter of fluid (in adults) per hour. Treatment with intravenous fluids for a few days and prevention of dehydration constitute effective treatment while an immune response is initiated.

Diarrhea and fluid loss result from the action of cholera toxin. Cholera toxin is an 87-kDa protein that is made of A and B subunits (AB_5). After cholera toxin binds to ganglioside G_{M1}, A subunits are taken into cells by endocytosis. The A subunit is proteolyzed to form two fragments, A_1 (22 kDa) and A_2 (5 kDa). A_1 catalyzes the ADP-ribosylation

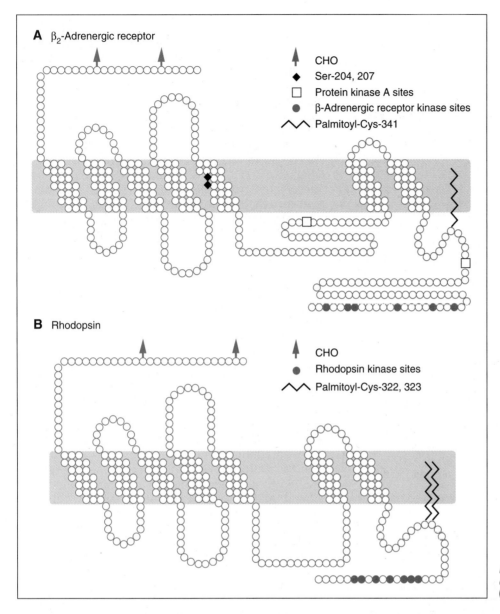

A β₂-Adrenergic receptor

↑ CHO
◆ Ser-204, 207
☐ Protein kinase A sites
● β-Adrenergic receptor kinase sites
〜 Palmitoyl-Cys-341

B Rhodopsin

↑ CHO
● Rhodopsin kinase sites
〜 Palmitoyl-Cys-322, 323

FIGURE 19-9. Topology of the β-adrenergic receptor (A) and rhodopsin (B).

of a specific arginine residue of αG_s proteins (Figure 19–14). This modification inhibits the GTPase activity of αG_s. As a result of this inhibition, αG_s remains in its activated state and continuously stimulates adenylyl cyclase activity and elevates

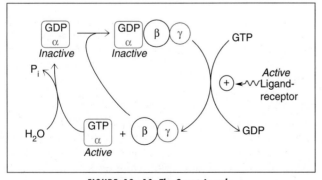

FIGURE 19-10. The G-protein cycle.

cellular cyclic AMP levels. Elevated cyclic AMP in intestinal cells results in the secretion of large quantities of fluid.

Bordetella pertussis is a gram-negative bacterium that produces a toxin which results in whooping cough (pertussis). The disease is rare in the United States because of the effectiveness of pertussis vaccine, a component of the triad of diphtheria, pertussis, and tetanus (DPT) commonly used for childhood immunization. *Bordetella pertussis* multiplies in the epithelium of the respiratory tract and produces pertussis toxin and other biologically active factors that are responsible for the disease. Pertussis toxin is a heterodimeric protein like cholera toxin. Pertussis toxin catalyzes the ADP-ribosylation of a specific cysteine in αG_i (Figure 19–14). ADP-ribosylated αG_i cannot exchange GTP for bound GDP, and αG_i remains in a permanently inactivated state. Cells thus lose the capability of inhibiting adenylyl cyclase under physiological

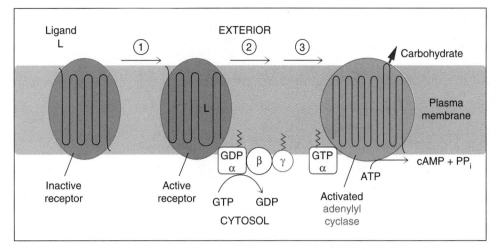

FIGURE 19–11. Regulation of adenylyl cyclase. *(1) Binding of the ligand to the receptor. (2) The activated receptor promotes exchange of GTP for GDP. (3) α-GTP activates adenylyl cyclase.*

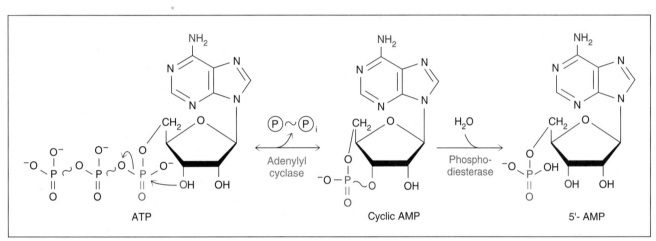

FIGURE 19–12. Cyclic AMP metabolism.

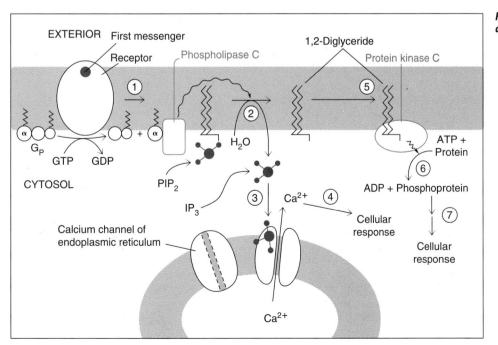

FIGURE 19–13. The phospholipase C and inositol lipid signaling pathway.

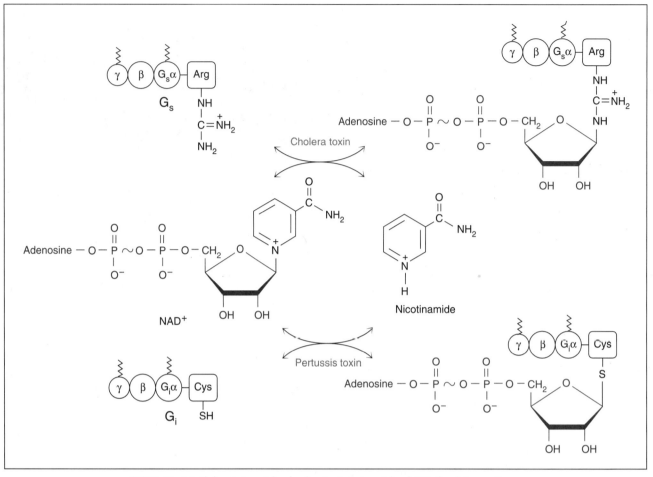

FIGURE 19–14. *Cholera toxin–catalyzed and pertussis toxin–catalyzed ADP-ribosylation reactions.*

conditions, and signal transduction is impaired. The disease is treated symptomatically and with erythromycin, to which *Bordetella pertussis* is sensitive. A third toxin that catalyzes the ADP-ribosylation of a G-protein is that of diphtheria. Diphtheria toxin catalyzes the ADP-ribosylation of EF-2, a G-protein that participates in translocation during mRNA-dependent protein synthesis (Figure 17–17). ◄

Dopamine Receptors

Dopamine receptors were initially classified as D_1 or D_2 according to whether they produced stimulation or inhibition of adenylyl cyclase, respectively. cDNA cloning experiments indicate the existence of additional dopamine receptors (Table 19–2). The genes corresponding to the various classes of dopamine receptor are located on five different chromosomes.

► Studies on the association of these varieties of receptor and various mental illnesses are in progress. Most drugs that are used in the treatment of schizophrenia, such as chlorpromazine, function as D_2-receptor antagonists. Amphetamine (a substance that increases synaptic dopamine concen-

trations) and bromocriptine (a dopamine agonist) produce experimental psychoses. ◄

Parkinson Disease

► This disorder, which is characterized by a shuffling gait or walk, tremor, rigidity, and weakness, is due to the degeneration of neurons of the dopaminergic nigrostriatal pathway in the brain. A 70% decrease of dopamine occurs prior to the onset of symptoms. Affected individuals are often treated early in the course of the disease with an MAO-B inhibitor such as deprenyl. Inhibition of MAO-B, which catalyzes the degradation of dopamine (and other biogenic amines), increases the effective concentrations of dopamine.

Parkinson disease is also treated with oral **L-dopa** administration. This substance is transported across the blood-brain barrier and serves as a substrate for dopamine biosynthesis in striatal cells. Because L-dopa is degraded in reactions catalyzed by aromatic amino acid decarboxylase outside the brain, carbidopa (Figure 19–3) is given concurrently with L-dopa. The hydrazine side chain ($-NHNH_2$) of carbidopa forms a covalent inhibitory complex with the pyridoxal phosphate of this decarboxylase. Carbidopa does not cross the blood-brain barrier and hence does not affect the conversion of dopa to dopamine in the brain. Although dopa is effective in early stages of the disease, the treatment becomes refractory or ineffective, and additional therapies are being sought. ◄

The **blood-brain barrier** was discovered when dyes were injected intravenously into animals to measure the extracellular space. These dyes crossed the capillary beds outside the nervous system, but they did not leave the circulation to enter the extracellular space of the brain. This finding led to the concept of the blood-brain barrier. Because of this barrier, hormones in the circulation do not affect the brain, and neurotransmitters released in the brain do not affect the remainder of the body.

ACETYLCHOLINE

Metabolism

Acetylcholine is formed in one step from acetyl-CoA (active acetate) and choline in a reaction catalyzed by **choline acetyltransferase** (Figure 19–15). Acetyl-CoA is an energy-rich compound, and acetylcholine is an energy-poor compound. The reaction proceeds with the loss of a high-energy bond and is exergonic. Following its secretion from nerve cells and interaction with its receptor to produce its physiological response, acetylcholine is inactivated by an exergonic hydrolysis reaction. The hydrolytic enzyme is **acetylcholinesterase.** Acetylcholinesterase, which is bound to plasma membranes, contains a serine group in its active site and is subject to inhibition by diisopropylfluorophosphate (Figure 19–16). **Diisopropylfluorophosphate** is an example of an irreversible enzyme inhibitor (Chapter 4). Diisopropylfluorophosphate and related agents have been used as insecticides and as agents in chemical warfare.

► There is evidence for a functional deficiency of acetylcholine in the brains of individuals with Alzheimer disease. This disease is characterized by neurofibrillary plaques and tangles observed histologically in brain. Tacrine, a long-acting acetylcholinesterase inhibitor, has been introduced for the treatment of Alzheimer disease. Only some affected individuals have a beneficial response, and more work is required to discover the pathogenesis of

this disorder and to design more effective treatments. ◄

Acetylcholine Receptors

Muscarinic Receptors

Acetylcholine receptors are divided into two major classes called nicotinic and muscarinic (Table 19–2). Muscarinic acetylcholine receptors, which are stimulated by a plant alkaloid called muscarine (Figure 19–17), interact with G-proteins. Responses to the muscarinic receptor can be excitatory or inhibitory and vary with cell type. Activation of the muscarinic receptor on the smooth muscle of the gut causes contraction and peristalsis. Activation of the muscarinic receptor on the heart decreases the heart rate (producing bradycardia). Like catecholamine receptors, acetylcholine muscarinic receptors trigger G-protein–linked changes in the metabolism of second messengers such as cyclic AMP, calcium, and diglyceride. The muscarinic receptor activates G_i but not G_s. As a result, activation of the muscarinic receptor can decrease cyclic AMP concentrations in target cells (Table 19–2).

► **Atropine** is a muscarinic receptor antagonist. Atropine is a widely used drug, especially in anesthesiology, because it diminishes pulmonary secretions. Muscarinic receptors are the effectors for acetylcholine at postganglionic parasympathetic cells. Poisoning with anticholinesterase drugs such as diisopropylfluorophosphate is treated with atropine injections. ◄

Nicotinic Receptors

Nicotinic acetylcholine receptors, which are stimulated by the plant alkaloid **nicotine,** function as ligand-activated ion channels. Acetylcholine is the endogenous ligand. Nicotinic receptors, which form sodium channels, promote depolarization and excitation of postsynaptic cells. *The nicotinic receptor contains several subunits each of which has four transmembrane segments, and four transmembrane segments are characteristic of all the ligand-activated ion channel receptors* that have been described thus far. The second transmembrane segments (M_2) form the ion channels. A diagram of the structure of the neuromuscular N_1 receptor is

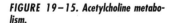

FIGURE 19–15. Acetylcholine metabolism.

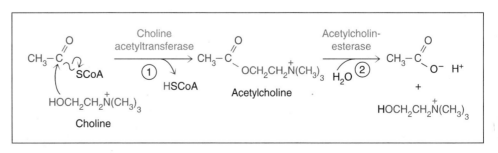

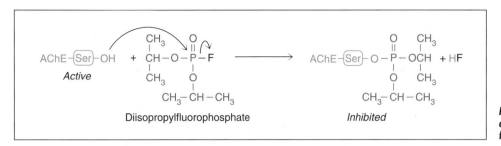

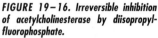

FIGURE 19–16. Irreversible inhibition of acetylcholinesterase by diisopropylfluorophosphate.

given in Figure 19–18. The nicotinic receptor at the neuromuscular junction consists of a pentamer composed of four different kinds of subunits. The embryonic form consists of $\alpha_2\beta\gamma\delta$-subunits, and the adult form consists of $\alpha_2\beta\epsilon\delta$-subunits. Each α-subunit binds acetylcholine, and receptor activation requires that both α-subunit sites be occupied. N_1 receptors (but not N_2 receptors) are inhibited by **d-tubocurarine,** the active substance in the poison called curare. Both muscarinic and nicotinic receptors are widespread in the brain.

▶ **Succinylcholine** is an acetylcholine analogue that is widely used as a muscle relaxant by anesthesiologists during surgery. The agent causes the muscle to remain in a depolarized state that is incapable of contracting. Succinylcholine and d-tubocurarine produce flaccid muscle paralysis by this same mechanism. Some individuals are very sensitive to the action of succinylcholine because they lack a circulating form of acetylcholinesterase called **pseudocholinesterase.** Owing to this increased sensitivity, succinylcholine produces paralysis of the diaphragm. Respiration must be maintained mechanically for several minutes to sustain life while the succinylcholine is slowly hydrolyzed by nonspecific esterases. The physiological role of pseudocholinesterase is a mystery, and individuals lacking it suffer no ill effects. ◀

Myasthenia Gravis

▶ This serious (grave) human disorder is characterized by skeletal muscle weakness. It is due to the development of antibodies (IgG) against the nicotinic receptor at the neuromuscular junction, and it is an example of an autoimmune disease. The receptor deficiency results from the degradation of the neuromuscular junction, followed by internalization of the receptor-antibody complex and destruction of the receptor. Myasthenia gravis is more common in women than in men. The disease often affects the ocular muscles and can lead to diplopia (double vision). The disorder is treated with acetylcholinesterase inhibitors such as pyridostigmine bromide (to prolong the response of existing receptor to acetylcholine), corticosteroids (to diminish the autoimmune response), and plasmapheresis (to remove the antibodies from blood plasma). ◀

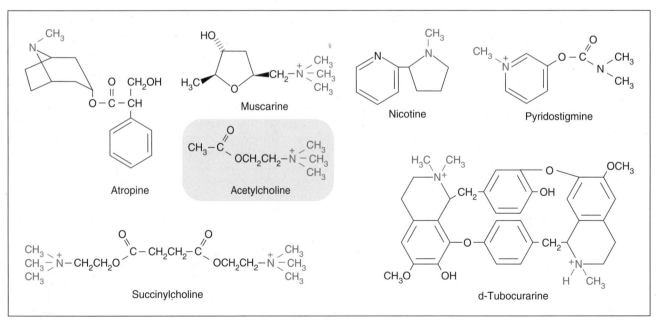

FIGURE 19–17. Acetylcholine and some of its congeners.

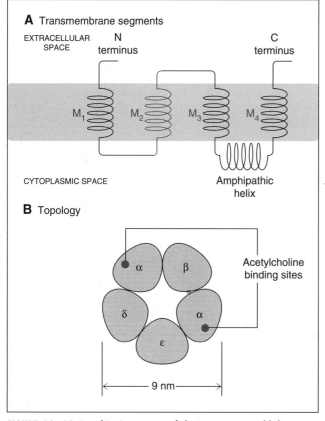

A Transmembrane segments

EXTRACELLULAR SPACE

N terminus

C terminus

M_1 M_2 M_3 M_4

CYTOPLASMIC SPACE

Amphipathic helix

B Topology

α β

δ α

ε

Acetylcholine binding sites

9 nm

FIGURE 19–18. A and B. Organization of the N_1 nicotinic acetylcholine receptor of the neuromuscular junction.

SEROTONIN

Serotonin is found in mast cells, platelets, enterochromaffin cells of the gut, and brain. The pathway for serotonin biosynthesis from tryptophan, an essential dietary amino acid, involves two steps. First, tryptophan reacts with tetrahydrobiopterin and oxygen to form 5-hydroxytryptophan, water, and dihydrobiopterin in a reaction catalyzed by **tryptophan hydroxylase** (Figure 19–19). This reaction is analogous to the phenylalanine hydroxylase (Figure 13–23) and tyrosine hydroxylase (Figure 19–5) reactions, and all three reactions are highly exergonic and physiologically irreversible. The three hydroxylase enzymes have similar amino acid sequences, and each uses tetrahydrobiopterin and oxygen as substrates. Second, 5-hydroxytryptophan undergoes an exergonic decarboxylation catalyzed by **aromatic amino acid decarboxylase** to form serotonin or 5-hydroxytryptamine (5-HT). This enzyme is the same enzyme that converts L-dopa to dopamine. The rate-limiting step in serotonin synthesis is catalyzed by tryptophan hydroxylase, the first and committed step in the pathway.

Different neurons synthesize serotonin and each of the three catecholamines. The idea that a single neuron synthesizes a single neurotransmitter is called Dale's law (named for Sir Henry Dale). Some cells, however, can synthesize and release a classical neurotransmitter and a neuropeptide neurotransmitter. Neurons in the brain stem synthesize serotonin (a classical neurotransmitter) and enkephalin (a neuropeptide). Neurons can synthesize a single classical neurotransmitter at one time, but the identity of the neurotransmitter may differ during development and in the mature neuron. The foundation of Dale's law has eroded, if not crumbled.

To terminate its action as a first messenger in brain, serotonin is taken up by serotonergic nerve cells by a sodium-dependent high-affinity uptake process. Its transport protein contains 12 transmembrane segments. The 12-transmembrane-segment motif is a property of many transport proteins. Several types of receptors for serotonin exist (Table 19–2).

Serotonin is a substrate for monoamine oxidase A (converting the amino group to an aldehyde). The aldehyde is converted to **5-hydroxyindoleacetic acid** (5-HIAA) following the oxidation of the aldehyde in a reaction catalyzed by aldehyde oxidase (Figure 19–6).

▶ Urinary 5-HIAA is used as a diagnostic test for diseases associated with excessive production of serotonin, as observed in carcinoid syndrome. This rare syndrome results most commonly from the excessive production of serotonin by enterochromaffin cells of the small bowel. Surgical excision of the isolated tumor is the treatment of choice. ◀

Serotonin plays a role in arousal, sleep-wake cycles, and mood alterations such as mental depression. Lysergic acid diethylamide (LSD), an analogue of serotonin, produces hallucinations. Psychoactive drugs have actions on serotonin metabolism.

▶ Tricyclic antidepressants including desipramine and imipramine, drugs that are used in the treatment of mental depression, inhibit both norepinephrine and serotonin uptake (norepinephrine more than serotonin). Fluoxetine (Prozac) and sertraline (Zoloft), other clinically effective antidepressants, are more effective inhibitors of serotonin than of norepinephrine uptake. Monoamine oxidase inhibitors, which are also used to treat mental depression, increase brain serotonin and catecholamine levels. Lithium salts are used in the treatment of some individuals with manic depression. Therapeutic concentrations of lithium inhibit inositol-4-phosphate phosphatase (Figure 12–7). ◀

Serotonin is converted to melatonin in the pineal gland. The first reaction involves the transfer of the acetyl group from energy-rich acetyl-CoA to form N-acetylserotonin in an exergonic process. The second reaction involves the transfer of the methyl group from the energy-rich S-adenosylmethionine to form melatonin (Figure 19–19). The concentration of melatonin is greatest at night and decreases in light, but its function is unknown.

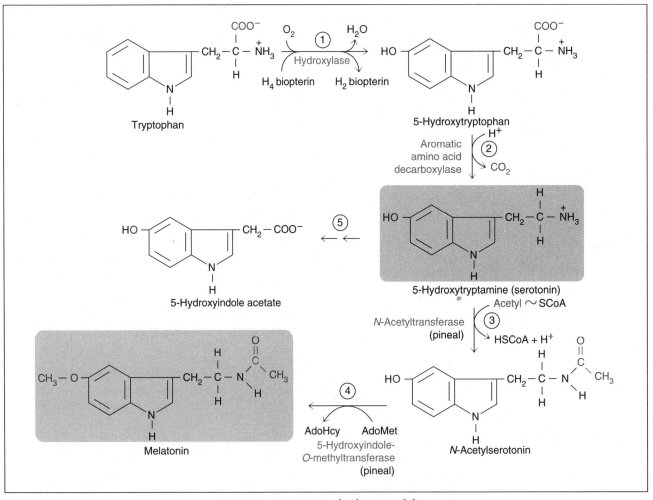

FIGURE 19–19. *Serotonin and melatonin metabolism.*

GABA

The metabolism of GABA, the chief inhibitory neurotransmitter of the brain, requires the cooperation of glia and GABAergic neurons. **Glutamate decarboxylase,** found in GABAergic neurons, catalyzes the exergonic conversion of glutamate to GABA (Figure 19–20). Glutamate decarboxylase contains pyridoxal phosphate as cofactor.

▶ Infants in the 1950s who were inadvertently fed milk formulas that lacked pyridoxal phosphate developed seizures. Medical scientists postulated that the seizures were due to a deficiency of GABA, the chief inhibitory neurotransmitter. This is noteworthy because questions about seizures that resulted from inadequate dietary pyridoxine in milk formulas have occurred in numerous biochemistry, pharmacology, and pediatrics examinations over the years. ◀ GABA can undergo an isoergonic transamination to produce succinate semialdehyde. Following a reaction with NAD⁺, the semialdehyde is converted to succinate.

Glia, which are supporting cells of the central nervous system, do not transmit an action potential. Following its release from a neuron, GABA dif-

fuses postsynaptically, interacts with its receptor, and hyperpolarizes the postsynaptic cells. GABA diffuses from the synaptic region and is taken up by GABAergic neurons or glia. The vesicles of GABAergic neurons can take up cytosolic GABA and subsequently release it again by calcium-dependent exocytosis. The metabolism of GABA by glia is more intricate. Glia convert GABA to succinate semialdehyde in an isoergonic reaction catalyzed by **GABA transaminase;** α-ketoglutarate and glutamate are the other reactant and the product, respectively. Glutamate is converted to glutamine in an exergonic reaction catalyzed by **glutamine synthetase,** and glutamine is transported to the neuron. Following the exergonic hydrolysis of glutamine to glutamate as catalyzed by **glutaminase,** GABA is synthesized in a reaction involving glutamate decarboxylase. The activity of glutamine synthetase is very high in brain. For many years this high activity was a mystery. After the discovery of its role in GABA metabolism, the role of the large activity of glutamine synthetase in the central nervous system was clarified.

There are two types of GABA receptor, denoted GABA$_A$ and GABA$_B$. The **GABA$_A$ receptor,** which is

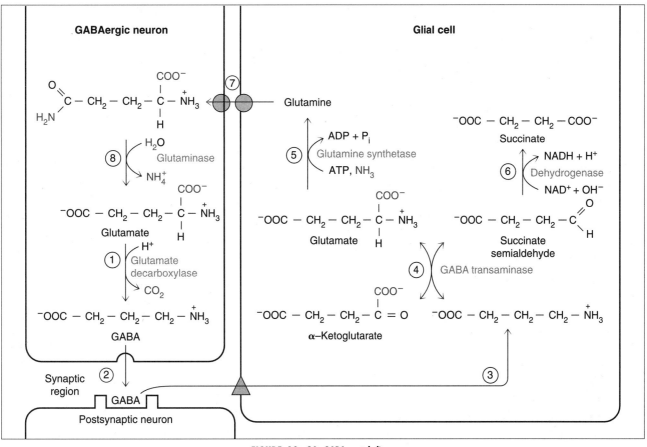

FIGURE 19-20. GABA metabolism.

the more prevalent form, functions as a ligand-gated chloride channel. Increasing chloride conductance from outside to inside the neuron produces hyperpolarization (more negative intracellular electromotive potential) and decreases nerve excitability. The $GABA_A$ receptor contains two GABA-binding sites. The receptor consists of up to five different subunits called α, β, γ, δ, and ρ. Each subunit has four transmembrane segments and resembles the nicotinic acetylcholine receptor (Figure 19–18).

▶ $GABA_A$ receptors contain allosteric binding sites for diazepam (Valium; an anxiolytic drug) and barbiturate (a sleep-inducing drug and an anticonvulsant used in the treatment of epilepsy). Both agents increase the effects of GABA on the receptor. There are suggestions that ethanol exerts some of its effects via the $GABA_A$ receptor. ◀ The **$GABA_B$ receptor** is linked to G-proteins. Targets of these G-proteins include adenylyl cyclase, which is inhibited, and potassium and calcium channels. The $GABA_B$ receptor lacks diazepam- and barbiturate-binding sites.

GLYCINE AND GLUTAMATE

Glycine is the chief inhibitory neurotransmitter in the spinal cord. Its action parallels that of GABA in

the brain. The finding that an ordinary and not specialized compound, such as glycine or glutamate, can function as a neurotransmitter was a surprise. Glycine is packaged in secretory vesicles and is released by calcium-dependent exocytosis. Its receptor, like the GABA receptor, increases chloride flux and hyperpolarizes the postsynaptic neuron. The glycine receptor structures resemble those of the $GABA_A$ receptors. Glycine is transported back into its neurons by high-affinity sodium-dependent transport proteins.

Glutamate is the chief excitatory amino acid in the brain. After interacting with its receptors, glutamate's action is ended by sodium-dependent high-affinity uptake. Most glutamate is taken up by glia, converted to glutamine, and translocated back to glutamatergic cells. Some glutamate is taken up directly by the cells that released it. Glutamate can be transported into vesicles and rereleased.

An intricate variety of receptors that mediate the actions of glutamate have been described, and these are given for general reference in Table 19–2. Most of these receptors are ligand-activated cation channels and promote neuronal depolarization. Two classes of receptor, however, are called metabolotropic because they interact with G-proteins. The most studied glutamate receptor is the **NMDA receptor.** Its name is based on its activation by *N*-methyl-D-aspartate, a pharmacological agent.

The NMDA receptor is unusual because both glutamate and glycine are required for its activation. The glycine-binding site differs from that of the inhibitory glycine receptor. This receptor is a ligand-gated sodium and calcium channel. The calcium conductance by the NMDA channel is greater than that of other glutamate (AMPA and kainate; see below) receptors. The NMDA receptor is postulated to play a role in learning, memory, and synaptic plasticity, and calcium has a key role in these processes. The family of glutamate receptors has a topology similar to that of the nicotinic, $GABA_A$, 5-HT_3, and glycine receptors.

The **AMPA receptors** resemble the NMDA receptors in topology but differ in pharmacologic specificity. *The AMPA receptor is responsible for most "fast" synaptic transmission in the brain and spinal cord.* The kainate receptors also resemble the NMDA and AMPA receptors but differ in their pharmacologic specificity. Several metabolotropic glutamate receptors, which possess seven transmembrane segments and interact with G-proteins, have been described.

HISTAMINE

The conversion of histidine to histamine occurs in one step (Figure 19–21). The reaction is catalyzed by **histidine decarboxylase,** a pyridoxal phosphate–containing enzyme that differs from aromatic amino acid decarboxylase. This reaction is an exergonic decarboxylation (PRINCIPLE 6 OF BIOENERGETICS). Histamine is released from synaptic vesicles by exocytosis and interacts with its receptors. In contrast to amino acids and the biogenic amines, a high-affinity sodium-dependent transport system for histamine does not exist in brain, and histamine is inactivated metabolically. In brain, histamine undergoes an exergonic methylation (*S*-adenosylmethionine is the methyl donor) followed by oxidation to methylimidazole acetate. **Histamine *N*-methyltransferase** is located postsynaptically. In peripheral tissues, histamine is metabolized to imidazole acetaldehyde and imidazole acetate (Figure 19–21).

There are three classes of histamine receptor, denoted H_1, H_2, and H_3 (Table 19–2). Because histamine H_1 receptor antagonists are sedative, histamine has been suggested to play a role in sleep-wake cycles and arousal.

▶ H_1 receptor antagonists such as diphenhydramine are used in the treatment of allergic responses and for symptomatic treatment of upper respiratory illnesses. Diphenhydramine is an over-the-counter drug. H_2 receptor antagonists such as cimetidine are prescription drugs that are used in the treatment of peptic ulcers. These therapies are directed at histamine functioning as a local mediator and not as a neurotransmitter. ◀

OPIOID PEPTIDE BIOSYNTHESIS

More than 50 neuropeptides have been described in central and peripheral neurons. Neuropeptides are synthesized by mRNA-dependent protein synthesis followed by proteolytic processing reactions. Opioids are one class of neuropeptides, and this class of compounds has morphine-like actions. β-Endorphin, methionine-enkephalin, leucine-enkephalin, and dynorphin are examples (Table 19–2).

These opioid peptides are cleavage products of three distinct genes and their encoded proteins. β-Endorphin is derived from **proopiomelanocortin** (**POMC,** pronounced "pom see"). This peptide is processed by proteolysis to yield ACTH, four forms of melanocyte-stimulating hormone (MSH), and **β-endorphin** (Figure 19–22). The **enkephalins** (the name means "in the head") are pentapeptides that are derived from proenkephalin (Figure 19–22) by proteolytic processing. The ratio of methionine-enkephalin to leucine-enkephalin is 6/1 in the precursor. The distribution of proenkephalin is much greater than the name implies. It is synthesized in the peripheral nervous system, gut, adrenal medulla, and various regions of the central nervous system. **Dynorphins** are opioid peptides that are synthesized from a third precursor called preprodynorphin. These substances contain leucine-enkephalin as part of their structure, but the dynorphins exist as independent entities. They are found in both the central and peripheral nervous systems. The genes for each of the three classes of opioids have been characterized, and the prepropeptide for each is expressed by two exons (Figure 19–22).

All three of the opioid propeptides have signal sequences that must be removed cotranslationally as described in Chapter 18. The bioactive peptide segments are surrounded by paired basic amino acid residues in the precursor proteins. Conversion of the propeptides to the final products is catalyzed by prohormone convertases and carboxypeptidase H, as described for insulin (Chapter 18). Several receptors for the opioids have been characterized pharmacologically (Table 19–2). These peptides are inactivated extracellularly by proteolytic cleavage and not by reuptake.

NITRIC OXIDE AND CYCLIC GMP

Nitric oxide, which is a gas with the formula NO, was shown to be a signaling molecule in the late 1980s. This compound is generated in a variety of cells including endothelium, smooth muscle, cardiac muscle, macrophages, and cells of the central nervous system. The compound was known for 20 years as the **endothelium-derived relaxation factor** (EDRF). Nitric oxide is derived from arginine and molecular oxygen in a reaction that involves

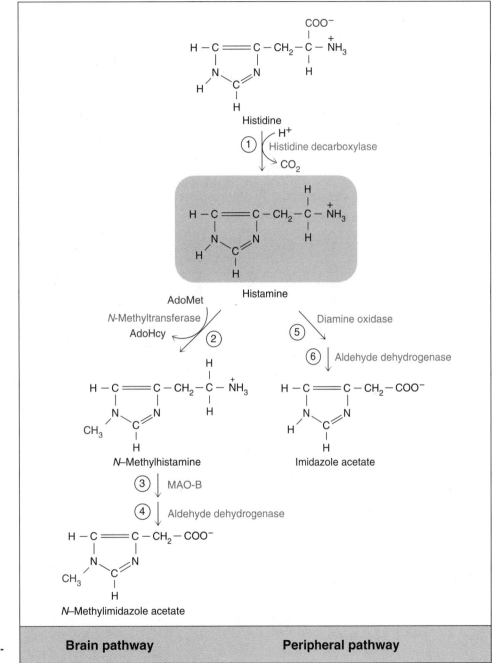

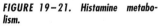

FIGURE 19–21. *Histamine metabolism.*

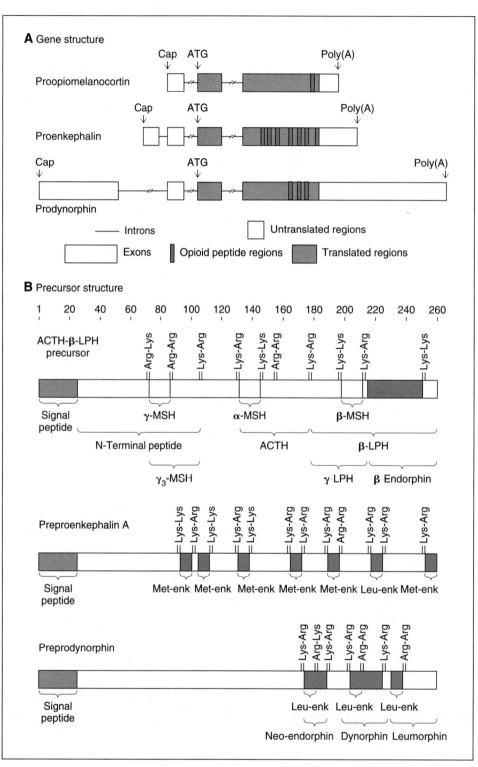

FIGURE 19–22. A and B. Opioid peptide gene structure and processing. *ACTH-β-LPH, adrenocorticotropic hormone–β-lipotropin; Leu-enk, leucine enkephalin; MSH, melanocyte-stimulating hormone; Met-enk, methionine-enkephalin.*

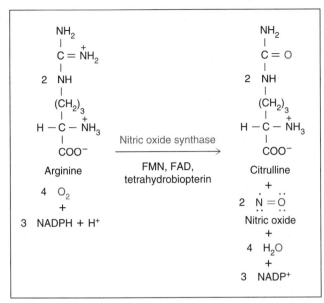

FIGURE 19–23. Biosynthesis of nitric oxide from arginine.

▶ Some bacterial endotoxins and cytokines activate transcription of the inducible form of nitric oxide synthase. The enzyme is induced in vascular smooth muscle cells, vascular endothelium, myocardium, and other cells. Induction of NO synthase underlies the production of shock (hypotension) observed in septicemia and during anti-tumor therapy with some cytokines because NO and cyclic GMP produce vasodilation. ◀ The inducible form of nitric oxide synthase, in contrast to the neuronal and constitutive enzymes, is active in the absence of calcium.

In contrast to adenylyl cyclase, an integral plasma membrane enzyme, guanylyl cyclase exists in two forms: particulate and soluble. The action of nitric oxide is to stimulate the soluble form of guanylyl cyclase. The soluble form of guanylyl cyclase contains a heme group to which nitric oxide binds. **Guanylyl cyclase** catalyzes the conversion of GTP to 3′,5′-cyclic GMP (Figure 19–24). This process is analogous to cyclic AMP formation.

The chief action of cyclic GMP in nonretinal cells is to activate protein kinase G. In contrast to protein kinase A, protein kinase G does not dissociate into regulatory and catalytic subunits. The enzyme is activated allosterically by cyclic GMP, as indicated by equation 19.1.

$$E_2 + 4 \text{ cyclic GMP} \rightleftharpoons E_2 \cdot \text{cyclic GMP}_4 \qquad (19.1)$$
$$\textit{Inactive} \qquad\qquad \textit{Active}$$

Protein kinase G is a serine/threonine protein kinase. In contrast to the large number of substrates known for protein kinase A, the physiological substrates for protein kinase G are largely unknown. Cyclic GMP is metabolized and inactivated by exergonic hydrolysis in a reaction catalyzed by **cyclic nucleotide phosphodiesterase** (Figure 19–24). There are several phosphodiesterases in cells, which are listed in Table 19–3 for general reference.

The use of nitric oxide as a first messenger in the brain and elsewhere has several unusual aspects. First, the compound is a gas. Second, ni-

NADPH (Figure 19–23). The products include nitric oxide, citrulline, water, and NADP⁺. The nitric oxide molecule contains an unpaired electron and is a free radical; this accounts for the requirement of *five electrons* and not an even number of electrons per molecule of NO formed. **Nitric oxide synthase** is a P-450 type of heme protein that contains FMN and FAD and is stabilized by tetrahydrobiopterin.

There are at least three forms of nitric oxide synthase including neuronal, constitutive, and inducible forms. The neuronal and constitutive (present in endothelium) forms of nitric oxide synthase are activated by calcium/calmodulin. Acetylcholine, acting via muscarinic receptors on vascular endothelial cells, increases nitric oxide synthase activity following activation of phospholipase C via G_p. The generation of inositol trisphosphate and the consequent elevation of cytosolic calcium activates NO synthase.

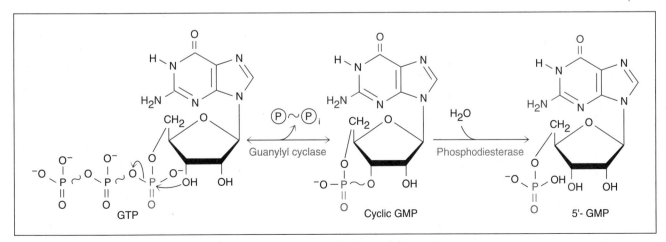

FIGURE 19–24. Cyclic GMP metabolism.

TABLE 19–3. Classification of Cyclic Nucleotide Phosphodiesterases

Family	Properties
I	Stimulated by calcium/calmodulin; low affinity for substrate.
II	Stimulated by cyclic GMP; low affinity for substrate
III	Inhibited by cyclic GMP; high affinity for substrate
IV	Unregulated; high affinity for cyclic AMP
V	Stimulated by retinal transducin; high affinity for cyclic GMP

tric oxide diffuses freely and is not packaged in secretory vesicles. It has the potential to diffuse from its site of synthesis and influence its surrounding cells (a paracrine effect). Nitric oxide is very unstable and breaks down spontaneously within a few seconds. Recent evidence suggests that **carbon monoxide** also functions as a neurotransmitter in brain. This substance is formed during the metabolism of heme as catalyzed by heme oxygenase (Figure 24–14). Carbon monoxide interacts with and activates soluble guanylyl cyclase. In contrast to nitric oxide, which breaks down rapidly, carbon monoxide is stable.

THE RHODOPSIN–CYCLIC GMP CASCADE

The two types of photoreceptor cells in the retina are the rods and cones. The three million cone cells in the human retina function in bright light and are responsible for color vision. The hundred million rod cells function in dim light and do not perceive color. The outer segment of the rod contains about 1000 disks that are packed with rhodopsin, the photoreceptor molecule. The rod outer segment is connected to the inner segment by a ciliated structure (Figure 19–25). The plasma membrane of rod cells contains cation channels through which sodium flows in the dark to keep the cell depolarized. Light closes these channels indirectly and the cell becomes hyperpolarized with a negative intracellular voltage as the sodium current is decreased.

The photochemical reactions that rhodopsin undergoes are illustrated in Figure 2–21. The carboxyl terminus of rhodopsin, which was the first membrane protein to be identified as a seven-transmembrane segment protein, occurs on the cytosolic side of the disk, and the amino terminus occurs on the inside of the disk (Figure 19–9). The cytosolic side of **rhodopsin** transmits the excitation signal to an enzymatic cascade. The *cis* to *trans* isomerization of retinal, bound to opsin by a Schiff-base linkage, is the primary event in visual excitation. Activated rhodopsin interacts with transducin, a G-protein. **Transducin** consists of α-, β,- and γ-subunits that resemble those of G_s and G_i. GTP exchanges for GDP, and αG_t activates cyclic GMP phosphodiesterase.

Cyclic GMP phosphodiesterase of the retina is a

protein that consists of three subunits, also called α, β, and γ. αG_t-GTP forms a complex with the γ-subunit of phosphodiesterase. Dissociation of the γ-subunit leaves the $\alpha\beta$ heterodimer, the active form of the enzyme (Figure 19–26). The cation channel is maintained in its open state by cyclic GMP. Because of the rhodopsin-transducin–mediated increase in phosphodiesterase activity, cyclic GMP levels fall and the cation channel is closed. This produces hyperpolarization of the plasma membrane of the rod cell. There are two hypotheses that relate hyperpolarization of the rod cells to visual excitation. First, cells next to the rod cells are influenced by changes in membrane potential, and intercellular communication is electrotonic. Second, less neurotransmitter (glutamate) is released because of hyperpolarization, and the

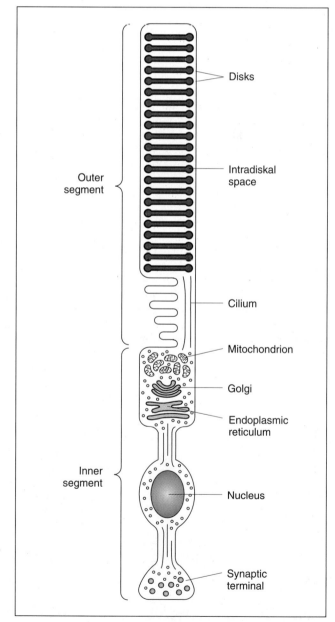

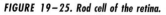

FIGURE 19–25. Rod cell of the retina.

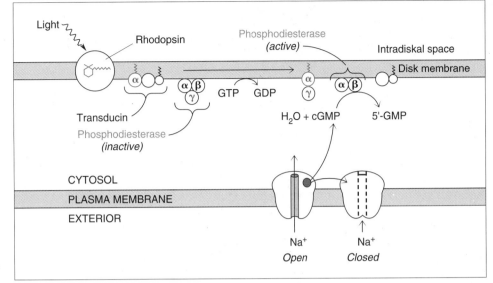

FIGURE 19–26. *Role of transducin in activating cyclic GMP phosphodiesterase in retina.*

postjunctional cell receives less excitatory neurotransmitter. The rod cell releases excitatory neurotransmitter in the dark, and light decreases the release of transmitter.

SUMMARY

Extracellular signaling molecules are required to coordinate the development and activities of the many cells and cell types present in humans. These extracellular signaling molecules are called first messengers and include neurotransmitters, hormones, and growth factors. The catecholamine neurotransmitters are dopamine, norepinephrine, and epinephrine. Tyrosine hydroxylase, which catalyzes the first and rate-limiting reaction in the pathway for catecholamine biosynthesis, is the main regulatory enzyme. The catecholamines bind to adrenergic receptors that possess seven transmembrane segments and interact with G-proteins. G-proteins are heterotrimeric proteins that associate with various effectors including adenylyl cyclase and phospholipase C.

Tryptophan hydroxylase catalyzes the first step in serotonin biosynthesis. Tryptophan hydroxylase, tyrosine hydroxylase, phenylalanine hydroxylase, and nitric oxide synthase require the participation of tetrahydrobiopterin. Acetylcholine is formed in one step from acetyl-CoA (active acetate) and choline in a reaction catalyzed by choline acetyltransferase. Acetylcholinesterase contains an active site serine residue and is responsible for inactivating acetylcholine. Muscarinic receptors are metabolotropic and nicotinic receptors are ligand-gated ion channels. Each subunit of a ligand-gated ion channel contains four transmembrane segments.

GABA, the chief inhibitory neurotransmitter of the brain, is synthesized from glutamate in a reaction catalyzed by glutamate decarboxylase. The cofactor for glutamate decarboxylase and aromatic amino acid decarboxylase is pyridoxal phosphate. The $GABA_A$ receptor is a ligand-gated ion channel that conducts chloride and leads to hyperpolarization of the postsynaptic cell. Glutamate is the chief excitatory transmitter of the brain. The glutamate AMPA receptor is responsible for most "fast" neurotransmission in brain.

The opioid peptides are synthesized by mRNA-dependent protein synthesis followed by proteolytic processing reactions. Opioids are compounds possessing morphine-like actions. These substances include methionine-enkephalin, leucine-enkephalin, β-endorphin, and dynorphin.

The main classes of plasma membrane receptors that recognize hydrophilic first messengers include ligand-gated ion channels (nicotinic acetylcholine, glutamate, GABA, glycine, and $5\text{-}HT_3$) and G-protein–associated receptors (muscarinic acetylcholine, α- and β-adrenergic, dopamine, serotonin, and opioid receptors) that can activate or inhibit adenylyl cyclase or can activate phospholipase C. Second messengers include cyclic AMP, cyclic GMP, diglyceride, inositol trisphosphate, and calcium. Cyclic AMP, cyclic GMP, and diglyceride activate their cognate protein kinases. Protein kinase C is the enzyme that is activated by diglyceride. Both protein kinase C and calmodulin-dependent protein kinases require calcium for the expression of activity.

The two fundamental mechanisms for terminating the action of neurotransmitters are metabolism and uptake. Acetylcholine and neuropeptides are inactivated by hydrolysis, and histamine is inactivated by methylation. The other neurotransmitters including dopamine, norepinephrine, serotonin, glutamate, GABA, and glycine are inactivated by transport into neuronal cells (or glia in the case of GABA and glutamate). Dopamine, norepinephrine, epinephrine, and serotonin are substrates for monoamine oxidase. Catechol-*O*-methyltransferase catalyzes a reaction of various catechols with

S-adenosylmethionine to form the methylated derivative. Homovanillate (HVA) is the chief metabolite of dopamine, and vanillylmandelate (VMA) is the chief metabolite of norepinephrine and epinephrine.

Nitric oxide, a gaseous first messenger, is formed from arginine and oxygen. This compound functions as a neurotransmitter in the brain and as a local mediator in nonneuronal cells. This compound activates soluble guanylyl cyclase. The chief action of cyclic GMP in nonretinal cells is the activation of protein kinase G. Light activates rhodopsin and transducin in the retina. Transducin is a heterotrimeric G-protein that activates cyclic GMP phosphodiesterase. αG_t-GTP removes the γ-subunit of cyclic GMP phosphodiesterase, and the heterodimeric $\alpha\beta$ complex catalyzes the hydrolysis of cyclic GMP. The action of cyclic GMP in retina is to activate sodium channels and depolarize rod cells.

Destruction of cyclic GMP leads to rod cell hyperpolarization.

SELECTED READINGS

Bloom, F.E., and D.J. Kupfer (eds.). *Psychopharmacology: The Fourth Generation of Progress.* New York, Raven Press, 1995.

Dohlman, H.G., J. Thorner, M.G. Caron, and R.J. Lefkowitz. Model systems for the study of seven-transmembrane-segment receptors. Annual Review of Biochemistry 60:653–688, 1991.

Gingrich, J.A., and M.G. Caron. Recent advances in the molecular biology of dopamine receptors. Annual Review of Neuroscience 16:299–321, 1993.

Kaziro, Y., H. Itoh, T. Kozasa, M. Nakafuku, and T. Satoh. Structure and function of signal-transducing GTP-binding proteins. Annual Review of Biochemistry 60:349–400, 1991.

Moncada, S., and A. Higgs. The L-arginine-nitric oxide pathway. New England Journal of Medicine 329:2002–1212, 1993.

Siegel, G.J., B.W. Agranoff, R.W. Albers, and P.B. Molinoff (eds.). *Basic Neurochemistry,* 5th ed. New York, Raven Press, 1994.

CHAPTER TWENTY

HORMONES AND

GROWTH FACTORS

The life so short, the craft so long to learn.
—HIPPOCRATES

SIGNAL TRANSDUCTION

The coordinate regulation of cellular and intercellular activities plays a pivotal role in differentiation, development, cell maintenance, and regulation of fuel and energy metabolism. Most of this coordination is mediated by extracellular signaling molecules, or first messengers, that alter intracellular processes. The field of endocrinology (the study of hormones) is interdisciplinary and can be considered from the viewpoints of biochemistry, cell biology, physiology, and clinical medicine. The mechanisms of selected hormones and growth factors are described in this chapter from a biochemical perspective.

Signal transduction is the process by which an extracellular signal produces intracellular signals that mediate physiological responses. Transduction refers to the conversion of one signal to another. For example, glucagon, a hormonal extracellular signal, activates intracellular signals that produce glycogenolysis in liver cells. Glucagon, the first messenger, mediates the generation of intracellular cyclic AMP, a second messenger, and the activation of protein kinase A (Chapter 10). Protein kinase A elicits a cascade that results in the activation of the chief glycogenolytic enzyme (phosphorylase) and inhibition of the chief glycogenic enzyme (glycogen synthase). This process constitutes a cyclic AMP signal transduction pathway, the first signal transduction pathway to be elucidated.

Extracellular signaling molecules are either hydrophilic or lipophilic. Hydrophilic extracellular signaling molecules interact with receptors that are integral membrane proteins. Several receptors for hydrophilic first messengers, acting via G-proteins, alter adenylyl cyclase or phospholipase C activity (Chapter 19). A variety of other mechanisms for signal transduction at the plasma membrane are illustrated in Figure 20–1. Lipophilic extracellular signaling molecules interact with intracellular receptors that alter gene transcription, and these are considered later in this chapter.

HYPOTHALAMUS AND PITUITARY

Hypothalamic Neurohormones

The hypothalamus secretes hormones that are carried to the anterior pituitary by the hypophyseal portal venous system where these hormones act by stimulating or inhibiting the secretion of the anterior pituitary hormones. Thyrotropin-releasing hormone, the first hypothalamic hormone whose structure was determined, regulates thyrotropin (thyroid-stimulating hormone) secretion. Secretion

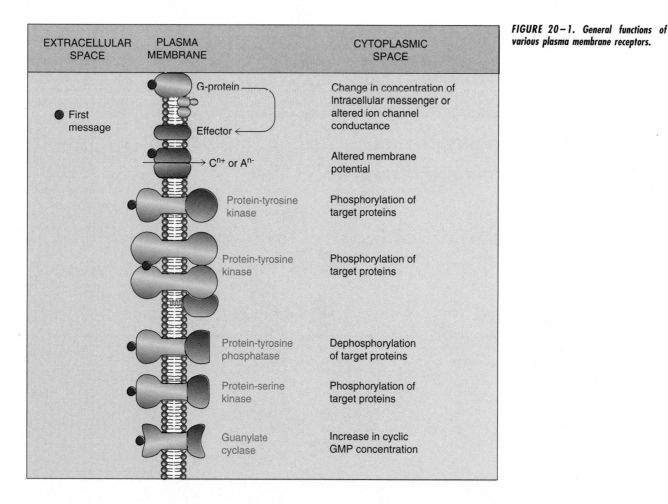

FIGURE 20–1. General functions of various plasma membrane receptors.

TABLE 20–1.   Hormones of the Hypothalamus and Anterior Pituitary

Hypothalamic Hormone	No. of Amino Acids	Pituitary Hormone Affected
Corticotropin-releasing hormone (CRH)	41	Adrenocorticotropic hormone (ACTH)
Gonadotropin-releasing hormone (GnRH = LHRH = FSHRH)	10	Luteinizing hormone (LH) and follicle-stimulating hormone (FSH)
Growth hormone–releasing hormone (GHRH)	44	Growth hormone (GH)
Growth hormone release-inhibiting hormone (somatostatin)	14	Growth hormone (GH)
Thyrotropin-releasing hormone (TRH)	3	Thyrotropin (thyroid-stimulating hormone, TSH)

of thyrotropin-releasing hormone by the hypothalamus is regulated, in turn, by circulating thyroid hormones (T_3 and T_4). Thyrotropin-releasing hormone, a tripeptide, is the smallest peptide that is produced by mRNA-dependent synthesis and post-translational processing. The hypothalamic hormones and the anterior pituitary hormones that they control are listed in Table 20–1.

Anterior Pituitary Hormones

The hormones of the anterior pituitary, which are under control of the hypothalamus, coordinate the activities of many target cells. ▶ Loss of anterior pituitary function (panhypopituitarism) results in atrophy of the thyroid, gonads, and adrenal cortex. Nitrogen and mineral balance are also adversely affected. ◀ Growth hormone, prolactin, and chorionic somatomammotropin (produced by the placenta) are a family of homologous protein hormones. Each of these hormones has growth-promoting and lactogenic (milk-producing) activity.

Growth hormone is the most abundant hormone in the anterior pituitary, and its content is 100 to 1000 times that of the other hormones. Growth hormone plays a primary role in controlling postnatal growth. Growth hormone's physiological effects are more extensive than suggested by its name. It is essential for carbohydrate, lipid, nitrogen, and mineral metabolism. Growth hormone has direct effects on glucose transport, differentiation of adipocytes, and cytochrome P-450 activity in liver cells.

The growth-promoting effects of growth hormone are indirect (Table 20–2). Nearly all growth-promoting effects of growth hormone are due to a peptide called **insulin-like growth factor–1.** Insulin-like growth factors–1 and –2 are known as **somatomedins.** Insulin-like growth factor–1, which is produced by the liver, increases amino acid transport into cells, promotes protein synthesis and a positive mineral balance, and stimulates lipolysis in adipose tissue. Insulin-like growth factor–1 antagonizes the effects of insulin by stimulating gluconeogenesis and hyperglycemia. The physiological roles of insulin-like growth factor–2 are uncertain.

▶ Growth hormone excess in children and adolescents results in **gigantism,** and in adults results in **acromegaly.** Individuals with increased growth hormone levels (because of a pituitary tumor) fail

TABLE 20–2.   Selected Hydrophilic First Messengers That Interact with Cell-Surface Receptors

First Messenger	Origin	Comments
Adrenocorticotropic hormone (ACTH)	Anterior pituitary	39-Amino-acid peptide stimulates adrenal cortex to produce cortisol
Angiotensin II, III	Plasma	Octapeptide and heptapeptide promote aldosterone synthesis and secretion from the adrenal cortex and produce arteriolar constriction
Atrial natriuretic peptide	Atria	28-Amino-acid peptide promotes vasodilatation, diuresis, and natriuresis by cyclic GMP–dependent mechanisms
Calcitonin	C cells of thyroid	32-Amino-acid peptide decreases serum calcium
Epinephrine	Adrenal medulla	Produces glycogenolysis and lipolysis in responsive cells. Increases cardiac contractility
Follicle-stimulating hormone (FSH)	Anterior pituitary	α-Chain, 92 amino acids; β-chain, 118 amino acids. Stimulates estrogen synthesis by the ovarian follicle cells
Glucagon	Pancreatic α-cells	29-Amino-acid polypeptide stimulates hepatic gluconeogenesis, glycogenolysis, ketogenesis, and adipocyte lipolysis
Growth hormone	Anterior pituitary	191-Amino-acid polypeptide stimulates release of insulin-like growth factors 1 and 2 by liver
Insulin	Pancreatic β-cells	A Chain, 21 amino acids; B chain, 30 amino acids. Anabolic hormone stimulates glucose uptake in extrahepatic cells. Stimulates lipid synthesis and inhibits lipolysis in adipose cells. General stimulation of protein synthesis
Insulin-like growth factor–1	Liver	70-Amino-acid polypeptide stimulates skeletal growth and replication of fibroblasts, hemopoietic, and epithelial cells
Luteinizing hormone (LH)	Anterior pituitary	α-Chain, 92 amino acids; β-chain, 115 amino acids. Stimulates estrogen and progesterone synthesis in ovarian follicle cells; stimulates androgen synthesis in Sertoli cells of the testis
Parathyroid hormone	Parathyroid	84-Amino-acid polypeptide increases serum calcium and decreases phosphate. Stimulates calcium and phosphate resorption from bone
Thyrotropin	Anterior pituitary	α-Chain, 92 amino acids; β-chain, 112 amino acids. Stimulates release of thyroxine from thyroid gland

to suppress growth hormone in response to glucose administration. Growth hormone–deficient individuals fail to increase growth hormone in response either to arginine or L-dopa administration or to hypoglycemia. These metabolic challenges are used for diagnostic purposes. The somatotropic effects of growth hormone are closely related to insulin-like growth factor–1. Individuals with normal growth hormone levels who lack insulin-like growth factor–1, exhibit major growth retardation and develop into **pygmies.** Individuals who lack insulin-like growth factor–2 exhibit normal growth.

Growth hormone deficiency severely retards growth in infants. **Growth hormone–deficient dwarfs** respond to injections of human growth hormone. Growth hormones from other species, in contrast to insulin (Chapter 3), are ineffective in humans. Treatment of growth hormone deficiency in hypopituitary dwarfs requires human growth hormone, which for many years was derived painstakingly from cadavers. Supplies were necessarily limited, and not all affected individuals could be treated. Growth hormone isolated from human tissue was a source of viral pathogens, and this method of deriving the hormone was discontinued.

Recombinant human growth hormone now provides a safe and plentiful supply of this therapeutic agent. The production of human growth hormone is achieved by linking human growth hormone cDNA to a bacterial promoter in a plasmid. The hormone is produced in *Escherichia coli* and is purified. The current production procedure involves a plasmid with a bacterial signal sequence (Chapter 18) that directs the hormone into the periplasmic space. The molecule resulting from bacterial signal peptidase action lacks the amino terminal methionine and is called Met-less human growth hormone. Fortunately the hormone possesses full biological activity. Secretion into the periplasmic space aids in hormone purification. ◄

Prolactin, produced by pituitary lactotropes, contains 198 amino acids. Pituitary lactotropes increase in size and number during pregnancy. Prolactin is involved in breast development and lactation. The function of human **chorionic somatomammotropin,** the third member of this group, is unknown. Pregnancies in which the fetus and placenta lack the gene for this hormone result in infants that develop normally in utero and postpartum. The levels of this hormone in blood are 100 times higher than those of other polypeptide hormones. The placenta produces about 1 gram of chorionic somatomammotropin daily during late pregnancy (a prodigious amount of hormone). This hormone may sustain important functions that are redundant and are provided by growth hormone and prolactin.

Thyrotropin, luteinizing hormone, follicle-stimulating hormone, and chorionic gonadotropin are glycoprotein hormones that consist of two subunits: the α-subunits are identical, and the β-subunits differ (Table 20–2). These hormones employ cyclic AMP as their intracellular second messenger (Table 20–3). A single gene encodes the α-subunit, and different genes encode the four β-subunits. The α- and β-subunits contain N-linked oligosaccharides.

Thyrotropin increases iodide transport into thyroid cells and T_3 and T_4 biosynthesis via cyclic AMP–dependent mechanisms. Thyrotropin secretion is regulated by thyrotropin-releasing hormone via phospholipase C activation. ► Thyrotropin-releasing hormone injections can be used to distinguish between hypothyroidism of pituitary or hypothalamic origin. Thyrotropin-releasing hormone is not useful therapeutically because its half-life in the circulation is only 4 minutes. ◄

Adrenocorticotropic hormone (ACTH; corticotropin) activates adenylyl cyclase in its target cells. This leads to the increased rate of conversion of

---

TABLE 20–3.   Some First Messengers That Alter Cyclic AMP in Target Cells

First Messenger	Target Cell	Metabolic Response
Increases cyclic AMP		
ACTH	Adrenal cortex	Increase in cortisol synthesis
Calcitonin	Osteoclasts	Inhibition of osteoclastic activity
Epinephrine	Muscle	Increase in glycogenolysis
Epinephrine, glucagon	Adipose	Increase in triglyceride hydrolysis
Follicle-stimulating hormone and luteinizing hormone	Ovarian follicle	Increase in estrogen and progesterone formation
Glucagon	Liver	Increase in glycogenolysis and gluconeogenesis
Norepinephrine	Juxtaglomerular cells of the kidney	Secretion of renin
Parathyroid hormone	Bone	Increase in calcium resorption
Thyrotropin	Thyroid	Secretion of thyroxine
Vasopressin	Kidney	Increase in water reabsorption (V_2 receptor)
Decreases cyclic AMP		
Acetylcholine	Smooth muscle	Contraction (M_2 receptor)
Angiotensin II	Adrenal cortex	Aldosterone synthesis in adrenal
Enkephalin	Brain	Behavioral effects (δ-opioid receptor)
Norepinephrine	Smooth muscle	Contraction (α_2-adrenergic receptor)
Somatostatin	Bone and muscle	Altered growth

cholesterol (C_{27}) to pregnenolone (C_{21}). ACTH also promotes adrenal cortical growth, RNA, and protein synthesis. ▶ Overproduction of ACTH by the pituitary results in excessive production of adrenal steroid hormones and **Cushing syndrome.** Affected individuals exhibit negative nitrogen balance, sodium retention, glucose intolerance or overt diabetes mellitus, increased plasma fatty acids, and decreased circulating lymphocytes and eosinophils. Affected individuals have muscle wasting and truncal obesity. A deficiency of glucocorticoid production by the adrenal cortex results in **Addison disease.** Increased secretion of adrenocorticotropic hormone often occurs in Addison disease as part of a compensatory feedback process. Increased levels of ACTH often increase skin pigmentation because ACTH includes the sequence of **melanocyte stimulating hormone** (Figure 19–22). ◀

Posterior Pituitary Hormones

The posterior pituitary, which is embryologically distinct from the anterior pituitary, is a neuroendocrine gland. Vasopressin and oxytocin are nonapeptides produced in the posterior pituitary gland by mRNA-dependent protein synthesis and post-translational processing. Each is transported within the neuroendocrine cells in association with a carrier protein named neurophysin. **Vasopressin** and **neurophysin I** are co-released by calcium-dependent exocytosis. **Oxytocin** and **neurophysin II** are co-released from a different cell type. The neurophysins lack physiological effects. Oxytocin stimulates uterine contraction, and this compound is used pharmacologically to induce childbirth. Oxytocin also plays a role in milk ejection.

Vasopressin is also called antidiuretic hormone. Its most important physiological function is to promote the reabsorption of water in the distal renal tubules, an effect that is mediated by cyclic AMP. Dehydration results in the secretion of vasopressin from the posterior pituitary. ▶ Primary **diabetes insipidus** usually results from destruction of the posterior pituitary as a result of trauma, tumor, or infection. This form of diabetes results from the inability to concentrate urine with the consequent excretion of large volumes of dilute urine. Heredi-

tary **nephrogenic diabetes insipidus** is due to a defect in the vasopressin receptor in the kidney. Acquired diabetes insipidus can be produced by lithium used in the treatment of manic depression. ◀ The action of vasopressin in the kidney is mediated by cyclic AMP via a V_2 receptor (Table 20–3). Vasopressin also activates glycogenolysis in the liver via activation of phospholipase C via a V_1 receptor (Table 20–4). Vasopressin is found in the brain, where it functions as a neuropeptide.

HORMONES AND CALCIUM METABOLISM

Calcium is the most abundant mineral in humans (Table 2–1). Calcium is important in the regulation of cellular metabolism and as a structural component of the skeleton. Calcium ion regulates many important physiological processes including exocytosis, secretion of neurotransmitters and hormones from secretory vesicles, muscle and nerve cell excitability, and blood coagulation. Intracellular calcium functions as an intracellular second messenger. There are two main sources of intracellular calcium. Calcium is derived from intracellular stores such as the endoplasmic reticulum in response to inositol 1,4,5-trisphosphate (Figure 19–13). Plasma membrane calcium channels also allow calcium to move down its gradient from the extracellular to the intracellular compartment. There are two mechanisms for keeping the intracellular calcium concentration low ($\approx 0.1\ \mu M$). Calcium ATPases translocate calcium from the cytosol into the endoplasmic reticulum or outside the cell. A sodium-calcium exchange protein in the plasma membrane translocates calcium ion to the cell exterior in exchange for extracellular sodium ion, an antiport process. The intracellular sodium is then transported out of the cell by the sodium/potassium-ATPase, or sodium pump.

Many intracellular effects of calcium are mediated by a calcium-binding protein called calmodulin. **Calmodulin,** which is a ubiquitous protein containing 148 amino acids, has four calcium-binding sites. After binding calcium, the protein undergoes a conformational change and can interact with and alter activity of target proteins. There is a family of calcium/calmodulin–dependent protein

---

TABLE 20–4.   Some First Messengers That Activate Phospholipase C Activity in Target Cells

First Messenger	Cell	Metabolic Response
Acetylcholine	Exocrine pancreas	Secretion of digestive enzymes
Acetylcholine	Salivary gland	Secretion of amylase
Acetylcholine	Pancreatic β-cells	Secretion of insulin
Angiotensin II	Adrenal glomerulosa, arteriole	Aldosterone production, arteriolar contraction
Norepinephrine	Liver	Glycogenolysis (α_1-adrenergic receptor)
Thrombin and serotonin	Blood platelets	Aggregation, cytokine secretion
Thyrotropin-releasing hormone	Thyrotropes	Secretion of thyroid-stimulating hormone
Vasopressin	Liver	Glycogenolysis (V_1 receptor)

kinases (I, II, and III) whose activity is stimulated by the calcium/calmodulin complex (Table 18–1). Moreover, the δ-subunit of phosphorylase kinase is calmodulin. Calcium/calmodulin also activates class I cyclic AMP phosphodiesterase (Table 19–3) and some forms of adenylyl cyclase. The interaction of two second messengers such as calcium and cyclic AMP, as described here, is called **cross talk.**

Besides its important role in signal transduction, calcium serves an important structural role in the body. Bone and teeth, which contain 99% of the total body calcium, consist of a deposit of calcium-phosphate as **hydroxyapatite** ($Ca_{10}(PO_4)_6(OH)_2$). The regulation of extracellular calcium is intricate and involves parathyroid hormone, calcitonin, and calcitriol. Parathyroid hormone and calcitriol action increases plasma calcium. Calcitonin decreases plasma calcium. Three organ systems that participate in calcium homoeostasis include intestine, kidney, and bone.

An important role of **calcitriol** in calcium metabolism is to stimulate intestinal absorption of calcium and phosphate. This hormone increases the synthesis of a calcium-binding protein called **calbindin** by increasing transcription of its gene in intestinal cells. Calcitriol increases calcium and phosphate reabsorption in the kidney. This hormone increases the synthesis of osteocalcin, the most abundant noncollagenous protein found in bone, by increasing its transcription in osteoblasts. **Osteocalcin** participates in bone mineralization. Osteocalcin contains γ-carboxyglutamate residues that are added by posttranslational modification involving vitamin K (Figure 18–20).

The conversion of 7-dehydrocholesterol to calcitriol, the active hormone, is illustrated in Figure 2–22. The last step of the pathway, C^1-hydroxylation, is rate-limiting. This reaction occurs in the proximal renal tubules and is under the control of parathyroid hormone and the cyclic AMP second messenger system.

Parathyroid hormone increases plasma calcium. Parathyroid hormone receptor, which occurs in osteoblasts and kidney, is a seven-transmembrane-segment receptor that activates adenylyl cyclase via G_s (Figure 19–10). Parathyroid hormone action leads to bone resorption. Osteoblasts, which produce bone, contain parathyroid hormone receptors. Osteoclasts, which resorb bone, lack the receptor. It is postulated that parathyroid hormone promotes the release of a local mediator from the osteoblast that stimulates the osteoclast to resorb bone. Parathyroid hormone also activates renal 1α-hydroxylase to increase calcitriol formation by cyclic AMP–dependent mechanisms. Low plasma calcium stimulates the release of parathyroid hormone.

Calcitonin decreases plasma calcium. It decreases bone and calcium resorption by inhibiting osteoclastic activity via the cyclic AMP second messenger system. High plasma calcium stimulates the release of calcitonin.

Alkaline phosphatase appears to participate in hydroxyapatite formation by generating phosphate by hydrolysis. ▶ Serum alkaline phosphatase levels are elevated in various bone diseases such as the invasion of bone by cancer (metastasis) and Paget disease of the bone. Serum alkaline phosphatase levels increase physiologically during skeletal growth in adolescence. A family of growth factors that sustain bone, cartilage, and dentin formation was discovered in the 1980s and called bone morphogenetic proteins. These are one example of a large family of growth and differentiation promoting agents that are undergoing tests in a variety of clinical situations. Because of their emerging importance, many of these are listed for reference in Table 20–5. The mechanism of signal transduction of several of these factors is considered later in this chapter. ◀

GLUCAGON

Glucagon promotes glycogenolysis, gluconeogenesis, and lipolysis. The glucagon receptor is a seven-transmembrane-segment protein that interacts with G_s and activates adenylyl cyclase. Glucagon and cyclic AMP increase gluconeogenesis in liver by increasing the transcription and synthesis of phosphoenolpyruvate carboxykinase, an important enzyme of gluconeogenesis (Chapter 10). Protein kinase A catalyzes the phosphorylation and inactivation of pyruvate kinase in liver. This phosphorylation decreases glycolysis while gluconeogenesis is activated. Glucagon activates hormone-sensitive lipase in adipose cells via the cyclic AMP second messenger system. Of all the first messengers listed in Table 20–3 that activate adenylyl cyclase, glucagon and epinephrine are the most helpful to commit to memory. The metabolic defects observed in diabetes mellitus are in large part related to the unopposed actions of glucagon (Chapter 25).

INSULIN, GROWTH FACTORS, AND PROTEIN PHOSPHORYLATION

Insulin binds to its plasma membrane receptor on target cells. The **insulin receptor** consists of two pairs of two subunits that are bound in β-α-α-β linkage by three disulfide bonds (Figure 20–2). The α-subunits are extracellular and bind insulin. The cytoplasmic domain of the β-subunit possesses protein-tyrosine kinase activity. The receptor for insulin-like growth factor–1 resembles that of insulin with two pairs of α- and β-subunits. In contrast, the receptors for epidermal growth factor (Figure 20–2) and nerve growth factor consist of a single polypeptide chain with an external domain, a single transmembrane segment, and an internal domain with protein-tyrosine kinase activity.

Insulin receptors are found in most human cells,

TABLE 20–5.   Selected First Messengers That Function as Growth and Differentiation Factors

Factor	Source	Function
Diverse Cell Types		
Acidic fibroblast growth factor	Brain, retina, kidney	Stimulates many cells
Basic fibroblast growth factor	Brain, liver, kidney, and many tumors	Stimulates many cells
Bone morphogenetic proteins 2A, 2B, and 3	Bone	Initiate bone and cartilage formation
Epidermal growth factor	Unclear	Stimulates proliferation of many cells
Platelet-derived growth factor	Platelets, endothelium, and glia	Stimulates cells of mesenchymal origin
Hematopoietic and Lymphoid Effectors		
Erythropoietin	Kidney and liver	Stimulates erythrocytosis
Granulocyte colony-stimulating factor	Multiple cell types	Stimulates granulocyte production
Granulocyte-macrophage colony-stimulating factor	Many cells	Stimulates macrophage and granulocyte production
Interferon-α	Macrophages	Induces proteins that inhibit viral and some tumor cell replication
Interferon-β	Fibroblasts	Induces proteins that inhibit viral and some tumor cell replication
Interferon-γ	T lymphocytes, macrophages	Induces proteins that inhibit viral replication
Interleukin-1α and β	Macrophages	Stimulates interleukin-6 synthesis, mediates inflammation
Interleukin-2	Activated T cells	Stimulates T and B lymphocytes
Interleukin-3	Activated T cells	Stimulates production of most hematopoietic cells
Interleukin-5	Activated T cells	Stimulates IgA production
Interleukin-6	T cells, macrophages, fibroblasts	Stimulates B cell differentiation and proliferation, stimulates hepatocytes
Interleukin-7	Bone marrow stromal cells	Stimulates B cell progenitors
Interleukin-8	Macrophages, endothelium	Stimulates neutrophils
Transforming growth factor-α	Macrophages	Stimulates proliferation of many cells Homologous to epidermal growth factor
Transforming growth factor-β	Platelets and many other cells	Stimulates some cells and inhibits others
Tumor necrosis factor-α	Macrophages	Inhibits tumors; pyrogenic; activates T cells
Nervous System Effectors		
Ciliary neurotropic factor	Uncertain	Promotes neuronal survival
Nerve growth factor	Uncertain	Promotes neuronal survival

even those not considered as traditional insulin target cells. The insulin receptor gene is located on the short arm of chromosome 19 (the insulin gene is on chromosome 11). The receptor, like insulin itself, is synthesized as a single-chain polypeptide in the rough endoplasmic reticulum. After formation of an intramolecular disulfide bond that will hold the two subunits together, the precursor polypeptide is cleaved to form α- and β-subunits. The connecting peptide of the insulin receptor is only four amino acids in length, much shorter than the 31-amino-acid connecting peptide of insulin (Figure 18–3). A disulfide bond forms between two α-chains to form the tetramer. One form of the insulin-receptor $\alpha\beta$ unit has 1370 amino acids. Alternative splicing adds 36 bases and produces a mature $\alpha\beta$ unit of 1382 amino acids. Both forms of receptor are expressed in all cells in about equal amounts. The significance of these two forms is uncertain. The insulin receptor undergoes constant turnover with a half-life of 7–12 hours. When insulin binds to its receptor, it activates protein-tyrosine kinase activity. The insulin cascade is intricate. Insulin promotes the phosphorylation of proteins that regulate intermediary metabolism, metabolite transport, and transcription of 60 or more genes.

Because insulin, other hormones, and growth factors operate through protein-tyrosine kinase signal transduction in a parallel fashion, we consider a general mechanism in detail. Signal transduction pathways that involve growth factors and protein-tyrosine kinases were studied in diverse organisms including yeast, fruit flies, worms, and mammals. The pathways and their components, which are remarkably similar in such diverse organisms, have led to a nomenclature that is daunting because names originating from one system were applied to others.

The Ras cycle participates in the insulin cascade. **Ras** is of a family of three proteins called H, K, and N (Harvey, Kirsten, and neural) that are encoded by genes on three different chromosomes. Ras, which consists of a single polypeptide chain with a molecular mass of 21 kDa, is a G-protein and possesses GTPase activity. The proteins exist in an active state with bound GTP and an inactive state with bound GDP. **GEF** (guanine nucleotide exchange factor; pronounced "gee ee eff") is required for the exchange of GTP for GDP to produce the activated state (Figure 20–3). **GAP** (GTPase activating protein; pronounced "gee aa pee") converts Ras from the on to the off state by accelerating the hydrolysis of GTP. Ras is a prominent par-

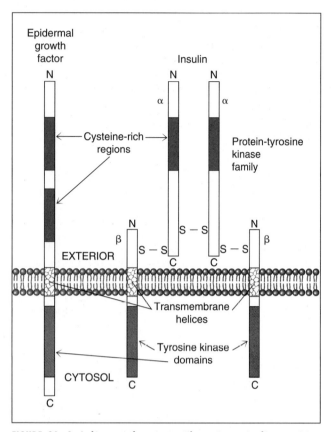

FIGURE 20-2. Architecture of receptors with protein-tyrosine kinase activity. C, carboxyl terminus; N, amino terminus.

thus mek is a dual-specificity protein kinase. Erk is a serine/threonine protein kinase that mediates the phosphorylation of transcription factors such as Jun and Fos, the *r*ibosomal small subunit protein *S*6 *k*inase (Rsk), and other proteins (Figure 20-4). (An alternative name for Erk is MAP kinase, where MAP represents mitogen-activated protein.) The Raf-Mek-Erk triad represents a protein kinase cascade that is downstream from Ras and is important in signal transduction. A **cascade** represents a series of regulatory reactions in which one enzyme acts on another in series.

Insulin stimulates glycogenesis in muscle, and this is antagonized by cyclic AMP that is generated in response to epinephrine. Insulin action promotes the dephosphorylation and activation of glycogen synthase and inactivation of glycogen phosphorylase. The dephosphorylation of these enzymes is catalyzed by the catalytic subunit (C) of phosphoprotein phosphatase-1, a serine/threonine phosphatase. Agents that activate the cyclic AMP second messenger system, such as epinephrine, promote the phosphorylation of glycogen synthase and glycogen phosphorylase (Figure 10-4). The antagonistic effects of cyclic AMP and the insulin protein-tyrosine kinase cascade are related to the phosphorylation of Raf (Figure 20-4) and the regulatory subunit of phosphoprotein phosphatase-1 (Figure 20-5).

Phosphoprotein phosphatase-1 is bound to gly-

ticipant in signal transduction in all nucleated cells. Moreover, mutant Ras proteins occur in about 20% of all human cancers (Chapter 21).

All known protein-tyrosine kinases undergo phosphorylation in their cytoplasmic domains in reactions catalyzed by the protein-tyrosine kinase; this process is called autophosphorylation. **Grb2** (*g*rowth factor *r*eceptor-*b*ound protein 2; pronounced "grab too") binds to the phosphorylated insulin receptor or to phosphorylated insulin receptor substrate-1 and becomes allosterically activated. Grb2 binds to proteins by an **SH2 domain** that specifically recognizes protein-tyrosine phosphate. SH2 is *s*rc *h*omology domain 2, first described in a protein-tyrosine kinase called Src (for sarcoma). Grb2 forms a complex with guanine nucleotide exchange factor or **GEF** via protein-proline binding **SH3 domain** to cause activation. Activated GEF interacts with and allosterically activates Ras by promoting the exchange of GTP for GDP (Figure 20-3).

Ras·GTP forms a complex with Raf, and Raf is allosterically activated. Raf is a protein-serine/threonine kinase that catalyses the phosphorylation of a threonine residue of **Mek,** thereby activating this enzyme. Mek also undergoes an intramolecular autophosphorylation on one of its tyrosine residues. Mek, in turn, catalyzes the phosphorylation of **Erk** (*e*xtracellular-signal *r*egulated *k*inase) on threonine and tyrosine residues, and

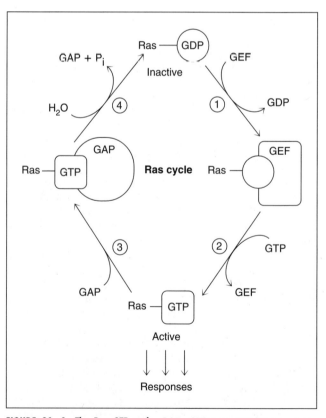

FIGURE 20-3. The Ras GTP cycle. GAP, GTPase activating protein; GEF, guanine nucleotide exchange factor.

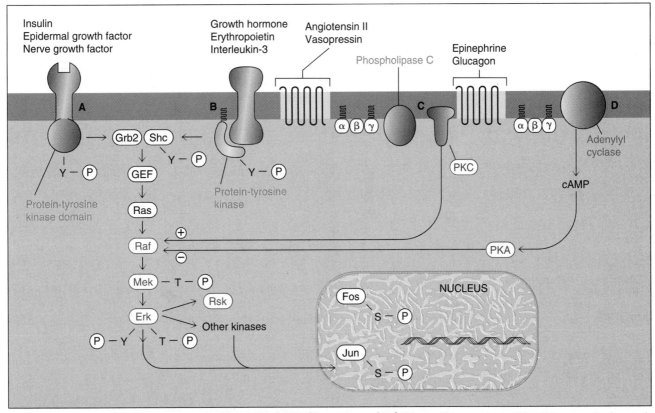

FIGURE 20–4. Overview of signal transduction involving protein-tyrosine kinases, Ras, and Raf. *The insulin receptor and insulin receptor substrate-1 activate Grb2 allosterically. Other protein-tyrosine kinases phosphorylate Shc, which activates Grb2. T, threonine; Y, tyrosine.*

cogen by a protein called **GBP** (for glycogen-binding protein, pronounced "gee bee pee"), the regulatory subunit. GBP contains two serine-acceptor phosphorylation sites. Phosphorylation of site 1, which activates phosphoprotein phosphatase–1, is catalyzed by insulin-stimulated ribosomal protein 6-kinase (Rsk, pronounced "risk"), an enzyme that is near the end of the insulin-activated cascade (Figure 20–4). As a result of Rsk-catalyzed phosphorylation, phosphatase–1 is activated (Figure 20–5) and glycogen synthase and phosphorylase are dephosphorylated. As a result of the overall process, insulin promotes glycogen synthesis.

Let us now consider the intricate mechanism of the epinephrine antagonism of insulin action. Protein kinase A, which is activated by the cascade initiated by epinephrine, catalyzes the phosphorylation of site 2 of GBP, the glycogen-binding protein. As a result, phosphoprotein phosphatase–1 dissociates from GBP and is inactivated (Figure 20–5). The activating effect of site 1 phosphorylation is abolished by site 2 phosphorylation. This results in the dissociation of C from GBP and glycogen and a decrease in glycogen synthase and phosphorylase dephosphorylation. Protein kinase A catalyzes the phosphorylation of sites 1 and 2 of the glycogen-binding protein; the resulting phosphatase is inactive. After adrenergic stimulation ceases, phosphoprotein phosphatase 2A catalyzes the dephosphorylation of site 2 and the formation of active phosphoprotein phosphatase–1.

A classic physiological effect of insulin is to increase the rate of glucose transport into muscle and adipocytes. This effect occurs within seconds after insulin binds to its receptor. Glucose transporters, which contain 12 transmembrane segments, have been studied by cDNA analysis. These are called GLUT1, GLUT2, GLUT3, GLUT4, GLUT5, GLUT6, and GLUT7, based upon the order of discovery (GLUT = *glucose transporter*). *GLUT4, which occurs in muscle and adipocytes, is insulin responsive.* GLUT4 occurs in the plasma membrane and in endocytosed plasma membrane vesicles. Following insulin stimulation and protein-tyrosine autophosphorylation, intracellular GLUT4 proteins are recruited to the plasma membrane and thereby increase the rate of glucose transport. Epinephrine and cyclic AMP attenuate the insulin-stimulatory effect. The GLUT4 transporter contains protein kinase A phosphorylation sites that account for this antagonistic effect.

Raf Protein Kinase Cascade

Insulin, epidermal growth factor, and nerve growth factor receptor protein-tyrosine kinases activate Ras and the Raf protein kinase cascade in their target cells. Still other mechanisms exist for activating the Raf cascade (Raf-Mek-Erk). For example, first messengers that lead to the activation of protein kinase C can activate the Raf cascade. Re-

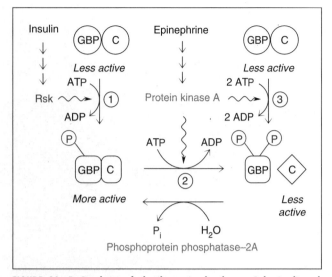

FIGURE 20–5. *Regulation of phosphoprotein phosphatase–1 by insulin and glucagon action. C, catalytic subunit of phosphoprotein phosphatase–1; GBP, glycogen-binding protein subunit of phosphoprotein phosphatase–1.*

ceptors that are linked to phospholipase C result in the generation of diglyceride and inositol trisphosphate. Diglyceride activates protein kinase C, which catalyzes Raf-serine phosphorylation and thereby activates Raf (Figure 20–4). This initiates signaling through the Raf-Mek-Erk cascade. The activation of Raf by Ras and by protein kinase C differs. Activation by Ras is produced allosterically and does not involve phosphorylation. Activation by protein kinase C involves covalent phosphorylation of Raf.

Protein-tyrosine kinases can activate this cascade by a process that bypasses Ras. Following the autophosphorylation of a protein-tyrosine kinase, phospholipase C$_\gamma$ binds to the phosphotyrosine by its SH2 domain; phospholipase C$_\gamma$ is activated following its phosphorylation at tyrosine. Phospholipase C$_\gamma$ catalyzes the generation of inositol trisphosphate and diglyceride and the activation of protein kinase C. Following the phosphorylation and activation of Raf by protein kinase C, the cascade is activated. The phospholipase C pathway provides a second mechanism for protein-tyrosine kinases to activate the Raf-Mek-Erk cascade.

Protein-tyrosine kinases also catalyze the phosphorylation of **phosphatidylinositol-3-kinase.** Phosphatidylinositol-3-kinase, which contains an SH2 domain, is an enzyme that catalyzes the phosphorylation of the 3-hydroxyl group of phosphatidylinositol 4,5-bisphosphate. This phosphorylation is distinct from the traditional phosphatidylinositol phosphate pathway that involves the 4- and 5-hydroxyl groups (Figure 12–7). The function of phosphatidylinositol 3,4,5-trisphosphate and its derivatives in signal transduction, however, is an enigma.

▶ People with diabetes mellitus were treated for 50 years with insulin extracted from the pancreas of pigs or cows. These hormones are effective in humans, but they differ slightly in primary structure from human insulin, and there is the possibility, observed occasionally, that the hormones are immunogenic and elicit an antibody response. To avoid this potential problem, genetic engineering was used to produce authentic human insulin in bacteria. The cDNAs corresponding to the A chain and B chain were expressed separately in *E. coli.* The chains were purified, combined, and oxidized to form disulfide bonds and the two-chain active form of insulin. Human insulin has supplanted the use of animal insulin in therapeutics in the United States. ◀

Cytokine Signal Transduction

Cytokines, which are listed in Table 20–5 for general reference, are proteins that regulate proliferation, differentiation, and functions of various cells. There are several varieties of growth factor, cytokine, and hormone receptors (Table 20–6). (1) The ligand-recognition protein possesses a transmembrane domain and an intracellular protein-tyrosine kinase intracellular domain. Examples include the epidermal growth factor and insulin receptors (Figure 20–2). (2) The transmembrane receptor, a single polypeptide, lacks an intracellular domain that has recognizable enzymatic activity. This class of receptor includes erythropoietin, granulocyte colony-stimulating factor, and growth hormone receptors for which signal transduction involves activation of membrane-associated intracellular protein-tyrosine kinases that do not form part of the receptor (nonreceptor protein-tyrosine kinases). (3) The receptor consists of two transmembrane proteins, which are required to produce a high-affinity binding site for the stimulatory ligand, with intracellular domains without enzymatic activity. Such receptors can activate nonreceptor protein-tyrosine kinases. Many of these receptors, including those for several interleukins, consist of a common subunit and a unique subunit. The common subunit may be responsible for transducing signals from different first messengers along a common pathway that produces a shared response. (4) Other receptors, such as the prototypical CD45 receptor of immune cells, are made of transmembrane proteins that possess extracellular ligand-binding domains and intracellular protein-tyrosine phosphatase activity, a receptor protein-tyrosine phosphatase (Figure 20–1). (5) Still other receptors, such as the transforming growth factor-β receptor, are transmembrane proteins that possess extracellular ligand-binding domains and intracellular protein-serine/threonine kinase activity, a receptor protein-serine/threonine kinase. (6) The receptor for atrial natriuretic peptide consists of an extracellular recognition domain, a single transmembrane segment, and an intracellular domain with guanylyl cyclase activity.

TABLE 20–6. Plasma-Membrane Receptor Signal Transduction Mechanisms

Class	Coupling Mechanism	Examples
G-protein receptor	Receptor couples with adenylyl cyclase, phospholipase C, or ion channel via G-protein	Glucagon, epinephrine, acetylcholine
Ion channel receptor	Ligand activates transmembrane ion channel	Acetylcholine (Na^+, nicotinic), GABA (Cl^-)
Receptor protein-tyrosine kinase	Cytoplasmic domain of receptor has protein-tyrosine kinase activity	Insulin, epidermal growth factor, platelet-derived growth factor
Nonreceptor protein-tyrosine kinase	Receptor couples with membrane-associated cytoplasmic protein-tyrosine kinase	Growth hormone, prolactin, interleukin-3, interleukin-5
Receptor protein-tyrosine phosphatase	Cytoplasmic domain of receptor has protein-tyrosine phosphatase activity	CD45 of immune cells
Receptor protein-serine/threonine kinase	Cytoplasmic domain of receptor has protein-serine/threonine kinase activity	Transforming growth factor-β, bone morphogenetic proteins
Receptor guanylate cyclase	Cytoplasmic domain of receptor has guanylate cyclase activity	Atrial natriuretic peptide

Receptor and Nonreceptor Protein-Tyrosine Kinases

Epidermal growth factor and its protein-tyrosine kinase receptor (Figure 20–2) have been extensively studied. After binding epidermal growth factor, two monomeric receptors form a dimeric complex to initiate signal transduction. The receptor undergoes autophosphorylation as one member of the dimer phosphorylates the other, and vice versa. Such ligand-induced receptor dimerization and protein-tyrosine phosphorylation are characteristic of several receptor protein-tyrosine kinases. Following epidermal growth factor receptor autophosphorylation, a protein called **Shc** (pronounced "schick") binds to receptor phosphotyrosines via SH2 domains. Shc is phosphorylated by the growth factor receptor protein-tyrosine kinase, and phosphorylated Shc binds to a proline-containing motif in Grb2 to initiate GEF and Ras activation. Shc and several other adaptor proteins contain SH2 and SH3 domains that recognize protein-tyrosine phosphate and protein-proline motifs, respectively.

Erythropoietin is a cytokine that interacts with red blood cell progenitors to promote differentiation. Its receptor is a single transmembrane protein that lacks protein-tyrosine kinase or other enzyme activity. The erythropoietin receptor activates a membrane-associated nonreceptor protein-tyrosine kinase called JAK2 (Janus kinase 2) to initiate signal transduction. JAK2 is also involved in growth hormone, prolactin, granulocyte colony-stimulating factor, granulocyte-macrophage colony-stimulating factor, interleukin-3, and interleukin-5 signal transduction. Events downstream from JAK activation include the phosphorylation of STAT (signal transducers and activators of transcription) proteins.

▶ Individuals with end-stage renal disease, who are deficient in erythropoietin, are often anemic. Erythropoietin is scarce and has never been purified from animal tissues in amounts adequate for therapeutic use. Because this cytokine is a glycoprotein, mature erythropoietin cannot be expressed in bacteria, since they lack the machinery to glycosylate proteins. Erythropoietin has been expressed in mammalian cells in culture and has been purified. This agent is used for the treatment of anemic individuals with end-stage renal disease and has decreased the need for transfusions. Erythropoietin infusion, used in tens of thousands of people in the United States, has dramatically improved their sense of well-being and quality of life.

Many of the growth and differentiation factors listed in Table 20–5 have been produced by recombinant DNA methods and are being tested in a variety of clinical conditions. For example, interleukin-2 and interferon-α have been used to treat a variety of cancers. Granulocyte and granulocyte-macrophage colony-stimulating factors are used to promote white blood cell production in individuals undergoing cancer chemotherapy. Bone morphogenetic factors have been used for promoting bone fracture healing and for regenerating bone in periodontal disease. Various cytokines are being tested in AIDS (an immunodeficiency) and arthritis (an inflammatory disease). ◀

The receptors for cytokines belong to several subfamilies. One subfamily of receptors, which corresponds to interleukin-3, interleukin-5, and granulocyte-macrophage colony-stimulating factor, consists of a cytokine-specific α-subunit and a common β-subunit. The α-subunits are single-transmembrane-segment glycoproteins of molecular mass of about 70 kDa with a short (50-amino-acid) cytoplasmic domain. The β-subunit is a single transmembrane segment glycoprotein of about 130 kDa and a large cytoplasmic domain without any known motif of signaling proteins. The α- and β-subunits are required to form a high-affinity cytokine binding site. The β-subunit is required for signal transduction. Another subfamily of receptors, which corresponds to interleukin-6 and ciliary neurotropic factor, possesses distinct α-subunits and a common β-subunit called gp130 (a glycoprotein of molecular mass of 130 kDa). Another subfamily of receptors, which corresponds to interleukin-2, consists of three subunits called α, β, and γ.

A large subfamily of cytokine receptors consists of one polypeptide with an external ligand-recognition domain, a transmembrane segment, and a cytosolic domain. The interleukin-8 receptor is in the seven-transmembrane-segment family of receptors that interact with G proteins that activate phospholipase C. Only experts know the detailed composition of these various receptors, and more information is anticipated. These receptors lack known enzyme activities.

Receptors that lack a recognizable catalytic intracellular domain are postulated to activate intracellular membrane–associated protein-tyrosine kinases. Whether other mechanisms are involved in their signal transduction, such as activation of membrane-associated protein-tyrosine phosphatase, remain to be established. The activated protein-tyrosine kinases may activate Ras, phospholipase C_γ, phosphatidylinositol-3-kinase, STAT, or other signaling pathways.

Protein Phosphatases

Protein phosphatases catalyze the exergonic hydrolysis of phosphate covalently attached to proteins. As a result of protein kinase and phosphatase action, phosphorylation-dephosphorylation is a reversible process that permits the cyclic activation and inactivation of protein function. **Protein-tyrosine phosphatases** are divided into three classes based upon their cellular location. Some of these enzymes consist of proteins with an extracellular recognition domain, a transmembrane segment, and an intracellular catalytic domain. The CD45 protein of immune cells is an example of a receptor protein-tyrosine phosphatase. Binding of appropriate ligand to the ectocellular domain activates cytosolic phosphatase activity. Another class of protein-tyrosine phosphatase is tethered to the interior of the plasma membrane and contains an intracellular catalytic domain. These phosphatases have the potential to be regulated by transmembrane receptors. The third class of protein-tyrosine phosphatases are cytosolic.

CD45 participates in the signal transduction process that follows antigenic activation of the T cell receptor for antigens. The CD45 protein family consists of several members that are all products of a single complex gene on chromosome 1. This gene codes for 34 exons, three of which are alternatively spliced, to generate up to eight different mRNAs and protein products. The ectocellular recognition domain contains between 400 and 500 residues, and the interior domain contains more than 700 amino acids, the largest interior domain identified among all integral membrane proteins.

CD45 participates in T cell activation and proliferation. The role of CD45, a phosphatase, is to activate a Src-like protein-tyrosine kinase called Lck (pronounced "lack"). When tyrosine-505 of Lck is autophosphorylated, its protein-tyrosine kinase activity for other substrates is abolished. CD45 catalyzes the dephosphorylation of tyrosine-505, thereby increasing protein-tyrosine kinase activity for protein substrates. Downstream events include activation of the transcription factor Fos, increased transcription of several cytokine genes, and cell proliferation. These events may result from the activation of the phospholipase C_γ and the Raf cascade as illustrated in Figure 20–4. The mechanism of CD45 illustrates a paradoxical strategy for signal transduction: a protein-tyrosine phosphatase stimulates a protein-tyrosine kinase.

Protein-serine/threonine phosphatases so far described are cytosolic enzymes. Protein-serine/threonine phosphatases are classified as type 1 or type 2 based upon their sensitivity to inhibition by protein phosphatase inhibitor–1 (Table 20–7. This inhibitor is a protein that is a substrate for protein kinase A and is active only in its phosphorylated form (Figure 10–14). The number of protein-tyrosine phosphatases greatly exceeds that of protein-serine/threonine phosphatases.

Besides the protein-tyrosine and protein-serine/threonine phosphatases, dual-specificity phosphatases exist. Human **HVH1 phosphoprotein phosphatase** is a dual-specificity protein phosphatase. It catalyzes the dephosphorylation of threonine and tyrosine residues in Erk. These threonine and tyrosine residues are phosphorylated by Mek, a dual-specificity protein kinase. Mek and HVH1 provide activities required for the interconversion of active and inactive Erk.

Receptor Protein-Serine/Threonine Kinases

Transforming growth factor-β receptors are transmembrane protein-serine/threonine kinases. The substrates for such protein kinases have not been determined. Bone morphogenetic proteins are members of the transforming growth factor-β family, and some of their receptors are homologous to transmembrane protein-serine/threonine kinases. This contrasts with protein kinase A, protein kinase G, and calcium/calmodulin-dependent protein kinases, which occur in the cytosol. Protein kinase C is a cytosolic protein that is activated at the plasma membrane. The nonactivated enzyme is

TABLE 20–7. Protein-Serine/Threonine Phosphatases

Enzyme	Inhibition by Phosphoprotein Phosphatase Inhibitor–1	Activated by Calcium/calmodulin
Phosphoprotein phosphatase–1	+	−
Phosphoprotein phosphatase–2A	−	−
Phosphoprotein phosphatase–2B	−	+
Phosphoprotein phosphatase–2C	−	−

soluble. Generation of diglyceride occurs at the interior of the plasma membrane where the active enzyme functions.

ATRIAL NATRIURETIC PEPTIDE

Atrial natriuretic peptide is synthesized, stored, and secreted by the atria. The heart is a nonclassical endocrine gland. Atrial natriuretic peptide promotes sodium and water excretion by the kidney and produces arteriolar muscle relaxation and vasodilatation. The receptor for atrial natriuretic peptide is a protein of about 1000 amino acid residues and one transmembrane segment. The ectocellular domain recognizes atrial natriuretic peptide, and *the intracellular domain of the atrial natriuretic peptide receptor possesses guanylyl cyclase activity* (Figure 20–1). The regulation of this membrane-associated guanylyl cyclase is controlled directly by the stimulatory ligand and does not involve G-proteins. The metabolism of cyclic GMP (Figure 19–24) and the activation of protein kinase G are considered in Chapter 19. Phosphorylation of proteins by protein kinase G leads to the physiological responses. The nature of the protein substrates responsible for the actions of atrial natriuretic peptide has not been elucidated.

RENIN AND ANGIOTENSIN

Angiotensin II and III Production

The renin-angiotensin system plays a pivotal role in the regulation of arterial pressure. The biosynthesis of angiotensin II and angiotensin III, the active forms of this hormone, is illustrated in Figure 3–14. **Angiotensinogen,** the prohormone, is synthesized by the liver and released into the circulation. Angiotensinogen contains more than 400 amino acids. **Renin,** a proteolytic enzyme with an active-site aspartate-like pepsin, is secreted into the circulation by the juxtaglomerular cells of the renal afferent arterioles. Renin is synthesized as an inactive proenzyme. Both prorenin (406 amino acids) and renin (340 amino acids) occur in the circulation at a ratio of 10/1. The mechanism for the conversion of prorenin to renin is unknown, and the function of circulating prorenin, if any, is obscure. Norepinephrine released from the postganglionic sympathetic fibers interacts with the juxtaglomerular cells of the kidney via a β_1-adrenergic receptor that activates adenylyl cyclase. Cyclic AMP promotes both renin transcription and release.

Renin catalyzes the hydrolytic cleavage of **angiotensin I,** a decapeptide, from angiotensinogen. Angiotensin I is converted to **angiotensin II,** an active octapeptide hormone, by an exergonic hydrolysis reaction that removes a dipeptide from the carboxyl end. The reaction is catalyzed by **angioten-sin converting enzyme** (ACE). Angiotensin converting enzyme, which is a protein containing 1278 amino acids and an ionic zinc cofactor, is found in endothelial cells throughout the circulation. Proline is one residue removed from the site of hydrolysis, and proline is a substrate specificity determinant. An amino peptidase catalyzes the hydrolytic removal of aspartate to yield **angiotensin III,** Angiotensin II and III are degraded by angiotensinases. Each of the hydrolysis reactions of angiotensin metabolism are exergonic (PRINCIPLE 5 OF BIOENERGETICS). Besides its function as a hormone, the renin-angiotensin system is operative in brain and plays a role in thirst. Angiotensin is thus a neuropeptide.

Hypertension

▶ Primary hypertension is a common malady of unknown etiology affecting tens of millions of people in the United States. Several classes of drugs are used in the treatment of hypertension, and the **ACE inhibitors** are one of the mainstays of therapy. **Captopril** and **enalapril** are two of many agents that are competitive inhibitors (Figure 4–6) of angiotensin converting enzyme (Figure 20–6). A serum esterase catalyzes the hydrolytic removal of the ethyl group from enalapril to produce enalaprilate, the active competitive inhibitor. Note that both drugs are proline derivatives. The prolyl group of the drug binds to that portion of the active site of angiotensin converting enzyme that ordinarily binds the prolyl group of angiotensin I. These agents decrease the proteolytic conversion of angiotensin I to angiotensin II.

Angiotensin II is a potent vasoconstrictor and promotes the formation of aldosterone. Aldosterone, a steroid hormone, promotes sodium retention. ACE inhibitors decrease peripheral vasoconstriction and decrease aldosterone synthesis. The fall in arterial pressure in hypertensive individuals treated with ACE inhibitors results chiefly from a decrease in peripheral vascular resistance. The ACE inhibitors are prescribed to millions of individuals for the treatment of hypertension and congestive heart failure.

Another major class of antihypertensive drug is the **β-adrenergic receptor blocker** such as acebutolol. It is likely that β-adrenergic receptor antagonists decrease arterial pressure by several mechanisms. These mechanisms include inhibition of renin release, a process that is mediated via β_1-adrenergic receptors. β-Blockers decrease arterial pressure by decreasing heart rate and cardiac output. **α-Adrenergic antagonists** such as doxazosin are used in the treatment of hypertension. α-Adrenergic antagonists are vasodilators that decrease peripheral vascular resistance and arterial pressure.

Another drug that acts by adrenergic mechanisms is **α-methyldopa.** This compound is metabo-

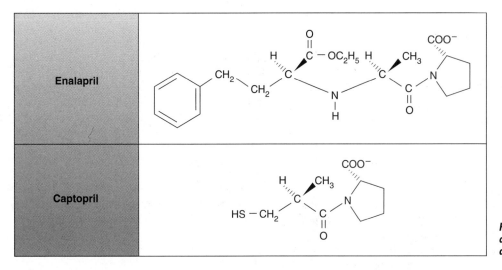

FIGURE 20–6. Captopril and enalapril, competitive inhibitors of angiotensin converting enzyme.

lized by tyrosine hydroxylase, aromatic amino acid decarboxylase, dopamine β-hydroxylase, and phenylethanolamine N-methyltransferase (Figure 19–5) to produce norepinephrine and epinephrine analogues in brain that attenuate the effects of sympathetic nervous system activity.

Calcium channel blockers are another group of drugs that are used to treat hypertension. Diltiazem and verapamil bind to and inhibit calcium channels throughout the cardiovascular system. These compounds, by decreasing the amount of calcium influx into arteriolar cells, relax smooth muscle and decrease peripheral vascular resistance. The calcium channel blockers are often effective in hypertensive individuals with low plasma renin levels.

Nitroglyccrin and **sodium nitroprusside** decompose in water to form nitric oxide. Nitric oxide operates via a cyclic GMP mechanism to produce vasodilation and to reduce arterial pressure. Nitric oxide initiates this process by activating the soluble form of guanylate cyclase (Chapter 19). Nitroglycerin and sodium nitroprusside are potent vasodilators and are used to relieve symptoms of cardiovascular disorders. Sodium nitroprusside injections are used to treat hypertensive crises. Nitroglycerin relieves the pain of angina pectoris by dilating coronary arteries. ◄

STEROID HORMONE ACTION

Steroid hormones play a vital role in growth, development, and regulation of metabolism (Table 20–8) and their structures are illustrated in Figure 12–31. Steroid hormones, in contrast to biogenic amines and peptide hormones, are synthesized and released on demand and are not stored in cells. Steroid hormones in the circulation are bound to transport glycoproteins that are synthesized by the liver. Four transport proteins have been characterized. **Corticosteroid-binding globulin** transports cortisol and progesterone. **Sex steroid hormone–**

binding globulin transports testosterone and estradiol. **Thyroid-binding globulin** transports thyroid hormone. **Vitamin D–binding globulin** binds to 25-hydroxycholecalciferol (a prohormone) with greater avidity than it binds to calcitriol (the hormone).

Steroid hormones, calcitriol, thyroid hormones (T_3 and T_4), and retinoate (retinoic acid) exert their physiological effects by altering gene expression. This process involves intracellular receptors that recognize these first messenger molecules. Two receptors have been described for thyroid hormone (α and β) and three for retinoic acid called RAR α, β, and γ. A second family of retinoate receptors, which bind 9-*cis* retinoate in preference to all-*trans* retinoate, have been described.

TABLE 20–8. Lipophilic First Messengers That Bind to Cytosolic/Nuclear Receptors

Class	Source	Action
Steroids		
Androgen	Testis	Sustains anabolism and male secondary sex characteristics
Estrogen	Ovary	Promotes uterine and breast growth and development; other anabolic effects on bone; increases serum HDL
Glucocorticoid	Adrenal	Stimulates gluconeogenesis; promotes catabolism
Mineralocorticoid	Adrenal	Promotes sodium reabsorption by the kidney
Progestin	Ovary	Promotes uterine growth and sustains female secondary sex characteristics
Vitamin D_3 (calcitriol)	Skin, liver, kidney	Induces calbindin synthesis in the gut and promotes calcium absorption
Nonsteroids		
Retinoate derivatives	Diet	Promote growth, differentiation, and epithelial homeostasis
Thyroid hormone (T_3 and T_4)	Thyroid	Promotes growth and development and many metabolic activities

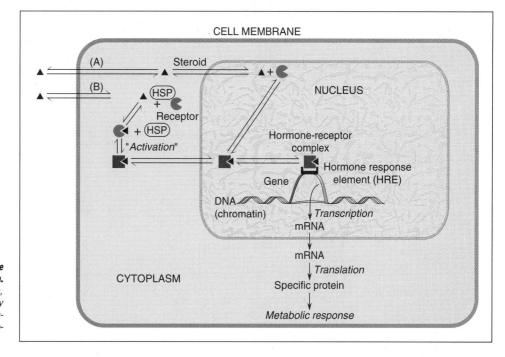

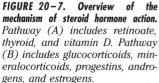

FIGURE 20–7. Overview of the mechanism of steroid hormone action. *Pathway (A) includes retinoate, thyroid, and vitamin D. Pathway (B) includes glucocorticoids, mineralocorticoids, progestins, androgens, and estrogens.*

Because the natural ligand was unknown, this second family of receptors was named RXR (retinoid X receptor). Target cells express receptors for one or more of these first messenger molecules. Nearly all nucleated human cells, for example, have receptors for glucocorticoids and thyroid hormone. In contrast, the distribution of the receptors for the other hormones is more restricted.

These lipophilic first messengers enter cells by diffusion. The hormones bind to their specific receptor in target cells. The retinoate, thyroid hormone, and vitamin D receptors are localized in the nucleus. The true steroid hormone receptors are localized initially in the cytosol. The cytosolic steroid hormone receptors bind heat shock proteins. Heat shock proteins are present in all nucleated cells under physiological conditions, but this fact is not reflected by their name, which instead reflects a property used in their discovery. These abundant proteins, which stabilize the free receptor, are released when the receptor binds its steroid hormone. **Heat shock proteins** are induced by various stresses including heat, and they have a variety of physiological functions. As chaperones, heat shock proteins assist protein folding and stabilization.

Following the interaction of the hormone with the receptor, the complex undergoes a conformational change (activation). Glucocorticoid, androgen, estrogen, aldosterone, and progesterone receptors, which bind hormone in the cytosol, are translocated into the nucleus.

Following activation, the receptor-hormone complexes dimerize and interact with specific sequences of DNA called **hormone response elements.** This interaction increases or decreases transcription of the target genes (Figure 20–7). For example, glucocorticoids enhance the transcription

of hepatic phosphoenolpyruvate carboxykinase (Figure 10–2) and tyrosine aminotransferase (Figure 13–24), enzymes that are gluconeogenic or that provide substrates for gluconeogenesis. Glucocorticoids also decrease transcription of osteocalcin gene expression in osteoblasts. ► This action in osteoblasts accounts in part for the demineralization of bone that occurs in Cushing disease (excessive production of glucocorticoids). ◄

The steroid hormone response elements consist of imperfect hexanucleotide palindromes separated by a spacer, provided as general information in Table 20–9. That several different classes of ster-

TABLE 20–9. The Steroid Superfamily of Receptors and the DNA Nucleotide Sequences of the Corresponding Hormone Response Elements

Extracellular Signal	Response Element (RE)	DNA Sequence
Steroids		
		←—— ——→
Androgen, glucocorticoid, mineralocorticoid, and progestin	GRE	GGTACA-NNN-TGTTCT
Estrogen	ERE	AGGTCA-NNN-TGACCT
Nonsteroids		
		←—— ——→
Retinoate (α, β, and γ)	RRE (β)	GTTCAC-NNNNN-GTTCAC
Thyroid hormone α	TRE (α)	AGGTCA-TGACCT
Thyroid hormone β	TRE (β)	GATCA-NNNNNN-TGACC
Vitamin D$_3$ (calcitriol)	DRE	GACTCA-TGAACG

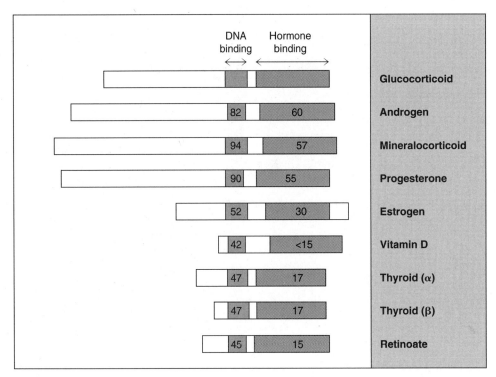

FIGURE 20–8. *Comparison of the steroid-thyroid superfamily of receptors. The numbers represent the percent amino acid identity with the glucocorticoid receptor.*

oid hormones possess the same regulatory element indicates that other factors are involved in determining specificity. Hormone response elements are generally upstream or 5′ to the promoter of a target gene. The hormone response elements modulate the frequency of transcription initiation. These effects may occur with variable positions relative to the start site, and they may occur with different orientations (from 5′ to 3′ and vice versa in different responsive genes). Hormone response elements resemble **enhancer elements** (increasing transcription) or **silencer elements** (decreasing transcription). Genes that are controlled by several hormones possess hormone response elements corresponding to each of the effective hormones. The activated hormone-receptor complex binds to hormone response elements with higher affinity than it binds to other regions of DNA.

We now consider the structure and domains of the various receptors in the steroid family. These receptors contain a hormone binding motif at the carboxyl terminus, an adjacent DNA-binding motif that binds to and recognizes the hormone responsive element, and a variable amino-terminal motif (Figure 20–8). The steroid hormone receptors each contain two classical zinc-finger motifs per polypeptide. Zinc fingers, which consist of two β-strands and an α-helix, are regions of a protein that consist of two cysteines and two histidines bound to zinc (Figure 3–23). These motifs, which are in the DNA-binding region of the receptor, interact with DNA. Part of the hormone-binding motif is involved also in receptor dimerization.

SUMMARY

Hydrophilic first messengers initiate signal transduction at the plasma membrane after binding to their receptor. First messengers often initiate the production of second messengers via G-protein interaction. These second messengers include cyclic AMP, cyclic GMP, diglyceride, inositol trisphosphate, and calcium. Hydrophilic first messengers also activate protein-tyrosine kinase, protein-tyrosine phosphatase, and protein-serine/threonine kinase activities. Signal transduction generally involves a cascade of reactions involving networks of components. The interaction of one signal transduction system with another involves cross talk. Lipophilic first messengers enter the cell and initiate signal transduction after interacting with an intracellular receptor that acts as a transcription factor.

Hypothalamic peptide hormones regulate the secretion of target hormones in the anterior pituitary. Growth hormone is secreted by the anterior pituitary. This hormone promotes the production of somatomedins (insulin-like growth factors–1 and –2) by the liver, and insulin-like growth factor-1 action is responsible for postnatal skeletal growth. ACTH stimulates glucocorticoid production in the adrenal cortex via a cyclic AMP mechanism. The glycoprotein hormones of the anterior pituitary, which consist of thyroid-stimulating hormone, follicle-stimulating hormone, and luteinizing hormone, are made of common α-subunits and distinct β-subunits. These hormones also act by cyclic AMP signal transduction.

The regulation of extracellular calcium is intricate and involves parathyroid hormone, calcitonin, and calcitriol. Parathyroid hormone and calcitriol action increase plasma calcium, and calcitonin decreases plasma calcium. The absorption of calcium from the intestine is regulated by calcitriol, and its role is controlling the level of calbindin. Parathyroid hormone acts on its target cells (osteoblasts and kidney) by increasing cyclic AMP production.

Glucagon and insulin have many antagonistic effects. Glucagon, which has a seven-transmembrane-segment receptor, operates through a cyclic AMP system via G-proteins. Insulin's receptor, in contrast, contains two α-subunits (exterior) and two transmembrane β-subunits. The β-subunits possess protein-tyrosine kinase activity. Insulin and other hormones and growth factors activate Ras. Grb2 and GEF are involved in Ras activation. Ras is a G-protein. Ras activates a Raf-Mek-Erk protein kinase cascade. Mek is a dual-specificity protein kinase that phosphorylates threonine and tyrosine residues of Erk. HVH1 is a dual-specificity protein-threonine and protein-tyrosine phosphatase that acts on Erk. Protein kinase A catalyzes the phosphorylation and inactivation of Raf.

Several hormones (growth hormone, prolactin) and cytokines (interleukins-3 and -5) possess receptors that interact with intracellular nonreceptor protein-tyrosine kinases. The transforming growth factor-β receptor is a protein-serine/threonine kinase. CD45, an immune cell receptor, is a transmembrane protein with an external ligand recognition domain and a cytosolic protein-tyrosine phosphatase domain. The receptor for atrial natriuretic peptide is a transmembrane protein with an external ligand recognition domain and a cytosolic guanylyl cyclase domain.

Prorenin and renin are released from juxtaglomerular cells following stimulation of the β_1-adrenergic receptor by norepinephrine. Renin, a proteolytic enzyme, catalyzes the hydrolysis of angiotensinogen to produce angiotensin I, a decapeptide. ACE catalyzes the hydrolysis of angiotensin I, which is inactive, to angiotensin II. A peptidase catalyzes the conversion of angiotensin II to angiotensin III. ACE inhibitors are widely used in the treatment of hypertension.

The steroid hormone family of first messenger molecules acts by altering gene expression. These hormones include the steroid hormones, calcitriol, thyroid hormones (T_3 and T_4), and retinoate. These hormones possess intracellular receptors. Following the formation of the hormone-receptor complex, the activated receptor alters the transcription of target genes. These genes contain hormone response elements that are recognized by the hormone-receptor complex. The true steroid hormone receptors are located initially in the cytosol; receptors for the other hormones of this family (thyroid hormone, retinoate, and vitamin D) are located in the nucleus. Each receptor possesses a ligand-recognition motif, a DNA-zinc-finger binding motif, and a variable motif. The receptor binds to DNA as a dimer.

SELECTED READINGS

Brown, E.M. Extracellular Ca²⁺ sensing, regulation of parathyroid cell function, and the role of Ca²⁺ and other ions as extracellular (first) messengers. Physiological Reviews 71:371–411, 1991.

Chinkers, M., and D.L. Garbers. Signal transduction by guanylyl cyclases. Annual Review of Biochemistry 60:553–575, 1991.

D'Andrea, A.D. Cytokine receptors in congenital hematopoietic disease. New England Journal of Medicine 330:839–846, 1994.

Egan S.E., and R.A. Weinberg. The pathway to signal achievement. Nature 365:781–783, 1993.

Kelly, P.A., S. Ali, M. Rozakis, L. Goujon, M. Nagano, I. Pellegrini, D. Gould, J. Djiane, M. Edery, J. Finidori, and B.C. Postel-Vinay. The growth hormone/prolactin receptor family. Recent Progress in Hormone Research 48:123–164, 1993.

Wilson, J.D. and D.W. Foster (eds.). *Williams Textbook of Endocrinology,* 8th ed. Philadelphia, W.B. Saunders Company, 1992.

CHAPTER TWENTY-ONE

CANCER, ONCOGENES, AND TUMOR SUPPRESSOR GENES

Tumors destroy man in a unique and appalling way, as flesh of his own flesh, which had somehow been rendered proliferative, rampant, predatory and ungovernable.

—PEYTON ROUS

Discovery is our business.

—CHARLES B. HUGGINS

Cancer is a disease characterized by uncontrolled cell proliferation. Of the more than 100 types of cancer, those of the lung, breast, and colorectum account for 44% of all forms of new cases per year in the United States (Table 21–1). Lung cancer, which is highly correlated with cigarette smoking, is responsible for more deaths than any other form of cancer. Cigarette smoking and other environmental factors, moreover, are associated with the majority of cancers. Major advances in molecular medicine, which are described in this chapter, have shed light on the pathogenesis of cancer at the biochemical level.

Let us define a few fundamental terms. A **tumor** is a swelling or mass. Tumors are divided into two categories based upon the potential to spread. **Benign tumors** are localized and lack the capability to invade adjacent tissue or to **metastasize** (spread) to other locations in the body. **Malignant tumors** have the capacity to invade adjacent tissue and to metastasize to other locations in the body. Surgical removal of a malignant tumor, if performed early, can prevent metastasis. Such tumors, if left in place, will eventually invade, metastasize, and kill the host. The term cancer, which implies malignancy, is derived from Greek *karkinos,* which means crab. A **neoplasm** is a new growth. Neoplasia, a general term, refers to benign and malignant tumors, leukemias, and lymphomas.

▶ Benign tumors, if they are removed, are usually nonlethal. Mature brain cells and heart cells are terminally differentiated and do not divide. Moreover, tumors that are derived from brain or heart cells are rarely, if ever, malignant and do not metastasize. Brain tumors that are benign can be lethal, however, if they are in a critical location and cannot be removed. ◀ The inherent inability of neuronal and myocardial cells to divide probably limits their ability to form malignant neoplasms.

Cancers are classified according to the tissue and cell type from which they arise. **Carcinomas** are cancers that arise from the epithelial tissue of the ectoderm or endoderm. **Sarcomas** are cancers that arise from the mesoderm. **Leukemias** and **lymphomas,** which arise from mesoderm, are usually classified separately from sarcomas because of their distinctive clinical courses. Acute denotes sudden onset of symptoms; chronic denotes gradual onset. A glossary of terms used in this chapter appears in Box 21–1.

The development of cancer is a multistep process, and the probability of developing cancer increases with age. Fewer than 8000 cancers of the 1 million cases diagnosed yearly in the United States occur in children. Cancer, however, is responsible for 10% of children's deaths. Leukemias and lymphomas account for about half of all childhood cancers. Acute lymphocytic leukemia, the most common childhood cancer, was fatal in 95% of affected children in 1960. Because of major advances in chemotherapy, up to 75% of children with acute lymphocytic leukemia are now cured.

BIOCHEMISTRY OF CANCER CELLS

The essential changes that transform normal cells into cancer cells are due primarily to somatic cell mutations. *Several somatic mutations are required to produce cancer, and this concept is called the multistage theory of carcinogenesis.* These mutations involve the production of growth-promoting cellular oncogenes (cancer-causing genes) and the inactivation of tumor suppressor genes (Figure 21–1). Between two and seven somatic cell mutations are required for the initiation and progression of various malignant neoplasms. Cancer begins when a single cell begins to proliferate abnormally. The neoplasm, derived from a single cell, is a clone. This altered cell divides to form two abnormally proliferating cells, which in turn divide, and so on. Additional somatic cell mutations in the progeny cells can produce more aggressive and rapidly proliferating cells (progression).

Otto Warburg, a physician and student of Emil Fischer, observed that nearly every type of cancer cell that forms a solid tumor produces more lactate than its normal counterpart. This increased production of lactate is called the Warburg effect. Warburg's most celebrated student, Hans Krebs, also a physician, performed some of these experiments on anaerobic glycolysis in neoplastic cells. Tumor cells contain a fetal form of phosphofructokinase that is insensitive to inhibition by ATP and citrate, and this accounts for their increased lactate production.

Neoplastic cells secrete angiogenesis factors that stimulate the development of blood vessels to supply the tumor. Basic fibroblast growth factor (Table 20–5), which stimulates endothelial cell proliferation, is one angiogenesis factor produced by tumors. Tumors produce metalloproteases and collagenases that facilitate the invasion of adjacent

TABLE 21–1. Cancer Incidence and Mortality in the United States*

Cancer Site	New Cases per Year	Mortality (Deaths per Year)
Lung	157,000 (15%)	142,000 (28%)
Colorectum	155,000 (15%)	61,000 (12%)
Breast	151,000 (14%)	44,000 (9%)
Prostate	106,000 (10%)	30,000 (6%)
Bladder	49,000 (5%)	10,000 (2%)
Uterus	47,000 (5%)	10,000 (2%)
Lymphomas	43,000 (4%)	20,000 (4%)
Oral cavity	31,000 (3%)	8,000 (2%)
Pancreas	28,000 (3%)	25,000 (5%)
Leukemias	28,000 (3%)	18,000 (4%)
Skin	28,000 (3%)	9,000 (2%)

*Data from American Cancer Society, *Cancer Facts and Figures,* 1990. Nonmelanoma skin cancers (about 600,000 cases per year) and carcinomas of the uterine cervix diagnosed *in situ* (about 50,000 cases per year) are excluded from incidence data.

BOX 21-1　GLOSSARY OF SOME TERMS USED IN DESCRIBING CANCERS

abl: A gene that encodes a protein-tyrosine kinase and is translocated in chronic myelogenous leukemia.

Adenocarcinoma: A malignant tumor arising from glandular epithelium.

Adenoma: A benign tumor arising from glandular epithelium.

Aflatoxin B_1: A potent liver carcinogen found in contaminated peanuts and grains.

Alkylating agents: Compounds that form covalent bonds with biological molecules such as DNA.

Aneuploidy: An abnormal number of chromosomes.

Apoptosis: A particular type of cell death that differs from anoxic cell death.

*bcl*2: A gene translocated in follicular B cell lymphomas that inhibits programmed cell death.

Benign tumor: A tumor that remains confined to its original location and does not invade adjacent tissue or metastasize to distant body sites.

Burkitt lymphoma: A non-Hodgkin B cell lymphoma associated with Epstein-Barr virus infection and translocation of the c-*myc* gene.

Cancer: A malignant tumor.

Carcinogen: A cancer-inducing agent.

Carcinoma: A malignant tumor of epithelial cells.

Cellular oncogene: An oncogene formed by mutation, rearrangement, or excessive expression of a protooncogene owing to dysregulation or increased gene copy number.

Hodgkin disease: A type of lymphoma.

Leukemia: A general term for malignant proliferation of leukocytes.

Lymphoma: A general term for malignant proliferation of lymph and reticuloendothelial cells.

Malignant tumor: A tumor that is capable of invading surrounding normal tissue and metastasizing to distant body sites.

Melanoma: A cancer of the pigment-producing cells of the skin.

Metastasis: Spread of cancer cells to distant body parts.

Neoplasm: An abnormal growth of cells.

Oncogene: A gene capable of producing one or more characteristics of cancer cells.

Papilloma: A tumor projecting from an epithelial surface.

Papillomaviruses: A family of tumor viruses that induce papillomas and carcinomas.

Philadelphia chromosome: An abbreviated human chromosome 22 formed by translocation of *abl* from chromosome 9; occurs in chronic myelogenous leukemias.

Polyp: A tumor projecting from an epithelial surface.

Protooncogene: A normal cellular gene, usually associated with growth and cell division, that can convert to an oncogene.

Retinoblastoma: A childhood eye tumor.

Rhabdomyosarcoma: A neoplasm of skeletal muscle cells.

Rous sarcoma virus: A transforming retrovirus in which the first oncogene was identified.

Sarcoma: A neoplasm of mesodermal tissue.

Squamous cell carcinoma: A cancer of flat epithelial cells.

Tumor suppressor gene: A gene that inhibits tumor development.

Tumor virus: A virus that induces neoplasia.

Viral oncogene: An oncogene present in a tumor virus.

Wilms tumor: A childhood kidney cancer.

---

structures. The digestion of collagen and the basement membrane facilitates the invasion of lymphatics and capillaries and the metastasis of tumors to distant sites. ▶ Specific types of tumors metastasize to characteristic tissues or organs. Prostate cancer, for example, characteristically spreads to bone. Elevation of serum acid phosphatase (from neoplastic prostate cells) and alkaline phosphatase (from bone) occurs in this disorder. Breast and lung cancers commonly metastasize to brain. Sometimes the symptoms produced by the metastatic lesion are the first indication that a malignancy has developed. The first indication of a metastatic brain tumor, for example, might be a seizure or a change in personality. ◀

The immune system plays a primary role in the body's defense against malignancy. Although a tumor is derived from the body's own cells and is expected to possess proteins that are recognized as self and nonantigenic, neoplastic cells can express antigens that are not recognized as self. These cells can often be eliminated by the immune system. ▶ One experimental treatment strategy for cancer is the administration of agents that stimulate the immune system, such as interleukin-2 (Table 20–5). Evidence that the normal immune system plays a crucial role in eliminating cancer-

ous cells is that individuals who are immunocompromised have a much greater incidence of malignancy than those with normal immune systems. Immunosuppression can result from AIDS or immunosuppressive drugs that are administered to organ transplant recipients. ◀

CARCINOGEN METABOLISM

Chemical carcinogens are compounds that produce cancer. Carcinogens are found in tobacco smoke, food contaminants, and solvents used in industry and manufacturing (Figure 21–2). Aflatoxin B_1 is produced by certain strains of the mold *Aspergillus flavus* that have contaminated peanuts and grains. This contamination, which is favored in hot and moist climates, occurs predominantly in Africa and Asia. Dietary components, especially in the presence of high concentrations of nitrite (NO_2^{1-}), may yield low levels of nitrosamines. Carcinogenic nitrosamines also occur in tobacco smoke. Nitrosonornicotine, for example, is derived from nicotine (Figure 21–2).

Chemical carcinogens are **direct** or **indirect acting.** The direct-acting carcinogens react with nucleophilic groups in nucleic acids. The indirect-

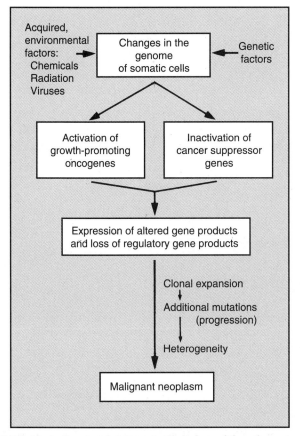

FIGURE 21–1. *Flow chart depicting a simplified scheme of the pathogenesis of* **cancer.** *Reproduced, with permission, from R.S. Cotran, V. Kumar, and S.L. Robbins (eds.).* Robbins Pathologic Basis of Disease, *5th ed. Philadelphia, W.B. Saunders Company, 1995, p. 258.*

acting carcinogens must be metabolized to **ultimate carcinogens.** Examples of indirect-acting carcinogens are polycyclic aromatic hydrocarbons (benzo[*a*]pyrene, aflatoxin B_1) and amines.

The process for converting the indirect-acting agents to the ultimate carcinogen involves oxidations catalyzed by the cytochrome P-450 electron transport system (Table 1–1). The first step in the conversion of benzo[*a*]pyrene to the direct carcinogen involves a reaction of the aromatic compound with molecular oxygen and NADPH to produce an epoxide, $NADP^+$, and water. The oxidation of organic compounds by molecular oxygen is exergonic (PRINCIPLE 8 OF BIOENERGETICS). Water adds to the epoxide to produce a diol. Most of the diols that are formed are chemically nonreactive and harmless, such as the 4,5-diol (Figure 21–3). Diols react with UDP~glucuronate, and the resulting glucuronides are excreted in the urine. The 7,8-diol undergoes a second cytochrome P-450–mediated epoxidation to produce an ultimate carcinogen (Figure 21–3). The epoxide oxygen makes the attached carbon electrophilic, which promotes the formation of a covalent bond with nucleic acids. The amino group of guanine is especially reactive in this process. Such modifications lead to base substitutions during DNA replication and to breaks in the DNA backbone that can produce more extensive genetic rearrangements.

This knowledge of the requirement for oxidative metabolism was used in the development of the Ames test for carcinogens (named for Bruce Ames, the originator). Each test compound is first incubated with a liver extract that contains the components of the cytochrome P-450 oxidation system. This mixture is incorporated into a histidine-free medium that is inoculated with a strain of *Salmonella* with a mutation in the locus that encodes the enzymes of the pathway for histidine biosynthesis. These bacteria are ordinarily unable to grow on histidine-free media. Revertants that result from the action of mutagenic agents, however, are able to produce colonies on histidine-free media. Essentially all known carcinogens are revealed as mutagens in this test. All carcinogens are mutagens, but not all mutagens are carcinogens. If the result of the Ames test is positive and a compound acts as a mutagen, then the compound can be subjected to more extensive testing to determine whether it is a carcinogen.

Chemicals such as dimethylnitrosamine alone are effective carcinogens. Other chemicals, however, require auxiliary agents to augment their carcinogenicity. For example, if mouse skin is painted with benzo[*a*]pyrene, only a few tumors develop even with multiple treatments. If a single exposure to benzo[*a*]pyrene is followed by multiple applications of phorbol myristoyl acetate, which is not a carcinogen, tumors will develop. Benzo[*a*]pyrene is called an **initiator,** and the phorbol ester is called a **tumor promoter.** Tumor promoters are not mutagens, and they fail to produce tumors alone. Tumor promoters are compounds that are required to induce a neoplasm following the application of a tumor initiator. The development of tumors in humans can involve the participation of multiple agents, and this intricacy can confound the study of the mechanism of neoplastic transformation and epidemiological studies.

Tumor promoters alter gene expression and stimulate cell division. The action of phorbol esters is mediated by the activation of protein kinase C. Phorbol esters resemble diglyceride (Figure 21–4) and activate protein kinase C. Protein kinase C can activate the Raf-Mek-Erk cascade. This cascade is activated by growth factors that lead to cell proliferation (Figure 20–4). Increased activity of this signal transduction pathway provides a mechanism for the action of phorbol ester as a tumor promoter.

CAUSES OF HUMAN NEOPLASIA

Environmental Factors

▶ There is great variation in the incidence of various cancers throughout the world. When people migrate to a new locale, they usually acquire the cancer incidence profile of the population at their new home within a generation. Thus, the en-

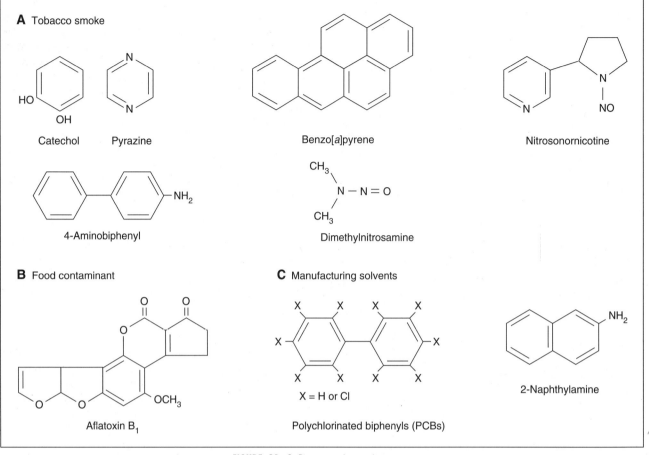

A Tobacco smoke

Catechol   Pyrazine

Benzo[a]pyrene

Nitrosonornicotine

4-Aminobiphenyl

Dimethylnitrosamine

B Food contaminant

Aflatoxin B$_1$

C Manufacturing solvents

X = H or Cl

Polychlorinated biphenyls (PCBs)

2-Naphthylamine

FIGURE 21–2. Representative carcinogens.

vironment can play a major role in the pathogenesis of malignant transformation.

Polycyclic hydrocarbons are implicated in the causation of human lung and skin cancers. Tobacco smoke is the predominant cause of cancer mortality in the United States and many other nations, and tobacco smoke contains several carcinogens, including polycyclic hydrocarbons. Perhaps a third of all cancer deaths in the United States are directly attributable to tobacco use, and this is the largest single preventable cause of cancer. The risk of lung cancer rises in proportion to the duration and amount of tobacco smoked. Cigarette smoking also increases the risk of other cancers, including those of the oral cavity, pharynx, esophagus, larynx, bladder, stomach, and uterine cervix.

Occupational exposures have long been recognized as causes of cancer. One of the most celebrated correlations was made by Percival Pott, a London physician, in 1775. He reported that scrotal cancer occurred with increased incidence in young men who, as children, worked as chimney sweeps. Carcinogens occurred in the soot that accumulated in the scrotal folds. Protective clothing and regular bathing resulted in a marked decline in the incidence of this cancer. Medicinal agents are also carcinogens. Many drugs that are used in cancer chemotherapy are mutagenic and can produce cancer, particularly leukemia.

Ionizing radiation from radioactive chemicals and

x-rays can produce cancer in humans. Leukemia can occur several years after exposure to high levels of radioactivity emanating from nuclear bombs or from major radioactive spills from nuclear power generators. High energy x-rays and γ-rays produce point mutations (a change in a single nucleotide) and chromosome breaks. Chromosome breaks can lead to large deletions of DNA. Reactive oxygen intermediates such as hydroxyl free radicals (Figure 5–4) are generated by the action of ionizing radiation, and these are thought to produce the observed chromosomal fragmentation and mutation.

Cancer risk increases in proportion to the radiation dose. Ultraviolet irradiation from sunlight is the major cause of skin carcinomas and melanomas, and the incidence increases with greater exposure. We note in Chapter 2 that radioiodine is used for the treatment of hyperthyroidism. The risks are low enough that this treatment can be used in people of childbearing age, but this medical decision was the result of painstaking efforts on the part on many experts. ◄

DNA Viruses

Both DNA and RNA viruses can produce tumors. DNA tumor viruses cause cell transformation by altering the types of proteins made in the cell.

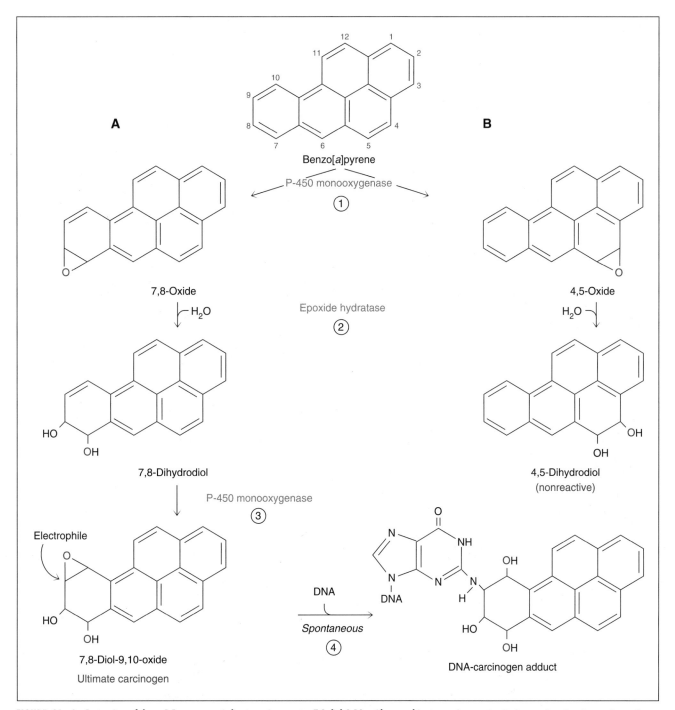

FIGURE 21–3. Conversion of benzo[a]pyrene, an indirect carcinogen, to 7,8-diol-9,10-oxide, an ultimate carcinogen. A. *Pathway for the formation of an ultimate carcinogen.* B. *Pathway for the formation of a noncarcinogenic metabolite.*

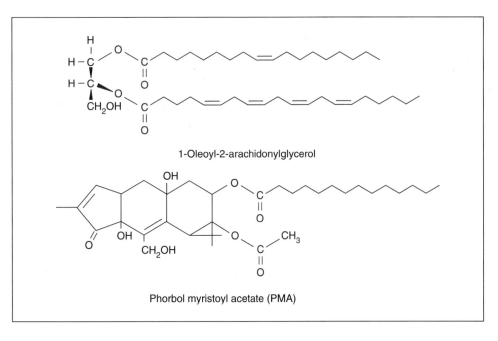

1-Oleoyl-2-arachidonylglycerol

Phorbol myristoyl acetate (PMA)

FIGURE 21–4. Comparison of diglyceride and phorbol myristoyl acetate, a tumor promoter. *Both compounds activate protein kinase C.*

Tumor viruses carry discrete genetic elements, called oncogenes, that are responsible for the virus's ability to transform cells. An oncogene (Greek *onkos,* "tumor") is a gene whose product leads to neoplasia.

How the oncogenes of viral DNAs produce the transformed cancerous state is still a mystery. One idea is that viral oncoproteins bind to tumor suppressors such as RB1 (named originally for retinoblastoma). By complexing with and inactivating a tumor suppressor, loss of negative regulators of cell proliferation contributes to the development of the neoplastic state.

▶ Epstein-Barr virus is a herpes-like DNA virus (Table 1–4) that produces two types of neoplasms in humans including Burkitt lymphoma (common in certain parts of Africa), a primary cancer in children, and nasopharyngeal carcinoma (common in southern China). In the United States, Epstein-Barr virus produces infectious mononucleosis in adolescents and young adults. It leads to cancer rarely in the United States, and then only in individuals who are immunocompromised. This suggests that infection by Epstein-Barr virus is only one of several steps required to produce malignant transformation.

Hepatitis B virus, which is responsible for serum hepatitis, is the most common virus linked to cancer in the United States. Hepatitis B virus, a DNA virus, is associated with liver cancers (hepatomas) and is responsible for 500,000 cancer deaths worldwide per year. The primary hepatitis B infection occurs about 25 years before the liver cell malignancy becomes manifest. Most hepatitis B virus carriers, however, never develop hepatomas. Although the virus has a DNA genome, it goes through an RNA intermediate like a retrovirus. The mechanism of malignant transformation produced by hepatitis B is unknown, although the usual suspects for malignant transformation have been examined.

Two papillomaviruses, which are DNA viruses that produce cutaneous warts, are associated with more than 80% of all invasive human cervical carcinomas (Table 21–2). Papillomaviruses replicate as extrachromosomal circular DNA in human cells. ◀

RNA Viruses

The first tumorigenic virus was discovered by Peyton Rous early in the 20th century. Rous sarcoma virus produces sarcomas in chickens. The virus also transforms cells of other species in cell culture. This virus uses RNA as the genome, and it is a retrovirus with a DNA intermediate that integrates into the host genome as a provirus (Figure

TABLE 21–2. Viruses Associated with Human Cancers

Virus	Type of Cancer
DNA Viruses	
Hepatitis B	Hepatocellular carcinoma
Human papillomaviruses	Cervical carcinoma, squamous cell skin carcinoma
Epstein-Barr virus*	Burkitt lymphoma and other B cell lymphomas, nasopharyngeal carcinomas
RNA Retroviruses	
Human T cell lymphotropic virus (HTLV-1)	Adult T cell leukemia
Human immunodeficiency virus† (HIV-1 and HIV-2)	Kaposi sarcoma, lymphomas

*Rarely a causative agent of the corresponding disorders in the United States.

†Immunosuppression allows neoplasm to develop.

16–33). The *src* (pronounced "sark") oncogene of Rous sarcoma virus encodes a protein-tyrosine kinase. Moreover, this was the first protein-tyrosine kinase to be discovered. The insulin and epidermal growth factor receptors possess protein-tyrosine kinase activity (Table 20–6). Insulin, epidermal growth factor, other growth factors, and oncogenes can stimulate cell proliferation.

The *src*-gene protein kinase leads to the phosphorylation of several proteins in transformed cells. These include enzymes of the glycolytic pathway such as enolase, phosphoglycerate mutase, and lactate dehydrogenase. These enzymes are easy to identify because they are abundant cellular proteins. Their activities, however, are unchanged in cells transformed with Rous sarcoma virus, and phosphorylation of these proteins may be adventitious and related neither to the pathogenesis of malignant transformation nor to the Warburg effect. A more plausible mechanism of action of *src*-gene protein kinase involves the activation of the Raf-Mek-Erk cascade to stimulate proliferation (Figure 20–4).

The *src*-gene protein kinase catalyzes the phosphorylation of vinculin, a cytoskeletal protein. Vinculin connects actin, a contractile protein, with the plasma membrane. In transformed or neoplastic cells, vinculin is distributed diffusely throughout the cell. Phosphorylation of vinculin by the *src*-gene protein kinase influences the distribution of vinculin in the transformed state, and this might produce the altered cell morphology characteristic of neoplastic cells.

Oncogenes are often named with a three-letter italic designation. For example, *src* is an oncogene that produced *sarc*omas in chickens. The corresponding gene product or protein (Src) is designated by the same three letters in Roman type beginning with a capital letter. Members of a related family of oncogenes may be given letters or numbers to distinguish between them. There are many examples of investigators cloning the same gene in apparently unrelated research projects, each naming the gene for an important characteristic and deriving a three-letter designation. This has generated a daunting nomenclature. The *erb*B2 and *neu* genes, for example, are the same gene. The viral form of an oncogene is labeled with the prefix "v" as in v-*src* (pronounced "vee-sark"). Viral oncogenes are not involved in virus replication, only in malignant transformation. The oncogenes from retroviruses were derived from normal cellular genes or protooncogenes. *Protooncogenes, despite their ominous-sounding name, are normal genes that participate in physiological processes.*

Cellular protooncogenes are highly conserved in evolution. All organisms from insects to humans have a homologue of chicken v-*src* and its normal counterpart, the *src* protooncogene. Moreover, the nucleotide sequences of the chicken and human protooncogenes are 90% identical. This degree of homology suggests that these genes play crucial and conserved roles in the biochemistry of signal transduction and cell proliferation. The *ras* protooncogenes of the rat have two homologues in yeast, and rat *ras* protooncogenes can function in yeast.

RNA tumor viruses are not involved in most neoplastic disorders that affect humans. **Human T cell lymphotropic virus** (HTLV), the only neoplastic disorder in humans that is caused by a retrovirus, is associated with a T lymphocytic neoplasia that occurs in people living in southern Japan. The provirus (the DNA complementary to the viral RNA genome that is integrated into the chromosomal DNA) is present in tumor cells but is not usually present in nonneoplastic cells. The time between infection and malignant transformation is long, and most carriers, moreover, do not develop the lymphoma. The virus does not integrate at specific sites of chromosomes, nor does it have to integrate near protooncogenes to participate in malignant transformation. The basis of the carcinogenicity, however, is a mystery.

MECHANISMS OF NEOPLASTIC TRANSFORMATION

Cellular Oncogenes

Because DNA tumor virus and retrovirus oncogenes are responsible for a minority of neoplasms in humans, oncologists have focused on nonviral, nontransmissible cellular oncogenes. Cellular oncogenes result from amplification, overexpression, or mutation of normal cellular genes, and they are not the result of viral infection. Carcinogens or radiation can promote the mutation of protooncogenes into cellular oncogenes. Although many cellular oncogenes are named after the animal retrovirus that led to their discovery, cellular oncogenes, which are not derived from a virus, occur in humans. Cellular oncogenes occur in many different types of cells, and their distribution is much broader than is suggested by the names reflecting their discovery. For example, the *ras* oncogene, initially found in sarcomas, is also present in many leukemia cells and carcinomas.

Proteins that participate in controlling cell growth include (1) growth factors, (2) receptor protein-tyrosine kinases, (3) nonreceptor protein-tyrosine kinases, (4) Ras, (5) protein-serine/threonine kinases, (6) nuclear proteins and transcription factors, and (7) a mitochondrial protein. These loci are illustrated in Figure 21–5, and examples are listed in Table 21–3 for general reference.

A growth factor oncogene (*hst*) that is related to fibroblast growth factor is amplified (present in increased copy number) in some human breast carcinomas. Increased expression of this growth factor can stimulate cells that bear its receptor and contribute to malignant transformation. The

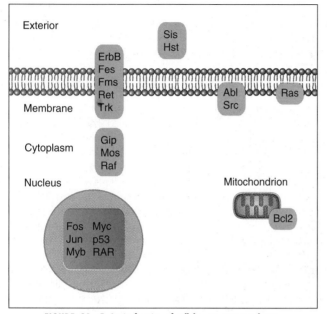

FIGURE 21–5. *Loci of action of cellular oncogene products.*

genes for growth factor receptors become oncogenes when they are amplified and overexpressed or mutated so that the receptor remains active even without its bound ligand. The *erb*B2 or *neu* protooncogene, a homologue of the epidermal growth factor receptor, is amplified in some breast and ovarian carcinomas. DNA rearrangements that result in the loss of the extracellular domain of receptor protein-tyrosine kinases lead to unregulated activity of the intracellular catalytic domain. The *ret* and *trk* (pronounced "track") oncogenes, which are produced by this mechanism, occur in some human thyroid carcinomas.

The *src* oncogene, first described in the Rous sarcoma virus, is a nonreceptor protein-tyrosine kinase. The *mos* and *raf* oncogenes have protein serine/threonine kinase activity. Mutations that lead to constitutively active protein-tyrosine or

protein-serine/threonine kinase activity can lead to neoplastic transformation.

The receptor and nonreceptor protein-tyrosine kinases catalyze the phosphorylation of phospholipase C_γ, one of the isoenzymes of phospholipase C. The stimulation of diglyceride and inositol trisphosphate formation catalyzed by phospholipase C represents one plausible mechanism by which growth factors and oncogenes produce their effects. Protein-tyrosine kinases can activate the Raf signal transduction pathway to produce their growth stimulatory effects. Downstream targets of this pathway include the AP-1 transcription factor that is made up of Fos and Jun (Figure 20–4). Dividing cells make many proteins at different rates than do quiescent cells. The idea that nuclear oncogene products are transcription factors is prevalent.

A much studied group of intracellular transducers includes the G-protein oncogene products. The most celebrated and perhaps most widespread cellular oncogene is *ras* (first described in a *rat* sarcoma). The *ras* oncogenes are related to normal cellular genes, and Ras proteins occur in all nucleated cells. The first protooncogene of this type to be discovered was H-*ras* based upon its homology to a viral oncogene (H refers to the Harvey virus, named for the discoverer). Additional *ras* protooncogenes and oncogenes include K-*ras* (Kirsten) and N-*ras* (neural). The three protooncogenes, although they encode similar proteins, are found on three different chromosomes.

ras oncogenes occur in about 25% of all human neoplasms, but this association is neither necessary nor sufficient to produce a particular neoplasm. Although 90% of human pancreatic carcinomas possess *ras* oncogenes, 10% occur without this oncogene. *ras* oncogenes occur in about half of all colon carcinomas. Most human neoplasms contain more than one oncogene, and these neoplasms often lack normal tumor suppressor genes. These characteristics fit the multistage theory of carcinogenesis. Selected examples are provided for general information in Tables 21–4 and 21–5.

A *ras* protooncogene can be converted to a *ras* oncogene by a single missense mutation. The *ras* cellular oncogene was discovered in a human bladder carcinoma. Activation of the *ras* protooncogene resulted from the substitution of valine for glycine at codon 12. This mutation reduces Ras GTPase activity. Reduced GTPase activity results in a pro-

TABLE 21–3. Function of Oncogene and Tumor Suppressor Gene Products

Cellular Function	Oncogene	Tumor Suppressor Gene
Cell adhesion		*DCC*
Cell survival		*bcl*2
Cyclin-dependent protein kinase inhibitor		*MTS*1
Growth factor	*hst, sis*	
Growth factor receptors	*erb*B2/*neu, fes, fms, ret, trk*	
Intracellular signal transduction	*gip, mos, raf*	*NF1*
Nuclear receptors	*RAR*	
Transcriptional regulation	*E2A, fos, jun, myb, myc*	*RB1, p53, WT1*

TABLE 21–4. Representative Tumors That Can Exhibit Multiple Gene Alterations in Adults

Tumor	Oncogene	Tumor Suppressor Gene
Breast carcinoma	*c-myc, erb*B2/*neu*	*RB1, p53*
Colorectal carcinoma	K-*ras*	*DCC, MCC, p53*
Lung carcinoma	K-*ras, c-myc, l-myc, n-myc*	*RB1, p53*

TABLE 21–5. Representative Oncogenes and Tumor Suppressor Genes in Neoplasms in Children

Neoplasm	Oncogene	Tumor Suppressor Gene
Leukemia	abl, fms, myb, myc, K-ras, N-ras, src	
Wilms (kidney)	myb, myc	WT1
Neuroblastoma	myb, myc, N-ras, src	
Retinoblastoma	myc, src	Rb1
Osteosarcoma	sis, src	Rb1

tein that is maintained in its active state (Figure 20–3). Ras proteins have a farnesyl group attached at the carboxyl terminus and are found at the inner side of the cell's plasma membrane (Figure 18–17). Inhibition of Ras farnesylation is a potential target for cancer chemotherapy.

Benign tumors can possess an activated *ras* protooncogene. Thus, activation of *ras* is not sufficient for malignant transformation. This result fits the multistage theory of carcinogenesis, which states that more than one somatic cell mutation is required to produce cancer cells. This finding also suggests that activation of *ras* may be an early event in malignant transformation, at least in some neoplasms.

myc is a celebrated nuclear oncogene product. *myc* protooncogene mRNA levels are low in quiescent cells. If such cells are stimulated with a mitogen such as platelet-derived growth factor, *myc* mRNA levels increase within an hour. Myc proteins are labile and exhibit a half-life of 20 minutes or so. Although it was one of the first cellular nuclear oncogene products to be described, its function is still a riddle. The *myb* and *ski* oncogene products resemble *myc*, and their function remains to be established.

Protooncogene Translocation and Amplification

Changing the location of a gene in chromosomes (translocation) can alter its regulation. Increased expression of a normal protooncogene can lead to malignant transformation. Human cells ordinarily have 23 pairs of chromosomes with well-defined structures, but tumor cells are usually aneuploid (i.e., they have an abnormal number of chromosomes, generally too many) and often contain translocations. These chromosomal abnormalities can be observed in chromosome spreads by light microscopy.

Malignant transformation in **chronic myelogenous leukemia** is related to the translocation of the *abl* protooncogene from its normal position on chromosome 9 to chromosome 22. *abl* encodes a protein-tyrosine kinase (Table 21–6). The **Philadelphia chromosome,** resulting from this translocation, is the fused product of a piece of chromosome 9 attached to the large fragment of chromosome 22 (Figure 21–6). The abbreviated chromosome 22, or Philadelphia chromosome, received attention because it can be easily identified (Figure 21–6A). Following translocation, hnRNA/mRNA is synthesized from a template derived originally from chromosomes 9 and 22. The translocation is a strong diagnostic indicator of chronic myelogenous leukemia.

A second example of a chromosomal transloca-

TABLE 21–6. Representative Oncogenes Associated with Human Neoplasia

Oncogene	Oncogene Function	Activation Mechanism	Representative Neoplasm
abl	Nonreceptor protein-tyrosine kinase	Translocation	Chronic myelogenous leukemia
bcl2	Cell survival	Translocation	Follicular B cell lymphoma
erbB2/neu	Truncated EGF receptor	Amplification	Breast and ovarian carcinomas
fes	Receptor protein-tyrosine kinase (ligand unknown)	?	Lymphocytic and myelogenous leukemias
fms	Macrophage colony-stimulating factor receptor protein-tyrosine kinase	?	Mammary and renal cell carcinoma
hst	Fibroblast growth factor	?	Breast
c-myc	Nuclear protein	Amplification	Burkitt and other B cell lymphomas, breast and lung carcinomas
n-myc	Nuclear protein	Amplification	Neuroblastoma, retinoblastoma, small cell lung carcinoma
l-myc	Nuclear protein	Amplification	Colon, lung, and small cell lung carcinomas, B cell lymphoma, promyelocytic leukemia
myb	Nuclear protein	?	Colon carcinoma, acute myelogenous leukemia, lymphocytic leukemia
raf	Protein-serine/threonine kinase	?	
RAR	Retinoic acid receptor	Translocation	Acute myelogenous leukemia
H-ras	Signal transduction	Point mutation	Thyroid carcinoma
K-ras	Signal transduction	Point mutation	Colon, lung, pancreatic, and thyroid carcinomas
N-ras	Signal transduction	Point mutation	Acute lymphocytic and myelogenous leukemias, thyroid carcinoma
ret	Growth factor receptor	DNA rearrangement	Thyroid carcinoma
src	Nonreceptor protein-tyrosine kinase	?	Brain tumors, leukemia, osteosarcoma, retinoblastoma, and rhabdomyosarcoma
trk	Receptor protein-tyrosine kinase of nerve growth factor	DNA rearrangement	Colon and thyroid carcinoma
sis	Truncated PDGF receptor	?	Osteosarcoma

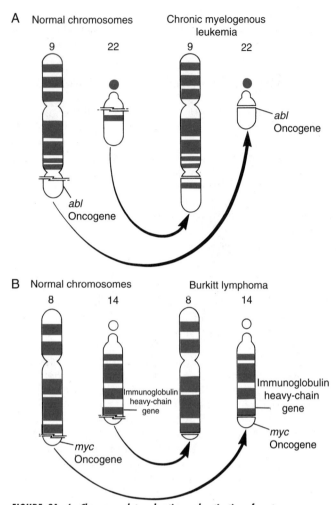

FIGURE 21–6. Chromosomal translocation and activation of protooncogenes.
A. *Chronic myelogenous leukemia* B. *Burkitt lymphoma. Reproduced, with permission, from R.S. Cotran, V. Kumar, and S.L. Robbins (eds.).* Robbins Pathologic Basis of Disease, *5th ed. Philadelphia, W.B. Saunders Company, 1995, p. 264.*

tion involves the *myc* protooncogene in **Burkitt lymphoma.** The c-*myc* protooncogene is translocated from chromosome 8 to chromosome 14, which carries the antibody heavy-chain genes (Figure 21–6B). Burkitt lymphoma, which is associated with Epstein-Barr virus infection, is a neoplasm of B lymphocytes. The antibody genes are actively transcribed in B cells.

Translocation of the c-*myc* protooncogene next to active antibody genes increases the transcription of c-*myc*, and an increase in transcription and translation of the protooncogene accounts in part for the malignant transformation. DNA sequence analysis of the translocated c-*myc* gene in Burkitt lymphoma shows that translocation occurs without mutation in the protein coding sequence. This result supports the hypothesis that altered expression of a normal cellular protooncogene can play a role in at least one step of malignant transformation.

Most of the cytogenetic changes associated with malignant transformation were described in leukemias because of the ready accessibility of cells for analysis. One form of acute promyelocytic leukemia is related to the translocation of the retinoate receptor (*RAR*) gene from chromosome 15 to 17. Translocation can lead to genetic overexpression.

Amplification of segments of DNA in individual chromosomes provides another mechanism for overexpression. Forty percent of human neuroblastomas, for example, contain up to 200 copies of the n-*myc* gene. c-*myc* is amplified in some lung carcinomas, and *neu* is amplified in some breast carcinomas.

Tumor Suppressor Genes

Mutations or deletions of tumor suppressor genes can participate in neoplastic transformation. Tumor suppressor gene products block abnormal growth and malignant transformation. Tumor suppressor genes are recessive, and both copies of normal diploid suppressor genes must undergo mutation to allow for malignant transformation. This is in contrast to dominant cellular oncogenes in which mutation of only one copy of a protooncogene is required. (The abbreviations of the tumor suppressor genes are pronounced letter by letter.)

Retinoblastoma (*RB1*) Gene

▶ Retinoblastoma is a rare childhood malignancy involving the retina. Hereditary (40%) and sporadic (60%) forms occur. In the heritable form, the child inherits one mutant gene at the retinoblastoma locus (*RB1*) on chromosome 13q through the germline. Retinoblastoma is produced by mutation of the remaining *RB1* gene. If a somatic cell mutation of the only normal copy of *RB1* occurs, malignant transformation can result (Figure 21–7). There often are multiple tumors in hereditary retinoblastoma, and both eyes can be affected. This is due to the possibility of mutations occurring in more than one retinoblast, and each tumor represents a clone that is derived from a single cell. Not all individuals, however, develop even one tumor because the somatic cell mutation involving the target gene is random.

The retinoblastoma gene product is expressed in many tissues besides the retina including osteoblasts, fibroblasts, and skin. There is an increased probability that individuals with the hereditary form of retinoblastoma will develop tumors at secondary sites. In the sporadic form of the disorder, both *RB1* alleles become inactivated by mutations that occur in a single cell (Figure 21–7). Because this is uncommon, multiple tumors in the sporadic form are rare. ◀

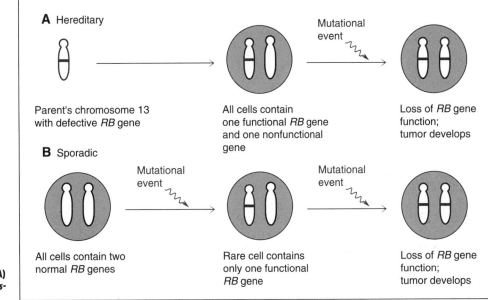

A Hereditary

Parent's chromosome 13 with defective *RB* gene

Mutational event

All cells contain one functional *RB* gene and one nonfunctional gene

Loss of *RB* gene function; tumor develops

B Sporadic

Mutational event

All cells contain two normal *RB* genes

Mutational event

Rare cell contains only one functional *RB* gene

Loss of *RB* gene function; tumor develops

FIGURE 21–7. Development of (A) hereditary and (B) sporadic retinoblastoma.

The *RB1* gene is entirely or largely deleted in many retinoblastoma tumors. The retinoblastoma gene product is a nuclear protein with a molecular mass of 105 kDa. The protein becomes heavily phosphorylated as cells begin to duplicate their DNA in the S phase of the cell cycle; otherwise, the protein is lightly phosphorylated. The lightly phosphorylated retinoblastoma gene product inhibits cell division, and the heavily phosphorylated form is less inhibitory. The most likely point at which the retinoblastoma gene protein exerts its effect is the G_1-S transition in the cell cycle (Figure 1–7). Unphosphorylated retinoblastoma gene protein binds to transcription factors and may alter the expression of genes involved in cell cycle regulation. Active retinoblastoma gene protein turns off the expression of the nuclear protooncogene *myc*, and this may be one mechanism for inhibiting cell division.

WT1 and *NF1* Genes

Wilms tumor is a kidney tumor involving tumor suppressor genes. This tumor, like retinoblastoma, is expressed during childhood and occurs in sporadic (90%) and hereditary (10%) forms. The genesis of Wilms tumor is associated with loss or deletion of DNA. The mechanisms of neoplastic transformation are more complex and involve two gene loci on chromosome 11 and a third that is not yet localized. One gene product, from the *WT1* locus, functions in the regulation of kidney and gonadal development and in the genesis of Wilms tumor. WT1, which contains four zinc finger motifs (Figure 3–23), binds to DNA at target sequences and regulates the transcription of specific genes. WT1 can suppress the transcription of selected growth factors, and this action may account, in part, for its tumor suppressor activity.

▶ Von Recklinghausen neurofibromatosis occurs with a frequency of 1 in 3000 births. Half of these represent new mutations, making this one of the most commonly mutated genes in the general population. Multiple tumors occur in affected individuals, the most common being the subcutaneous neurofibromas that are composed of proliferating neurites, Schwann cells, and fibroblasts. The tumors in 97% of affected individuals are benign. ◀ This autosomal dominant trait maps to the long arm of chromosome 17. This gene and the dystrophin gene are among the largest known. The *NF1* gene is 270–390 kb in length, the mRNA is 11–13 kb, and the NF1 protein (**neurofibromin**) is 330 kDa. The large size of the gene, which is responsible for the large number of mutations, has hindered its characterization. Mutations found thus far include translocations, deletions, insertion of an Alu sequence (Table 15–1) into an intron, and point mutations. It is uncertain whether both alleles must be mutated for transformation to occur. The *NF1* gene is expressed in many normal tissues, and it is unclear why only particular cell types are susceptible to the effects of mutation.

Analysis of the coding region of *NF1* has revealed significant homology to GAP, the GTPase activating protein that converts active Ras to its inactive form (Figure 20–3). The *NF1* gene product activates Ras-dependent GTP hydrolysis. A decline in GTPase activity of *NF1* in neurofibromatosis may lead to increased Ras activity, and this can lead to neoplastic transformation via the downstream Raf signal transduction pathway (Figure 20–4).

p53 Gene

p53 is a tumor suppressor with a molecular mass of 53 kDa, hence its name. The *p53* gene is found on the short arm of chromosome 17. The *p53* gene is inactivated by point mutations, and normal p53 protein can be inactivated by forming complexes with cellular proteins or by proteolysis. Oncoproteins produced by human papillomavirus, for example, trigger degradation of p53. Loss of p53 function occurs in 70% of colorectal cancers, 50% of lung cancers, and 40% of breast cancers. *Alteration of p53, which occurs in about half of all human neoplasms, is one of the most common biochemical findings in human neoplasia.* (Alteration of Ras, which occurs in about 25% of all human tumors, also is common).

Eighty percent of *p53* mutations are missense mutations causing one amino acid to be substituted for another. This is in contrast to the *RB1* and *WT1* genes, in which deletions predominate. Sequence changes can occur from exposure to agents that damage DNA such as electrophilic carcinogens. p53 is present in low levels in normal cells. As a result of missense mutations, the half-life of p53 increases from minutes to hours, and the amount of detectable p53 (of mutant form) increases. This result is of practical benefit in the immunochemical analysis of tumors.

p53 is usually localized in the nucleus and can be phosphorylated. p53 binds to DNA, and mutant forms fail to bind. p53 can put the brakes on cell growth and division, prevent the unruly amplification and mutation of DNA, and push cells into a programmed self-destruct pathway called apoptosis. **Apoptosis** (Greek "dropping off") is the normal and programmed destruction of cells during embryogenesis, development, and adult life. Disruption of apoptosis can promote inappropriate cell survival and the development of cancer and is yet another mechanism for neoplastic transformation. The suppression of cell death by mutant *p53* can lead to cancer. Normal p53 can also turn on the synthesis of p21, a protein that inhibits cyclin-dependent protein kinase. As a result of inhibiting this kinase, the cell is unable to pass a checkpoint in the cell division cycle (see below).

Transformation to the malignant state requires mutations in several genes, and this multistep pathway often involves production of oncogenes and elimination of tumor suppressor genes. Loss of both the *RB1* and *p53* tumor suppressor genes and activation of protooncogenes to oncogenes has been demonstrated in some breast and lung carcinomas (Table 21–4).

Other Tumor Suppressor Genes

Familial adenomatous polyposis (FAP) is an autosomal dominant condition in which many polyps develop in the colon during the second and third decades of life. All affected individuals will develop carcinoma of the colon unless it is removed. This disorder is responsible for only 1% of all cases of colon cancer. The *FAP* locus is on the long arm of chromosome 5. Two genes (*APC* and *MCC*) have been implicated in this disease. The functions of

the *a*deomatous *p*olyposis *c*oli and *m*utated in colorectal *c*ancer genes are a mystery.

DCC (*d*eleted in *c*olorectal *c*ancer) is another tumor suppressor gene. Its gene product resembles cell adhesion molecules. **Cell adhesion molecules** are integral membrane proteins that are involved in cell-cell and cell-matrix interactions. Inactivation of *DCC* may result in reduced cell adhesion, thereby contributing to the development of the potential to metastasize and produce malignancy. Inactivation of *DCC* usually occurs late in colorectal carcinogenesis along with the capacity to invade surrounding normal tissue.

The *bcl*2 gene contributes to the development of lymphomas by blocking programmed cell death. The gene product is located in the inner mitochondrial membrane. The cellular mechanisms involved in apoptosis and the role of *bcl*2 gene in this process are unknown. Table 21–3 provides, for general reference, a list of various oncogenes and tumor suppressor genes and their function.

CYCLINS AND CELL CYCLE CONTROL

The cell cycle consists of four phases (G_1, S, G_2, and M). Quiescent cells are considered to be in G_0 phase (Figure 1–7). Mitosis (nuclear division) is closely followed by cytokinesis (cytoplasmic division). Together they constitute the M phase. Mitosis is relatively brief, lasting 1–2 hours. The nonmitotic phase of the cell cycle is called interphase. The cell duplicates its contents, both nuclear and cytoplasmic during interphase. DNA synthesis occurs in the S phase between two gaps, G_1 and G_2. During the cell division cycle, the cell passes through a number of checkpoints or transition points at which progression to the next stage can be promoted or halted. Checkpoints make cell division responsive to external conditions such as nutrients and growth factors. An orderly progression through the cell cycle ensures that mitosis, for example, starts only after all of the DNA has been replicated.

The most important checkpoint in the cell cycle occurs at the initiation of DNA replication. If the conditions for cell division are unfavorable, the cell becomes arrested in G_1. A group of proteins called G_1 **cyclins** accumulate during G_1 and participate in the pathway to initiate DNA synthesis. A second group, called **M cyclins,** participate in the pathway to initiate mitosis. Cyclins, a family of proteins with molecular masses ranging from 30 to 50 kDa, function by activating their cognate protein kinases. Human cells possess at least a dozen homologous protein-serine/threonine kinases that were discovered because of the activation of the parent enzyme by cyclins. Although the levels of the cyclin-dependent protein kinases are constant throughout the cell cycle, their activities are regulated. A G_1 **cyclin–dependent protein kinase** catalyzes the phosphorylation of proteins that initiate the S

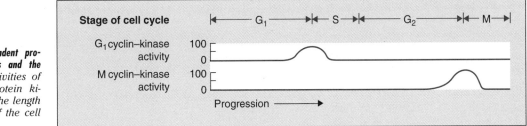

FIGURE 21–8. Cyclin-dependent protein-serine/threonine kinases and the cell division cycle. The activities of the cyclin-dependent protein kinases are relative, and the length of time of each stage of the cell cycle is not to scale.

phase of the cell cycle (Figure 21–8). After this checkpoint is passed, proteases destroy the activating cyclins and G₁ cyclin–dependent protein activity declines.

A different protein kinase, **M cyclin–dependent protein kinase,** is responsible for traversing the G_2-M checkpoint. There is an increased synthesis of cyclin M before M phase. Cyclin M associates with its kinase, but the latter becomes phosphorylated at specific tyrosine and threonine residues by other protein kinases that maintain inhibition, even in the presence of activating cyclins. To pass this checkpoint, **p54 phosphatase** catalyzes the dephosphorylation of threonine and tyrosine and the activation of M cyclin–dependent protein kinase. The activated kinase initiates mitosis by catalyzing the phosphorylation of acceptor proteins. Cyclin M is degraded by proteolysis, and the kinase is thereby inactivated following destruction of the activator. The process is repeated during the next cell division. The substrates for M cyclin–dependent protein kinase include (1) histone H1, promoting chromosomal condensation; (2) nuclear laminins, causing dispersal of the nuclear membrane; (3) nucleolin, arresting ribosome synthesis; and (4) myosin-light-chain kinase, promoting cytokinesis.

p53 participates in the cell cycle regulatory scheme. p53 directs the transcription of p21, a protein of molecular mass of 21 kDa that binds to the cyclin-dependent kinases and inhibits them. This action halts the cell cycle before the cell is committed to divide. The delay allows the cell to repair DNA before dividing, thus preventing replication of damaged DNA. If p53 is nonfunctional, permanent somatic mutations can result during replication of damaged DNA, and such mutations can contribute to the multistage pathway of neoplastic transformation. MTS1 (multiple tumor suppressor 1) is a16-kDa protein that acts by inhibiting cyclin-dependent kinases. Mutations of *MTS1* occur in a wide variety of tumors.

CANCER CHEMOTHERAPY

▶ Cancer is a family of diseases, and each type of cancer has its characteristic clinical course. Clinicians often classify neoplastic diseases by stages, from localized to extensively spread. The course of treatment often depends upon the stage of the disease. Moreover, a single cancer cell can lead to relapse and subsequent death of the host. All cancer cells must therefore be removed or killed to achieve a cure. The four main treatments used in cancer therapy are chemotherapy, surgery, symptomatic treatment, and x-irradiation. It is common to combine treatments such as surgery with irradiation or chemotherapy.

Studies have shown that treatment with a single drug, with rare exceptions, is unable to produce either significant remission or cure of cancer. In this section, we consider the action of selected drugs used in the treatment of various neoplasms. Our aim is to understand the biochemical basis for their action. Representative examples of the major classes of drugs and the disorders that they have been used to treat are provided for general information in Table 21–7, and their loci of action are illustrated in Figure 21–9.

Successful treatment of tumors with drugs and radiation depends upon the greater sensitivity of neoplastic cells to the treatment than that of normal cells. Proliferating cells, such as neoplastic cells, are generally more sensitive to these agents than are quiescent cells. Sensitivity differences between neoplastic and normal cells are sometimes marginal, however, and toxicity (killing of normal cells) is a common problem. Cells that normally proliferate rapidly include hair follicle cells, cells of the hematopoietic system (both red and white cells), and cells that line the gut. Temporary loss of hair is a common side effect of cancer chemotherapeutic agents. Anemia (decreased red blood cell mass) and decreased resistance to infection result from inhibition of hematopoiesis by cancer chemotherapeutic agents and radiation. Abdominal pain and diarrhea are a manifestation of inhibition of enterocyte proliferation by cancer chemotherapeutic agents. ◀

Alkylating Agents

Nitrogen mustards (Figure 21–10) react with bases in nucleic acids. The term "mustard" refers to blisters that these agents produce on skin. The parent compounds, in water, form an electrophile that reacts with biological nucleophiles. The reaction of N^7 of guanine with mechlorethamine is illustrated in Figure 21–11. The modified base can pair abnormally during replication and lead to mu-

TABLE 21–7. Classes of Major Antineoplastic Agents

Class	Representative Diseases
Alkylating Agents	
Cisplatin	Head and neck, lung, ovary, and testis carcinomas
Chlorambucil	Chronic lymphocytic leukemia, lymphomas
Cyclophosphamide	Leukemias, lymphomas, and breast, cervix, lung, ovary, and testis carcinoma
Melphalan	Multiple myeloma and breast and ovary carcinomas
Antimetabolites	
Cytosine arabinoside	Acute lymphocytic and acute myelogenous leukemias
Fluorouracil	Breast, gastrointestinal tract, and head and neck carcinomas
Hydroxyurea	Chronic myelogenous leukemia
Mercaptopurine	Leukemias
Methotrexate	Acute lymphocytic leukemia, choriocarcinoma, osteosarcoma, and breast, head and neck, and lung carcinomas
Thioguanine	Leukemias
Antibiotics	
Bleomycin	Head and neck, lung, skin carcinomas, and lymphomas
Actinomycin D	Rhabdomyosarcoma and Wilms tumor in children, choriocarcinoma in women, metastatic testicular carcinoma in men, and Kaposi sarcoma
Daunorubicin	Acute lymphocytic and acute myelogenous leukemias
Doxorubicin	Various sarcomas, lymphomas, acute leukemias, and breast, lung, and stomach carcinomas
Plant Derivatives	
Etoposide, teniposide	Lymphomas, Kaposi sarcoma, and breast and lung carcinomas
Vinblastine	Lymphomas, breast and testis carcinomas
Vincristine	Lymphomas, acute lymphocytic leukemia, Wilms tumor
Biological Response Modifiers	
Interferon-α	Non-Hodgkin lymphomas, Kaposi sarcoma, chronic myelogenous and hairy cell leukemias, and ovary and bladder carcinomas
Enzyme	
Asparaginase	Acute lymphocytic leukemia
Sex Hormone Antagonists	
Diethylstilbestrol	Prostate carcinoma
Flutamide	Prostate carcinoma
Tamoxifen	Breast carcinoma

tation, or it can be eliminated from DNA, leading to chain scission or DNA fragmentation. Cross-linking of DNA chains can also occur. Alkylating agents disturb cell growth, mitosis, differentiation, and cell function. More rapidly dividing cells are susceptible to the action of these agents. In slowly dividing cells, DNA repair processes can reverse the effects of DNA modification. Nitrogen mustards are mutagenic and carcinogenic.

Cisplatin is the only heavy metal compound used as a cancer chemotherapeutic agent. The hydrolytic removal of chloride is responsible for the generation of the active form of the drug (Figure 21–12). This complex can react with DNA and produce both intrastrand and interstrand cross-links. N^7 of guanine is a reactive portion of DNA, and cross-linking of two adjacent guanines on the same strand is common. As a result of chemical modification, changes in DNA conformation and inhibition of DNA synthesis occur. Modification is opposed by enzymatic DNA repair; the relative rates of modification and repair determine cytotoxicity. Cisplatin is mutagenic.

Antimetabolites

Literally thousands of purine and pyrimidine analogues have been tested for cancer chemothera-

peutic effects. **Cytosine arabinoside** differs stereochemically from cytidine at the 2′ hydroxyl group (Figure 21–13). Cytosine arabinoside is converted to the triphosphate by three successive reactions with ATP and is incorporated into DNA. Cytosine arabinoside triphosphate is not a potent inhibitor of DNA polymerase, but the DNA strands that have cytosine arabinoside incorporated are unstable, which leads to breaks in these DNA strands.

5-Fluorouracil (5-FU) must be converted to its monophosphate before any effect on cellular metabolism occurs. Orotate phosphoribosyltransferase, one of the two activities of the UMP synthase complex of pyrimidine synthesis (Figure 14–4), catalyzes the reaction of PRPP with fluorouracil. Fluorouridine monophosphate can be converted sequentially to the diphosphates and triphosphates in reactions involving ATP. Fluorouridine triphosphate can be incorporated into RNA, and this incorporation diminishes the posttranscriptional processing and physiological activity of RNA. Fluorouridine diphosphate can be converted to fluorodeoxyuridine diphosphate as catalyzed by ribonucleotide reductase. Fluorodeoxyuridine monophosphate, derived from precursors, is a **suicide inhibitor** of thymidylate synthase (Figure 14–13). Suicide inhibition requires the generation of an active species, during an abortive catalytic cycle, that reacts with and inactivates the enzyme. The

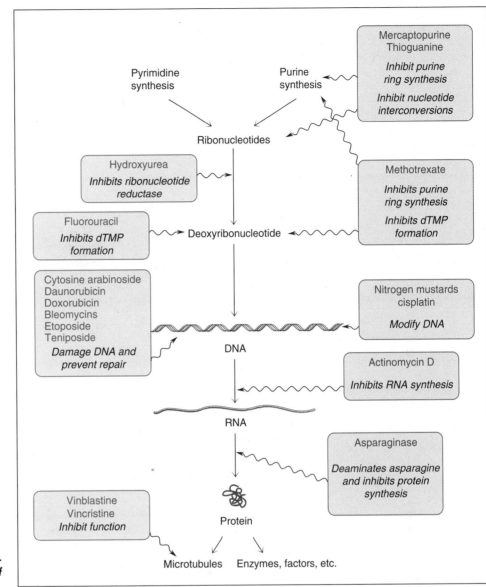

FIGURE 21–9. Sites of action of selected drugs used in the treatment of cancer.

FIGURE 21–10. Nitrogen mustards.

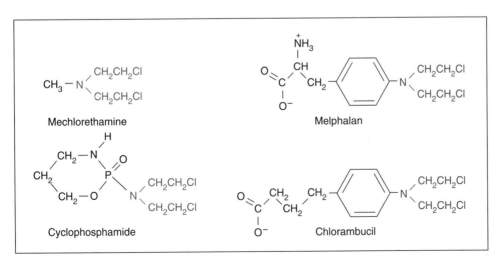

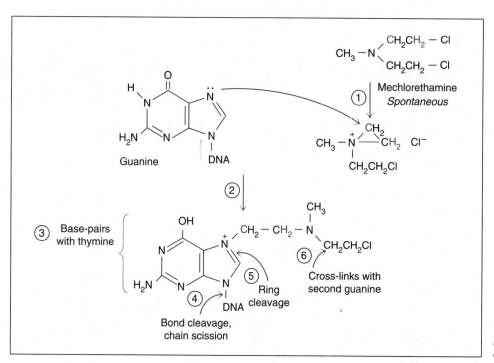

Guanine   DNA

③ Base-pairs with thymine

⑤ Ring cleavage

④ Bond cleavage, chain scission

① Mechlorethamine *Spontaneous*

⑥ Cross-links with second guanine

FIGURE 21–11. The reaction of mechlorethamine with guanine.

FIGURE 21–12. Cisplatin.

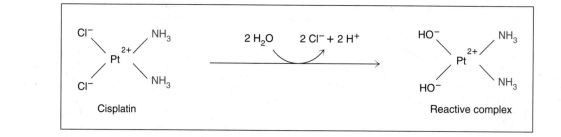

Cisplatin   Reactive complex

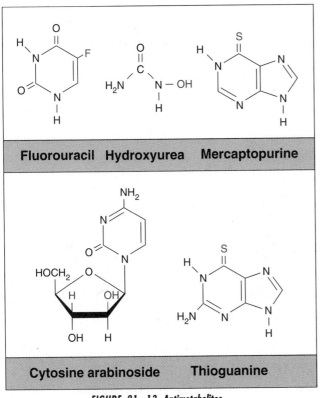

FIGURE 21–13. Antimetabolites.

clinical efficacy of fluorouracil is due to its incorporation into RNA and to inhibition of thymidylate synthase.

Hydroxyurea, which is an inhibitor of ribonucleoside diphosphate reductase, is a chemical scavenger that destroys an active site protein-tyrosyl free radical intermediate. Hydroxyurea decreases the formation of deoxyribonucleoside precursors of DNA.

Mercaptopurine and **thioguanine** are converted to the nucleoside 5'-phosphate following a reaction with PRPP catalyzed by HGPRT (Figure 14–17). 6-Thioinosine monophosphate (formed from mercaptopurine) and 6-thioguanosine monophosphate inhibit the rate-limiting step in purine biosynthesis, which is catalyzed by PRPP-glutamine amidotransferase. These monophosphates also inhibit the conversion of IMP to AMP and GMP. The deoxynucleoside triphosphates of mercaptopurine and thioguanine are incorporated into cellular DNA and produce cellular toxicity in a delayed manner after drug exposure.

▶ **Methotrexate,** an antifolate, produced the first striking remission in leukemia and the first cure of a solid tumor, a choriocarcinoma. A cure implies that every single cancer cell was killed. Later treatments have been even more impressive with higher, potentially lethal, doses followed by "rescue" of the host by treatment with leucovorin (Figure 13–34). ◀

Tetrahydrofolate derivatives are required for purine and thymidylate biosynthesis (Figures 14–8 and 14–12). *Methotrexate is an inhibitor of dihydro-folate reductase,* which catalyzes the conversion of dietary folate to di- and tetrahydrofolate. Dihydrofolate is also generated in the thymidylate synthase reaction where methylenetetrahydrofolate acts as a reductant and methyl group donor (Figure 14–12). Methotrexate prevents the regeneration of tetrahydrofolate from dihydrofolate. Leucovorin, the drug used in the rescue process, is at the tetrahydrofolate stage of reduction. Thymidylate synthesis is more sensitive to tetrahydrofolate depletion than is purine synthesis. Cell killing, however, proceeds more efficiently when both thymidylate and purine synthesis are inhibited.

Antibiotics

Actinomycin D, also called dactinomycin, is a peptide derivative (Figure 16–34) that was one of the first antibiotics isolated from *Streptomyces* in the 1940s. *Actinomycin D inhibits DNA-dependent RNA synthesis.* Actinomycin D intercalates with DNA between two adjacent G-C base pairs. This antibiotic binds to the DNA template and inhibits the elongation reactions of RNA synthesis; DNA synthesis is less sensitive.

Daunorubicin and **doxorubicin** are anthracycline antibiotics that are among the newer cancer chemotherapeutic agents. As antitumor agents, the anthracycline agents are matched only by alkylating agents in terms of their clinical usefulness. These compounds, which have a planar anthraquinone nucleus attached to an amino sugar (Figure 21–14), bind to DNA by intercalation (insertion between adjacent base pairs). The rings insert between base pairs and lie perpendicular to the long axis of the DNA double helix. The amino sugar, with the positively charged amino group, binds electrostatically to the phosphate backbone. These agents inhibit both DNA and RNA biosynthesis. Moreover, these compounds are mutagenic and produce breaks in DNA in a process that involves topoisomerase II (Figure 15–18). Topoisomerase II forms phosphodiesters through protein-tyrosine residues with the backbone of DNA during the catalytic cycle. Topoisomerase II thereby creates discontinuities in DNA during its catalytic cycle, and daunorubicin and doxorubicin abort complete catalysis and thereby produce aberrant DNA cleavage.

Bleomycins are a family of complex hydrophilic glycopeptides. Bleomycins cause chromosomal breaks, fragmentation, and translocations. These modifications involve the cooperative interaction of the antibiotic, ferrous iron, and oxygen. Reactive oxygen intermediates (superoxide and hydroxyl free radicals, Figure 5–4) are formed and react preferentially with phosphodiester bonds between guanine and a pyrimidine of DNA. The action of bleomycins resembles that of ionizing radiation because of the generation of hydroxyl free radicals. Free bases are released from DNA, causing strand

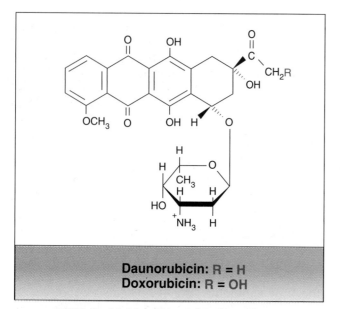

Daunorubicin: R = H
Doxorubicin: R = OH

FIGURE 21–14. *Daunorubicin and doxorubicin antibiotics.*

breaks. Cells with chromosomal aberrations with breaks, gaps, fragments, and translocations accumulate in the G_2 phase of the cell cycle.

Plant Alkaloids

Etoposide and **teniposide** (Figure 21–15A), which are derived from the mandrake plant, cause topoisomerase II to cleave DNA in an aberrant reaction. The action of these two agents resembles that of daunorubicin and doxorubicin.

Vincristine and **vinblastine** are derived from the periwinkle plant. These *Vinca* alkaloids are composed of two paired multiringed systems linked by a carbon-carbon bridge. They are alkaloids because they contain basic nitrogen (Figure 21–15B). They are cytotoxic because they bind to tubulin. Tubulin, a protein heterodimer, is soluble and exists in equilibrium with the polymerized form that makes microtubules. Microtubules form the spindle along which chromosomes migrate during mitosis, and they play a vital role in maintaining cell structure. The *Vinca* alkaloids prevent polymerization and promote the disassembly of microtubules. These compounds produce metaphase arrest during mitosis, leading to cell death.

Biological Response Modifiers

▶ The immune system plays a primary role in the body's defense against cancer. Stimulation of the immune system by interleukin-2 and a variety of other cytokines (Table 20–5) is used to treat various neoplasms. Interferon α is an agent that promotes differentiation and is used in the treatment of lymphomas, leukemias, and carcinomas (Table 21–7). ◀

FIGURE 21–15. *Plant derivatives used in cancer chemotherapy.*

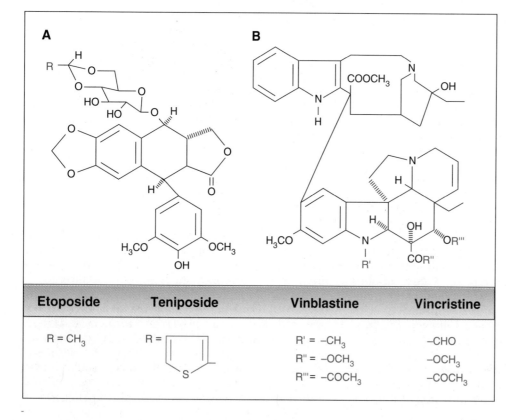

Etoposide	Teniposide	Vinblastine	Vincristine
R = CH₃	R = (thiophene)	R' = –CH₃	–CHO
		R'' = –OCH₃	–OCH₃
		R''' = –COCH₃	–COCH₃

Asparaginase

Many normal cells synthesize asparagine in amounts sufficient for protein synthesis. Biosynthesis involves a reaction between aspartate, glutamine (the amide donor), and ATP (which undergoes a pyrophosphate split) as catalyzed by asparagine synthetase (Figure 13–30). Many neoplastic cells require an exogenous source of asparagine for protein synthesis. Asparaginase catalyzes the hydrolysis of asparagine to aspartate and ammonia (Figure 13–6). Asparaginase, isolated and purified from *Escherichia coli* or from *Erwinia carotovora,* when injected, catalyzes the degradation of extracellular asparagine and thereby deprives cells of this amino acid. Deficiency of a single amino acid in a cell prevents protein synthesis and causes cell death.

▶ There is a striking synergism of asparaginase and other drugs such as methotrexate or cytosine arabinoside. Because asparaginase is a foreign protein, it is antigenic and allergic reactions can occur. The enzymes from *E. coli* and *E. carotovora* are not immunologically cross reactive. The *Erwinia* enzyme is used in individuals who develop antibodies to the *E. coli* enzyme. ◀

Sex Hormone Antagonists

A substantial body of evidence indicates that hormones play an auxiliary role in neoplastic transformation. One idea is that excessive hormonal stimulation of the target organ increases the number of cell divisions; random genetic errors accumulate during the process of repeated cell division and can lead to neoplastic phenotypes. Cancers of hormone-responsive tissues account for more than 20% of newly diagnosed cancers in the United States. In prostate carcinoma, the goal is to remove androgen stimulation and in breast carcinoma, estrogen stimulation. These therapies will be effective only if the tumor cells contain the corresponding steroid hormone receptor (Chapter 20).

▶ The development of the field of hormonal control of cancer is largely due to the work of Charles B. Huggins. Huggins shared the Nobel prize in Medicine or Physiology with Peyton Rous in 1966. Prostatic cancer commonly spreads to the skeleton, and the morbidity of skeletal pain can be incapacitating. Localized prostate cancer is treated with surgery or irradiation. Metastatic prostate cancer is treated by eliminating androgens. Huggins initially treated patients by bilateral orchiectomy (removal of the testes). The first patient treated by Huggins with orchiectomy lived for several years and died of a myocardial infarction. The lives of many individuals are enhanced as pain subsides or disappears during this palliative treatment.

Affected individuals are now treated more commonly with synthetic estrogens such as diethylstilbestrol that act as indirect androgen antagonists. Diethylstilbestrol decreases luteinizing hormone secretion and withdraws the stimulus for testosterone production. Serum acid phosphatase is elevated in patients with metastatic prostate cancer (Chapter 4). Serum enzyme levels decrease following the removal of androgen stimulation during successful treatment.

Carcinoma of the breast is treated by surgical extirpation, irradiation, and chemotherapy, depending upon the extent of the disease. Cancer of the breast that has metastasized is often treated by antiestrogens such as tamoxifen. Tamoxifen binds to estrogen receptors but does not activate them. As a result, these receptors cannot be activated by estrogen. Tumors that contain estrogen receptors are likely to respond to this treatment. The amount of estrogen receptor in the primary tumor removed during surgery is often measured to determine the likelihood that the tumor will respond to antiestrogens. It is common for tumors to respond initially to endocrine control and then to become independent of hormones following receptor loss. ◀

Drug Resistance

Tumors can develop resistance to multiple unrelated drugs such as vincristine, actinomycin D, doxorubicin, and etoposide. The *MDR1* (multiple drug resistance) gene product can be responsible. The gene product, called P-glycoprotein, contains about 1300 amino acids and consists of two portions each with six transmembrane segments and an ATP-binding site (for a total of 12 transmembrane segments and two ATP-binding sites per polypeptide chain). The protein functions as an ATP-dependent efflux pump. P-glycoprotein, moreover, occurs in many intrinsically drug-resistant solid tumors such as colon, kidney, liver, and pancreas. The physiological function of this transporter is to pump hydrophobic substances from cells. Natural substrates may include toxic compounds from the environment. P-glycoprotein is related to the cystic fibrosis transmembrane regulator (CFTR) that transports chloride out of cells (Figure 22–12). Other mechanisms can produce drug resistance.

DIET AND CANCER

Epidemiological studies indicate that high dietary fat increases the incidence of cancer of the colon, rectum, and breast. Confounding factors include total caloric intake, the composition of fat (saturated, monounsaturated, polyunsaturated), and obesity. Several international studies indicate that breast cancer is associated with high fat intake, even when corrected for caloric intake. The

National Cancer Institute of the United States recommends that dietary fat account for 30% or fewer calories of total intake. The average caloric content of American diets consists of about 40% fat. The biochemical mechanisms for the production of cancer by dietary fat are unclear.

There is an inverse correlation between fiber intake and colorectal cancer and also breast cancer in women. Fiber is the dietary component of plants that is resistant to digestion by human enzymes. Fiber includes insoluble cellulose and a variety of other soluble and insoluble plant products. The National Cancer Institute of the United States recommends that fiber intake be increased to 20–30 grams daily. The biochemical mechanisms for the beneficial effects of dietary fiber are an enigma.

Some epidemiological studies suggest an inverse relationship between cancer incidence and intake of foods high in several antioxidant nutrients such as β-carotene, ascorbate, and vitamin E. β-Carotene and vitamin E (tocopherol) are lipids that dissolve in membranes. Ascorbate, in contrast, is a hydrophilic vitamin. These antioxidants may function as scavengers of reactive oxygen intermediates that are generated from ionizing irradiation produced by natural sources including radium, radon, uranium, and [210]polonium (found in cigarette smoke).

SUMMARY

Malignant transformation of cells to produce cancer is a multistep process that involves somatic cell mutations. Chemical carcinogens are direct or indirect acting. Direct-acting carcinogens react with nucleic acids. Indirect-acting carcinogens must be metabolically converted to ultimate carcinogens by the cytochrome P-450 system. The Ames test uses liver extracts to convert potential indirect-acting carcinogens to the ultimate carcinogen, followed by a test for mutagenicity using a *Salmonella* histidine-requiring strain.

Tumor promoters are compounds that are required to induce a tumor following the application of a tumor initiator. Tumor promoters stimulate cell division. An oncogene is a gene whose product participates in neoplastic transformation. The oncogene of Rous sarcoma virus encodes a protein-tyrosine kinase, the first to be discovered. The normal cellular genes, which are progenitors of oncogenes, are called protooncogenes.

Several types of proteins participate in control of cell growth: growth factors, growth factor receptor protein-tyrosine kinases, nonreceptor protein-tyrosine kinases, Ras, intracellular serine/threonine protein kinases, and nuclear proteins. Cellular oncogenes have been described that have each of these functions. Ras is a GTP-binding protein that is implicated in several types of human cancers. Oncogenic *ras* can be derived from the normal cellular protooncogene by a mutation involving a single nucleotide change. In chronic myelogenous leukemia, malignant transformation is related to the translocation of the *abl* protooncogene from its normal position on chromosome 9 to chromosome 22. The Philadelphia chromosome is an abbreviated chromosome 22 that represents one product of this reciprocal translocation.

Tumor suppressor gene products block abnormal growth and malignant transformation. The best-characterized suppressor genes are the retinoblastoma gene and the *p53* genes. These tumor suppressors are localized in the nucleus and alter transcription of genes that are required for cell division or that inhibit cell division. Alterations in *p53,* a tumor suppressor, occur in about half of all human neoplasms. Alterations in *ras,* an oncogene, occur in about one fourth of all human neoplasms.

The sites of action of the various compounds used in cancer chemotherapy include those antimetabolites that inhibit purine synthesis, including mercaptopurine, thioguanine, and methotrexate. Agents that inhibit deoxyribonucleotide formation include hydroxyurea and fluorouracil. Methotrexate is a competitive inhibitor of dihydrofolate reductase, and fluorouracil is converted to an agent that is a suicide inhibitor of thymidylate synthase. Agents that modify DNA by alkylation include the nitrogen mustards and cisplatin. Incorporation of cytosine arabinoside into DNA produces abnormal DNA. Agents that modify DNA by interacting with topoisomerase II include antibiotics (bleomycin, daunorubicin, doxorubicin) and plant alkaloids (etoposide, teniposide). Actinomycin D inhibits RNA synthesis, and asparaginase inhibits protein biosynthesis indirectly. The *Vinca* alkaloids disrupt microtubule function and mitosis. Sex hormone antagonists are used in the treatment of cancer of the breast and prostate.

SELECTED READINGS

Brugge, J., T. Curran, E. Harlow, and F. McCormick (eds.). *Origins of Human Cancer.* Cold Spring Harbor, New York, Cold Spring Laboratory Press, 1991.

Carbone, D.P., and J.D. Minna. Antioncogenes and human cancer. Annual Review of Medicine 44:451–464, 1993.

Cooper, G.M. *Elements of Human Cancer.* Boston, Jones and Bartlett Publishers, 1992.

DeVita, V.T., Jr., S. Hellman, S.A. Rosenberg (eds.). *Cancer: Principles and Practice of Oncology,* 4th ed. Philadelphia, J.B. Lippincott Company, 1993.

Franks, L.M., and N.M. Teich (eds.). *Introduction to the Cellular and Molecular Biology of Cancer,* 2nd ed. Oxford, Oxford University Press, 1991.

Harris, C.C., and M. Hollstein. Clinical implications of the p53 tumor-suppressor gene. New England Journal of Medicine 329:1318–1327, 1993.

Huggins, C. Two principles in endocrine therapy of cancers: Hormone deprival and hormone interference. *Cancer Research* 25:1163–1167, 1965.

Lippman, M.E., and Swain, S.M. Endocrine-responsive cancers of humans. *In* J.D.Wilson and D.W. Foster (eds.). *Williams Textbook of Endocrinology,* 8th ed. Philadelphia, W.B. Saunders Company, 1992, pp. 1577–1597.

Rustgi, A.K., and D.K. Podolsky. The molecular basis of colon cancer. Annual Review of Medicine 43:61–68, 1992.

MEMBRANE

TRANSPORT

It is easier to explain biochemistry in terms of transport than it is to explain transport in terms of biochemistry.

—PETER MITCHELL

Clinical medicine would be child's play if the clinical picture resulting from a particular etiologic agent were always identical. Learning clinical medicine is largely learning how to cope with variability in clinical expression.

—VICTOR A. MCKUSICK

The plasma membrane and various intracellular membranes play a crucial role in cellular metabolism. The plasma membrane is the boundary between the cell interior and exterior, and the intracellular concentrations of ions and metabolites differ from those of the exterior. The lipid bilayer, of which cell membranes are composed, is impermeable to most polar molecules. This property prevents the escape from the cell of essential metabolites, most of which are polar, ionized, or both polar and ionized. A variety of mechanisms are responsible for the flux of essential components into and out of cells.

Translocases are integral membrane proteins, and they traverse the entire membrane bilayer. Many translocase proteins cross the cell membrane from inside to outside several times (a dozen times for several glucose transporters). In ordinary metabolite transport, the chemical nature of the transported metabolite is unchanged during translocation. The translocation of glucose into cells is an example of such a transport process. In rare cases, metabolites are chemically changed during translocation across membranes, and this process is called **group translocation** to distinguish it from transport. One process of amino acid transport, for example, results in the formation of a γ-glutamyl derivative of the amino acid during translocation. Humans expend an appreciable portion of their metabolic energy on transport. Perhaps one quarter of the total expended chemical energy in resting individuals is used to maintain ion gradients.

Besides the plasma membrane, which all living systems possess, animal cells also possess intricate intracellular membranes. Membranes surround the nucleus and define intracellular organelles such as mitochondria, lysosomes, and peroxisomes. The organelles and endoplasmic reticulum account for the vast preponderance of the total membrane of typical human cells (Table 1–1). Indeed, the plasma membrane constitutes only about 1% of the total cellular membrane of nucleated cells. Membranes are indispensable for the energy transduction processes within the mitochondrion, and many translocases shuttle metabolites into and out of the mitochondrion (Table 9–1).

GENERAL CHARACTERISTICS

Oxygen, carbon dioxide, urea, and ethanol are among the few biological substances that can diffuse across biological membranes (Figure 22–1). For ions, larger polar molecules such as glucose, and charged molecules such as amino acids, glucose 6-phosphate, and ATP, special transport systems effect translocation. The rate of transport by simple diffusion is a linear function of the solute concentration and does not exhibit saturation. In contrast, transport that is mediated by protein

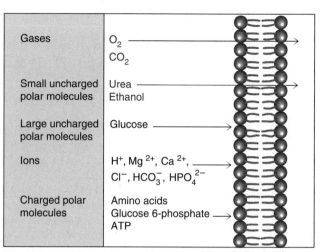

FIGURE 22–1. Differential permeability of lipid bilayers and biological membranes.

translocases exhibits saturation. The initial rate of transport is a hyperbolic function of solute concentration (Figure 22–2). This hyperbolic relationship means that a defined number of proteins mediate transport, and this number limits the rate of transport and explains **saturation kinetics** reflected by the rectangular hyperbola.

Transport proteins are called **translocases, permeases, carriers,** and **porters.** Transport systems are either active or passive. **Active transport** can

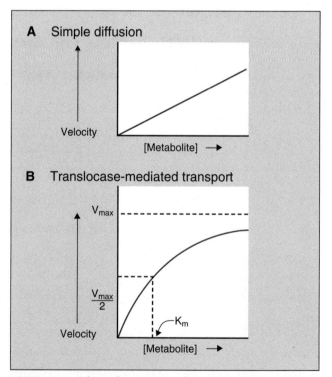

FIGURE 22–2. Velocity of transport as a function of substrate concentration. A. *Simple diffusion.* B. *Translocase-mediated transport.* V_{max} represents the maximal velocity when the carrier is saturated. K_m is the substrate concentration at 1/2 of the V_{max}. K_m is sometimes called K_t (for transport).

move an ion or metabolite against its electrochemical gradient. Transport of protons from the parietal cells of the stomach (pH ≈7) into the gastric juice (pH ≈1) occurs against a concentration gradient of 1 million. Such processes require energy. Active transport systems, moreover, are generally unidirectional. In **primary active transport,** an exergonic chemical process drives the transport process directly. The sodium/potassium-ATPase, or sodium pump, in the plasma membrane is an example of a primary active transport process. In **secondary active transport,** the energy to drive transport is generated independently of the transport process. In the transport of amino acids in the kidney, for example, sodium moves down its electrochemical gradient and sustains amino acid transport. The sodium gradient, however, is produced by an independent process: the sodium/potassium-ATPase. Sodium-driven amino acid transport represents secondary active transport.

Passive transport by facilitated diffusion, which does not require energy, translocates substances down their electrochemical gradient. The direction of transport is from higher to lower concentration. Facilitated diffusion involves translocases and exhibits saturation kinetics and metabolite specificity. The properties of saturation and metabolite specificity are analogous to characteristics that enzymes exhibit. The molecular basis for these properties is dependent on the ability of proteins to recognize metabolites in the same way that an enzyme recognizes its substrates.

The transport of a substance into a cell by facilitated diffusion is an example of **uniport.** Glucose is transported into erythrocytes by a uniport mechanism. When two substances are cotransported from one side of a membrane to the other, such as sodium and an amino acid, the process is called **symport** (Figure 22–3). When the transport of a substance in one direction is coupled to the transport of another substance in the opposite direction, the process is termed **antiport.** For example, a translocase within the inner mitochondrial membrane transports ATP from inside to outside the mitochondrion in exchange for ADP. This process, which is specifically inhibited by atractyloside, is an example of an antiport system. Both ATP and ADP move down their concentration gradient during this process. The movement of phosphate from the mitochondrial exterior to interior can be considered as a symport process; a proton and phosphate formally move into the mitochondrion. The chemical mechanism, however, differs from this process. Phosphate moves into the mitochondrion and hydroxide moves out of the mitochondrion in an antiport process.

FACILITATED DIFFUSION

Glucose does not cross lipid bilayers by simple diffusion. Human cells contain translocases that transport glucose. The **glucose translocase** in the erythrocyte and most other cells (except kidney and intestine) recognizes and transports glucose by facilitated diffusion. The process is called facilitated diffusion because there is no requirement for an external source of energy. Transport of glucose into the erythrocyte is ATP-independent and sodium ion–independent. The source of energy for transport is a glucose gradient. The glucose translocase transports glucose down its concentration gradient.

The glucose translocase of the erythrocyte is an integral membrane protein with a molecular mass of 45 kDa. Seven subclasses of sodium-independent glucose transporter have been studied by cDNA analysis. These are called GLUT1 through GLUT7, based upon the order of discovery (GLUT, *glu*cose *t*ransporter). GLUT1 is the erythrocyte glucose transporter, and GLUT4, which occurs in muscle and adipocytes, is insulin responsive (Chapter 20). The other glucose transporters are found in a variety of cells. The GLUT family of glucose transporters contain 12 transmembrane segments. These transmembrane segments form a channel through which D-glucose is translocated. The channel is not simple, or molecules smaller than glucose could pass through it. Rather, glucose binds to the active site of the translocase and induces a conformational change (Figure 22–4). Glucose is then released on the cell interior. The protein assumes its original conformation and is ready to transport another molecule of glucose.

A translocase is required for transport by facilitated diffusion. Metabolites can cross a membrane in either direction; the route is determined by the concentration gradient. Under physiological conditions, glucose is transported into the erythrocyte. Once glucose is inside the red blood cell, it is phosphorylated to form glucose 6-phosphate by the hexokinase reaction. This keeps the concentration of glucose somewhat lower on the inside of the cell than on the outside of the cell so that net transfer occurs from the cell exterior to interior. The first product of glucose metabolism, glucose 6-phosphate, is not a substrate for glucose translocase. Phosphorylation of glucose locks the ionic metabolite in the cell.

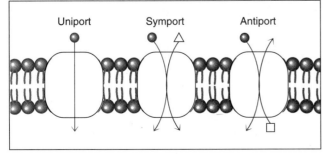

FIGURE 22–3. Uniport, symport, and antiport.

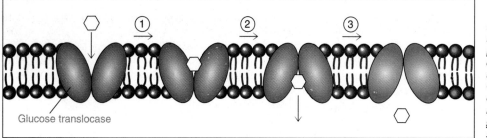

FIGURE 22–4. Scheme for the translocation of glucose by a glucose transporter. The glucose transporter is an integral membrane protein that exists in two conformations. Glucose binds to the transporter on one side of the membrane; following a conformational change, glucose dissociates on the other side of the membrane.

PRIMARY ACTIVE TRANSPORT

Cells expend considerable energy in maintaining ion gradients between the intracellular and extracellular compartments. Cells maintain a higher intracellular potassium concentration and a lower intracellular sodium concentration when compared with the extracellular compartment. Cells also maintain a calcium gradient (outside > inside). Intracellular calcium concentration is maintained between 0.1 and 5.0 μM, and extracellular calcium is on the order of 2–4 mM. The calcium concentration gradient is thus more than a thousand. Besides these ion gradients, some animal cells sustain pH gradients. Parietal cells in the stomach, for example, secrete gastric juice that contains about 0.1 M HCl (pH $\approx$ 1). The proton concentration in gastric juice is about one million–fold greater than that found in gastric cells.

Besides the intracellular and extracellular differences in pH, various organelles also maintain pH gradients. Lysosomes, for example, maintain a proton gradient with respect to the cytosol. The cytosolic pH is maintained close to 7.4. The pH inside the lysosome, on the other hand, is maintained near 5.

Sodium/Potassium-ATPase

The intracellular concentration of sodium is low relative to the extracellular concentration. Physiologists named the process that established this ionic gradient the **sodium pump.** The intracellular concentration of potassium is high relative to the extracellular concentration. The extent of these ionic gradients is somewhat greater than 10. We now consider the **sodium/potassium-ATPase** responsible for maintaining these two ion gradients.

The sodium/potassium-ATPase is a tetramer consisting of two dissimilar subunits; its composition is $\alpha_2\beta_2$ and its total molecular mass is 270 kDa. Both subunits are transmembrane proteins (Figure 22–5). The small β-subunit (40 kDa) is a glycoprotein with one transmembrane segment, and its function is unknown. The large α-subunit (95 kDa), which contains eight transmembrane segments, reacts with ATP and contains the binding sites for sodium, potassium, ouabain (pronounced "wahbane"), and the other cardiotonic steroids including digitalis. Ouabain is a specific inhibitor of the sodium/potassium-ATPase (see later).

The following steps describe the mechanism of the sodium/potassium-ATPase (Figure 22–6). (1) Three sodium ions in the cell interior bind to the enzyme (E_1), and (2) ATP phosphorylates the α-subunit of the enzyme in a functionally isoergonic process. The enzymic aspartyl-phosphate bond is initially energy rich. (3) The enzyme, which undergoes a conformational change to form E_2, delivers the three sodium ions to the exterior of the cell. The phosphate remains linked to the same aspartyl group, but its standard free energy of hydrolysis is of the low-energy variety ($E_1 \sim P \rightarrow E_2 - P$). The protein alters the standard free energy of hydrolysis of the acylphosphate. (4) Potassium binds to the exterior of the sodium/potassium-ATPase and is transported to the interior. (5) The enzyme undergoes an exergonic hydrolytic de-

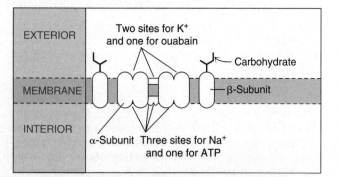

FIGURE 22–5. Architecture of the sodium/potassium-ATPase.

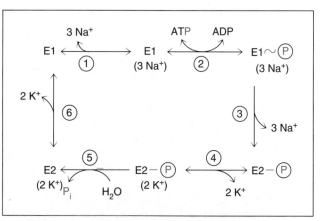

FIGURE 22–6. Ion transport by the sodium/potassium-ATPase.

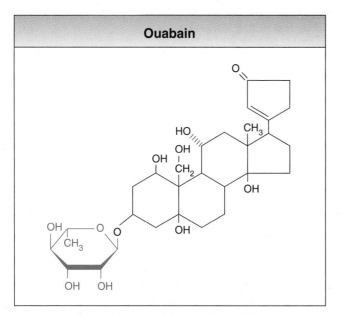

Ouabain

FIGURE 22-7. Ouabain, a cardiac glycoside.

phosphorylation reaction, and (6) two potassium ions are released inside the cell. The enzyme reverts to the original E_1 conformation.

The energy of the sodium/potassium-ATPase changes in a graded fashion to accomplish the transfer of the two sets of ions. Sodium is transported against an electrochemical gradient, and potassium is transported against a concentration gradient. (The intracellular electrical potential is negative.) The net transport process is electrogenic because the number of positive ions transported to the exterior exceeds the number of positive ions transported to the interior.

▶ **Ouabain** is one member of a group of cardiotonic (heart stimulant) steroids that inhibit the sodium/potassium-ATPase (Figure 22–7). Digitalis is the prototypical cardiotonic steroid found empirically to be effective in the treatment of congestive heart failure. Digitalis and its congeners increase the strength and force of cardiac muscle contraction. The therapeutic effects of digitalis are related to secondary changes in calcium concentrations that result from inhibition of the sodium/potassium-ATPase. The inhibition of cardiac sodium/potassium-ATPase increases intracellular sodium. Intracellular sodium exchanges with extracellular calcium by an antiport process and increases the intracellular calcium. This increase in intracardiac calcium is responsible for the augmentation of myocardial contraction that is produced by digitalis. ◀   The role of intracellular calcium in regulating skeletal and cardiac muscle contraction is described in Chapter 23.

Calcium-ATPase

Calcium ions subserve many processes in human cells. The release of hormones and neurotransmit-

ters from cells, for example, occurs by exocytosis in a calcium-dependent fashion. The contraction of muscle is triggered by an increase in intracellular calcium concentration. The calcium concentration of a muscle cell increases from about 0.1 μM (resting) to about 5 μM following excitation.

The relaxation of skeletal muscle requires the transport of calcium from the cytoplasm of muscle cells (sarcoplasm) into a specialized and abundant sarcoplasmic reticulum membrane system. An associated **calcium-ATPase** decreases the concentration of calcium in the sarcoplasm and promotes skeletal muscle relaxation. The activity of calcium-ATPase in the sarcoplasmic reticulum is very high. In fact, calcium-ATPase accounts for about 80% of the integral membrane protein of the sarcoplasmic reticulum. The lumen of the sarcoplasmic reticulum contains an acidic glycoprotein named **calsequestrin,** which binds up to 40 moles of Ca^{+2} per mole of protein. Calsequestrin serves as a repository for calcium transported into the sarcoplasmic reticulum. The total calcium content of the sarcoplasmic reticulum may be as high as 10 millimoles per kilogram.

Calcium-ATPase consists of a single polypeptide with a molecular mass of 100 kDa. Calcium-ATPase is phosphorylated analogously to the sodium/potassium-ATPase. For each mole of ATP hydrolyzed, two moles of calcium are transported into the sarcoplasmic reticulum. The mechanism for transport is similar to that proposed for the sodium/potassium-ATPase. The binding of two moles of calcium to the calcium-ATPase in the cytosol promotes the phosphorylation of the enzyme by ATP. As with the sodium/potassium-ATPase, a β-carboxylate of a specific aspartyl group is phosphorylated. This acylphosphate is energy rich. The enzyme undergoes a conformational change and releases the two calcium ions within the sarcoplasmic reticulum. Concomitant with these changes, the enzyme is converted from an E_1 conformation to an E_2 conformation. The acylphosphate bond is now energy poor. The acylphosphate is hydrolyzed in an exergonic reaction and is converted from the E_2 state to the original E_1 state.

Based upon genetic analysis of complementary DNA, calcium-ATPase consists of 10 transmembrane segments, and it thus differs from the sodium/potassium-ATPase, which has eight in the α-subunit and one in the β-subunit. Cells other than muscle cells contain calcium-ATPase. It is found in plasma membranes and pumps calcium out of the cells.

Class P, V, and F ATPases

We have thus far considered transport by facilitated diffusion by the glucose translocase, and the active transport of sodium-potassium and calcium by ion-related ATPases. The ion-related ATPases are called **class P ATPases** because this group of enzymes proceeds through a *p*hosphorylated

TABLE 22–1. P, V, and F Ion-Translocating ATPases

ATPase	Membrane	Class
Na$^+$/K$^+$	Plasma	Class P ATPases consist of transmembrane polypeptides that form a covalent *p*hospho-enzyme (denoted by P) as part of their reaction cycle
Ca^{2+}	Sarcoplasmic reticulum, plasma	
H$^+$/K$^+$	Plasma	
H$^+$	Lysosomes, endosomes, secretory vesicles	Class V ATPases are H$^+$ transporters found in the membranes of acidic *v*esicles (denoted by V). Class V ATPases do not form a phospho-enzyme intermediate during catalysis
H$^+$	Inner mitochondrial	Class F ATPases consist of about 20 polypeptides and contain a membrane-bound (F$_O$) complex as well as an extrinsic (F$_1$) segment that synthesizes ATP from ADP and P$_i$. Class F ATPases do not form a phosphoenzyme intermediate during catalysis

(**phospho-aspartyl**) covalent intermediate. Proton/potassium-ATPases have been described that are also in this class (Tables 22–1 and 22–2).

The **class V** (for *v*esicle) **ATPases** transport protons. These enzymes acidify intracellular organelles such as lysosomes by pumping protons against a concentration gradient of 2 pH units or more. These enzymes are energized by ATP as it undergoes hydrolysis to ADP and P$_i$. The class V enzymes do not form a covalent phosphate linkage, and their mechanism thereby differs from that of the class P enzymes. The molecular properties of the class V enzymes also differ from those of the class P and class F enzymes. The class V enzymes are composed of three to five polypeptides.

The **class F ATPases** are the familiar F$_O$F$_1$ synthases that play a central role in the generation of ATP by oxidative phosphorylation (Figure 9–13). These enzymes do not possess a detectable phospho-enzyme intermediate. The class F ATPases contain about 20 different polypeptides. Some of these polypeptides form a transmembrane segment (F$_O$), a stalk, and a globular ATP synthase (F$_1$). Based on complementary DNA sequence analysis, the molecular structures of the class F ATPases differ from those of the class P and class V ATPase activities.

SECONDARY ACTIVE TRANSPORT

The transport of sodium and potassium by the sodium/potassium-ATPase is an example of primary active transport. ATP reacts with the translocase and energizes active transport directly. In secondary active transport, ATP provides the energy for transport indirectly. One mechanism for performing this function is to use the energy of an ion gradient to energize transport. For example, metabolites in some cells are cotransported with sodium. The sodium/potassium-ATPase uses the energy of ATP to establish a sodium gradient. The concentration of sodium exterior to the cell is high, and that in the interior of cells is low. Sodium can move down its electrochemical gradient in an exergonic process, and sodium can drive the cotransport of glucose in an endergonic direction (Figure 22–8). The cotransport of sodium and glucose is an example of symport (Figure 22–3).

The sodium-dependent glucose transporters occur only in kidney and intestine. The kidney transporter is responsible for the reabsorption of glucose from the glomerular filtrate into the circulation, and the intestinal transporter is responsible for the absorption of glucose and galactose (but not fructose) from the gut into the circulation. The sodium-independent glucose transporters (GLUT1 through GLUT7) that translocate glucose by facilitated diffusion have a much wider tissue distribution including the erythrocyte, brain, liver, muscle, adipocyte, kidney, and intestine. Some kidney and intestinal cells contain both sodium-dependent and sodium-independent glucose transporters. The two classes of transporter are nonhomologous. The sodium-independent forms possess 12 transmembrane segments, and the sodium-dependent trans-

TABLE 22–2. Characteristics of Metabolite Transport Systems

Ion or Metabolite	Polarity of Pump	Energy Coupling	Location
Na$^+$/K$^+$	Out-in	Primary active (ATP) (Na$^+$/K$^+$-ATPase)	All animal cells
Ca^{2+}	Out	Primary active (ATP) (Ca^{2+}-ATPase)	Sarcoplasmic reticulum, plasma membrane
H$^+$/K$^+$	Out-in	Primary active (ATP) (H$^+$/K$^+$-ATPase)	Apical plasma membrane of stomach epithelial cells
H$^+$	Out	Primary active (electron transport)	Mitochondrion
Glucose	None	Facilitated diffusion	Most cells
Glucose	In	Secondary active (Na$^+$ cotransport)	Gut, kidney
HCO$_3^-$-Cl$^-$	None	Facilitated diffusion (anion channel)	Erythrocytes and stomach epithelium
ATP-ADP	None	Facilitated diffusion	Mitochondrion
P$_i$-OH$^-$	None	Facilitated diffusion	Mitochondrion

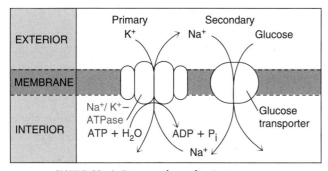

FIGURE 22–8. Primary and secondary active transport.

porters possess 11 transmembrane segments. Moreover, there are two classes of sodium-dependent glucose transporters that differ in the stoichiometry of transport. One form cotransports one sodium and one glucose molecule and occurs in the proximal tubule of the kidney and in the intestine. The second form transports two sodium ions per glucose. The second form can transport glucose against a higher glucose concentration gradient and is found in the distal tubule of the kidney.

The transport of glucose through the intestinal epithelia is intricate. Beginning in the lumen, glucose is transported through an epithelial cell and is released into the blood (Figure 22–9). Sodium and glucose are cotransported by a sodium-glucose symport system through the apical membrane of the epithelial cell. This is an example of secondary active transport. The epithelial cell's sodium ion concentration is maintained at low levels through the action of the sodium/potassium-ATPase. The transport of glucose through the basal membrane is mediated by facilitated diffusion under the aegis of a glucose transporter (GLUT5).

SECRETION OF ACIDIC GASTRIC JUICE

The stomach secretes gastric juice that contains nearly 0.1 M HCl. Acid denatures ingested proteins

and makes them more susceptible to the action of proteases. The chief proteolytic enzyme in the stomach is pepsin. This enzyme has a pH optimum of about 1, a rare enzyme property.

Four protein components are required for the generation of hydrochloric acid from parietal cells: (1) a chloride-bicarbonate antiport protein, (2) a chloride channel protein, (3) a potassium channel protein, and (4) a proton/potassium-ATPase. The mechanism for the secretion of HCl is illustrated in Figure 22–10. Carbon dioxide generated by Krebs cycle activity or derived from the blood reacts with water to form carbonic acid in a reaction catalyzed by carbonic anhydrase. Carbonic acid dissociates (nonenzymatically) into HCO_3^- and H^+. The intracellular bicarbonate (HCO_3^-) exchanges for plasma chloride (Cl^-). This exchange is negotiated by an anion antiport protein.

Chloride crosses a protein channel in the apical surface of gastric parietal cells and is released into the stomach (Figure 22–10). The main source of energy for the secretion of protons is the ATP that sustains a proton/potassium-ATPase. This ATPase is a class P enzyme (Table 22–1). The proton/potassium-ATPase pumps two protons in exchange for one potassium ion. This pump is electrogenic (more positive charges are pumped out of than into the cell). The electrogenic nature of the pump sustains the transport of chloride through its channel in an electropositive direction. The proton/potassium-ATPase (and the sodium/potassium-ATPase present in the cells) maintains a high intracellular potassium concentration. Potassium is released into the stomach through a protein that functions as a potassium channel; the diet also provides potassium in the stomach lumen.

▶ Gastric and duodenal ulcers are common maladies in the United States. They are produced in part by the excessive secretion of hydrochloric acid. Ulcers were treated with antacids for many years, but the use of histamine H_2-receptor antagonists has become prevalent. Histamine is produced in the oxyntic glands of the stomach. These cells possess gastrin and muscarinic acetylcholine recep-

FIGURE 22–9. Absorption of glucose through the intestine. *Sodium moves down its concentration gradient with glucose by symport through a carrier located in the apical membrane (toward the intestinal lumen). Glucose is transported through the basal membrane (toward the bloodstream) by facilitated diffusion. Apical refers to the top of the cell, and basal refers to the bottom of the cell in relation to the cell's binding to the wall of the intestine.*

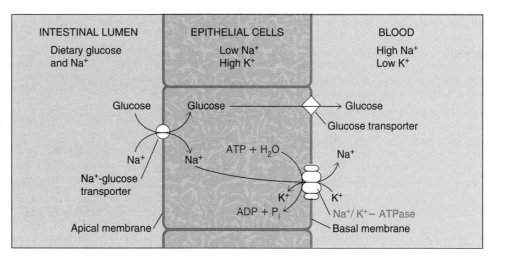

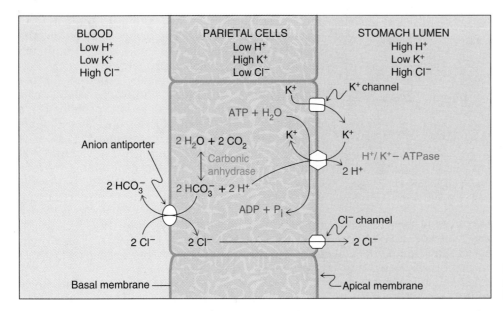

FIGURE 22–10. Secretion of hydrochloric acid (H^+ and Cl^-) by the parietal cells of the stomach.

tors that stimulate histamine release. Parietal cells of the stomach possess histamine H_2-receptors that are blocked by antagonists such as cimetidine. Parietal cell histamine receptors activate adenylyl cyclase, and cyclic AMP plays a role in hydrochloric acid secretion. Calcium also regulates HCl production. Omeprazole, an inhibitor of the proton/potassium-ATPase, is also used for the treatment of ulcers. The use of the histamine antagonists has revolutionized the treatment of peptic ulcers, and the relative effectiveness of antihistamines and the proton pump inhibitors is under study. The role of bacterial infection (*Helicobacter pylori*, Table 1–3) in producing ulcers and the efficacy of antibiotic treatment is another avenue of therapy. ◄

γ-GLUTAMYL CYCLE FOR AMINO ACID TRANSPORT

Glutathione is a tripeptide (γ-glutamylcysteinylglycine) found in animals and bacteria (Figure 22–11). Glutathione plays a role in amino acid transport in the nephron and jejunum. The amino acid is modified as a result of translocation across a membrane, and this process is classified as a **group translocation** reaction. The peptide bond between glutamate and cysteine is not that of the α-carboxyl group of glutamate but rather is that of the γ-carboxylate. Glutathione synthesis is catalyzed by two enzymes, and each reaction involves the orthophosphate split of ATP to ADP and P_i. Let us consider the reactions involved in amino acid translocation and in glutathione biosynthesis.

The concentration of glutathione intra- and extracellularly is appreciable (approaching millimolar). Glutathione reacts with the amino acid to be transported to form the γ-glutamyl amino acid and cysteinylglycine (Figure 22–11). The reaction is catalyzed by a membranous γ-glutamyl transpeptidase. The transpeptidation reaction is isoergonic, and no exogenous chemical energy is required. In a concerted step, the γ-glutamyl amino acid and cysteinylglycine are transported into the cell. The process is not simple transport, owing to the conversion of the amino acid on the exterior to the glutamyl adduct during the group translocation. The best substrates for the transpeptidase include cystine, glutamine, and methionine.

Cysteinylglycine, the other product, is transported into cells and is hydrolyzed. This hydrolysis makes the transport process exergonic. An intracellular γ-glutamyl cyclotransferase catalyzes the cyclization of the glutamyl residue to form 5-oxoproline with the concomitant release of the amino acid. This reaction involves the displacement of the amino acid by the α-amino group of glutamate. Although cyclization reactions occur with a decrease in entropy, formation of five- and six-membered organic rings is a facile process. The energy of ATP, and two water molecules, is required to open the 5-oxoproline ring. One water is necessary for the cleavage of the oxoproline to yield glutamate, and the second is required for the conversion of ATP to ADP and P_i. This completes the reactions involved in the transport of the amino acid.

Next let us consider the pathway for glutathione biosynthesis (Figure 22–11). ATP reacts with glutamate to form γ-glutamyl∼phosphate (an energy-rich acylphosphate) as an enzyme-bound intermediate, and ADP. The γ-glutamyl∼phosphate undergoes a nucleophilic attack by the amino group of cysteine to displace phosphate and form γ-glutamyl-cysteine (with a resulting energy-poor peptide bond). This dipeptide reacts with ATP and glycine (perhaps by an analogous mechanism) to form glutathione, ADP, and P_i.

The energetics of the complete transport process requires the expenditure of three ATP mole-

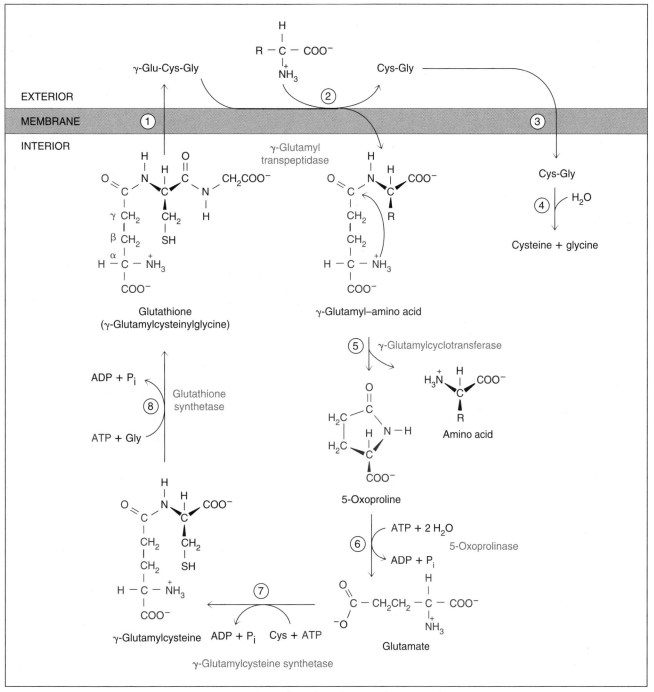

FIGURE 22–11. *The γ-glutamyl amino acid transport cycle.*

cules for the transport of a single amino acid. Two are required for glutathione biosynthesis, and the third is required for conversion of 5-oxoproline to glutamate. The transport of amino acids by this mechanism is not bioenergetically trivial.

The γ-glutamyl cycle is restricted to only a few cell types including the nephron and jejunum. Most amino acids are transported into cells by sodium-dependent translocases. Transporters exist for several families of amino acids including (1) small nonpolar, (2) large nonpolar and aromatic, (3) glycine and proline, (4) acidic, and (5) basic amino

acids. The absence of the transporter for large nonpolar and aromatic amino acids results in **Hartnup disease,** and the absence of the transporter for basic amino acids produces **cystinuria.** Rare human disorders of the γ-glutamyl transport cycle have also been described.

CHLORIDE TRANSPORT AND CYSTIC FIBROSIS

▶ The most common disorder of metabolite transport is that of cystic fibrosis. The clinical fea-

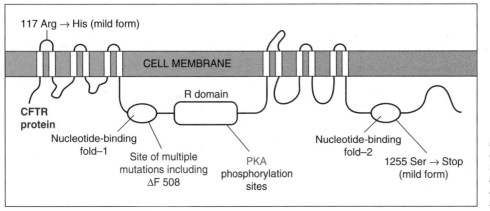

117 Arg → His (mild form)

CELL MEMBRANE

R domain

CFTR protein

Nucleotide-binding fold–1

Site of multiple mutations including ΔF 508

PKA phosphorylation sites

Nucleotide-binding fold–2

1255 Ser → Stop (mild form)

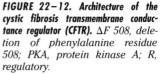

FIGURE 22–12. *Architecture of the cystic fibrosis transmembrane conductance regulator (CFTR).* ΔF 508, *deletion of phenylalanine residue 508; PKA, protein kinase A; R, regulatory.*

tures of cystic fibrosis are dominated by the respiratory tract, where obstruction of the airways by thick, sticky mucus and subsequent infection, especially with *Pseudomonas* species, occurs. Affected individuals usually do not survive into their fourth decade, and the median life span is ≈ 30 years. This life span is increasing because of better control of infections with antibiotics. Ninety-eight percent of males and 90% of females are infertile.

Cystic fibrosis is accompanied by an increase in sweat chloride concentration, and this finding was undoubtedly made by an astute parent or physician by taste. Sweat chloride values in cystic fibrosis are generally greater than 60 milliequivalents per liter. The pulmonary secretions are thick, and recurrent infections are one result. The hallmark of cystic fibrosis is chronic pulmonary disease. There is also a deficiency of pancreatic enzymes (lipase, trypsin, chymotrypsin) and improper digestion. Current management includes chest percussion to promote mucus drainage, DNAse treatment by aerosol to decrease the viscosity of pulmonary mucus, antibiotic treatment, and pancreatic enzyme replacement. Therapeutic DNAse is the human enzyme produced by genetic engineering.

The incidence of this hereditary disease is about 1 in 2000 Caucasian live births, making it one of the more common autosomal recessive diseases. Cystic fibrosis is rare in other races. The carrier frequency is about 1 in 22. The gene product is called CFTR (for *c*ystic *f*ibrosis *t*ransmembrane conductance *r*egulator). This protein was discovered in 1989 during research on the disease's etiology and mechanism.

The cystic fibrosis gene spans about 230 kilobases on chromosome 7q31 and contains 27 exons (Table 16–5). The highest mRNA levels for CFTR occur in the pancreas, salivary glands, sweat glands, gut, and reproductive tract. The gene product is a large integral membrane protein of 170 kDa. The protein has 12 transmembrane segments, a regulatory (R) domain that contains sites for phosphorylation by protein kinase A (PKA), and two intracellular ATP-binding domains called nucleotide-binding folds (NBF-1 and NBF-2) as shown in Figure 22–12. CFTR is related to proteins

that participate in active transport across membranes including the P-glycoprotein that accounts for multiple drug resistance to cancer chemotherapeutic agents (Chapter 21).

Mutations that cause cystic fibrosis are variable and include missense, nonsense, and frameshift mutations having small insertions or deletions, and point mutations that affect splicing. The most common mutation (70% of all cases) results in the deletion of phenylalanine 508. The clinical heterogeneity of the disorder arises, at least in part, from allelic heterogeneity. It has been suggested that carriers of the cystic fibrosis gene are less sensitive to the effects of cholera toxin. Prenatal diagnosis using DNA analysis is possible, and such diagnostic tests are undergoing continual refinement (Figure 15–34).

CFTR plays a role in anion transport, and this function is affected by phosphorylation by protein kinase A. The normal efflux of chloride ions across respiratory epithelial cell membranes in response to elevated cyclic AMP is lacking in cystic fibrosis. Protein kinase A is activated, but protein kinase A fails to activate chloride conductance. Because mutations do not occur in the regulatory domain that contains the phosphorylation sites, the inability to respond to protein kinase A is an indirect effect. ◄

SUMMARY

Several mechanisms have evolved to translocate essential components into and out of cells and their organelles. Translocases are integral membrane proteins that traverse the membrane bilayer. Some translocases transport metabolites down a concentration gradient by facilitated diffusion, and external energy is not required. Active transport, on the other hand, requires energy. If ATP is the direct source of energy, the process is called primary active transport. If a gradient, produced by the action of ATP, sustains metabolite transport, the process is called secondary active transport. Group translocation refers to the condition in which the metabolite undergoes chemical modification during the translocation. The expenditure of an appreciable fraction (one-quarter) of basal energy for ion and metabolite transport is a key attribute of all organisms.

Most integral membrane enzymes that possess ATPase activity are involved in maintaining ion and pH gradients. These membrane components can be divided into three groups based upon the structure and mechanism of the enzyme. Class P ATPases are ion translocases that exhibit a covalent phosphorylated enzyme intermediate. Sodium/potassium-ATPase is the best characterized of this group of enzymes. Class V enzymes are found in vesicles and lysosomes and lack a phosphorylated enzyme intermediate. Class F enzymes are the ATP synthases in mitochondria. They consist of an F_O portion within membranes and an F_1 portion on the interior face of the membranes.

The class P transport proteins form an aspartyl-phosphate during the translocation process. This bond is initially high energy in nature (the E_1 conformation). The protein forms a low-energy form (the E_2 conformation). The sodium/potassium-ATPase was the first class P transport protein to be described. It transports three sodium ions out of and two potassium ions into cells during one cycle. Sodium/potassium-ATPase is inhibited by ouabain and other cardiotonic glycosides including digitalis. Other examples of the class P ATPase include the calcium-ATPase that sequesters intracellular calcium in the sarcoplasmic reticulum of muscle cells and the proton/potassium-ATPase responsible for secreting acid in the stomach. γ-Glutamyl transpeptidase participates in amino acid translocation in kidney and jejunum. This is a group translocation process due to the chemical modification of the substance transported.

Cystic fibrosis is the most common disorder that results from defective transport. The cystic fibrosis transmembrane regulator participates in chloride transport. A variety of mutations occur in the cystic fibrosis gene, and the gene was cloned before the nature of the gene product was known (positional cloning). A genetic disease and fundamental studies using the methodology of molecular biology led to the discovery of a physiological process.

SELECTED READINGS

Doohan, M.M., and H.H. Rasmussen. Myocardial cation transport. Journal of Hypertension 11:683–691, 1993.

Fuller, C.M., and D.J. Benos. CFTR! American Journal of Physiology 263:C267–286, 1992.

Lienhard, G.E., J.W. Slot, D.E. James, and M.M. Mueckler. How cells absorb glucose. Scientific American 266(January):86–91, 1992.

Meister, A., and A. Larsson. Glutathione synthetase deficiency and other disorders of the γ-glutamyl cycle. In C.R. Scriver, A.L. Beaudet, W.S. Sly, and D. Valle (eds.). *The Metabolic Basis of Inherited Disease,* 6th ed. New York, McGraw-Hill Book Company, 1989, pp. 855–868.

Sferra, T.J., and F.S. Collins. The molecular biology of cystic fibrosis. Annual Review of Medicine 44:133–144, 1993.

Silverman, M. Structure and function of hexose transporters. Annual Review of Biochemistry 60:757–794, 1991.

CHAPTER TWENTY-THREE

MUSCLE AND

CONNECTIVE TISSUE

The function of muscle is to produce motion.
—ALBERT SZENT-GYORGYI

The three classes of muscle are skeletal, cardiac, and smooth. Skeletal and cardiac muscle are called **striated muscle** because of their striped microscopic appearance, which **smooth muscle** lacks. The mechanism of force generation by these three types of muscle is similar. The connective tissue tendons and ligaments that tether muscle to bones and joints are the agents that effect the forces generated by muscle. Connective tissue also plays a pivotal role in maintaining the structure of tissues and organs.

Collagen, elastin, proteoglycans, and glycoproteins make up the extracellular matrix. The matrix is a dynamic milieu in which cells differentiate, develop, move, and organize into tissues. Collagen gives tissues and organs their tensile strength. Elastin, as its name suggests, is responsible for the extensibility and recoil of lung, blood vessels, and some ligaments. Proteoglycans serve important structural and functional roles as the extracellular matrix of tissues throughout the body. Fibronectin, a glycoprotein, connects cells with the proteoglycans of the extracellular matrix.

MUSCLE

Ultrastructure

The striations of skeletal muscle appear as alternating light and dark bands (Figure 23–1). The dark bands are the **A bands** (*a*nisotropic) and contain the thick filaments of myosin. The A bands also contain the thin filaments that overlap the thick filaments. The light bands are the **I bands** (*i*sotropic) and contain thin filaments. Muscle and muscle fasciculi (bundles) are made up of units called muscle fibers, and muscle fibers are made up of myofibrils (Figure 23–2). Myofibrils, in turn, are composed of a repeating series of sarcomeres. Sarcomeres extend from one Z disk to the next. Actin thin filaments are attached to the **Z disk.**

Electron micrographs of transverse sections of the sarcomere reveal additional structural details. Sections through the I band show an array of thin filaments (Figure 23–2F). Sections through the central portion of the H zone of the A band show an array of thick filaments only (Figure 23–2G). Sections through the A band show that each thick filament is surrounded by a hexagonal array of thin filaments, and each thin filament is surrounded by three thick filaments (Figure 23–2I). Electron micrographs reveal cross-bridges from the thick to thin filaments, and **cross-bridges** are central to the sliding filament model of muscle contraction.

The sliding filament hypothesis rationalizes the structures of relaxed and contracted muscles. During contraction, the sarcomeres shorten and the Z disks come closer together. The A band maintains a constant length in the contracted state, but the I band shortens. The lengths of the thin and thick filaments also do not change. The sliding filament

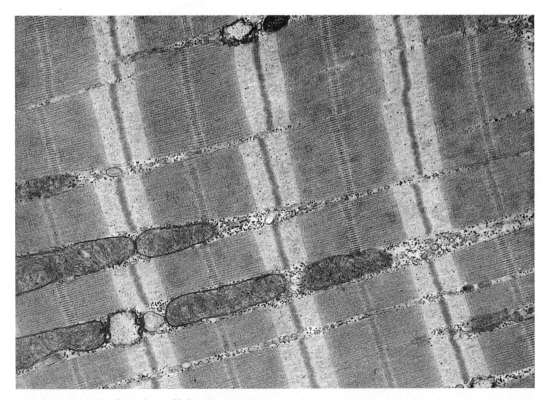

FIGURE 23–1. *Electron micrograph of muscle myofibrils. The myofibrils are in register and produce the characteristic striations. Note the mitochondria lying between the myofibrils. The dark bands are A (anisotropic) bands that contain myosin (and actin). The light bands are I (isotropic) bands containing actin. Reproduced, with permission, from D.W. Fawcett. The Cell. Philadelphia, W.B. Saunders Company, 1981, p. 235.*

SKELETAL MUSCLE

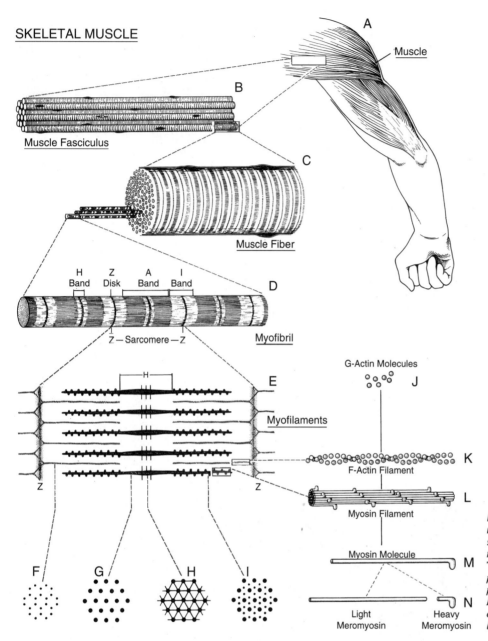

FIGURE 23–2. The hierarchy of skeletal muscle organization—from muscle to myosin. *Reproduced, with permission, from W. Bloom and D.W. Fawcett.* A Textbook of Histology. *Philadelphia, W.B. Saunders Company, 1986, p. 282. Drawing by Sylvia Colard Keene. Heavy and light meromyosin are produced artificially by proteolytic digestion of myosin* in vitro.

hypothesis states that the fibers of the thin filament, attached to the Z-disk structure at each end of a sarcomere, are pulled toward the center of the sarcomere by the thick filaments of the A band (Figure 23–3).

Proteins

Myosin makes up about 60% of the total protein in skeletal muscle. It consists of two identical heavy chains (230-kDa molecular mass each), two essential light chains (16- to 20-kDa molecular mass each), and two regulatory light chains (also 16- to 20-kDa molecular mass each). Myosin possesses ATPase activity. *Myosin is the site of energy transduction where the chemical energy of ATP is converted into mechanical energy.*

Myosin contains a globular domain at the amino terminus and a long, rod-like tail segment at the carboxyl terminus of its heavy chain. The rod-like portion results from the coiling of the α-helix of one heavy chain about the α-helix of the other heavy chain to form a coiled coil. Tail segments of several myosin molecules assemble to form thick filaments (Figure 23–2L, M). Each globular region contains an essential light chain and a regulatory light chain (Figure 23–4). The appearance of nonglobular myosin is dependent upon the direction of viewing, and this is by definition anisotropic. *Myosin is the chief protein component of the A (anisotropic) band.*

Actin (42-kDa molecular mass) is the second major protein of muscle. Actin is also a preeminent protein in all other cells. Actin exists as a monomeric or G (globular) form. Several G-actin mono-

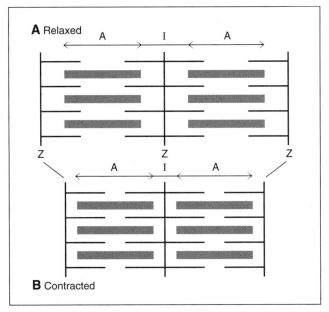

FIGURE 23–3. *Diagrammatic structure of sarcomeres in the relaxed (A) and contracted (B) states.*

mers form helical filaments (F, filamentous actin) and occur as such in the thin filaments of skeletal muscle (Figure 23–2). Fourteen actin molecules form one turn of the helical filament. The interaction of the myosin heads and actin filaments is responsible for the generation of force.

Tropomyosin (70-kDa molecular mass) is a long, thin molecule composed of two different protein subunits of molecular mass of 33 kDa and 37 kDa. Tropomyosin interacts with seven actin molecules in the thin filament (Figure 23–5) and blocks the interaction of actin and myosin in the resting state. Tropomyosin occurs with **troponin,** consisting of three different types of subunit. **Troponin I** inhibits the interaction of actin and myosin through the action of tropomyosin. **Troponin C** binds *calcium* reversibly. **Troponin T** interacts with *t*ropomyosin. These components are listed in Table 23–1.

Contraction

Striated Muscle

Myosin ATPase activity plays a central role in the conversion of chemical energy to mechanical energy. ATPase activity resides in the globular domain of heavy meromyosin (Figure 23–2). Under resting conditions, tropomyosin sterically blocks the interaction of actin with myosin. Following an increase in sarcoplasmic calcium concentration from about 0.1 to 5 μM, troponin C forms a complex with calcium and undergoes a conformational change. Tropomyosin is displaced by the troponin-calcium complex, and actin forms a complex with myosin. This interaction stimulates myosin ATPase activity and promotes force generation. When the calcium concentration falls, troponin C releases calcium, assumes its initial conformation, and promotes the relative movement of tropomyosin which, in turn, inhibits actin and myosin interaction.

The cyclic association and dissociation of actin and myosin is related to ATP hydrolysis as described in the following scheme. A complex of actin and myosin reacts with ATP; actin is displaced, and myosin binds ATP (Figure 23–6). ATP is hydrolyzed to form ADP + P_i and an energized state of myosin. Surprisingly, this hydrolysis occurs before any force generation. The complex, however, is energized like an extended spring. This energized component then interacts with actin to form a complex of actin·myosin·(ADP + P_i). Myosin generates force and is transformed from an energized to a de-energized state. ADP + P_i is discharged, leaving an energy-poor actin·myosin complex.

The following describes the **sliding filament mechanism for muscle contraction** (Figure 23–7). (1) ATP is required to dissociate actin from myosin. This allows myosin to move relative to the thin filament. (2) Hydrolysis of ATP produces energized myosin. In response to a nerve impulse, calcium is

FIGURE 23–4. *Architecture of myosin.*

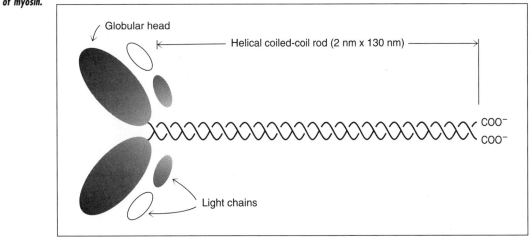

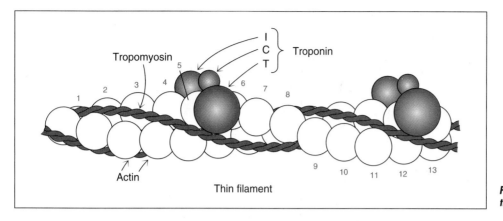

Tropomyosin

Troponin

I
C
T

5

1 2 3 4

6 7 8

9 10 11 12 13

Actin

Thin filament

FIGURE 23-5. Protein components of the thin filament.

released from the sarcoplasmic reticulum, and calcium triggers muscle contraction. Calcium ions, acting through troponin and tropomyosin, allow energized myosin·(ADP + P_i) to interact with actin. (3) The head of myosin tilts and moves a chain of filamentous actin molecules relative to the thick filament by a rachet-like process. During this event, the thin filament moves about 12 nm (the length of two actin monomers) relative to the thick filament. (4) ADP and P_i are discharged, and myosin binds ATP and the cycle repeats. This cycle occurs up to eight times per second for the duration of a single contraction.

At the end of a contraction, the sarcoplasmic reticulum no longer releases but actively removes calcium from the sarcoplasm. This process involves calcium ATPase activity of the sarcoplasmic reticulum as described in Chapter 22. When the calcium concentration decreases, calcium dissociates from troponin C and tropomyosin moves to inhibit the interaction of actin and the myosin head. The interaction of actin and myosin is required for force generation in both striated and smooth muscle.

Smooth Muscle

Smooth muscle lacks the microscopic striations exhibited by skeletal and cardiac muscle. This difference between smooth and striated muscle is due to the lack of regular arrays of ordered thin and thick filaments. Smooth muscle possesses actin and myosin but in less ordered fashion than the corresponding components of striated muscle. Smooth muscle contraction, like that of striated muscle, is regulated by alterations in the levels of intracellular calcium. Smooth muscle, unlike striated skeletal and cardiac muscle, lacks a well-defined sarcoplasmic reticulum. The rates of change of cytosolic calcium levels are much slower in smooth muscle than in striated muscle. This permits a slow, steady response in contractile tension. *Smooth muscle, moreover, lacks the troponin system and utilizes protein phosphorylation to initiate and sustain contraction.*

The interaction of nonphosphorylated smooth muscle myosin and actin is disallowed. Initiation of contraction is the result of phosphorylation of regulatory myosin light chains; cessation of contraction is the result of the dephosphorylation of these myosin light chains. These reactions are catalyzed by **myosin-light-chain kinase** and **phosphoprotein phosphatase,** respectively (Figure 23-8). Following phosphorylation of the myosin light chains, myosin can interact with actin and generate force. Following dephosphorylation of the regulatory myosin light chain, interaction between actin and myosin is inhibited and contraction ceases.

Myosin-light-chain kinase is a protein kinase with restricted specificity because it catalyzes only the phosphorylation of a specific serine residue near the amino terminus of the regulatory myosin light

---

TABLE 23-1. Protein Components of Muscle

Component	Relative Molecular Mass (kDa)	Structure	Function
Myosin	540	Two heavy chains	ATPase
		Two essential light chains	Thick filament
		Two regulatory light chains	
Actin	42	Globular monomeric actin forms filamentous actin	Interacts with myosin to generate force
		Fourteen monomers per turn of the helix	Thin filament
Tropomyosin	70	Two coiled subunits extend the length of 7 actin monomers	Blocks binding of actin to myosin
Troponin	76	Troponin I, 21 kDa	Controls *i*nhibition by tropomyosin
		Troponin T, 37 kDa	Binds *t*ropomyosin and troponin C
		Troponin C, 18 kDa	Binds Ca^{2+}

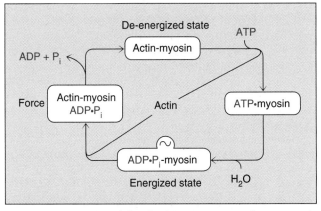

FIGURE 23–6. Overview of the role of ATP in energy transduction in muscle contraction.

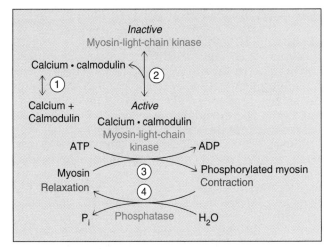

FIGURE 23–8. Regulation of smooth muscle contraction.

chain. Myosin-light-chain kinase is regulated by calcium in combination with calmodulin. **Calmodulin** received its name because it alters or modulates physiological and biochemical effects in response to calcium. Calmodulin is a low-molecular-mass protein (16 kDa) that binds up to four molecules of calcium. Free calmodulin does not activate myosin-light-chain kinase. The calcium·calmodulin complex, however, activates myosin-light-chain kinase and leads to smooth muscle contraction.

High-Energy Phosphates

Muscle, like other tissues, derives its chemical energy from ATP generated by glycolysis and oxi-

dative phosphorylation. In contrast to most other tissues, however, muscle requirements for ATP can rapidly change. During maximal activity, mammalian skeletal muscle uses ATP at the rate of about 1 mol per kilogram per minute. The content of ATP, however, is 3–5 mmol per kilogram of muscle. This is the amount of ATP required for 10 contractions, and this quantity of ATP would be depleted in about one second of intense activity. Creatine phosphate makes a substantive contribution in maintaining sarcoplasmic ATP.

Skeletal and cardiac muscle (and brain) contain significant amounts (25 mmol/kg of muscle) of **creatine phosphate.** This phosphoramidate (P~N) serves as a storage form of high-energy phosphate.

FIGURE 23–7. Myosin-ATPase energy transduction cycle of muscle contraction.

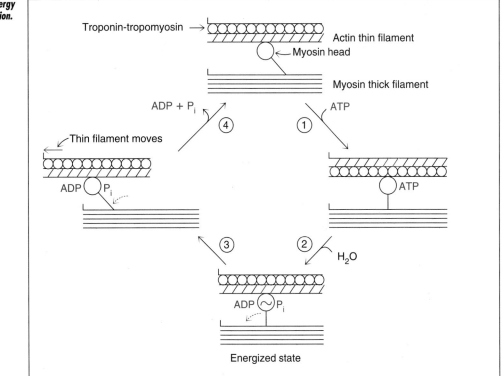

The only physiological reaction of phosphocreatine is the transfer of its phosphoryl group to ADP to generate ATP and creatine. It does not donate its phosphoryl group to other acceptors, and there are no known creatine phosphatases. The levels of creatine phosphate exceed those of ATP in resting muscle by a factor of five. **Creatine phosphokinase** catalyzes the reversible transphosphorylation between creatine phosphate and ADP (Figure 4–13).

Muscle and other tissues regenerate ATP from ADP as catalyzed by **adenylate kinase.** The original name given to this enzyme was **myokinase** because it was first isolated from muscle. Adenylate kinase catalyzes a reaction between two molecules of ADP to yield ATP and AMP in an isoergonic process. Besides capturing the residual energy of ADP in utilizable form, adenylate kinase generates AMP, which is an activator of the phosphofructokinase reaction, and thereby promotes glycolysis. During recovery, adenylate kinase and creatine phosphokinase reactions can use newly formed ATP (from glycolysis and oxidative phosphorylation) to convert AMP to ADP and creatine to creatine phosphate (Figure 23–9).

Let us consider the differential role of glycolysis and oxidative phosphorylation in various muscles. Skeletal muscle consists of both red and white muscle types. **Red muscle** is pigmented owing to a relatively high content of mitochondrial cytochromes and myoglobin. Red muscle and cardiac muscle have a higher rate of oxidative phosphorylation than white muscle. The external muscles of the eye are almost purely red muscle. **White muscle,** in contrast, contains small amounts of cytochromes. The soleus muscle, attached to the Achilles tendon, is an example of white muscle. White muscle uses glycolysis for most of its energy production. Some muscles such as the gastrocnemius (the calf muscle of the leg) contain both red and white muscle fibers. Red muscle uses fatty acids as a major fuel; fatty acids are metabolized by β-oxidation to acetyl-CoA. Acetyl-CoA is then completely degraded to carbon dioxide and water by the combined action of the Krebs cycle and oxidation phosphorylation with the attendant formation of ATP. Ketone bodies (acetoacetate and β-hydroxybutyrate) are also used by red muscle. White muscle, in contrast, uses glycogen and glucose as major fuels.

Following creatine phosphate and ATP utilization, the increased content of ADP controls the operation of the Krebs cycle in red muscle by activating isocitrate dehydrogenase allosterically. Enhanced production of NADH with the availability of ADP and P_i will increase oxidative phosphorylation. In active white muscle, adenylate kinase generates AMP. AMP activates glycogen phosphorylase and phosphofructokinase and accordingly accelerates the rate of glycolysis (Table 25–1). The δ-subunit of phosphorylase kinase is calmodulin, and this enzyme is activated by calcium. Release of calcium from the sarcoplasmic reticulum triggers muscle contraction and activates glycogenolysis. This dual regulation by calcium provides an instructive example of the metabolic logic of the cell (PRINCIPLE 9 OF BIOCHEMISTRY).

With limited oxygen, for example, during a sprint, considerable lactate is produced in muscle by anaerobic glycolysis and is released into the bloodstream. Following this exertional period, humans consume considerably greater oxygen than during resting periods. This extra oxygen consumed is termed the **oxygen debt.** Oxygen debt corresponds to the oxidation of some of the lactate produced. These oxidation reactions occur in the liver, and energy derived from oxidation of some lactate is used for the conversion of the remaining lactate to glucose by gluconeogenesis (Chapter 10). Glucose is stored in liver as glycogen or is released and transported to muscle (and other tissues). Transport of lactate from muscle to the liver and the return transport of glucose from the liver to muscle is called the **Cori cycle,** described by Carl and Gerty Cori.

Duchenne Muscular Dystrophy

▶ Muscular dystrophy is a severe disorder that occurs with relentless clinical deterioration. Muscular dystrophy is an X-linked recessive disease (Table 16–5) that occurs almost exclusively in males (about 1 per 3000 live births). It is characterized by muscle weakness, onset at 3–5 years of age, and death by the third decade. Death is due to respiratory failure and its complications. Affected individuals exhibit elevated serum creatine phosphokinase levels. Most carrier mothers (70%) have elevated serum creatine phosphokinase levels. Before the development of genetic probes, serum enzyme levels were used to assess the carrier state. A small proportion (8%) of carrier

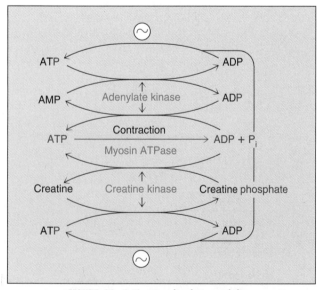

FIGURE 23–9. Creatine phosphate metabolism.

women exhibit abnormal muscle weakness in adult life. Muscular dystrophy is due to an abnormality of the structural gene for **dystrophin** that results in reduced levels or absence of this protein. Dystrophin helps maintain the integrity of muscle fibers.

The muscular dystrophy gene is located on Xp21. The gene is extremely large (2300 kb) and spans 1.5% of the X chromosome. The large size may be related to the 100-fold higher mutation rate of this gene as compared with most other genes. One-third of those with muscular dystrophy have new mutations, and two-thirds have carrier mothers. Two-thirds of the mutations are deletions, and 5% involve duplications. The gene has 79 exons, and dystrophin is a 430-kDa protein. The gene product is most abundant in skeletal and cardiac muscle, and lesser amounts are found in brain. Prenatal diagnosis is possible for 90% of offspring of known female carriers. Its presence or absence in offspring can be determined by amniocentesis or chorionic villus sampling and Southern blot analysis or by multiplex PCR (Chapter 15). There is no specific therapy. ◄

CONNECTIVE TISSUE

Connective tissue consists of four major components: collagen, elastin, proteoglycans, and glycoproteins. Various mesenchymal cells including fibroblasts, osteoblasts, chondroblasts, and odontoblasts are responsible for the synthesis of these substances. Collagen is the major protein of tissues requiring high tensile strength such as blood vessels, bone, cornea, ligaments, sclera, skin, tendons, and the dentine and cementum of teeth. Elastin, with rubber-like properties, occurs in distensible structures such as arteries and lungs. Proteoglycans and glycoproteins connect cells and other connective tissue elements in the extracellular matrix.

Collagen

Structure and Biosynthesis

Collagen, which is the major macromolecule of connective tissue, is the predominant human protein and accounts for one-third of all protein by mass. Human collagen consists of more than a dozen different types of molecules composed of more than two dozen genetically distinct α-chains. The role and function of all the collagen types have not been determined. Type I collagen, a fibrillar collagen, accounts for 90% of all collagen by mass. Type IV collagen, which forms meshes and not fibrils, is important because it forms basement membranes.

The most distinguishing property of collagen is that each α-chain forms a **left-handed helix** with three amino acid residues per turn. Three left-

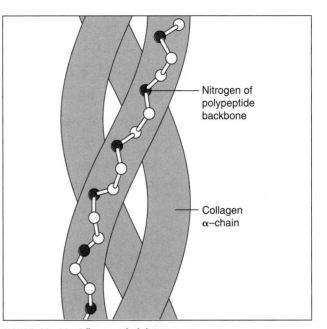

FIGURE 23–10. Collagen triple helix. *Only the polypeptide backbone (carbonyl carbon, α-carbon, and nitrogen) is illustrated.*

Nitrogen of polypeptide backbone

Collagen α–chain

handed helical polypeptides combine to form a **right-handed triple helical molecule,** which is a long (300 nm) and narrow (1.5 nm) rope-like structure (Figure 23–10). *Every third residue of collagen is glycine,* another distinguishing feature. The sequence of the main body of collagen is Gly-X-Y, where X and Y are residues other than glycine. Glycine is the only amino acid small enough to exist at the central core of a triple helix. Of the 1050 residues per chain, about 100 X residues are proline, about 100 Y residues (10%) are 4-hydroxyproline, and 10–50 Y residues (1–5%) are 5-hydroxylysine. Because no rotation is possible between the α-carbon and nitrogen of proline and hydroxyproline, the high content of these amino acids promotes the formation of a left-handed α-chain helix.

Collagen genes contain many exons (about 40). Various genes span from 20 to 40 kilobases. The genes are dispersed among nine chromosomes. The primordial collagen exon contains 54 nucleotides and corresponds to (Gly-X-Y)₆. More than half the exons contain 54 nucleotides; many exons consist of two primordial units, and occasional exons consist of three primordial units. Nonhelical portions of collagen are represented by several exons not related to the primordial unit. Collagen types are denoted by Roman numerals, as in α1(I) for type I collagen. Greek letters and arabic numerals refer to different chains of the various collagen types (Table 23–2). Type V collagen, for example, can contain combinations of three different chains that are designated α1(V), α2(V), and α3(V).

The collagen helix is stabilized in fibrillar structures and other meshworks through 5-hydroxylysine–derived cross-links. Moreover, hydroxylysine residues serve as *O*-linked attachment

TABLE 23-2. Selected Types of Collagen*

Collagen Type	Chain	Chromosomal Location	Procollagen Molecule	Tissue Distribution	Associated Anchorage Protein	Cell-Surface Receptor	Associated Proteoglycans
I	$\alpha 1(I)$	17	$[\alpha 1(I)]_2 \alpha 2(I)$	Skin, tendon, bone, arteries, and nearly all others	Fibronectin	Integrin	Chondroitin sulfate, dermatan sulfate
	$\alpha 2(I)$	7					
II	$\alpha 1(II)$	12	$[\alpha 1(II)]_3$	Cartilage, vitreous	Fibronectin	Integrin	Chondroitin sulfate
III	$\alpha 1(III)$	2	$[\alpha 1(III)]_3$	Skin, arteries, uterus, gut	Fibronectin	Integrin	Heparan sulfate, heparin
IV	$\alpha 1(IV)$	13	$[\alpha 1(IV)]_2 \alpha 2(IV)$	Basal lamina	Laminin	Laminin	Heparan sulfate, heparin
	$\alpha 2(IV)$	13	$[\alpha 1(IV)]_3$				
			$[\alpha 2(IV)]_3$				

*More than 12 types are currently known.

sites for one or two carbohydrate residues (glucose, galactose, or glucosylgalactose). The hydroxyl groups of 5-hydroxyproline stabilize collagen by forming hydrogen bonds. Variations occur in the amino acid sequence of the α-chains, resulting in structural components of the same size but with slightly different properties. These α-chains combine to form the various types of collagen found in tissues. The fundamental unit of type I collagen consists of two $\alpha 1$-chains and one $\alpha 2$-chain.

Although collagen functions outside the cell, its synthesis begins intracellularly and is completed extracellularly. Synthesis requires mRNA-dependent protein synthesis and several posttranslational reactions. Collagen is synthesized as **preprocollagen α-chains** in the rough endoplasmic reticulum. The signal peptide, which is remarkably long (about 100 amino acids) is cleaved by hydrolysis, yielding **procollagen α-chains.** Prolyl and lysyl hydroxylation requires oxygen, α-ketoglutarate, and ascorbate substrates (Figure 18–18). A few hydroxylysine residues of each chain are glycosylated. Intrachain disulfide bonds form that connect carboxyterminal portions of three chains together. Disulfide bond formation aligns the three chains so that the physiological triple helix forms. Without proper alignment, abnormal triple helix formation can occur. The **procollagen** triple helix is formed in the Golgi. *Triple helix formation begins at the carboxyl terminus and extends to the amino terminus in a zipper-like process.* Procollagen has a central region of triple helix surrounded by nonhelical amino and carboxyterminal extensions, or propeptides. Procollagen is secreted from the fibroblast (Figure 23–11). **Procollagen amino-terminal protease** and **procollagen carboxyterminal protease** are extracellular enzymes that catalyze the hydrolytic removal of amino and carboxyterminal fragments of the nascent triple helix, yielding tropocollagen. **Tropocollagen** is the mature building block of collagen.

Tropocollagen molecules spontaneously form regular, parallel arrays that become connected and stabilized by cross-linking reactions that result in **collagen.** Cross-links form from ϵ-aldehyde groups derived from lysine and hydroxylysine residues and ϵ-amino groups of other lysine or hydroxylysine residues in tropocollagen. Tropocollagen that

has combined into fibrils is the substrate for lysyl oxidase, an enzyme that operates extracellularly. **Lysyl oxidase** requires pyridoxal phosphate and copper for activity. The products of the reaction include the aldehyde form of lysine (Figure 23–12) or hydroxylysine. The main cross-links in collagen include **hydroxylysyl pyridinoline** and **hydroxylysinonorleucine** (Figure 23–13). (The nor of norleucine means without a methyl radical $-CH_3$.) Lysyl oxidase is the only enzyme known to be required for cross-linking. After formation of the aldehyde, cross-linking occurs nonenzymatically. The chemistry of these reactions has not been deciphered.

Collagenopathies

▶ Osteogenesis imperfecta and Ehlers-Danlos syndrome are genetic diseases involving collagen. Four types of osteogenesis imperfecta and 10 types of Ehlers-Danlos syndrome, which are clinically and biochemically heterogeneous, are recognized by clinicians. One abnormal allele is sufficient to produce disease, and these disorders are autosomal dominant inherited diseases. These are rare maladies, and only specialists know their detailed characteristics by rote. We consider a few salient features.

Osteogenesis imperfecta (brittle bone disease) is characterized by bone fragility that results from various mutations of **type I collagen.** Other signs and symptoms pointing to connective tissue disease include abnormalities of teeth and conductive hearing loss due to abnormalities of the middle ear bones. Type I osteogenesis imperfecta results from mutations that prevent splicing and formation of preprocollagen mRNA. Half the normal amount of preprocollagen $\alpha 1(I)$ mRNA and polypeptide result from the normal allele; no mature message or polypeptide results from the mutant allele. Osteogenesis imperfecta types II, III, and IV involve point mutations that involve glycine residues in the triple helical domain. Such mutations prevent normal helix formation. These three types are distinguished by their clinical picture, which in turn is due to the particular glycine of type I collagen that is mutated. Osteogenesis imperfecta type II is lethal in the neonatal period and is usually the result of a new point mutation not inherited from the parents. Type III and IV phenotypes of osteo-

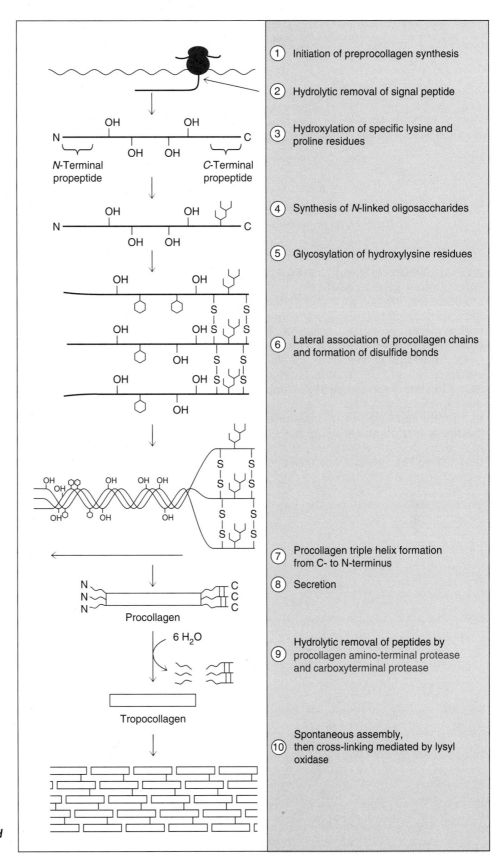

1. Initiation of preprocollagen synthesis
2. Hydrolytic removal of signal peptide
3. Hydroxylation of specific lysine and proline residues
4. Synthesis of N-linked oligosaccharides
5. Glycosylation of hydroxylysine residues
6. Lateral association of procollagen chains and formation of disulfide bonds
7. Procollagen triple helix formation from C- to N-terminus
8. Secretion
9. Hydrolytic removal of peptides by procollagen amino-terminal protease and carboxyterminal protease
10. Spontaneous assembly, then cross-linking mediated by lysyl oxidase

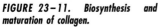

FIGURE 23–11. *Biosynthesis and maturation of collagen.*

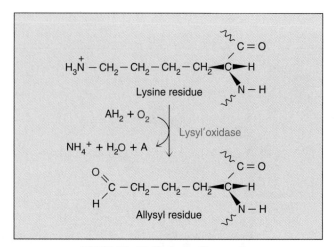

FIGURE 23–12. The lysyl oxidase reaction.

Ehlers-Danlos syndrome is a group of 10 generalized connective tissue disorders characterized by skin fragility, skin hyperextensibility, and joint hypermobility. The genetic basis is heterogeneous. The type VI syndrome results from decreased activity of **lysyl hydroxylase.** The majority of cross-linking reactions involves protein-hydroxylysine and its aldehyde derivative so that lysyl hydroxylase deficiency decreases the normal pattern of cross-linking.

Ehlers-Danlos type VII usually results from mutations that alter the amino acid sequence of one chain of type I procollagen so that it is not recognized by procollagen amino-terminal protease. Procollagen cannot be processed normally in the type VII disease, and abnormal collagen results. Ehlers-Danlos type IX disease is due to a mutation affecting the incorporation of copper into **lysyl oxidase,** and normal cross-linking is diminished. The biochemical basis of the other types of Ehlers-Danlos syndromes is unknown. The collagenopathies range from the nonsevere to those that are incompatible with life. Treatment is symptomatic. ◄

genesis imperfecta result from point mutations involving other glycine residues.

The more severe forms of osteogenesis imperfecta are produced by glycine mutations on the carboxyterminal side of collagen. This greater severity is attributable to the formation of the triple helix from the carboxyl to amino terminus. The collagen is normal in type I osteogenesis imperfecta, but only about half the usual amount is produced. A portion of the type I collagen that forms in the three other types is abnormal and is degraded in a process called procollagen suicide. The clinical course of the type I disorder is generally less severe than that of the others.

Elastin

Elastin is the connective tissue protein responsible for the extensibility of lung, large arterial blood vessels, and some ligaments. Elastin is an abundant protein but not as prevalent as collagen or myosin. Elastin differs from collagen in several properties: there is only one gene for elastin, and

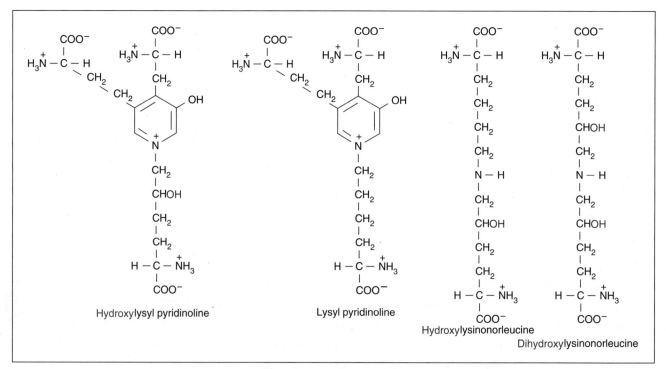

FIGURE 23–13. Collagen cross-links.

elastin lacks hydroxylysine, is not glycosylated, and does not form a triple helix. There are several types of elastin, and they are derived by alternative splicing of hnRNA to form different mature elastin mRNAs.

Elastin is synthesized as a soluble monomer of about 700 amino acids called **tropoelastin.** Tropoelastin is secreted from fibroblasts and other connective tissue cells. Specific lysine residues are deaminated to aldehydes in a reaction catalyzed by **lysyl** *oxidase,* the same copper-containing enzyme that acts on collagen. The resulting aldehyde groups participate in **desmosine** and **isodesmosine** formation, hallmarks of elastin (Figure 23–14). Desmosine cross-links are formed from three aldehyde groups derived from lysine and one unmodified lysine. A few elastin prolines are converted to hydroxyproline in a reaction catalyzed by prolyl hydroxylase. Mature elastin is insoluble and extremely stable. Elastin exhibits a variety of random coil conformations that permit it to stretch when tension is applied and to recoil when tension is removed.

Proteoglycans

Structure and Biosynthesis

The extracellular matrix is rich in proteoglycans. Proteoglycans have a widespread distribution in bone, cartilage, cornea, synovial fluid, teeth, and the vitreous of the eye. Proteoglycans, which bind

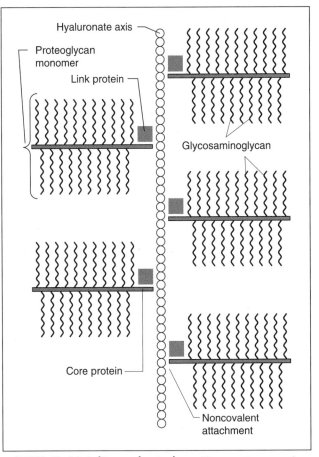

FIGURE 23–15. Architecture of proteoglycans. *The proteins are red.*

large amounts of water, form the gel-like extracellular matrix in which collagen and cells embed to form tissues. The lubricating properties of mucous secretions are due to proteoglycans. Proteoglycans consist of negatively charged polysaccharides (95% by mass) and proteins (5%). That carbohydrate is the main component is indicated by naming them as protein derivatives (proteo) of carbohydrate (glycans). The carbohydrate portion is composed of glycosaminoglycans (GAGs, formerly called mucopolysaccharides).

Proteoglycans are built on a polysaccharide axis of hyaluronate. Hyaluronate is unusual because it is not covalently linked to protein as are the other glycosaminoglycans. Many core proteins, which emanate laterally from the long, thin hyaluronate axis (Figure 23–15), are bonded to the axis by a **link protein.** Link proteins stabilize the **noncovalent** attachment of hyaluronate to core proteins. Many chondroitin sulfate and keratan sulfate chains are covalently attached to the core proteins, and the carbohydrates constitute the major mass of the molecule. The carbohydrate chains extend from the core protein and remain separated from each other by electrostatic repulsion. The proteoglycan structure resembles a bottle brush. The core protein also contains typical *N*-linked and *O*-linked carbohydrates.

The repeating units of glycosaminoglycans are

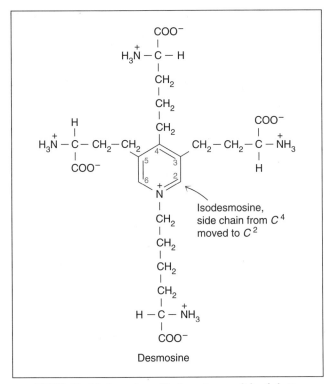

FIGURE 23–14. Desmosine and isodesmosine cross-links of elastin.

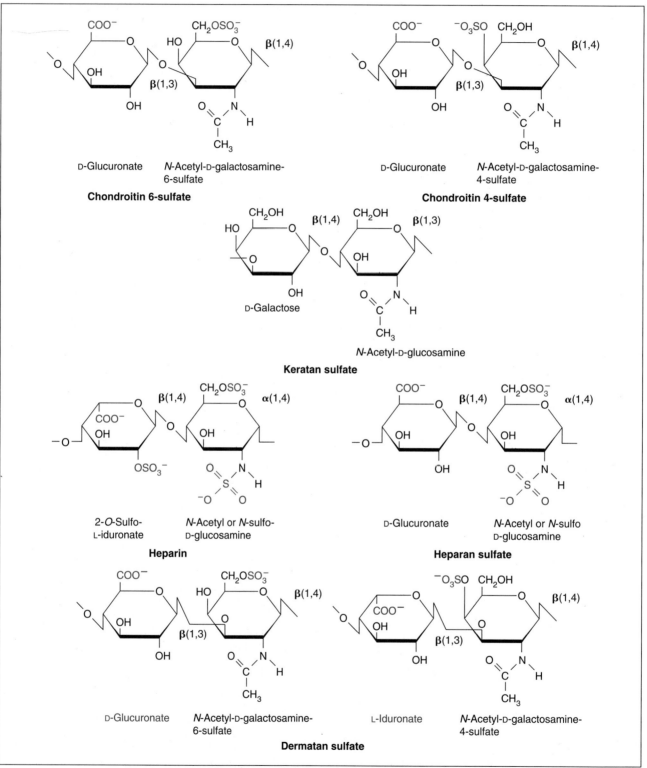

FIGURE 23–16. Repeating disaccharides of proteoglycans.

attached to the core protein by O-linked (the predominant form) and N-linked glycoside bonds. **Chondroitin sulfates, heparan sulfate, and dermatan sulfate** are covalently linked to the core protein by a β1-O-glycoside bond between xylose and protein-serine. Some molecules of keratan sulfate are covalently linked to the core protein by an α1-O-glycoside bond between N-acetylgalactosamine and threonine. Other molecules of **keratan sulfate** are attached to the core protein by a β1-N-glycosidic bond between GlcNAc and protein-asparagine. These linkage regions contain three or four carbohydrate residues to which the repeating units of disaccharides are attached.

The carbohydrate component of glycosaminoglycans found in proteoglycans is a long, unbranched heteropolysaccharide consisting of a repeating disaccharide unit. The components of the polysaccharide repeating units are illustrated in Figure 23–16 for general reference. The following simplifying generalizations can be made. One component of the repeating disaccharide unit consists of N-acetylglucosamine, N-acetylgalactosamine, or one of the sulfate derivatives. Except for keratan sulfate (with galactose), the second component consists of a uronate (either D-glucuronate or its 5-epimer, L-iduronate) with a negatively charged carboxylate. Excepting the hyaluronate axis, the polysaccharides of proteoglycans contain O-sulfate or N-sulfate esters. The sulfates and glucuronates account for the anionic nature of this group of complex carbohydrates. Owing to the large number of negative charges, the chains are extended because the electrostatic forces repel each other.

Chondroitin sulfates are the most abundant proteoglycans in humans, and the pathway for their biosynthesis illustrates the important principles for all classes of proteoglycans. The core protein is synthesized in the rough endoplasmic reticulum in an mRNA-dependent fashion (Figure 18–2). The three linking carbohydrates are added sequentially from activated UDP precursors in three sequential steps (Figure 23–17). Each step is catalyzed by a different transglycosylase.

The repeating disaccharide is made of glucuronate and N-acetylgalactosamine. The biosynthetic donors are the activated UDP-glucuronate and UDP-GalNAc. A glucuronyltransferase catalyzes the addition of glucuronate to the terminal galactosyl residue of the linkage region. Next, a galactosyltransferase catalyzes the addition to glucuronate. This process recurs many times to produce a chain of the repeating disaccharide. Each elongation reaction occurs with the loss of one high-energy bond and is exergonic (PRINCIPLE 2 OF BIOENERGETICS).

A sulfotransferase catalyzes a reaction involving the 4-hydroxyl group of the N-acetylgalactosamine of the repeating disaccharide to form the low-energy sulfate ester. Phosphoadenosylphosphosulfate is the activated donor of sulfate. These reactions, which take place with a decrease in the number of high-energy bonds (Figure 12–12), occur before the carbohydrate chain is completed. Synthesis of L-iduronate in dermatan sulfate, heparin, or heparan sulfate occurs after D-glucuronate has already been incorporated into the carbohydrate chain. **Uronosyl-5-epimerase** catalyzes the isoergonic epimerization of the D- to the L-sugar.

The sequence of the carbohydrate is determined by enzyme specificity and not by a template. The size of the carbohydrate chains is variable. Moreover, the location of the sulfates is variable in that not every 4-hydroxyl group receives a sulfate.

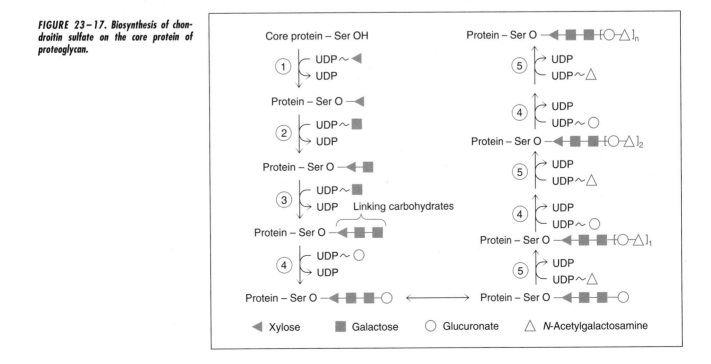

FIGURE 23–17. *Biosynthesis of chondroitin sulfate on the core protein of proteoglycan.*

Complex carbohydrate synthesis does not occur with the certitude of nucleic acid or protein biosynthesis.

Mucopolysaccharidoses

▶ Glycosaminoglycans are degraded in lysosomes. Several inherited mucopolysaccharide storage diseases are the result of deficient activities of lysosomal catabolic enzymes. Depending upon the deficiency, the catabolism of dermatan sulfate, heparan sulfate, or keratan sulfate may be blocked, singly or in combination. Chondroitin sulfate may also be involved. Undegraded glycosaminoglycan molecules accumulate in lysosomes. Their accumulation can result in cell, tissue, and organ dysfunction. Glycosaminoglycan fragments are excreted in the urine.

Some of these disorders are listed in Table 23–3 for general reference. The incidence of these rare disorders is about 1 in 100,000 live births. The chromosomal location of several of these enzymes has been identified, but the nature of the nucleotide changes has not yet been established. Only individuals who work with these diseases regularly know the eponyms and the corresponding enzyme defects by rote. These storage diseases are characterized by organomegaly, abnormal facies, and a chronic and progressive course. Except for Hunter syndrome (iduronate sulfatase deficiency), which is X-linked, they are transmitted in an autosomal recessive fashion. ◀

Glycoproteins

Glycoprotein biosynthesis is described in Chapter 18. The major noncollagenous glycoprotein of the extracellular matrix is **fibronectin.** Fibronectin is a 250-kDa dimer that is linked by a disulfide bridge. Fibronectin binds reversibly to the external face of the plasma membrane and interacts with other extracellular molecules including collagen. The cell-binding region of fibronectin binds to **integrin,** an $\alpha\beta$-protein complex that spans the plasma membrane. The fibronectin gene consists of more than 50 exons, and various forms of fibronectin are generated by alternative splicing of hnRNA.

Laminin is another glycoprotein in the extracel-

lular matrix that enables epithelial cells to attach to connective tissue. Laminin has high affinity for type IV collagen, a component of basement membranes.

SUMMARY

Myosin is the chief protein in muscle, and myosin possesses ATPase activity. Tropomyosin blocks the interaction of actin and myosin in resting striated muscle. The troponin system plays a regulatory role in triggering striated muscle contraction, and calcium is the activating agent. Following the interaction of calcium with troponin, tropomyosin no longer blocks the interaction of myosin and actin. Myosin moves relative to actin and generates force.

The sliding filament hypothesis has been invoked to rationalize the structures of relaxed and contracted muscles. During contraction, the sarcomeres shorten and the Z disks come closer together. The A-band length (corresponding to the myosin thick filaments) is constant in relaxed and contracted states, but the I band shortens during contraction. The lengths of the thin and thick filaments also do not change. The sliding filament hypothesis states that the fibers of the thin filament, attached to the Z-disk structure at each end of a sarcomere, are pulled toward the center of the sarcomere by the thick filaments of the A band.

Smooth muscle contraction, like that of striated muscle, is regulated by alterations in the levels of intracellular calcium. Initiation of contraction is the result of phosphorylation of the regulatory myosin light chains; cessation of contraction is the result of the dephosphorylation of myosin light chains. These reactions are catalyzed by myosin-light-chain kinase and phosphoprotein phosphatase, respectively. Phosphorylation of myosin light chains facilitates actin-myosin interaction that leads to force generation. Following dephosphorylation of the regulatory myosin light chain, interaction between actin and myosin is inhibited.

Skeletal and cardiac muscle (and brain) contains significant amounts of phosphocreatine. This phosphoramidate (P~N) serves as a storage form of high-energy phosphate. Muscle and other tissues can regenerate ATP from ADP by the adenylate kinase reaction. This enzyme catalyzes a reaction between two molecules of ADP to yield ATP and AMP in an isoergonic process. White muscle uses glycolysis for most of its energy production. Some muscles such as the gastrocnemius contain both red and white muscle fibers. Red muscle uses fatty acids as a major fuel; fatty acids are metabolized by β-oxidation to acetyl-CoA. The transport of lactate from the muscle to the liver and the return transport of glucose from the liver to muscle is called the Cori cycle.

TABLE 23–3. Enzyme Deficiencies in Selected Mucopolysaccharidoses*

Eponym	Enzyme Deficiency	Number
Hurler	L-Iduronidase	MPS I
Hunter	Iduronate sulfatase	MPS II
Sanfilippo A	Heparan-N-sulfatase	MPS III A
Sanfilippo B	α-N-Acetylglucosaminidase	MPS III B
Morquio A	Galactose-6-sulfatase	MPS IV A
Sly	β-Glucuronidase	MPS VII

*Fourteen have been described.

Collagen is the major macromolecule of connective tissue and the most abundant protein in humans, accounting for one-third of human protein by mass. The most distinguishing property of collagen is that three collagen α-chains form a triple helix. There are three amino acid residues per helical turn, and every third residue is glycine, since it is the only amino acid small enough to exist at the central core of a triple helix. The preponderance (90% by mass) of collagen in humans is type I collagen, a fibrillar collagen. Collagen is synthesized as preprocollagen α-chains in the rough endoplasmic reticulum where the triple helix forms. Triple helical procollagen is secreted from the cell. After cleavage of the amino and carboxyl termini, tropocollagen is the product. Interchain cross-linking of tropocollagen yields collagen.

Lysyl and prolyl hydroxylase catalyze the formation of hydroxylated residues of collagen in the endoplasmic reticulum. Hydroxylysine is a site of carbohydrate attachment and of cross-linking. In contrast, hydroxyproline forms hydrogen bonds that stabilize the triple helix. Allysine residues, which result from the action of lysyl oxidase extracellularly, cross-link tropocollagen to form collagen. Collagen cross-links include hydroxylysinonorleucine and hydroxylysyl pyridinoline. The collagenopathies are rare heterogeneous disorders including osteogenesis imperfecta and Ehlers-Danlos syndrome.

Some of the prolines of elastin, like collagen, are converted to hydroxyproline in a reaction catalyzed by prolyl hydroxylase. Elastin lacks hydroxylysine and is not glycosylated. Elastin does not consist of the glycine triad repeats and consequently cannot form the triple helix. Desmosine and isodesmosine, which are formed from allysine and lysine residues, are unique cross-links that are hallmarks of elastin.

Proteoglycans consist of acidic polysaccharides (95% by mass) and proteins (5%). Proteoglycans are built on a polysaccharide axis of hyaluronate. Many core proteins emanate laterally from the long, thin hyaluronate axis. A link protein stabilizes the hyaluronate–core protein complex by noncovalent means. Many chondroitin sulfate and keratan sulfate chains are covalently attached to the core proteins, and the carbohydrates constitute the major mass of the molecule. The various proteoglycans contain glycosaminoglycans made of characteristic repeating disaccharides. Their biosynthesis involves the addition of sugars from activated uridine nucleotide donors in exergonic reactions. Only one sugar unit is added at a time, and the specificity is determined by the glycosyltransferases. The mucopolysaccharidoses are a group of lysosomal diseases that are due to the accumulation of compounds that cannot be catabolized.

SELECTED READINGS

Bray, D. *Cell Movements.* New York, Garland Publishing, 1992.

Harrington, W.F., and M.E. Rodgers. Myosin. Annual Review of Biochemistry 53:35–73, 1984.

Huxley, H.E. The mechanism of muscle contraction. Science 164:1356–1366, 1969.

Lachman, R.S., G.E. Tiller, J.M. Graham, Jr., and D.L. Rimoin. Collagen, genes, and skeletal dysplasias on the edge of a new era: A review and update. European Journal of Radiology 14:1–10, 1992.

Neufeld, E.F., and J. Muenzer. The mucopolysaccharidoses. In C.R. Scriver, A.L. Beaudet, W.S. Sly, and D. Valle (eds.). *The Metabolic Basis of Inherited Disease,* 6th ed. New York, McGraw-Hill Book Company, 1989, pp. 1565–1587.

Prockop, D.J. Mutations in collagen genes as a cause of connective-tissue diseases. New England Journal of Medicine 326:540–546, 1992.

Yoewell, H.N., and S.R. Pinnell. The Ehlers-Danlos syndromes. Seminars in Dermatology 12:229–240, 1993.

CHAPTER TWENTY-FOUR

HEMOGLOBIN,

HEME, AND BLOOD

COAGULATION

Just as our present knowledge and practice of medicine relies on a sophisticated knowledge of human anatomy, physiology, and biochemistry, so will dealing with disease in the future demand a detailed understanding of the molecular anatomy, physiology, and biochemistry of the human genome. We shall have to have physicians who are as conversant with the molecular anatomy of chromosomes and genes as the cardiac surgeon is with the structure and workings of the heart and circulatory tree.

—PAUL BERG

Blood, which transports oxygen and carbon dioxide, consists of **cells** and **plasma.** When blood plasma clots, the liquid remaining is called the **serum.** The blood clot consists of fibrin, which is derived from fibrinogen. The percent, by volume, of the cellular component to the total volume of blood is called the **hematocrit.** The hematocrit reflects the red blood cell mass. ▶ The hematocrit is one of the most important laboratory values of clinical medicine. An individual with a low hematocrit is anemic, and anemias are common clinical entities. **Pernicious anemia,** caused by a deficiency of vitamin B_{12}, folate-deficiency anemia, and **iron-deficiency anemia** are described in Chapter 2. ◀

Erythrocytes are small (7 μm in diameter), biconcave, disk-shaped cells that have lost their nucleus, mitochondria, peroxisomes, and endoplasmic reticulum. *Erythrocytes, lacking mitochondria, derive their ATP from anaerobic glycolysis by converting glucose to lactate.* Erythrocytes also possess an active pentose phosphate pathway (Figure 7–12). NADPH generated by this pathway is responsible for the maintenance of reduced glutathione. Glutathione participates in the destruction of hydrogen peroxide in a reaction catalyzed by glutathione peroxidase (Figure 5–3).

HEMOGLOBIN

Structure

Hemoglobin is the key molecule of oxygen transport. Hemoglobin consists of four polypeptide chains and four heme groups; it is a dimer of dimers with two chains from the α-family and two chains from the β-family. The four chains are held together by noncovalent attractions. Each chain contains a heme group that binds a molecule of oxygen. Hemoglobin A, the principal hemoglobin in adults, consists of two α-chains and two β-chains as $\alpha_2\beta_2$. The α-chains contain 141 amino acid residues each and the β-chains 146 each. The levels of hemoglobin A_1, which result from nonenzymatic modification of hemoglobin A by glucose (Figure 7–5), are used to monitor the control of diabetes mellitus. Adults express hemoglobin A_2, a minor form that makes up about 2% of the total. Hemoglobin A_2, which contains δ-chains for β-chains, has the molecular structure $\alpha_2\delta_2$. The α- and β-

chains of hemoglobin consist of seven and eight helical regions (from A through H). An invariant histidine in all hemoglobins, called F8 or the proximal histidine, binds heme. F8 refers to the eighth residue of the F helix.

Genes for the α-gene family occur on chromosome 16, and those for the β-gene family occur on chromosome 11. Note that two identical α-genes (α1 and α2) per haploid genome encode for the α-chain of hemoglobin (Figure 24–1). Both genes are expressed, and the normal diploid genome consists of four α-genes designated αα/αα. This unusual pairing helps explain the mechanism for the production of **α-thalassemia,** a genetic disease that leads to a deficiency of α-chains, as considered later in this chapter. The Greek psi (ψ) designates pseudo genes (genes with mutations such that they cannot produce a functional protein) for α, β, and ζ (zeta) chains. Hemoglobin chain genes are developmentally expressed. α-Chain production begins in utero, but β-chain production does not occur until postpartum (Figure 24–2).

Cooperative Oxygen Binding

The concentration dependence of oxygen binding to myoglobin is expressed by a **rectangular hyperbola** (Figure 24–3). The rectangular hyperbola signifies oxygen's binding to identical sites, as expected, because myoglobin is a monomer (Figure 3–15). The concentration dependence of oxygen binding to hemoglobin is expressed by a **sigmoidal curve.** *The sigmoidal curve is diagnostic of positive cooperativity.* This is physiologically important because hemoglobin can bind and release more of its oxygen cargo over the physiological range of oxygen tension.

The structure of hemoglobin differs in the oxygenated and deoxygenated states. The quaternary structure of the oxygenated state is called the **R state** (for relaxed), and the conformation of the deoxygenated state is called the **T state** (for tense). Deoxyhemoglobin is tauter and more constrained than oxyhemoglobin because the T form contains eight more salt bridges between subunits than the R form. The transition from the R to T state involves large structural changes at the $\alpha_1\beta_2$ contacts and small changes at the $\alpha_1\beta_1$ contacts (Figure 24–4). Most of these interactions are hy-

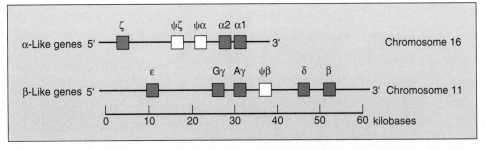

FIGURE 24–1. Location of the α-family and β-family of globin chains. ψ, psi, for pseudo; ζ, zeta.

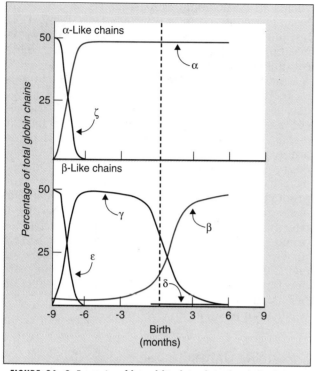

FIGURE 24-2. Expression of hemoglobin chains during human development.

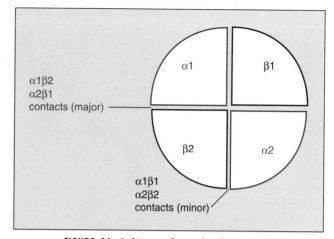

FIGURE 24-4. Diagram of α- and β-chain contacts.

sense and follows the molecular logic of the cell (PRINCIPLE 9 OF BIOCHEMISTRY). When erythrocytes pass through active tissues that are producing lactic acid, lactic acid serves as a signal that more oxygen is needed. The increased acidity causes the hemoglobin to release oxygen. This celebrated pH effect was discovered by the Danish physiologist Christian Bohr (father of the atomic physicist Niels Bohr) and is called the **Bohr effect.**

drophobic, but salt bridges and hydrogen bonds are also involved. Differences in quaternary structure of the R and T states are produced by the movement of the F8 histidine as oxygen binds or dissociates from heme. The F8 histidine alters the position of the F and H helices (Figure 24–5) and leads to altered contacts between the subunits.

The ability of hemoglobin to bind oxygen decreases with an increase in acidity; protons make hemoglobin dump oxygen (Figure 24–6). The pH dependence of oxygen binding makes physiological

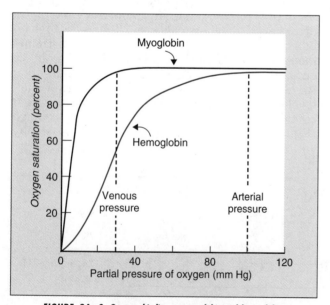

FIGURE 24-3. Oxygen binding to myoglobin and hemoglobin.

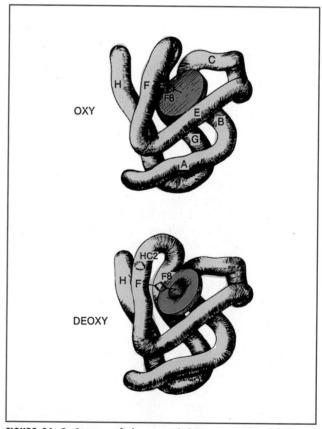

FIGURE 24-5. Structure of the oxy and deoxy states of a globin chain. Reproduced, with permission, from E.J. Benz, Jr. In J.B. Wyngaarden, L.H. Smith, Jr., and J.C. Bennett (eds.). Cecil Textbook of Medicine, 19th ed. Philadelphia, W.B. Saunders Company, 1992, p. 873.

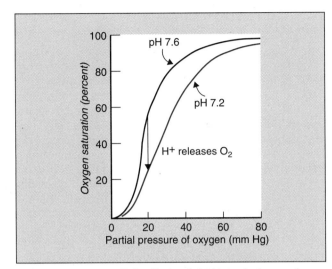

FIGURE 24–6. *Protons (Bohr effect) and 2,3-bisphosphoglycerate decrease oxygen binding to hemoglobin and shift the oxygen-binding curve to the right.*

Deoxyhemoglobin is a weaker acid (has greater proton affinity) than oxyhemoglobin (equation 24.1).

$$HHb^+ + O_2 \rightleftharpoons HbO_2 + H^+ \quad (24.1)$$
Weaker   Stronger
acid   acid

The difference in acidity is due to a difference in the pK_a values of the imidazole side chain of histidine 87 of the α-chains and histidine 92 of the β-chains. The average pK_a of these **histidines** of deoxyhemoglobin is slightly basic (7.9) and that for oxyhemoglobin is slightly acidic (6.7). At physiological pH, each mole of tetrameric deoxyhemo-

globin takes up about 2.8 moles of protons. This reversible uptake and release of protons is responsible for the isohydric transport of carbon dioxide as described later in this chapter.

2,3-Bisphosphoglycerate (Figure 7–10) occurs in the red cell. It binds preferentially to deoxyhemoglobin (Figure 3–16) and therefore promotes the release of oxygen from hemoglobin (2,3-bisphosphoglycerate makes hemoglobin dump oxygen). The concentrations of this allosteric regulator of hemoglobin increase when humans adapt to lower oxygen pressure at high altitudes.

Isohydric Transport of Carbon Dioxide

The erythrocyte and the circulatory system are responsible for the transport of carbon dioxide from the tissues to the lungs for expiration. Carbon dioxide transport is more intricate than oxygen transport. The term isohydric refers to a lack of change of pH in the process. Deoxyhemoglobin carries protons (Bohr effect) and accounts for isohydric transport.

Carbon dioxide is formed by reactions of the Krebs cycle. Carbon dioxide diffuses from the mitochondrion through the cell and interstitial space to the capillaries and into erythrocytes. As a small uncharged molecule, carbon dioxide can pass through membrane bilayers by diffusion. When inside the red cell, carbon dioxide combines with water to form carbonic acid in a reaction catalyzed by **carbonic anhydrase** (a zinc-containing enzyme). Carbonic acid dissociates to form a proton and bicarbonate (Figure 24–7).

FIGURE 24–7. *Isohydric transport of carbon dioxide by the circulation.* RBC, red blood cell.

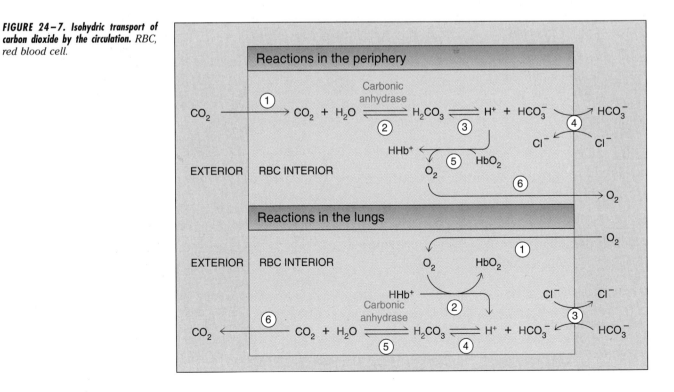

We consider the transport of bicarbonate and the hydrogen ion separately. Bicarbonate is transported in the blood plasma, and the proton is transported as a complex with hemoglobin. Bicarbonate from the red cell enters the blood through the **anion exchange protein** of the red cell membrane. The anion exchange protein is also called the **band 3 protein** because of the position that this prominent protein displays during electrophoresis of proteins of the red cell plasma membrane. The facilitated diffusion of bicarbonate occurs in exchange with plasma chloride to maintain ionic balance. Bicarbonate is transported by the plasma to the lung.

Let us consider the transport of hydrogen ions that are formed by the dissociation of carbonic acid. As hemoglobin releases its oxygen in the capillary bed, oxyhemoglobin is converted to deoxyhemoglobin. Deoxyhemoglobin, a weaker acid than oxyhemoglobin, binds 2.8 moles more protons per mole of hemoglobin than does oxyhemoglobin and transports them to the pulmonary capillaries.

Next we consider the generation of carbon dioxide that is expired. Deoxyhemoglobin is converted to oxyhemoglobin as the protein binds oxygen in the pulmonary capillaries (Figure 24–7). During this process, histidines release their bound protons, which can then combine with bicarbonate. Bicarbonate enters the red cell via the anion exchange protein as chloride leaves. Bicarbonate and protons combine to form carbonic acid. Carbonic anhydrase catalyzes the conversion of carbonic acid to carbon dioxide and water. Carbon dioxide diffuses from the cell into the capillary and into the expired air. The key elements of isohydric transport include carbonic anhydrase, anion exchange protein, and the greater affinity of deoxyhemoglobin than of oxyhemoglobin for protons.

Another mechanism for carbon dioxide transport involves the direct reaction of carbon dioxide with the amino terminal residues of hemoglobin to form **carbaminohemoglobin** (Figure 24–8). Each of the four amino terminal residues of hemoglobin can form this derivative. The reaction is spontaneous (nonenzymatic). Carbon dioxide is transported as carbaminohemoglobin ($\approx$10%), by isohydric transport ($\approx$85%), and in solution ($\approx$5%). Hemoglobin is required for both carbon dioxide and oxygen transport because these gases are only sparingly soluble in water.

Hemoglobinopathies

▶ Hemoglobinopathies are among the most common genetic diseases worldwide. There are two groups of genetic hemoglobinopathies. The first is due to mutations that alter the structure of the globin polypeptide, the most celebrated example of which is sickle cell anemia. Over 400 variants of hemoglobin have been described, and more than half produce clinically significant disease. The second group is associated with decreased synthesis of the globin chains. These disorders are called thalassemias. Sickle cell anemia, an autosomal recessive disease, results from a single nucleotide substitution in each allele of the β-chain. Both α- and β-thalassemia, on the other hand, can be due to a variety of mutations. ◀

Sickle Cell Anemia

▶ Sickle cell anemia is the cause of considerable mortality and morbidity in Africa and in every population where there has been migration of individuals of African descent. These individuals are homozygous for hemoglobin S expression. *Hemoglobin S differs from hemoglobin A by the conversion of $\beta 6$ Glu $\rightarrow$ Val.* This alteration is due to an A $\rightarrow$ T transversion in the triplet codon for the sixth residue of the β-globin chain. In concentrated hemoglobin solutions that are partially or fully deoxygenated, this mutation leads to polymerization of hemoglobin that causes cell deformity. The formula for sickle cell hemoglobin is $\alpha_2^A \beta_2^S$. A heterozygote with sickle cell trait is asymptomatic, accounting for the designation of the disease as autosomal recessive. A single blood cell of a heterozygote contains 60% $\alpha_2^A \beta_2^A$ and 40% $\alpha_2^A \beta_2^S$. The diagnosis of sickle cell anemia is possible in utero, and genetic tests are shown in Figures 15–37 and 15–38.

Because of the mutation, deoxyhemoglobin S aggregates and sickle-shaped cells form (Figure 24–9). This morphology leads to the reduced deformability of the red cell and its defective passage through the microcirculation. Vascular occlusion is the result. Such structural alterations lead to hemolysis and chronic anemia. Red cells usually spend one second or less in the capillary circulation. If cells containing hemoglobin S spend more time at reduced oxygen concentrations, sickling can occur.

Sickle cell anemia is characterized by a lifelong hemolytic anemia, the occurrence of acute or sudden exacerbations called crises, and a variety of complications resulting from an increased propensity to infection and the deleterious effects of repeated vascular blockage. Individuals with sickle cell anemia usually present during the first or second year of life. They exhibit a failure to thrive (a common expression used to indicate that something serious is affecting an infant) and repeated infections due to *Streptococcus pneumoniae* or *Haemophilus influenzae*.

Hemoglobin	Carbaminohemoglobin

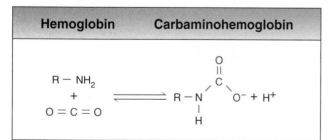

FIGURE 24–8. Transport of carbon dioxide as carbaminohemoglobin.

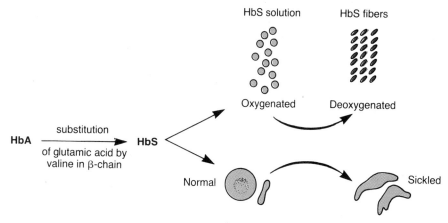

FIGURE 24–9. Hemoglobin S and formation of sickle cells. *Reproduced, with permission, from R.S. Cotran, V. Kumar, and S.L. Robbins.* Robbins Pathologic Basis of Disease, *5th ed. Philadelphia, W.B. Saunders Company, 1995, p. 593.*

The crises of sickle cell anemia can take many forms including chest or abdominal pain, bone infarction, and perhaps an underlying infection. Renal disease and retinopathy are characteristic of long-term disease. Therapy is supportive and includes treatment of infections, analgesics for pain, and transfusions, as required. Individuals with sickle cell trait exhibit greater resistance to malaria than those without the trait, and this characteristic accounts for the continued prevalence of sickle cell anemia in the population. Protection afforded in those with sickle cell trait is called **heterozygote advantage.** ◄

Thalassemias

► Thalassemias are a heterogeneous group of hemoglobinopathies in which the mutation reduces the level of synthesis of the α- or β-chains. The name is derived from Greek *thalassa* "sea," referring to the geographic distribution of many cases around the Mediterranean Sea. There are two main groups of diseases and several clinical pictures that bear specific names. *The main groups are the α-thalassemias, in which α-chain synthesis is impaired, and the β-thalassemias, in which β-chain synthesis is impaired.* Thalassemias are classified as α^+ and α^0 for some or no α-chain production and as β^+ and β^0 for some or no β-chain production.

Genetic disorders of α-globin production affect the formation of both fetal and adult hemoglobins (Figure 24–2). With complete deficiency of α-chain synthesis, the chains from the β-chain family form homotetramers. Hemoglobin with a γ_4 composition is called **hemoglobin Bart,** and hemoglobin with a β_4 composition is called **hemoglobin H.** These hemoglobins have high oxygen affinities and do not release oxygen to fetal tissues.

There are two identical genes for α-globin on each chromosome 16 for a total of four α-globin genes in a normal individual (Figure 24–1). Possible genotypes, listed in Table 24–1, indicate that humans can contain from zero to four normal α-globin genes. The approximate α-globin production is also indicated. The possession of two normal

genes is associated with a mild anemia and is called the α-thalassemia trait. Possession of one or no genes produces severe disease.

The most common forms of α-thalassemia are due to deletions, and these deletions are produced by unequal crossing-over during meiosis. Let us consider the mechanism. There are two identical α-globin genes on chromosome 16, and the flanking DNA sequences are highly homologous. This arrangement of tandem regions of homology in and around the α-globin genes facilitates misalignment, homologous pairing, and recombination between the α1 gene on one chromosome and the α2 gene on the other (Figure 24–10). As a consequence, gametes with only one gene can result. Thus, less α-chain is produced. The heterozygous state for α-thalassemia can be the result of either of two genotypes: α-/α- or $\alpha\alpha$/--.

β-Thalassemias share many features with the α-thalassemias. Decreased β-globin production and the imbalance of globin chain synthesis lead to precipitation of the excess α-chains and hemolytic anemia. The β-chain is expressed only in the postnatal period (Figure 24–2), and the onset of β-thalassemia is not apparent until a few months after birth. The levels of hemoglobin A_2 ($\alpha_2\delta_2$) and hemoglobin F ($\alpha_2\gamma_2$) are somewhat elevated in β-thalassemia.

Infants with homozygous β-thalassemia present with severe anemia before the age of 2. They exhibit jaundice, hepatosplenomegaly, and skeletal changes reflecting an increase in bone marrow vol-

TABLE 24–1.   Genotypes of α-Thalassemias

Clinical Condition (severity of disease)	Number of Functional α-Genes	Genotype	α-Chain Production (%)
Normal	4	$\alpha\alpha/\alpha\alpha$	100
Silent carrier (nil)	3	$\alpha\alpha/\alpha$-	75
α-Thalassemia (mild)	2	α-/α- or $\alpha\alpha$/--	50
Hemoglobin H disease (moderate)	1	α-/--	25
Hydrops fetalis (severe)	0	--/--	0

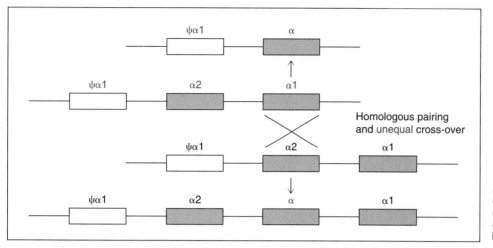

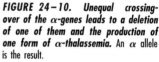

FIGURE 24–10. *Unequal crossing-over of the α-genes leads to a deletion of one of them and the production of one form of α-thalassemia.* An α allele is the result.

ume. These infants have **thalassemia major,** which may be of the more severe β^0 or the β^+ variety. In the former case, there is no detectable hemoglobin A, whereas some hemoglobin A is detectable in the latter case. Carriers of one β-thalassemia allele are clinically well and are said to have **thalassemia minor.** These individuals generally have higher levels of hemoglobin A_2, and this laboratory determination can aid in the diagnosis.

β-Thalassemias are usually due to single nucleotide substitutions rather than deletions. More than 80 different mutations produce β-thalassemia, and mutations include almost every conceivable type of abnormality that can reduce the synthesis of an mRNA or protein. These include promoter mutations that decrease transcription, cap site and initiator codon mutations, splicing mutations, frameshift mutations, nonsense mutations, and point mutations that produce unstable hemoglobin. In contrast to the α-thalassemias, deletions of DNA are a minor cause of the β-thalassemias. ◀

HEME

Biosynthesis

Heme is a tetrapyrrole that occurs in hemoglobin, myoglobin, and mitochondrial cytochromes, cytochrome P-450, catalase, peroxidases, tryptophan pyrrolase, prostaglandin endoperoxide synthase, and the soluble form of guanylate cyclase. Hemoglobin is quantitatively the most abundant heme protein in the body. Heme consists of iron bound to **protoporphyrin IX** (Figure 24–11). Isomer IX reflects the positions of the substituents on the protoporphyrin ring.

Protoporphyrin IX is derived from eight molecules each of **succinyl-CoA** and **glycine.** Heme synthesis is initiated within the mitochondrion (two steps), continues in the cytosol (three steps), and is completed within the mitochondrion (three steps). Figure 24–12 provides an overview of the pathway. The nomenclature of the porphyrins is

daunting, and only specialists know the structures by rote. Uroporphyrins were initially isolated from urine, and coproporphyrins were isolated from the feces, but these compounds can occur in all cells of the body.

The first and rate-limiting step in the biosynthesis of heme is catalyzed by δ-aminolevulinate synthase (ALA synthase), a pyridoxal phosphate enzyme. The amino group of glycine forms a Schiff base with pyridoxal phosphate. The α-carbon of glycine then reacts with the energy-rich thioester of succinyl-CoA to form a six-carbon intermediate and CoA (Figure 24–13). The intermediate undergoes an exergonic decarboxylation to produce δ-aminolevulinate. After exiting the mitochondrion, two molecules of δ-aminolevulinate combine in a reaction catalyzed by **porphobilinogen synthase** to produce porphobilinogen, a substituted pyrrole, and two water molecules. Four moles of porphobi-

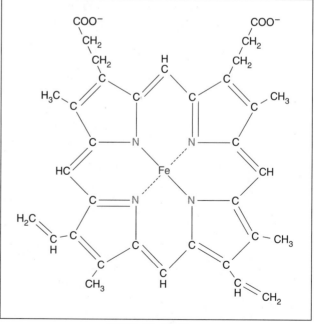

FIGURE 24–11. Heme.

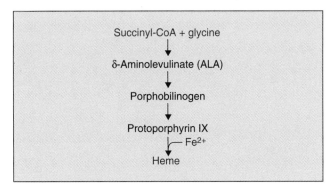

FIGURE 24-12. Overview of heme biosynthesis.

linogen condense to produce uroporphyrinogen III, a cyclic tetrapyrrole, and four ammonium molecules. This intricate process requires **uroporphyrinogen synthase** and **uroporphyrinogen III cosynthase. Uroporphyrinogen decarboxylase** catalyzes the conversion of substrate to form coproporphyrinogen III. During this process, four acetyl groups ($-CH_2COOH$) are converted to four methyl groups ($-CH_3$) and carbon dioxide during successive exergonic decarboxylation reactions.

Coproporphyrinogen III enters the mitochondrion. **Coproporphyrinogen oxidase** catalyzes the oxidative decarboxylation of each of two propionate side chains ($-CH_2CH_2COOH$) to carbon dioxide and vinyl side chains ($-CH=CH_2$). Molecular oxygen serves as the oxidant. **Protoporphyrinogen oxidase** catalyzes the conversion of methylene ($-CH_2-$) bridges, linking four tetrapyrroles, to methenyl ($-CH=$) bridges. Molecular oxygen is also the oxidant for these conversions. Finally, **ferrochelatase** catalyzes a reaction between protoporphyrin IX and ferrous iron to produce heme. Heme combines with its apoproteins to produce the final product. Loss of high-energy bonds, decarboxylation, and reactions of organic compounds with molecular oxygen make the overall pathway exergonic.

Degradation

Proteins undergo turnover, and the heme liberated during protein catabolism is metabolized. Heme is converted into various bile pigments (not to be confused with bile salts, which are cholesterol derivatives). Key intermediates include biliverdin (*verd* "green") and bilirubin (*ruber* "red"). Bilirubin can undergo a conjugation reaction to form bilirubin diglucuronide. Bilirubin is also converted to urobilin (isolated from urine) and stercobilin (isolated from feces).

The first step in heme degradation is catalyzed by **heme oxygenase,** an enzyme of the endoplasmic reticulum. The reactants include two moles of oxygen, one mole of NADPH, and ferric heme. Besides playing a role in heme degradation, this process generates carbon monoxide. **Carbon monox-**

ide may serve as a second messenger in brain analogous to nitric oxide (Figure 19–23). Heme is cleaved between the A and B rings to produce **biliverdin,** ferric iron, carbon monoxide, and water (Figure 24–14). Two atoms of oxygen occur in biliverdin, a third in carbon monoxide, and the fourth in water. The oxidation of organic compounds by molecular oxygen is exergonic and irreversible (PRINCIPLE 8 OF BIOENERGETICS). Biliverdin reacts with NADPH in a reaction catalyzed by **biliverdin reductase** to form **bilirubin.** Bilirubin, a lipophilic substance, is transported to the liver as a complex with albumin. Bilirubin reacts with two molecules of energy-rich UDP~glucuronate to form **bilirubin diglucuronide,** a hydrophilic energy-poor substance (Figure 24–14). Bilirubin diglucuronide is excreted in the bile.

Bilirubin diglucuronide can be hydrolyzed by bacterial enzymes (β-glucuronidases) in the large bowel to form free bilirubin. Bilirubin is reduced to colorless **urobilinogen** by bacterial flora. Most of the fecal urobilinogen is converted to **stercobilin,** a pigment that gives feces its brown color. A small portion of urobilinogen can be taken up from the gut, transported in the circulation, and excreted in the urine as **urobilin.** Urobilins impart the characteristic amber color to urine.

▶ When the blood contains excessive bilirubin, the sclerae of the eyes and the skin become yellow and the sign is called **jaundice.** Jaundice is not a disease *per se* but indicates an abnormal condition. Clinical chemistry laboratories commonly measure total bilirubin (bilirubin and bilirubin diglucuronide) and bilirubin diglucuronide. Historically, rapidly reacting or soluble bilirubin diglucuronide was called **direct bilirubin,** and the insoluble bilirubin was called **indirect bilirubin** as formerly measured by the van den Bergh reaction. The relative proportions of the direct and indirect van den Bergh bilirubin are helpful in pinpointing the mechanism for producing jaundice. Jaundice is classified as prehepatic, hepatic, and posthepatic. ◀

Abnormal Porphyrin Metabolism

▶ The porphyrias are a group of inherited and acquired disorders in which the activities of the enzymes of heme biosynthesis are partially deficient. These disorders are classified as hepatic or erythroid, depending on the principal site of expression of the disease. Deficiencies in seven of eight of the biosynthetic enzymes have been reported; δ-aminolevulinate synthase—the first enzyme of the pathway—is the only enzyme not associated with porphyria.

Acute intermittent porphyria, an autosomal dominant disorder, is the most common form of hepatic porphyria. This disease is due to a 50% reduction of **uroporphyrinogen synthase,** the third enzyme of the pathway. About 90% of individuals with this defect remain asymptomatic throughout

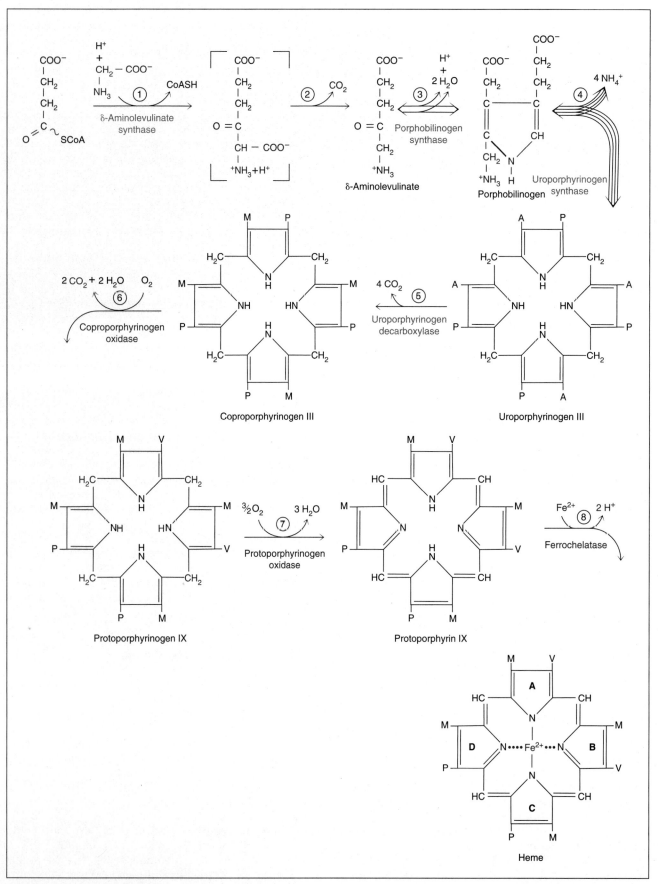

FIGURE 24–13. Heme biosynthesis. *One enzyme catalyzes steps 1 and 2. Reactions 3, 4, and 5 occur in the cytosol. The number of arrows indicates the number of substrates required for reaction. A, acetyl; M, methyl; P, propionyl; V, vinyl.*

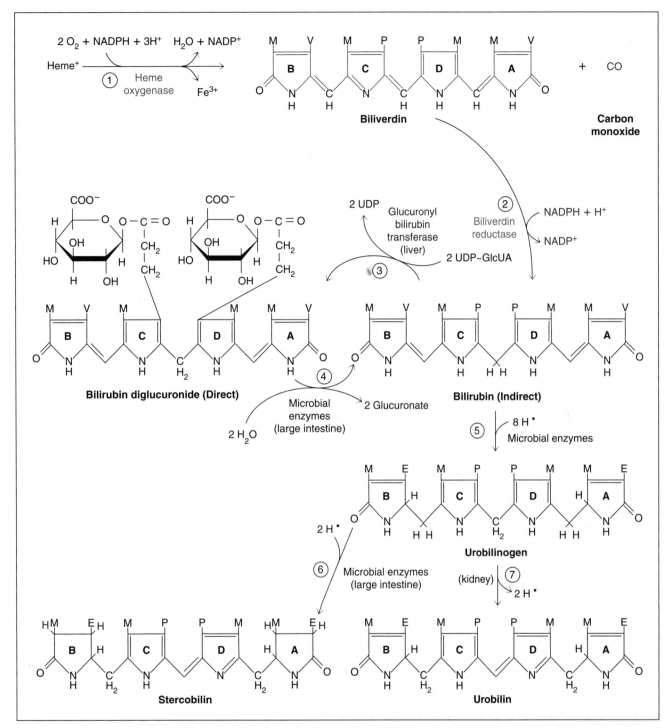

FIGURE 24–14. Heme degradation. *E, ethyl; M, methyl; P, propionyl; V, vinyl.*

life. The symptoms are quite variable and may involve the peripheral, autonomic, or central nervous system and usually include abdominal pain. The mechanism for the production of the symptoms is unclear. The incidence is between 5 and 10 per 100,000 in the United States. The gene is located on chromosome 11q23 (Table 16–5).

Porphyria cutanea tarda is the most common form of all of the porphyrias, with many thousands of cases worldwide. The disorder can be congenital or acquired. Symptoms of the acquired form occur in middle or late life. This disease is due to reduced hepatic **uroporphyrinogen decarboxylase** activity, a cytosolic enzyme and the fourth enzyme of the pathway. These individuals have photosensitivity, and the most common clinical finding is cutaneous lesions on the light-exposed areas of the hands, arms, and face. There is an increase in uroporphyrin I, formed nonenzymatically from a porphobilinogen metabolite, in the urine.

Lead poisoning results from a wide array of exposures that include lodged bullets, inhaled fumes, ingested contaminated food, and lead solubilized from glazes of utensils and linings of stills. In children, the primary source is ingestion of lead-based paint chips. The anemia that accompanies lead poisoning (plumbism) is in part the result of various inhibitory effects of lead on heme biosynthesis. Porphobilinogen synthase is most sensitive to lead, followed by ferrochelatase. Typical clinical manifestations are autonomic neuropathy causing abdominal pain and ileus (lead colic) and motor neuropathy (lead palsy). These symptoms are produced by advanced lead toxicity, but insidious nonspecific musculoskeletal and neuropsychiatric complaints are more prevalent. ◄

BLOOD CLOTTING

There is an exquisite balance between initiating and retarding blood clotting. Normal hemostasis (cessation of bleeding) requires interactions among blood vessels, platelets, monocytes, and blood coagulation proteins. Blood coagulation is initiated by substances in injured tissues and is propagated by a network of serine proteases with trypsin-like specificity (Table 4–2). These proteolytic factors contain a **catalytic triad** consisting of serine, histidine, and aspartate residues. Calcium and phospholipid are essential for blood coagulation. The coagulation reactions occur quickly but remain localized. Natural anticoagulation mechanisms also depend on serine proteases. After several days, moreover, fibrin clots are lysed by serine proteases and are replaced by connective tissue matrix molecules.

Two pathways initiate blood clotting: intrinsic (simple) and extrinsic (complicated). The **intrinsic pathway,** which may be initiated by an abnormal surface provided by damaged endothelium *in vivo* or glass *in vitro,* is so named because all components are present in blood; no exogenous component is required to initiate or propagate the reaction. In contrast, the **extrinsic pathway** requires an extravascular component (**thromboplastin** or **factor III**), which results when blood contacts any tissue because of injury. Many tissues express factor III. Both pathways merge at the common pathway (Figure 24–15). The **common pathway** involves the conversion of prothrombin to active thrombin, a serine protease. Thrombin catalyzes the conversion of fibrinogen to fibrin. These are the two most important steps of the process.

Blood clotting proteins are designated by Roman numerals and common names that are used interchangeably (Table 24–2). The numerals reflect the order of discovery and not their order in the overall process. Note, however, that factor VI is omitted from the blood clotting components. Fibrinogen, prothrombin, thromboplastin, and calcium,

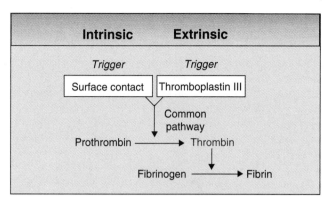

FIGURE 24–15. Overview of the extrinsic and intrinsic pathways of blood clotting.

rather than the Roman numerals, are the terms used by most hematologists.

Blood clotting involves a series of reactions in which the product of one process initiates a subsequent process, the product of which initiates still another. This scheme is called a **cascade.** The concepts of a blood clotting cascade and protein kinase cascades were formulated simultaneously in the 1960s. Blood clotting involves at least six distinct proteases with a serine residue at the active site (factors II, VII, IX, X, XI, and XII). These serine proteases exhibit trypsin-like specificity (hydrolyzing a peptide bond on the carboxyl side of a basic amino acid residue). Not all such peptide bonds are attacked by the factors, and the enzyme factors operate on selected targets in their specific substrates. During proteolysis, an inactive proenzyme (for example, factor XII) is converted to an active enzyme, designated by an "a" following the factor number (for example, XIIa). At the end of the blood clotting cascade, prothrombin (II) is converted to thrombin (IIa). The protein substrate for thrombin that results in clot formation is fibrinogen (factor I); fibrinogen is converted into a fibrin clot by proteolysis catalyzed by thrombin (factor IIa).

Four factors (III, IV, V, and VIII) function as auxiliary components in mediating specific conversions. Factor IV is calcium, and factors III, V, and VIII are proteins. Ca^{2+} is necessary for at least five steps in the clotting cascade (formation of IIa, VIIa, IXa, Xa, and XIIIa). The first four of these protein factors contain several γ-carboxyglutamyl residues that bind calcium. γ-Carboxyglutamate is a product of posttranslational modification and involves a vitamin K–dependent reaction (Figure 18–20).

Factor VIII is the famous **antihemophilic factor** associated with hemophilia A. ► Hemophilia A is an X-linked bleeding disorder associated historically with European royalty. Factor IX is called **Christmas factor.** The name is based on that of a person who had a disease resembling classical hemophilia, but whose biochemical lesion was shown to be different. Christmas disease is hemophilia B. ◄ Von Willebrand factor is found in plasma, in

TABLE 24-2. Properties of Blood Clotting Proteins

Factor	Common Name	Pathway	Function
I	Fibrinogen	Common	Forms fibrin clot
II	Prothrombin*†	Common	Generates fibrin from fibrinogen
III	Thromboplastin	Extrinsic	Activates X
IV	Calcium	Multiple	Activates II, VII, IX, X, and XIII
V	Proaccelerin	Common	Activates II (with Xa)
VII	Proconvertin*†	Extrinsic	Activates X (with III)
VIII	Antihemophilic factor	Intrinsic	Activates X (with IXa)
IX	Christmas factor*†	Intrinsic	Activates X (with VIII)
X	Stuart factor*†	Common	Activates II
XI	Plasma thromboplastin antecedent*	Intrinsic	Activates IX
XII	Hageman factor*	Intrinsic	Activates XI
XIII	Fibrin-stabilizing factor	Common	Cross-links fibrin
	Prekallikrein*	Intrinsic	Activates XII (with kininogen)
	Kininogen	Intrinsic	Activates XII (with kallikrein)
	Von Willebrand factor	Intrinsic	Stabilizes VIII; mediates platelet adhesion
	Platelet		Forms plug and initiates clotting

*Active form is a serine protease.
†Contains γ-carboxyglutamate.

platelet granules, and in subendothelial tissue. Von Willebrand factor performs two functions. It binds to receptors on the platelet surface and forms a bridge between the platelet and areas of vascular damage. Von Willebrand factor also binds to and stabilizes factor VIII. That a deficiency of any of these three factors (von Willebrand, VIII, IX) produces the same clinical manifestations illustrates that the three factors interact during blood clotting. Their functions are noted later.

Blood Clotting Cascade

Hemostasis involves many plasma proteins, platelets, and their interaction with the vascular endothelium. The intrinsic pathway is more intricate than the extrinsic pathway (Figure 24–16), and only experts know the entire cascade by rote. The main features of blood clotting can be summarized as follows. **Thromboplastin** (factor III) initiates the short extrinsic pathway. Factor VII has weak proteolytic activity that is augmented by thromboplastin. The intrinsic pathway includes several factors. Prekallikrein, XI, and XII are activated upon surface contact. Christmas factor (IXa) and antihemophilic factor (VIII) activate factor X. *Factors Xa and V, which are at the intersection of the intrinsic and extrinsic pathways, activate prothrombin.*

In the common pathway, thrombin catalyzes the proteolytic conversion of fibrinogen to fibrin. **Fibrinogen** consists of dimers of three different polypeptides $[(A\alpha)_2(B\beta)_2\gamma_2]$ and molecular mass of 340 kDa. Aα and Bβ each represent a single polypeptide chain. **Thrombin** catalyzes the hydrolysis of specific Arg-Gly bonds in each of the two Aα- and two Bβ-chains to form four small **fibrinopeptides** (two A and two B peptides) and fibrin (Figure

24–17). Fibrin spontaneously associates to form a loose fibrin clot. Thrombin also activates factor XIII by proteolysis to yield XIIIa. XIIIa, a transamidase, catalyzes cross-link formation between glutaminyl and lysyl residues (Figure 24–18). Although the amide bond of glutamine is not high energy in nature, the amide linkage provides a modicum of activation to energize the cross-linking reaction. Both intrinsic and extrinsic pathways appear to be activated upon vascular damage. Properties of the blood clotting factors are outlined in Table 24–2 for general reference.

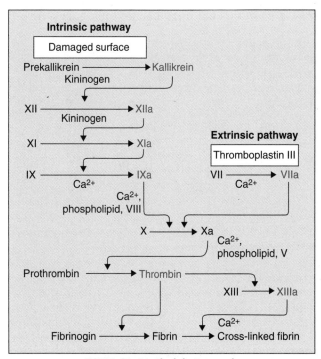

FIGURE 24-16. Blood clotting cascade.

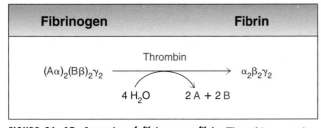

FIGURE 24–17. Conversion of fibrinogen to fibrin. *Thrombin, a serine protease, catalyzes the hydrolytic cleavage of A and B fibrinopeptides from fibrinogen.*

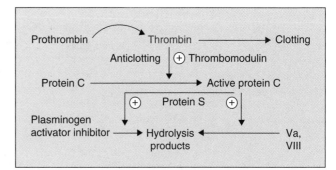

FIGURE 24–19. Activation and action of protein C.

Anticoagulants and Fibrinolysis

Antithrombin III and protein C are anticoagulants in blood. **Antithrombin III,** activated by heparin, binds and inhibits many serine proteases including thrombin and Xa, accounting for the anticoagulant effects of heparin. Antithrombin III is a suicide inhibitor. When thrombin or Xa attacks a specific Arg-Ser peptide bond of antithrombin III, a stable 1:1 complex containing the protease and antithrombin III forms. Blockade of the active site of thrombin or Xa by antithrombin III produces irreversible inhibition. Heparin increases the rate of formation of the antithrombin-protease complex 1000-fold.

Protein C, together with **protein S,** shuts off the coagulation pathway by inactivating factors VIII and Va by proteolysis. Protein C is converted to active protein C, a serine protease, by thrombin in a proteolysis reaction enhanced by thrombomodulin (Figure 24–19). **Thrombomodulin,** derived from endothelial cells, forms a complex with thrombin that produces a potent activator of protein C. Note that free thrombin catalyzes a key reaction in blood clotting, but thrombomodulin turns throm-

bin into an anticoagulant. Protein C regulates clotting as part of a servomechanism that limits the cascade and does not permit unrestrained coagulation.

The anticoagulant activity of catalytic protein C requires stimulatory protein S as cofactor (Table 24–3). The complex of activated protein C and protein S is readily formed on the endothelial cell surface. Protein S, which lacks a serine protease domain, is inactivated proteolytically by thrombin. Thrombin turns on protein C proteolytic activity directly and shuts off protein C activity indirectly by inactivating protein S. As a result, activity of the blood clotting cascade is finely tuned. *Antithrombin III and protein C–protein S limit the extent of clot formation.*

After tissue repair has abrogated the need for a clot, the clot is removed by fibrinolysis. **Plasmin,** a serine protease formed from plasminogen, is responsible for fibrinolysis. Plasmin catalyzes the hydrolysis of fibrin to produce **fibrin degradation products** (Figure 24–20). Like trypsin, plasmin attacks many peptide bonds on the carboxyterminal side of lysine or arginine. Soluble plasmin is inhibited by α_2**-plasmin inhibitor.** When bound to fibrin, however, plasmin is resistant to α_2-plasmin inhibitor. Binding of plasmin to fibrin or α_2-plasmin inhibitor is mutually exclusive. Factor XIIIa, besides cross-linking fibrin peptides, catalyzes the cross-linking of fibrin with α_2-plasmin inhibitor. This

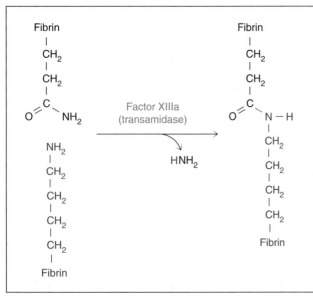

FIGURE 24–18. The cross-linking reaction of blood clotting catalyzed by factor XIIIa.

TABLE 24–3. Fibrinolytic Agents and Inhibitors of Blood Clotting

Component	Function
Antithrombin III	Inactivates thrombin and Xa; activated by heparin
Protein C*†	Inactivates Va and VIII
Protein S†	Activates protein C
Thrombomodulin	Complexes with thrombin to activate protein C
Plasminogen*	Lyses fibrin and other proteins
Tissue plasminogen activator (tPA)*	Activates plasminogen
Urokinase*	Activates plasminogen
α_2-Antiplasmin	Inhibits plasmin

*Active form is a serine protease.
†Contains γ-carboxyglutamate.

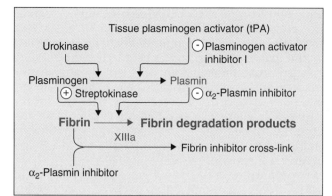

FIGURE 24–20. Activation of plasminogen by tissue plasminogen activator, urokinase, and streptokinase.

cross-linking makes fibrin more resistant to digestion by plasmin. The properties of α_2-plasmin inhibitor account for the specificity and efficiency of this protein as the principal inhibitor of fibrinolysis.

Tissue plasminogen activator (tPA) is a serine protease that catalyzes the conversion of plasminogen to plasmin by hydrolyzing a single peptide bond. Tissue plasminogen activator is synthesized and secreted by endothelium. Like the blood clotting pathway, the plasminogen pathway consists of a cascade (Figure 24–20). **Streptokinase** is a protein isolated from streptococci that, like tissue plasminogen activator, initiates fibrinolysis. Streptokinase *per se* lacks protease activity. Streptokinase forms a complex with plasminogen and activates its proteolytic activity. Activated plasminogen catalyzes the proteolytic activation of other plasminogen molecules to form plasmin, thereby initiating fibrinolysis. **Urokinase,** which is a family of serine proteases that are produced by the kidney and excreted in the urine, functions as a plasminogen activator. Urokinase is also found in the plasma. The relative efficacy of tissue plasminogen activator, streptokinase, and urokinase for the treatment of thrombotic diseases is under investigation.

▶ **Heparin** (by injection) is a short-acting anticoagulant with a rapid onset of action. **Coumarin** is a vitamin K analogue (Figure 2–23) that inhibits the vitamin K–dependent carboxylation of several blood-clotting factors (Figure 18–20); the coumarins require 12–24 hours to elicit an anticoagulant effect. Both heparin and coumarins (e.g., warfarin) are used clinically.

The following procedures are used to monitor various components of the blood clotting pathways. The instantaneous plugging of a hole in a blood vessel wall, primary hemostasis, is achieved by a combination of vasoconstriction and platelet adhesion and aggregation. The formation of a fibrin clot is not required. Measurement of the **bleeding time** is a sensitive laboratory index of primary hemostatic function. Bleeding time is elevated in people with von Willebrand disease and with thrombo-

cytopenia. Thrombocytopenia (low platelet count) is a common cause of abnormal bleeding. People with hemophilia have a normal bleeding time.

Activated partial thromboplastin time (aPTT) reflects the functional state of the intrinsic pathway. Therapeutic heparin treatment increases aPTT. Elevated aPTT occurs in hemophilias A and B. **Prothrombin time** reflects the functional state of both the extrinsic and the intrinsic pathways. A normal result requires adequate fibrinogen, prothrombin, and factors V, VII, and X. Because the biosynthesis of prothrombin and factors VII, IX, and X requires vitamin K, the prothrombin time is used to monitor coumarin therapy. ◀

Genetics of Coagulopathies

▶ Hemophilia A and hemophilia B (Christmas disease) are X-linked bleeding disorders (Table 16–5). Because of defective fibrin formation, affected individuals suffer joint and muscle hemorrhage, easy bruising, and prolonged bleeding from wounds. The incidence of both types is about 1 in 10,000 individuals and is similar in different parts of the world and in different races. Owing to the low reproductive fitness of individuals with hemophilia, about one-third of the mutant alleles are lost per generation. Because the number of affected individuals has been constant, about one-third of newly diagnosed cases are the result of new mutations. The genes for human factors VIII and IX are close to each other on the tip of the long arm of the X chromosome at q26-q27.

The gene for factor VIII is about 186 kb in size and consists of 26 exons and 25 introns. Factor VIII has sequences that are homologous to ceruloplasmin (a copper-containing oxidase in human plasma), but the significance of this surprising finding is unknown. The human factor VIII gene contains two notable features. It contains an unusually large exon of 3106 base pairs (average size for exons is 75 to 200 base pairs). The factor VIII gene contains an extremely large intron of 32,000 base pairs between exons 22 and 23. It might take hours to transcribe such a large gene into RNA. Liver cells are the main source of circulating factor.

Hemophilia A can be the result of one of several point mutations or deletions in the factor VIII gene. In hemophilia A and hemophilia B, diverse mutations give rise to the same clinical disorder. Many point mutations in hemophilia A occur in the recognition sequence for *Taq*I, TCGA, in the factor VIII gene. *Taq*I is a restriction enzyme (Box 15–1). The dinucleotide CG is a frequent site of methylation that produces 5-methylcytosine. Hydrolysis of 5-methylcytosine yields thymine and results in C→T transitions. The conversion of TCGA to TTGA in five of the seven *Taq*I sites in the factor VIII gene leads to the introduction of a stop codon. These *Taq*I sites appear to be mutational "hotspots." Besides point mutations, several deletions in the factor VIII gene have been observed. Deletions range from 2.5 kb to the entire gene. These deletions lead to severe disease. Insertion of L1, a family of long, interspersed repeats that are present throughout the human genome (Table 15–1), has occurred in exon 14 in unrelated families. This type of rearrangement represents a novel mechanism for the production of a mutation that leads to a disease, in this case hemophilia A.

Hemophilia B (Christmas disease) is due to mutations of the factor IX gene. The factor IX gene consists of eight exons and seven introns and is about 34 kb pairs in size. The introns range in size from 188 to 9473 nucleotides. Missense, nonsense, and splicing mutations of factor IX have been described. Single nucleotide mutations in the prepropeptide of factor IX have also occurred. The inability to correctly process the prepropeptide leads to the synthesis of defective molecules. The demonstration of multiple mutations ranging from no activity to partial activity helps explain the clinical variation in hemophilia B.

Von Willebrand disease is due to a mutation of the factor gene that is located on or near the tip of the short arm of chromosome 12. More than 20 variants of the disease have been described that are produced by point mutations, insertions, and deletions. In its commonest form, von Willebrand disease is transmitted as an autosomal dominant trait. The clinical course is variable. A mild form seems to reflect a quantitative deficiency of the factor, and a severe form seems to reflect the formation of an abnormal factor.

Individuals with hemophilias A and B have a prolonged activated partial thromboplastin time. The bleeding time is increased in von Willebrand disease. These diseases are treated with proteins prepared from human pooled plasma samples obtained from more than 2000 individual blood donors. Factor IX is stable, but factor VIII and von Willebrand factor are unstable. The possible and actual transmission of AIDS by such therapies was recognized in the 1980s. Preparation of these factors by recombinant DNA methods is under development. Factor VIII produced by recombinant DNA procedures has been approved for human use with the trade name Recombinate (for recombinate factor VIII). ◀

SUMMARY

Hemoglobin is a dimer of dimers with two chains from the α-family and two chains from the β-family. Hemoglobin A, the principal hemoglobin in adults, consists of two α-chains and two β-chains as $\alpha_2\beta_2$. The structure of hemoglobin differs in the oxygenated and deoxygenated states. The quaternary structure of the oxygenated state is called the R state (for relaxed) and the conformation of the deoxygenated state is called the T state (for tense).

Binding of oxygen to hemoglobin exhibits a sigmoidal concentration dependence. Such curves are diagnostic of positive cooperativity. The Bohr effect is the name ascribed to the acid-induced release of oxygen from hemoglobin. 2,3-Bisphosphoglycerate also causes hemoglobin to release oxygen. The isohydric transport of carbon dioxide is related to the increased ability of deoxyhemoglobin to bind protons. Carbonic anhydrase and the erythrocyte anion exchange protein also participate in the isohydric transport of carbon dioxide.

Protoporphyrin IX, the heme precursor, is derived from eight molecules each of succinyl-CoA and glycine. The first and rate-limiting step in the biosynthesis of heme is catalyzed by δ-aminolevulinate synthase (ALA synthase), a pyridoxal phosphate enzyme. Heme is degraded to biliverdin and bilirubin. Bilirubin can undergo a conjugation reaction to form bilirubin diglucuronide.

Blood clotting involves a series of reactions in which the product of one process initiates a subsequent process, the product of which initiates still another. This scheme is called a cascade. Blood clotting involves at least six distinct proteases with a serine residue at the active site (factors II, VII, IX, X, XI, and XII). These serine proteases exhibit trypsin-like specificity (hydrolyzing a peptide bond on the carboxyl side of a basic amino acid residue) but of a restricted nature. Four factors (III, IV, V, and VIII) function as auxiliary components in mediating specific conversions. Factor IV is calcium. Factor VIII is the famous antihemophilic factor associated with hemophilia A. Factor IX is called Christmas factor. Fibrin consists of three different polypeptides: $(A\alpha)_2(B\beta)_2\gamma_2$. Thrombin catalyzes the hydrolysis of four specific Arg-Gly bonds in the Aα- and Bβ-subunits of fibrinogen to form four small fibrinopeptides (two A and two B peptides) and fibrin. Hemophilia A and hemophilia B (Christmas disease) are X-linked bleeding disorders.

Anticoagulants and thrombolytic agents are required for the balance of physiological hemostasis. Antithrombin III, which is activated by heparin, is a natural anticoagulant that forms a stable complex with thrombin and factor Xa. Protein C (a catalyst) is activated by thrombin-thrombomodulin. Protein S (stimulatory factor)–protein C catalyzes the hydrolysis and inactivation of factors Va, VIII, and plasminogen activator inhibitor. Tissue plasminogen activator and urokinase catalyze the hydrolytic conversion of plasminogen to plasmin. Streptokinase activates the cryptic proteolytic activity of plasminogen. Plasmin catalyzes the hydrolysis of fibrin to produce fibrin degradation products. α_2-Plasmin inhibitor forms an inhibitory complex with plasmin.

SELECTED READINGS

Charache, S. Fetal hemoglobin, sickling, and sickle cell disease. Advances in Pediatrics 37:1–31, 1990.

Dickerson, R.E., and I. Geis. *Hemoglobin: Structure, Function, Evo-*

lution and Pathology. Benjamin/Cummings, Menlo Park, California, 1983.

Dyke, C., and M. Sobel. The management of coagulation problems in the surgical patient. Advances in Surgery 24:229–257, 1991.

Hess, D.C., R.J. Adams, and F.T. Nichols III. Sickle cell anemia and other hemoglobinopathies. Seminars in Neurology 11:314–328, 1991.

Mosher, D.F. Disorders of blood coagulation. In J.B. Wyngaarden, L.H. Smith, Jr., and J.C. Bennett (eds.). *Cecil Textbook of Medicine,* 19th ed. Philadelphia, W.B. Saunders Company, 1992, pp. 999–1017.

Paslin, D.A. The porphyrias. International Journal of Dermatology 31:527–539, 1992.

Ruggeri, Z.M., and J. Ware. Von Willebrand factor. FASEB Journal 7:308–316, 1993.

Stamatoyannopoulos, G., A.W. Nienhuis, P.W. Majerus, and H. Varmus. *The Molecular Basis of Blood Diseases,* 2nd ed. Philadelphia, W.B. Saunders Company, 1994.

Thompson, M.W., R.R. McInnes, and H.F. Willard. *Thompson and Thompson Genetics in Medicine,* 5th ed. Philadelphia, W.B. Saunders Company, 1991.

CHAPTER TWENTY-FIVE

INTEGRATION OF

METABOLISM

Perhaps the most important element of attitude is humility, because from it flows a self-critical mind and a continuous effort to learn and improve.

—HANS A. KREBS

By limiting our analysis to the behavior of single enzymes and simple pathways, we miss the point that in real life, thousands of enzyme reactions are occurring, and tens of metabolic pathways interact.

—PAUL A. SRERE

The activity of regulatory enzymes can be controlled by several mechanisms. For instance, enzymes may be regulated by **covalent modification** and noncovalently by **allosteric agents.** Enzyme levels may also be altered by changing the rates of synthesis or degradation. Increased synthesis is called **enzyme induction,** and decreased synthesis is called **enzyme repression.** Covalent modification and allosteric regulation occur rapidly (seconds to minutes), whereas changes in enzyme levels occur slowly (minutes to hours). Metabolic rates may also be controlled by substrate availability, product inhibition, and translocation of molecules from one cellular compartment to another. Likely sites for metabolic control are reactions that irrevocably commit a metabolite to a definite pathway. Control mechanisms, moreover, follow the molecular logic of the cell and make physiological sense (PRINCIPLE 9 OF BIOCHEMISTRY). Molecular logic enables one to predict whether a given metabolite will increase or decrease the activity of a pathway. For example, *ATP will inhibit energy-producing pathways, and ADP or AMP will activate energy-producing pathways.*

Besides enzymatic control, metabolism is coordinated at tissues and organs. Food is absorbed from the gut and distributed to various organs. Carbohydrates and amino acids are transported by the hepatic portal venous system to and through the liver. Lipids, in contrast, are transported from the gut via chylomicrons through the lymphatic system to the venous system as their cargoes are carried to cells. Metabolic fuels are stored for future use and are released for maintenance.

Insulin and glucagon play a pivotal role in metabolic homeostasis. These two hormones generally produce opposite physiological effects. **Insulin** is anabolic and promotes glycogen, triglyceride, and protein synthesis. **Glucagon** is catabolic and promotes glycogenolysis, lipolysis, and protein degradation. Before considering interorgan metabolism, let us review the control points of various metabolic pathways.

REGULATION OF MAINSTREAM METABOLIC PATHWAYS

Glycolysis and Gluconeogenesis

Hexokinase (all cells) and glucokinase (liver, β-cells of the pancreas) catalyze the first step in glucose metabolism to form glucose 6-phosphate. Glucose 6-phosphate occupies a central point of carbohydrate metabolism and can be converted to glycogen and other carbohydrates via UDP-glucose, to pentose phosphates, to lactate, to acetyl-CoA for oxidation or for fatty acid synthesis (Figure 25–1).

The three irreversible steps in glycolysis include the hexokinase, phosphofructokinase, and pyruvate kinase reactions. **Phosphofructokinase** catalyzes the main regulatory step in glycolysis (Table 25–1). Phosphofructokinase is activated allosterically by fructose 2,6-bisphosphate and AMP (Figure 25–2). AMP is formed from ADP by the adenylate kinase reaction; adenylate kinase is also called myokinase because of its special importance in muscle.

$$ADP + ADP \rightleftharpoons AMP + ATP \qquad (25.1)$$

This reaction converts ADP to ATP and simulta-

FIGURE 25–1. Overview of glucose and amino acid metabolism.

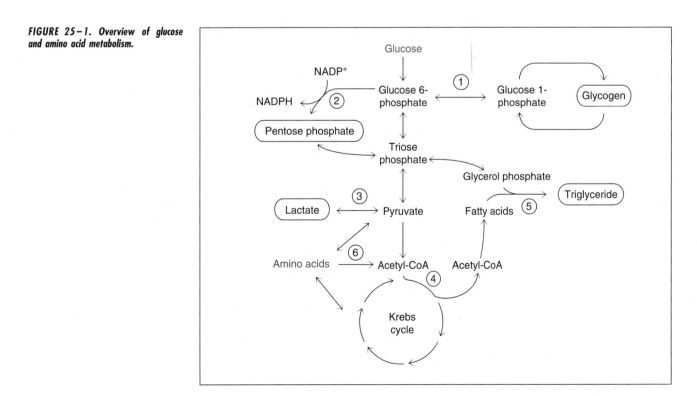

TABLE 25–1.   Sites of Control of Mainstream Metabolic Pathways

Pathway	Major Regulatory Enzymes	Activators	Inhibitors	Hormonal Effects	Comments
Glycolysis	Phosphofructokinase	Fructose 2,6-bisphosphate, AMP	Citrate (except liver), ATP	Glucagon cascade ↓ [fructose 2,6-bisphosphate]	Insulin cascade induces and glucagon cascade represses synthesis of enzymes of this pathway in liver
	Hexokinase Glucokinase		Glucose 6-phosphate Regulatory protein-fructose 6-phosphate		
	Pyruvate kinase	Fructose 1,6-bisphosphate	Alanine, ATP, fatty acyl-CoA	Glucagon cascade ↓ enzyme activity (liver only)	
Gluconeogenesis	Pyruvate carboxylase PEP carboxykinase	Acetyl-CoA			Glucagon, glucocorticoids, and epinephrine induce and insulin represses synthesis of enzymes of this pathway in liver
	Fructose-1,6-bisphosphatase		Fructose 2,6-bisphosphate, AMP	Glucagon cascade ↓ [Fructose 2,6-bisphosphate]	
	Glucose-6-phosphatase				
Glycogenesis	Glycogen synthase	High glucose 6-phosphate (not physiological)		Insulin cascade ↑; glucagon (liver) and epinephrine (muscle) cascades ↓	Insulin cascade induces
Glycogenolysis	Phosphorylase	AMP (muscle), Ca^{2+}	ATP, glucose (liver), glucose 6-phosphate (liver)	Glucagon cascade ↑; insulin cascade ↓	
Pentose phosphate pathway	Glucose-6-phosphate dehydrogenase				Insulin cascade induces; $NADP^+$ availability may be regulatory
Pyruvate dehydrogenase activity	Pyruvate dehydrogenase kinase		Kinase, activated by acetyl-CoA and NADH, inhibits dehydrogenase		Phosphorylation of pyruvate dehydrogenase is inhibitory
Krebs cycle	Isocitrate dehydrogenase	ADP			Substrate availability (acetyl-CoA, oxalacetate, and NAD^+) is important for the entire cycle
Lipogenesis	Acetyl-CoA carboxylase	Citrate	Fatty acyl-CoA	Insulin cascade ↑ (adipocyte); glucagon cascade ↓	Insulin cascade induces
Lipolysis	Hormone-sensitive lipase			Glucagon, epinephrine cascades ↑; Insulin cascade ↓	
β-Oxidation	Carnitine acetyltransferase–I		Malonyl-CoA		

neously generates an activator of glycolysis. This process occurs in exercising skeletal muscle when aerobic metabolism is unable to maintain ATP production by oxidative phosphorylation and from creatine phosphate. **AMP** signals a need for enhanced energy production by glycolysis. Generation of AMP is important in muscle but probably is not important in heart or liver under physiological conditions.

Fructose 2,6-bisphosphate is the main allosteric activator of phosphofructokinase and glycolysis. In liver, the glucagon cascade inhibits glycolysis by decreasing the concentration of **fructose 2,6-bisphosphate.** Glucagon, a hormone that promotes gluconeogenesis, elevates hepatic cyclic AMP and decreases the rate of glycolysis by decreasing fructose 2,6-bisphosphate. Regulation of the levels of fructose 2,6-bisphosphate by a polypeptide with both kinase and phosphatase activity is illustrated in Figure 7–11. Citrate levels are elevated when fatty acids are used as metabolic fuel in muscle

and extrahepatic cells. **Citrate** decreases phosphofructokinase activity allosterically. Citrate apparently lacks this effect in liver because glycolysis and citrate provide precursors for fatty acid synthesis in pathways that are conjointly active. **ATP** signals the lack of a need for glycolysis and energy production, and ATP is an allosteric inhibitor of phosphofructokinase (Figure 25–2). Regulation by ATP is important in muscle where levels of ATP are high during rest. Inhibition by ATP is overcome by high concentrations of fructose 6-phosphate.

Hexokinase and **glucokinase** catalyze a secondary regulatory step of glycolysis. Glucokinase in liver exhibits a high K_m for glucose (10 mM) and is not saturated by the concentrations of glucose that occur in the hepatic portal vein. Substrate availability thus plays a direct role in regulating the conversion of glucose to glucose 6-phosphate in liver. Hexokinase, which occurs in all cells, has a low K_m (30 μM) and is half-saturated at 0.56 mg/dL of glucose (1 mM = 18 mg/dL). Hexokinase, but not glu-

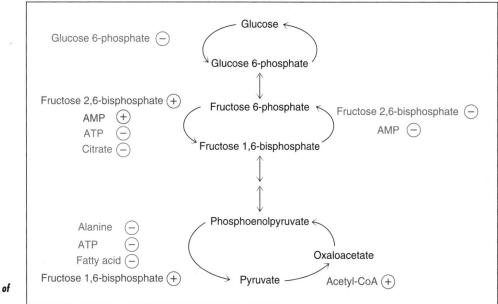

FIGURE 25-2. Allosteric regulation of glycolysis and gluconeogenesis.

cokinase, is inhibited by glucose 6-phosphate. The failure of glucose 6-phosphate to inhibit glucokinase permits glucokinase to metabolize large amounts of glucose during the well-fed state. The activity of glucokinase, however, is inhibited by a **regulatory protein-fructose 6-phosphate** complex. Fructose 6-phosphate is derived from glucose 6-phosphate by isomerization. In contrast, the regulatory protein-fructose 1-phosphate complex does not inhibit glucokinase. Fructose 1-phosphate (Figure 7–14), which occurs in liver after digestion of sucrose or ingestion of fruit, is a fructose metabolite. Ingesting fructose results in a metabolite that removes an inhibitor of glucokinase.

Liver pyruvate kinase catalyzes a secondary regulatory step of glycolysis. **Alanine,** a preferred substrate for liver gluconeogenesis, is an allosteric inhibitor of this step. Pyruvate kinase is also inhibited allosterically by **ATP** and long-chain **fatty acyl–CoA.** Fatty acyl–CoA provides an alternative fuel for oxidation, and ATP signals a large energy charge. **Fructose 1,6-bisphosphate,** formed by the rate-limiting enzyme of glycolysis, activates pyruvate kinase allosterically. The activity of pyruvate kinase is high compared with the activities of the other enzymes of glycolysis, and inhibition is probably more important than activation. Control of glycolysis (and other pathways) can be distributed over several steps (the distributive control of metabolism). Additional control points can include glucose transport and the enolase reaction.

The cyclic AMP second messenger system inhibits hepatic glycolysis by two parallel mechanisms. Active protein kinase A decreases the concentration of fructose 2,6-bisphosphate by phosphorylating phosphofructo-2-kinase/fructose-2,6-bisphosphatase, thereby decreasing the concentration of fructose 2,6-bisphosphate, an activator of phosphofructo-1-kinase. Protein kinase A also catalyzes the

phosphorylation and inhibition of liver pyruvate kinase (Table 25–2).

Let us now consider the regulation of gluconeogenesis and the conversion of pyruvate to glucose 6-phosphate and glucose. *Gluconeogenesis occurs in liver and kidney.* The glycolytic bypass reactions that are unique to gluconeogenesis include **pyruvate carboxylase, PEP carboxykinase, fructose-1,6-bisphosphatase,** and **glucose-6-phosphatase.** Acetyl-CoA levels play a reciprocal role in regulating pyruvate oxidation or gluconeogenesis. Pyruvate carboxylase requires **acetyl-CoA** as an allosteric activator, and acetyl-CoA promotes gluconeogenesis (Figure 25–2). Acetyl-CoA inhibits pyruvate dehydrogenase indirectly by activating pyruvate dehydrogenase kinase (Table 25–2). AMP and fructose 2,6-bisphosphate inhibit fructose-1,6-bisphosphatase allosterically. Note that fructose 2,6-bisphosphate and AMP have opposite effects on phosphofructokinase and fructose-1,6-bisphosphatase (Figure 25–2), and these reciprocal effects make physiological sense. Fructose 2,6-bisphosphate is the more important physiological regulator.

There are two schemes for gluconeogenesis based on **mitochondrial** and **cytosolic phosphoenolpyruvate carboxykinase.** With pyruvate or alanine as precursor, oxaloacetate is formed in the mitochondrion in a reaction catalyzed by pyruvate carboxylase, followed by reduction to malate, which is then transported to the cytosol. Cytosolic malate is reconverted to oxaloacetate, generating the cytosolic NADH required for gluconeogenesis, and the oxaloacetate is converted to phosphoenolpyruvate carboxykinase. With lactate as precursor, it is oxidized to produce cytosolic NADH and pyruvate. Pyruvate is taken up in the mitochondrion, and converted to oxaloacetate. Mitochondrial phosphoenolpyruvate carboxykinase catalyzes the

TABLE 25-2. Covalent Modification of Regulatory Enzymes*

Kinase Substrate	Kinase	Effect on Protein Substrate Activity	Comments
Acetyl-CoA carboxylase	AMP-dependent protein kinase	↓	Kinase activated by decreased energy charge
Branched-chain keto acid dehydrogenase†	Branched-chain keto acid dehydrogenase kinase	↓	Kinase activated by CoA products and NADH
Glycogen synthase	Protein kinase A and glycogen synthase kinase	↓	
Glycogen synthase kinase	AMP-dependent protein kinase	↓	Kinase activated by decreased energy charge
HMG-CoA reductase	AMP-dependent protein kinase	↓	Kinase activated by decreased energy charge
Hormone sensitive lipase	Protein kinase A	↑	
Pyruvate kinase (liver)	Protein kinase A	↓	
Phosphofructo-2-kinase/fructose-2,6-bis-phosphatase (liver)	Protein kinase A	↓/↑	
Pyruvate dehydrogenase†	Pyruvate dehydrogenase kinase	↓	Kinase activated by acetyl-CoA and NADH, phosphatase activated by calcium and insulin action
Phosphorylase	Phosphorylase kinase	↑↑	
Phosphorylase kinase	Protein kinase A	↑	

*Actions mediated by protein kinase A are antagonized by the insulin cascade.
†Mitochondrial.

formation of phosphoenolpyruvate, which is then translocated to the cytosol.

Glycogenesis and Glycogenolysis

The regulation of glycogen metabolism is intricate. *Glycogen synthase (biosynthesis) and glycogen phosphorylase (degradation) are the two important regulatory enzymes.* **Phosphorylase** is activated allosterically by **AMP** (muscle) and is inhibited by **glucose** (liver), **glucose 6-phosphate,** and **ATP** (Figure 25-3). High concentrations of glucose and glucose 6-phosphate signal the need for glycogenesis and not glycogenolysis. AMP, which is generated by myokinase, signals the need for catabolism and ATP production. The δ-subunit of phosphorylase kinase is calmodulin, and phosphorylase kinase is activated by calcium. **Calcium** triggers muscle contraction and phosphorylase kinase (and thus phosphorylase) activation simultaneously.

Besides these allosteric regulators, the two enzyme activities are altered by phosphorylation (Table 25-2). Glucagon (liver) and epinephrine (muscle), which activate the cyclic AMP cascade, concomitantly activate glycogenolysis and inhibit glycogenesis. Insulin has the opposite effects. Moreover, insulin induces glycogen synthase activity as part of its overall anabolic action. Insulin also induces **glucose-6-phosphate dehydrogenase** and **6-phosphogluconate dehydrogenase** to increase activity of the pentose phosphate pathway.

Pyruvate Dehydrogenase and Krebs Cycle

Next we consider the the regulation of the oxidation of pyruvate and acetyl-CoA. Pyruvate dehydrogenase is regulated by phosphorylation and dephosphorylation catalyzed by a mitochondrial kinase and phosphatase that operate only on this enzyme. Phosphorylation is inhibitory. **Pyruvate dehydrogenase kinase** is regulated allosterically. **Acetyl-CoA** and **NADH** (products) decrease pyruvate dehydrogenase activity by activating the kinase (Table 25-2). Note that acetyl-CoA has opposite effects on pyruvate carboxylase and pyruvate dehydrogenase activities (Figure 25-4). Acetyl-CoA promotes gluconeogenesis, and a lack of acetyl-CoA promotes production of acetyl-CoA by pyruvate dehydrogenase.

Isocitrate dehydrogenase is the chief regulatory enzyme of the Krebs cycle. It is activated allosterically by ADP (Table 25-1). **ADP** signals the need for enhanced generation of reducing equivalents for oxidative phosphorylation. The rate of oxidative phosphorylation under physiological conditions is controlled by substrate availability, and **ADP** is limiting.

Fatty Acid and Ketone Body Metabolism

Fatty acid and triglyceride synthesis occur chiefly in the liver. Insulin, which is anabolic, stim-

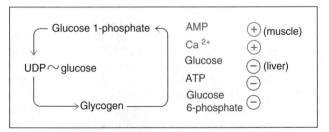

FIGURE 25-3. Allosteric regulation of glycogenolysis.

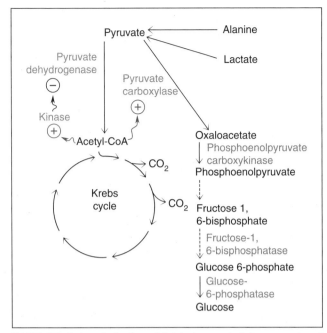

FIGURE 25–4. *Central role of acetyl-CoA in the control of gluconeogenesis and pyruvate oxidation.*

phorylation catalyzed by protein kinase A (Table 25–2). Lipolysis releases fatty acids and glycerol into the circulation. Fatty acids enter cells by diffusion and are converted to fatty acyl-CoA. Acyl-CoA is converted to acylcarnitine before entering the mitochondrion. Fatty acid synthesis and β-oxidation are differentially regulated. This is achieved at the intersection of malonyl-CoA and fatty acyl-CoA. **Carnitine acyltransferase–I** is inhibited by **malonyl-CoA,** a fatty acid precursor (Figure 25–5). Fatty-acylcarnitine enters the mitochondrion when fatty acid synthesis is not prevalent. *The transport of fatty-acyl groups into the mitochondrion is the rate-limiting process in β-oxidation.* Without fatty acid synthesis, there is little or no malonyl-CoA to inhibit the formation and translocation of fatty-acylcarnitine into the mitochondrion and β-oxidation proceeds. Furthermore, when the delivery of fatty acid and acyl-CoA exceeds the capacity of the Krebs cycle, acetyl-CoA is shunted into the pathway for ketone body production. Ketone body synthesis is thus regulated by acetyl-CoA availability. Ketone bodies diffuse from liver to the circulation

ulates these processes by induction of acetyl-CoA carboxylase and the fatty acid synthase complex. Insulin also antagonizes the opposite effects mediated by the cyclic AMP cascade. **Acetyl-CoA carboxylase** catalyzes the first and rate-limiting reaction in fatty acid biosynthesis. This cytosolic enzyme is activated by **citrate,** the carrier of two-carbon fragments from the mitochondrion to the cytosol. Acetyl-CoA carboxylase is inhibited by **fatty acyl-CoA,** a product of fatty acid synthesis (Figure 25–5). A low energy charge decreases acetyl-CoA carboxylase activity indirectly. When ATP is converted to ADP, and ATP generation is limited, AMP results (equation 25.1). AMP activates an **AMP-dependent protein kinase** (note AMP-dependent and *not cyclic* AMP–dependent) that catalyzes the phosphorylation and inactivation of acetyl-CoA carboxylase. AMP-dependent protein kinase also mediates the phosphorylation and inactivation of **glycogen synthase** and **HMG-CoA reductase** (Table 25–3). A rise in AMP, an activator of AMP-dependent protein kinase, serves as a signal to shut off anabolic responses. The generation of AMP leads to the inhibition of fatty acid, glycogen (Table 25–1), and cholesterol synthesis (Table 25–3), three anabolic responses.

Fatty acids are derived from triglyceride stored in adipocytes. Availability of fatty acids represents an important control point. **Hormone-sensitive lipase** in adipocytes is inhibited by insulin, an anabolic hormone. Moreover, *insulin inhibition of hormone-sensitive lipase occurs at insulin levels that are too low to stimulate glucose transport into adipocytes and muscle.* The inhibition of fatty acid release from adipocytes is thus a notable regulatory locus for insulin.

Hormone-sensitive lipase is activated by phos-

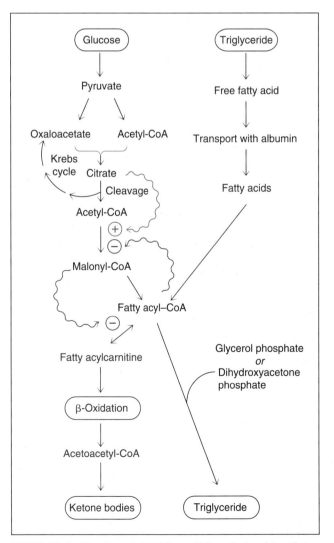

FIGURE 25–5. *Allosteric regulation of fatty acid biosynthesis and β-oxidation.*

TABLE 25–3. Sites of Control of Auxiliary Metabolic Pathways

Pathway	Regulatory Enzyme	Activators	Inhibitors	Hormonal Effects	Comment
Branched-chain keto acid dehydrogenase	Branched-chain keto acid dehydrogenase kinase		Kinase is activated by NADH and acyl-CoA and inhibits dehydrogenase	Insulin stimulates branched-chain amino acid transport into muscle	Phosphorylation by kinase is inhibitory
Cholesterol synthesis	HMG-CoA reductase				Cholesterol represses enzyme synthesis
Deoxynucleotide synthesis	Ribonucleotide reductase	ATP	dATP		Regulation by nucleotides is complex; enzyme is induced prior to S phase of cell cycle
Heme synthesis	δ-Aminolevulinate synthase		Heme		Heme represses enzyme synthesis
Purine nucleotide synthesis	PRPP amidotransferase	PRPP	AMP, GMP, IMP		
Pyrimidine synthesis	Carbamoyl-phosphate synthetase–II		UTP		
Urea cycle	Carbamoyl-phosphate synthetase–I	N-Acetylglutamate			N-Acetylglutamate synthase is activated by arginine

and are taken up and metabolized by extrahepatic cells.

Nitrogen Metabolism

The urea cycle eliminates excess ammonia. Ammonia is derived mainly from dietary amino acids that are not used promptly for protein synthesis. *Carbamoyl-phosphate synthetase–I catalyzes the rate-limiting step of the urea cycle.* **N-Acetylglutamate** is a positive allosteric effector, and this substance is required for the expression of activity. **N-Acetylglutamate synthase,** which catalyzes a reaction between acetyl-CoA and glutamate, is activated allosterically by **arginine.**

The branched-chain amino acids (valine, leucine, and isoleucine) are metabolized by **branched-chain keto acid dehydrogenase** (Figures 13–20, 13–21, and 13–22), a mitochondrial enzyme. This enzyme, which resembles pyruvate dehydrogenase in mechanism, is regulated by **branched-chain–keto acid dehydrogenase kinase** and **phosphatase.** The kinase is activated by the products of the dehydrogenase reaction including NADH and the corresponding acyl-CoA products. The rate-limiting reactions for pathways unrelated to main metabolic fuels are listed in Table 25–3.

ORGAN METABOLISM

Metabolic homeostasis requires the cooperation of several organs. The **liver** is situated between the intestine and the general circulation and plays a pivotal role in metabolic homeostasis. Liver has the greatest metabolic versatility of any organ (Table 25–4). It is the first organ exposed to amino

acid and carbohydrate nutrients from the intestine and to insulin and glucagon from the pancreas. Liver is the primary site of blood glucose regulation. Liver imports and stores glucose when it is provided during absorption, and it produces and exports glucose when extrahepatic cells require it.

TABLE 25–4. Organ Metabolism

Organ	Properties
Brain	Uses glucose as chief energy source. Can use ketone bodies only after a few days without food
Erythrocytes	Can use only glucose for metabolism. Lack mitochondria, and release lactic acid into the circulation
Intestine	Releases digested carbohydrate (glucose, galactose, fructose, mannose) into the portal vein. Releases alanine, citrulline, proline, and lactate derived from amino acids. Releases branched-chain amino acids and other essential amino acids, but little aspartate, asparagine, glutamate, or glutamine. Can use glutamine for energy production, and releases alanine derived from glutamine into the circulation. Forms chylomicrons for triglyceride and cholesterol uptake
Kidney	Uses glutamine for ammonia production. Uses glutamine for gluconeogenesis after a few days of fasting
Liver	Maintains blood glucose by glycogenolysis and gluconeogenesis. Contains glucose 6-phosphatase that enables it to release glucose into the circulation. Active in triglyceride, cholesterol, bile acid production. Exports cholesterol and triglyceride as VLDL. Takes up HDL during reverse cholesterol transport. Liver-derived proteins include albumin, the chief protein of blood, most transport proteins, and blood clotting factors. Insulin-responsive organ, except for glucose transport. Forms, but does not utilize, ketone bodies. Synthesizes urea
Muscle	Insulin-responsive glucose and amino acid transport systems. Uses fatty acids and ketone bodies for energy. Can perform anaerobic glycolysis for energy production. Takes up and transaminates branched-chain amino acids. Releases lactate, alanine, and glutamine. Lactate and alanine are used for hepatic gluconeogenesis

Liver can take up glucose and convert it to glycogen and fat. In the fed state in humans about 7.5% of the wet weight of the liver is glycogen. This decreases to less than 1% during fasting. Liver first releases stored glycogen, and then uses gluconeogenesis to maintain blood glucose. Substrates for gluconeogenesis include lactate and pyruvate released from erythrocytes and active skeletal muscle, alanine released from muscle, and glycerol released from adipocytes. Both glycolysis and gluconeogenesis can proceed simultaneously but in different tissues. Red cells metabolize glucose to lactate, while liver simultaneously converts lactate to glucose.

Liver is active in protein synthesis after a protein-containing meal, and liver protein is degraded to provide precursors for gluconeogenesis. Liver is also the site of urea production. The liver is the main organ of cholesterol homeostasis and is responsible for substantial triglyceride production. Liver releases about 180 g of glucose, 100 g of fat, and 14 g of albumin into the circulation daily.

Adipose tissue participates in the storage and provision of the body's metabolic fuel. During anabolism, adipocytes synthesize triglyceride from fatty acids delivered by chylomicrons from the intestine or VLDL from liver. Glucose and glycolysis provide dihydroxyacetone phosphate for triglyceride synthesis owing to the lack of glycerol kinase in adipocytes and their inability to use glycerol as substrate. Adipocytes contain an insulin-responsive glucose transporter (GLUT4). Glucose provides pyruvate for acetyl-CoA and malonyl-CoA for adipocyte fatty acid biosynthesis, which is quantitatively less important in adipose tissue than in liver. Adipocytes derive most of their energy from fatty acid oxidation. During catabolism, adipocytes hydrolyze triglyceride and release fatty acids.

A 70-kg adult contains about 28 kg of **skeletal muscle.** In the well-fed state, the glycogen content is about 1% as wet weight. Glycogen stores in muscle are greater than in liver because of muscle's greater mass. Since muscle lacks glucose-6-phosphatase, muscle glycogen is not directly available as a source of blood glucose. Muscle protein contributes amino acid–carbon substrates for gluconeogenesis during fasting or starvation. The two most important amino acids that are released by muscle are alanine and glutamine. Lacking a storage form of protein, the source of these amino acids is contractile protein. The cyclic process of

lactate production by muscle and other cells and gluconeogenesis in liver that provides glucose for extrahepatic cells is called the **Cori cycle.**

Myocardial metabolism differs from that of skeletal muscle. **Heart muscle** functions aerobically and uses fatty acids under ordinary conditions as the main fuel. Heart can also use ketone bodies, lactate, and pyruvate. Heart contains some glycogen, but little is used under ordinary conditions. Glycolysis is an important source of energy production in heart muscle during circumstances of impaired perfusion (coronary artery disease).

Brain is a constant user of metabolic fuels provided by other tissues. Brain uses about 20% of the total ATP produced in resting adults. Considerable energy is used to maintain ion gradients by the sodium/potassium-ATPase. The brain uses glucose almost exclusively as a source of energy. Brain does not contain appreciable glycogen, and lactate generation is nil. After a few days of fasting, brain can use ketone bodies as an oxidative substrate. Brain consumes about 120 g of glucose daily.

METABOLIC FUELS

Fuel metabolism varies greatly as a function of time between meals, meal composition, overnight fasting, prolonged fasting, starvation, and pathological conditions. The **well-fed state** of metabolism begins during the later stages of digestion and lasts a few hours. The **postabsorptive state** lasts from 6 to 12 hours after a meal and refers to the period during which the transition from the postprandial to the fasting state occurs. The **early-fasting state** occurs from 12 to 48 hours after a meal, and the **late-fasting state** extends from 2 to 10 days after the last meal. **Starvation** represents the lack of caloric intake for a period greater than 10 days. These states have distinctive metabolic characteristics.

The daily energy expenditure for a 70-kg person with a moderate level of physical activity is about 2500 kcal (Table 2–5). Healthy adults consist of about 20% body fat by weight. This corresponds to 135,000 kcal and is by far the largest energy reserve in the body (Table 25–5). Stores of glycogen and glucose would not suffice for one day's normal energy expenditure, but the amount of fat is adequate to supply calories for 40 days of starvation (100,000 kcal ÷ 2500 kcal per day). This 40-day pe-

TABLE 25–5.   Energy Reserves of a 70-Kg Human

Stored Fuel	Tissue	Grams	% Body Weight	Kilocalories
Fat	Adipose	11,000–15,000	16–21	100,000–135,000
Glucose	Body fluids	12	<1	48
Glycogen	Liver	70	<1	280
Glycogen	Muscle	280	<1	1120
Protein	Muscle	8,000–12,000	11–17	32,000–48,000

riod is an underestimate because the basal metabolic rate and energy expenditure decrease with starvation.

Carbohydrate Homeostasis

Carbohydrate accounts for 40–60% of dietary caloric intake; a judicious diet corresponds to the higher value (Figure 2–27). Absorbable dietary carbohydrate consists of glucose (80%), fructose (15%), galactose (5%), and small amounts of mannose. Fructose, galactose, and mannose are converted to glucose derivatives by the liver (Figures 7–13, 7–14, and 7–15). A temporary rise in plasma glucose occurs immediately following a meal containing carbohydrate, fat, and protein. Blood glucose can increase from about 4 mM (72 mg/dL) to 7 mM (126 mg/dL) within 2 hours. After 3–4 hours, blood glucose returns to its initial value (Figure 25–6). **Glucose** promotes insulin release from the pancreas. **Arginine** and **lysine** also stimulate insulin release, but they are not as effective as glucose. **Glucose** decreases glucagon secretion, but **arginine** and **alanine** stimulate it. Glucagon secretion is maintained when the meal contains both carbohydrate and protein. With a carbohydrate-rich, protein-poor meal, glucagon secretion decreases.

Red blood cells obtain their energy exclusively from glucose by glycolysis. Brain and nervous tissue use glucose as sole energy source, except during prolonged fasts. Although brain can use ketone bodies for about 50% of its energy during starvation, brain still requires glucose. Because of **brain** and **red blood cell** metabolism, blood glucose must always be available. Other cells can use fatty acids and ketone bodies as their primary source of metabolic energy.

Liver takes up about half the glucose that is delivered by the portal vein from the intestine after a meal, and the remainder is taken up by other cells. Hepatic **glycogen** synthesis is much more intricate than one might imagine and involves direct and indirect pathways. The **direct pathway** for liver glycogen synthesis in the fed state involves the conversion of glucose to glucose 6-phosphate, glucose 1-phosphate, and UDP-glucose. The **indirect pathway** for liver glycogen synthesis requires gluconeogenesis. Glucose that is not taken up by liver is transported from the circulation into all cells. Some glucose taken up by muscle and erythrocytes is converted to lactate. Lactate returns to the liver and is converted to glycogen, thus involving the indirect pathway (Figure 25–7A). The gluconeogenic-glycogen pathway accounts for a variable amount of glycogen synthesized in the well-fed state and may provide as much as half of the liver glycogen stores.

An insulin-initiated cascade promotes dephosphorylation of the inactive glycogen synthase–D to active glycogen synthase–I (Figure 20–5). The insulin cascade also decreases glycogen phosphorylase activity as a result of dephosphorylation of serine residues. This reciprocal regulation of **glycogen synthase** and **phosphorylase** promotes glycogenesis in liver and muscle. In muscle after feeding, about 50% of the glucose is completely oxidized, 35% is stored as glycogen, and 15% is released as lactate and alanine. Besides glycogen, liver converts excess glucose and lactate into **triglyceride.** VLDL transports triglyceride and cholesterol to extrahepatic cells.

Insulin stimulates **glucose transport** into muscle by recruiting **GLUT4** transporters from sequestered intracellular membranes to the plasma membrane. Muscle glycogen is restored in the well-fed state as a result of insulin-stimulated transport and glycogen synthase activity. Insulin stimulates glucose transport into adipocytes, which contain GLUT4 transporters. This increases the availability of dihydroxyacetone phosphate for triglyceride synthesis. Some glucose can also be converted into fatty acids in adipocytes, but most fatty acids derived from carbohydrate are generated by the liver and transported to adipocytes. Liver, β-cells of the pancreas, and erythrocytes contain **GLUT1** transporters (unresponsive to insulin).

The liver is responsible for most gluconeogenesis in the postabsorptive stage (6–12 hours without food), and the kidney becomes more prominent in the late fasting stage (4 days without food). The main sources of carbon atoms for gluconeogenesis include alanine (skeletal muscle), lactate and pyruvate (erythrocytes, exercising muscle),

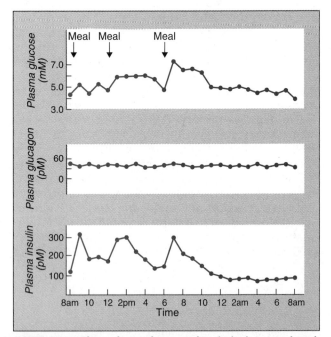

FIGURE 25–6. Plasma glucose, glucagon, and insulin levels in normal people eating a well-balanced diet. pM, picomoles/L (1 picomole is 1×10^{-12} mole). Data from Y. Tasaka, M. Sekine, M. Wakatsuki, H. Ohgawara, and K. Shizume. Levels of pancreatic glucagon, insulin and glucose during 24 hours of the day in normal subjects eating a well-balanced diet. Hormone and Metabolic Research 7:205–206, 1975.

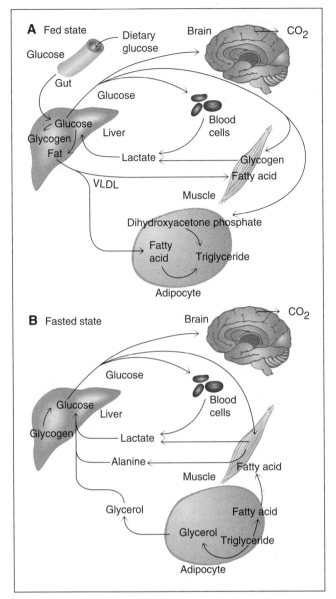

FIGURE 25–7. Carbohydrate metabolism. A. *Fed state.* B. *Fasted state.*

and glycerol (adipocytes). In sedentary people, about 15% of plasma glucose is derived from the lactate produced by erythrocytes and other cells. This percentage can increase if skeletal muscle produces additional lactate. Amino acids that are derived from proteolysis in liver and muscle furnish substrates for gluconeogenesis. Alanine is the primary amino acid released from muscle, and alanine is gluconeogenic. Hydrolysis of triglyceride in adipocytes releases fatty acids and glycerol. Adipocytes, lacking glycerol kinase, are unable to metabolize glycerol. It is transported to the liver where it is metabolized.

All body cells can use glucose as a partial source of metabolic energy during the fed state when circulating blood glucose is derived from intestinal absorption. This proportion decreases as the time since a meal increases. In the postabsorptive state

(from 6 to 12 hours after a meal), blood glucose is derived from liver glycogen and hepatic gluconeogenesis. In the early fasting state (from 12 to 48 hours), blood glucose is derived mainly from gluconeogenesis and the remainder from hepatic glycogen. In the late fasting state (from 2 to 10 days), gluconeogenesis provides almost all the blood glucose.

Only brain and erythrocytes require glucose as fuel. Other cells use fatty acids and ketone bodies. Even brain, at this stage, can derive some energy from ketone bodies. During starvation (greater than 10 days without food), the basal metabolic rate decreases. Otherwise, the pattern of metabolism resembles that of the late fasting state. Of the 125 g of glucose released per day by the liver during starvation, about 75% is used by the brain and the remainder by blood cells. About 35 g of lactate is produced per day by blood cells and is returned to the liver for gluconeogenesis. The other substrates for gluconeogenesis include about 75 g of protein (as amino acids) and 15 g of glycerol per day. **Glucagon** and **insulin** are important in the regulation of gluconeogenesis.

Lipid Homeostasis

Dietary **triglyceride** is transported from the intestine to various cells and organs in chylomicrons. Triglyceride is transported between organs as components of lipoproteins (Chapter 12). Excess dietary carbohydrate is converted into triglyceride in the liver (Figure 25–8). The liver synthesizes 50–100 g of triglyceride daily with normal food intake. Triglyceride is transported from the liver as VLDL (Figure 12–26). Lipoprotein lipase, which is required for the uptake of fatty acids from VLDL and chylomicrons, is induced by insulin.

Cells use glucose as a source of energy in the well-fed state, and most cells can use increasing amounts of fatty acid during postabsorptive states. Insulin, which is elevated after glucose absorption, inhibits lipolysis and the availability of free fatty acids as fuel. Hormone-sensitive lipase liberates free fatty acids and glycerol in the postabsorptive state (Figure 25–8). **Hormone-sensitive lipase** is activated directly following its phosphorylation as catalyzed by protein kinase A. Hormones that activate adenylyl cyclase in adipocytes include glucagon, epinephrine, and ACTH. Fatty acids are transported as a complex with albumin. The tissue uptake of fatty acids is proportional to their concentration in plasma and is therefore largely dependent on blood flow. During exercise, blood flow through the splanchnic bed is reduced and more fatty acids are available to skeletal muscle. Except nerve tissue and erythrocytes, tissues can metabolize fatty acids by β-oxidation and the Krebs cycle. Free fatty acid transport into cells occurs by simple diffusion and is not regulated. When extrahepatic cells are using fatty acids as substrate,

Intake and production	Storage and release	Utilization

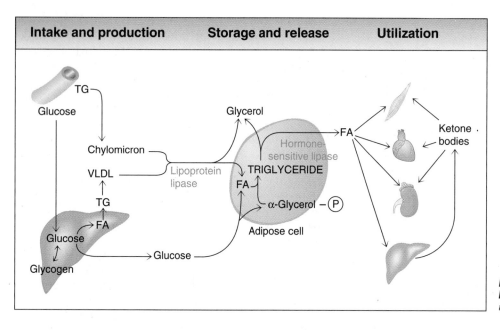

FIGURE 25–8. *Triglyceride metabolism. FA, fatty acid; TG, triglyceride.*

citrate levels increase and **citrate** inhibits phosphofructokinase and thus glycolysis (Table 25–1).

The rate-limiting step in fatty acid oxidation is the formation of fatty acylcarnitine. Carnitine acyltransferase I is inhibited by malonyl-CoA, the primary substrate of fatty acid synthesis (Figure 25–5). Because of low malonyl-CoA levels in response to a high glucagon-to-insulin ratio, fatty acid oxidation is favored. With an accumulation of acetyl-CoA in liver mitochondria in excess of that needed for energy production, **ketone body** synthesis is promoted. Ketone body synthesis occurs exclusively in liver (Figure 11–22). Ketone bodies diffuse from the liver into the circulation and are transported to other cells. Ketone bodies are metabolized in extrahepatic cells (Figure 11–23). During starvation, fatty acids provide about 75% and ketone bodies 25% of the fuel for non–glucose-requiring cells. After a week of fasting, brain can obtain up to half its energy from ketone bodies, thereby decreasing its need for glucose. The ability to use ketone bodies in lieu of glucose decreases the need to catabolize protein as a source of substrate for gluconeogenesis, and this strategy conserves muscle.

Protein and Nitrogen Homeostasis

Protein homeostasis differs from that of carbohydrate and lipid because protein does not serve as an energy storage form. Dietary protein is digested in the stomach and small intestine. Amino acids are absorbed into the portal vein. The outflow of amino acids into the portal vein does not reflect the amino acid composition of the ingested protein. Most amino acids released into the portal vein are metabolized preferentially by the liver with the exception of the branched-chain amino acids (**valine, leucine,** and **isoleucine**). The liver interconverts many amino acids and synthesizes

cellular and plasma proteins. Valine, leucine, and isoleucine account for 60% of the amino acids entering the circulation from the gut despite their 20% contribution to the total amino acids in a protein meal consisting of lean beef. These amino acids contribute to only 20% of the skeletal muscle protein, and excess amounts of branched-chain keto acid metabolites, derived by transamination, can be oxidized by muscle or transported to other cells.

Following a protein-containing meal, insulin secretion increases, and *insulin stimulates peripheral tissue uptake of amino acids and net protein synthesis.* Amino acid carbon skeletons in excess can be converted to carbohydrate and fat; excess nitrogen is converted to urea. Citrulline, formed in the intestine from protein-rich meals, is taken up by the liver. Citrulline is formed from glutamate and from amino acids that can be metabolized to glutamate. Glutamate is converted to glutamate semialdehyde (Figure 13–32), ornithine (Figure 13–15), and finally citrulline (Figure 13–9). Intestine lacks the complete urea cycle pathway. Citrulline and other amino acids are delivered simultaneously to the liver during absorption. **Citrulline** increases the activity of the urea cycle during periods of amino acid excess. This is an example of metabolic control through availability of a catalytic intermediate.

Branched-chain amino acids released from the intestine are metabolized preferentially by muscle (Figure 25–9A). Skeletal muscle is rich in the transaminases that operate on the branched-chain amino acids, but other cells contain only low activities of these enzymes. The branched-chain amino acids can be oxidized following transamination. If muscle **branched-chain keto acid dehydrogenase** is in its phosphorylated and inactive form, the keto acids are released into the circulation and are oxidized by other tissues including liver. The nitrogen derived from the branched-chain amino acids in

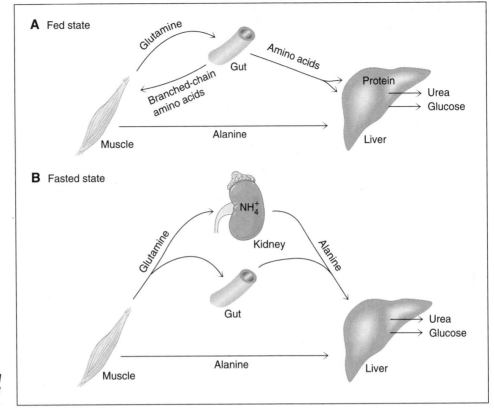

FIGURE 25-9. Protein and amino acid metabolism. A. *Fed state.* B. *Fasted state.*

muscle is donated from glutamate to pyruvate to yield alanine and α-ketoglutarate. The conversion of glucose to pyruvate and alanine increases the molar ATP yield for glycolysis from 2 (glucose to 2 lactate) to 5 (glucose to 2 alanine). Muscle contains the glycerol phosphate shuttle, and the two moles of NADH that are generated per mole of glucose can be transported into the mitochondrion for the production of three moles of ATP (1.5 moles per mole of cytosolic NADH).

Amino acids become the major source for glucose homeostasis after hepatic glycogen is depleted during fasting. The pattern of amino acids released from the muscle does not reflect the composition of muscle protein. **Alanine** and **glutamine** account for more than 80% of the amino acids released by muscle. Alanine is taken up by the liver and is converted to glucose by gluconeogenesis, and the nitrogen is converted to urea (Figure 25-9B). Glutamine is also released from muscle and is metabolized by intestine. Glutaminase catalyzes the hydrolytic generation of glutamate and ammonia (Figure 13-6). Glutamate is converted to alanine, and alanine (gluconeogenic) is transported to the liver.

In starvation, ketogenesis causes increased acid production (acetoacetate and β-hydroxybutyrate). As a consequence, increased ammonium ion is produced by the kidney from glutamine in a reaction catalyzed by glutaminase. The ammonium ion with its proton is excreted in the urine. Glutamate, produced concomitantly with ammonium ion, is

used for renal gluconeogenesis. As the length of fasting increases, gluconeogenesis diminishes in liver and increases in kidney as the need for ammonium increases. The chief nitrogen product during the fed state is urea. In fasting, total nitrogen excretion decreases. During starvation, urea excretion decreases and ammonium excretion increases, coinciding with the increased rate of renal gluconeogenesis.

DIABETES MELLITUS

▶ *Diabetes mellitus is the consequence of a relative or absolute deficiency of insulin.* It is characterized by hyperglycemia in the postprandial or fasting state. In its most florid forms, diabetes is accompanied by muscle-protein wasting and ketosis. Prolonged diabetes is complicated by nephropathy, retinopathy, and neuropathy. The clinical picture varies from an asymptomatic disorder (detected by abnormal blood glucose level found during a routine examination) to a fulminant condition with shock and coma.

The significance of insulin secretion and action with respect to human disease is underscored by the ranking of diabetes mellitus as the third leading cause of death and the leading cause of blindness in the United States. Diabetes elevates the risk of coronary artery disease fourfold or more. Diabetes ranks from third to eighth as a cause of death in countries outside the United States. **Type**

I, or **insulin-dependent, diabetes** is usually due to immunologic destruction of the β-cells of the islets and requires treatment with insulin injection. The failure to produce insulin is the primary pathogenic factor. Type I diabetes is also associated with the excessive production of acetoacetate and β-hydroxybutyrate and the development of acidosis. New cases of type I diabetes develop in 11,000 children annually in the United States. **Type II, or non-insulin-dependent, diabetes,** which is the more common form, is due to insensitivity to insulin (insulin resistance). Non-insulin-dependent diabetes is not associated with acidosis and does not usually require treatment by insulin injection. Most individuals with type II diabetes are obese, and weight reduction usually increases the response to insulin. No single causative factor for diabetes has been identified. Genetic background, autoimmunity, viral infection, and nutrition have been suggested.

Diabetes is characterized by changes in the metabolism of carbohydrate, fat, and protein (Table 25-6). Diabetes mellitus is characterized by **hyperglycemia** and **hyperlipidemia** (Table 12-5). Increased hepatic glucose production is the initial event in the development of fasting hyperglycemia in persons with non-insulin-dependent diabetes. Increased gluconeogenesis is driven by an elevated glucagon-to-insulin ratio with an induction of the enzymes of gluconeogenesis. Plasma levels of glucose observed in glucose tolerance tests in normal and diabetic individuals are provided in Table 10-2.

The elevated glucagon-to-insulin ratio in diabetes enhances triglyceride hydrolysis by **hormone-sensitive lipase** and thereby increases free fatty acid levels in plasma. There is increased uptake of fatty acids by the liver. Acetyl-CoA carboxylase

activity and malonyl-CoA concentrations are decreased in diabetes. Increased fatty acids and decreased malonyl-CoA result in increased β-oxidation of fatty acids and the generation of increased acetyl-CoA. As a result, pyruvate carboxylase for gluconeogenesis is stimulated and increased ketone body production occurs. Ketosis does not occur in non-insulin-dependent diabetes as it does in insulin-dependent diabetes. The reason for this difference is an enigma.

Increased uptake of fatty acids by liver is accompanied by increased re-esterification of glycerol and increased triglyceride synthesis and reassembly of triglyceride in VLDL, also contributing to hyperlipidemia. With severe insulin deficiency, however, there is decreased lipoprotein synthesis and decreased VLDL production. Failure to export triglyceride under these conditions produces a fatty liver. Decreased **lipoprotein lipase** activity in diabetes decreases uptake of fatty acids from VLDL and chylomicrons, also resulting in hypertriglyceridemia.

Insulin promotes **amino acid transport** into cells and **protein synthesis.** In contrast, diabetes increases protein catabolism. In diabetes, muscle releases increased amounts of alanine, thereby providing a substrate for gluconeogenesis and promoting hyperglycemia. Because of increased substrate availability, gluconeogenesis can account for greater than 30% of hepatic glucose production as compared with 15-20% in normal humans. Increased amino acid utilization increases urea production. Increased amino acid catabolism produces negative nitrogen balance and protein wasting. Increased ammonium ion is excreted in the urine during ketoacidosis.

With higher concentrations of glucose in diabetes, free intracellular glucose can be converted to sorbitol in a reaction catalyzed by **aldose reductase** (Figure 25-10). Aldose reductase is widely distributed and occurs in several cells that are prone to lesions in diabetes including nerve, lens, retina, and vascular endothelium. Excess sorbitol accumulates in cells unless it is converted to fructose as catalyzed by **sorbitol dehydrogenase.** Sorbitol accumulation contributes to the neuropathy, retinopathy, nephropathy, and cataracts characteristic of diabetes.

Insulin structure (Figure 3-17) and synthesis (Figure 18-3), its role in gluconeogenesis (Chapter 10), and its receptor and signal transduction pathways (Figure 20-4) are described elsewhere. The ϵ-amino groups of lysine residues and the free amino terminus of proteins can be glycosylated nonenzymatically (Figure 7-5). Formation of such derivatives may contribute to the common complications of diabetes mellitus. The chronically high blood and tissue levels of glucose may promote the modification of critical proteins in retina, kidney, peripheral nerves, and other cells. Such protein modifications are postulated to contribute to the pathogenesis of the complications of diabetes

---

TABLE 25-6. Metabolic Derangements in Diabetes Mellitus

Effect	Mechanism
Hyperglycemia	$\downarrow$ Glucose transport into muscle and adipocytes
	$\uparrow$ Gluconeogenesis
	Induction of pyruvate carboxylase, PEP carboxykinase, fructose-1,6-bisphosphatase, and glucose-6-phosphatase unopposed by insulin
	$\uparrow$ Alanine from muscle
	$\downarrow$ Glycogen synthase activity and glycogen storage
	$\uparrow$ Phosphorylase activity
	$\downarrow$ Conversion of glucose to fatty acids
Hyperlipidemia	$\downarrow$ Lipoprotein lipase and chylomicron and VLDL metabolism
	$\uparrow$ Hormone-sensitive lipase increases fatty acids in the circulation that promote reesterification in liver
Ketosis	$\uparrow$ Fatty acids in serum, promoting ketone body production
	$\downarrow$ Induction and activity of acetyl-CoA carboxylase and $\downarrow$ malonyl-CoA, allowing β-oxidation of fatty acids and provision of acetyl-CoA for synthesis
Muscle wasting	$\downarrow$ Amino acid transport into cells and $\downarrow$ protein synthesis
	$\uparrow$ Protein catabolism, providing alanine for gluconeogenesis and urea synthesis

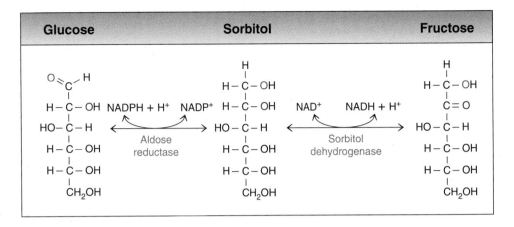

FIGURE 25-10. Sorbitol metabolism.

mellitus. The extent of glycosylation of hemoglobin to form hemoglobin A_1 (Figure 7-5) can be conveniently monitored and used to assess the control of hyperglycemia.

Insulin has been associated with several breakthroughs. It was the first protein whose primary structure was determined, and proinsulin was the first prohormone to be discovered. Moreover, insulin was the first protein produced by recombinant DNA techniques for use in human therapeutics. ◄

ETHANOL METABOLISM

Alcoholic beverages have been used since the dawn of history. Although often viewed as a stimulant, ethanol is a primary depressant of the central nervous system. Its neurochemical mechanism of action is unclear, but it has been suggested that ethanol augments stimulation of the GABA receptor. GABA is the chief inhibitory neurotransmitter in the brain, and ethanol increases the action of GABA by increasing chloride conductance (Table 19-2). Ethanol is absorbed rapidly from the stomach (25%) and intestine (75%) and is detected in the blood within minutes of ingestion. Ethanol diffuses across biological membranes and distributes to all cells and compartments of the body including the brain. Intestinal bacteria produce about 3 g of ethanol daily by fermentation, and blood ethanol is about 0.02 mM without alcohol intake. Bacteria decarboxylate pyruvate to produce acetaldehyde, and acetaldehyde is reduced by NADH to form ethanol. Blood levels of less than 5 mM (1 mM = 4.6 mg/dL) do not increase reaction time, impair critical faculty, or decrease motor control. Levels between 10 and 20 mM produce frank intoxication.

Ethanol is oxidized in two steps to acetate. The first step is catalyzed by **alcohol dehydrogenase** to form acetaldehyde (Figure 25-11). This enzyme, which occurs predominantly in liver, is a cytosolic enzyme with zinc as cofactor. The K_m of the enzyme for ethanol is about 1 mM, and the enzyme functions near saturation after moderate alcohol

(1 ounce) intake. The second step is catalyzed by **aldehyde dehydrogenase,** and acetate is the product. Mitochondrial aldehyde dehydrogenase, which exhibits a low K_m (10 μM) for acetaldehyde, is responsible for the conversion of most acetaldehyde to acetate. Cytosolic aldehyde dehydrogenase, which is a high K_m (1 mM) form, is less important. Most acetate is exported to extrahepatic tissues by the circulation, but a portion is metabolized by liver. Blood acetate levels without ethanol consumption are nil. Acetate is converted to acetyl-CoA by a short-chain fatty acid-activating enzyme that involves ATP and CoA and occurs with pyrophosphate production (Table 11-5). The energy

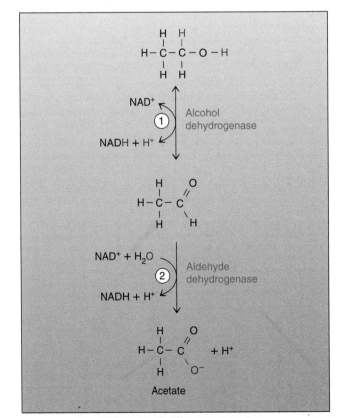

FIGURE 25-11. Ethanol metabolism.

content of ethanol (7 kcal/g) is between that of carbohydrate (4 kcal/g) and lipid (9 kcal/g).

Besides alcohol dehydrogenase, **cytochrome P-450** enzymes can catalyze ethanol oxidation according to the following equation.

$$CH_3CH_2OH + NADPH + H^+ + 2\ O_2 \rightarrow$$
$$CH_3CHO + 2\ H_2O_2 + NADP^+ \quad (25.2)$$

The K_m for the P-450 enzymes for ethanol is about 10 mM. Competition between drugs and ethanol for this enzyme complex can decrease the rates of drug metabolism. One of the cytochrome P-450 isozymes is induced by regular ethanol consumption. Because of enzyme induction, the metabolism of some drugs can be increased.

About 20% of ingested ethanol in men, and about 10% in women, is metabolized by the gastric mucosa. The liver, however, is the chief organ of ethanol metabolism. The rate of ethanol metabolism is 11 mL per hour by a 70-kg person (1 ounce $\approx$ 30 mL). This rate cannot be increased by physical activity or caffeine. The increase in the hepatic ratio of NADH/NAD$^+$ due to ethanol catabolism promotes the conversion of pyruvate (derived from alanine) to lactate and decreases lactate oxidation by NAD$^+$. As a result, ethanol metabolism decreases **gluconeogenesis** by decreasing the concentration of pyruvate. ▶ Alcoholic hypoglycemia can be the result. In liver, ethanol metabolism increases fatty acid synthesis by increasing substrate availability, and this may contribute to the development of a fatty liver. ◀ Gluconeogenesis from glycerol is unaffected by ethanol metabolism.

Acetaldehyde, the product of ethanol oxidation, is a reactive substance that forms covalent Schiff bases with the ϵ-amino groups of protein-lysine residues. Such modification may be deleterious. ▶ About half the Asian population has a mutant **aldehyde dehydrogenase** isoenzyme with reduced activity. After ethanol intake, affected individuals develop increased blood acetaldehyde levels and experience vasodilation with facial flushing, increased heart rate, and hypotension. Malnutrition is common in individuals with alcoholism. It can be the result of inadequate food intake or may be secondary to altered vitamin me-

tabolism. The most common deficiencies are those of **thiamine, folate,** and **pyridoxine.** Thiamine deficiency and **Wernicke encephalopathy** occur frequently in people with alcoholism. Aberrations in liver metabolism lead to hepatic **cirrhosis** owing to protein modification and to vitamin deficiencies.

Alcoholism (with tolerance and dependence) and alcohol abuse are leading public health problems that lead to cirrhosis, alcohol-related injuries, and deaths as a result of automobile accidents. Alcohol-abuse-related health-care costs account for more than 10% of total expenditures for health care in the United States. Ethanol has also been implicated in the development of birth defects in the **fetal alcohol syndrome.** The embryo and early fetus appear most sensitive to the effects of ethanol and its metabolites. Mental retardation in offspring has been attributed to ethanol ingestion by the mother during pregnancy, and ethanol is considered a major cause of mental retardation in the United States. The incidence of fetal alcohol syndrome ranges between 1 in 300 to 1 in 2000 live births. It occurs in one in three infants born to mothers with alcoholism. ◀

Selected Readings

Dinneen, S., J. Gerich, and R. Rizza. Carbohydrate metabolism in non-insulin-dependent diabetes mellitus. New England Journal of Medicine 327:707–713, 1992.

Kurland, I.J., and S.J. Pilkus. Indirect versus direct routes of hepatic glycogen synthesis. FASEB Journal 3:2277–2281, 1989.

Lieber, C.S. Biochemical and molecular basis of alcohol-induced injury to liver and other tissues. New England Journal of Medicine 319:1639–1650, 1988.

Linder, M.C. (ed.). *Nutritional Biochemistry and Metabolism with Clinical Applications,* 2nd ed. New York, Elsevier, 1991.

Shafrir, E., M. Bergman, and P. Felig. The endocrine pancreas: Diabetes mellitus. In P. Felig, J.D. Baxter, A.E. Broadus, and L.A. Frohman (eds.). *Endocrinology and Metabolism,* 2nd ed. New York, McGraw-Hill Book Company, 1988, pp. 1043–1178.

Sugden, M.C., M.J. Holness, and T.N. Palmer. Fuel selection and carbon flux during the starved-to-fed transition. Biochemical Journal 263:313–323, 1989.

Unger, R.H., and D.W. Foster. Diabetes mellitus. In J.D. Wilson and D.W. Foster (eds.). *Williams Textbook of Endocrinology,* 8th ed. Philadelphia, WB Saunders Company, 1992, pp. 1255–1333.

INDEX

Note: Page numbers in *italics* refer to illustrations;
page numbers followed by the letter t refer to tables.

515

SOME COMMON BIOCHEMICAL ABBREVIATIONS

A	adenine
ACAT	acyl-CoA cholesterol acyltransferase
ACE	angiotensin converting enzyme
ACP	acyl carrier protein
ACS	2-amino-3-carboxymuconate-6-semialdehyde
ADA	adenosine deaminase
AdoMet	S-adenosylmethionine
ADP	adenosine diphosphate
AIDS	acquired immunodeficiency syndrome
Ala	alanine
ALA	δ-aminolevulinate
ALT	alanine aminotransferase
AMP	adenosine monophosphate
APRT	adenine phosphoribosyl transferase
APS	adenosylphosphosulfate
Arg	arginine
Asn	asparagine
Asp	aspartate
AST	aspartate aminotransferase
ATP	adenosine triphosphate
ATPase	adenosine triphosphatase
AZT	3′-azido-2′,3′-dideoxythymidine
BMR	basal metabolic rate
bp	base pair
BPG	2,3-bisphosphoglycerate
C	cytosine
CaM	calmodulin
cAMP	cyclic AMP
cDNA	complementary DNA
CDP	cytidine diphosphate
cGMP	cyclic GMP
CMP	cytidine monophosphate
CoA or CoASH	coenzyme A
COMT	catechol-O-methyltransferase
CoQ	coenzyme Q (ubiquinone)
CPK	creatine phosphokinase
CRE	cyclic AMP response element
CT	computed tomography
CTP	cytidine triphosphate
Cys	cysteine
cyt	cytochrome
d	2′-deoxyribo-
Da	dalton
DAP	diaminopimelate
dd	dideoxy-
DHA	docosahexaenoate
DHF	dihydrofolate
DNA	deoxyribonucleic acid
DNase	deoxyribonuclease
Dol	dolichol
$\Delta\mathcal{E}^{o'}$	difference in standard reduction potential at pH 7.0
EF	elongation factor
$\mathcal{F}$	Faraday
FAD	flavin adenine dinucleotide (oxidized form)
$FADH_2$	flavin adenine dinucleotide (reduced form)
Fe-S	iron-sulfur
F_oF_1-ATPase	ATP synthase of mitochondrial membranes
FIGLU	N-formimino-L-glutamate
fMet	N-formylmethionine
FMN	flavin mononucleotide (oxidized form)
$FMNH_2$	flavin mononucleotide (reduced form)
5-FU	fluorouracil
G	guanine
$\Delta G^{o'}$	standard free energy change at pH 7.0
GABA	γ-aminobutyrate
Gal	galactose
GAP	GTPase activating protein
GDP	guanosine diphosphate
GGT	γ-glutamyl transpeptidase
Gla	γ-carboxyglutamate
Glc	glucose
GlcNAc	N-acetylglucose
GlcUA	glucuronate
Gln	glutamine
Glu	glutamate
GLUT4	glucose transporter 4 (insulin-responsive)
Gly	glycine
GMP	guanosine monophosphate
GSH	reduced glutathione
GSSG	oxidized glutathione
GTP	guanosine triphosphate
HDL	high-density lipoprotein
HETE	hydroxyeicosatetraenoate
HGPRT	hypoxanthine-guanine phosphoribosyltransferase
His	histidine
HIV	human immunodeficiency virus
HMG-CoA	3-hydroxy-3-methylglutaryl-CoA
hnRNA	heterogeneous nuclear RNA
HPETE	hydroperoxyeicosatetraenoate
HVA	homovanillate
IDL	intermediate-density lipoprotein
IF	initiation factor
IgG	immunoglobulin G
Ile	isoleucine
IMP	inosine monophosphate
IP_3	inositol-1,4,5-trisphosphate
ITP	inosine triphosphate
K_{eq}	equilibrium constant
K_m	Michaelis constant
kb	kilobase
kDa	kilodalton
KSase	β-ketoacyl-ACP synthase
LCAT	lecithin-cholesterol acyltransferase
LCR	locus control region
LDH	lactate dehydrogenase
LDL	low-density lipoprotein
Leu	leucine
LINE	long interspersed nuclear element
LT	leukotriene
Lys	lysine
Man	mannose